EXAMINATION IN PHYSICAL THERAPY PRACTICE

Screening for Medical Disease

EXAMINATION IN PHYSICAL THERAPY PRACTICE

Screening for Medical Disease

Edited by

William G. Boissonnault, M.S., P.T.

Partner and Therapist
Physical Therapy Orthopaedic Specialists, Inc.
Minneapolis, Minnesota

Clinical Instructor
Department of Physical Medicine and Rehabilitation
Program in Physical Therapy
University of Minnesota
Minneapolis, Minnesota

Assistant Professor
Institute of Graduate Physical Therapy
St. Augustine, Florida

Clinical Assistant Professor
Department of Rehabilitation Sciences
College of Allied Health Sciences
University of Tennessee–Memphis
Memphis, Tennessee

Churchill Livingstone
New York, Edinburgh, London, Melbourne, Tokyo

Library of Congress Cataloging-in-Publication Data
Examination in physical therapy practice : screening for medical
  disease / edited by William G. Boissonnault.
      p.   cm.
    Includes bibliographical references and index.
    ISBN 0-443-08738-5
    1. Physical therapy. 2. Diagnosis, Differential.
  I. Boissonnault, William G.
    [DNLM: 1. Physical Examination. 2. Physical Therapy.   WB 460
  E96]
  RM701.E9 1991
  615.8'2—dc20
  DNLM/DLC
  for Library of Congress   91-26796
                                                             CIP

© Churchill Livingstone Inc. 1991

Distributed in the United Kingdom by Churchill Livingstone, Robert Stevenson House, 1–3 Baxter's Place, Leith Walk, Edinburgh EH1 3AF, and by associated companies, branches, and representatives throughout the world.

Accurate indications, adverse reactions, and dosage schedules for drugs are provided in this book, but it is possible that they may change. The reader is urged to review the package information data of the manufacturers of the medications mentioned.

The Publishers have made every effort to trace the copyright holders for borrowed material. If they have inadvertently overlooked any, they will be pleased to make the necessary arrangements at the first opportunity.

Acquisitions Editor: *Leslie Burgess*
Copy Editor: *Christina Joslin*
Production Designer: *Patricia McFadden*
Production Supervisor: *Jeanine Furino*

Printed in the United States of America

First published in 1991   7 6 5 4 3 2 1

To my wife, Jill, and my children, Joshua and Eliya, who are my heart and soul, and to my parents, Gregory and Geneva Boissonnault, whose love and support have been a continuing source of strength

Contributors

David Arnall, Ph.D., P.T.
Assistant Professor, Physical Therapy Program, Northern Arizona University, Flagstaff, Arizona

Warren J. Bilkey, M.D.
Clinical Assistant Professor, Department of Physical Medicine and Rehabilitation, University of Minnesota Medical School—Minneapolis; Associate Medical Director, Chronic Pain Rehabilitation Program, Sister Kenny Institute, Minneapolis, Minnesota

Jill S. Boissonnault, M.S., P.T.
Therapist, Physical Therapy Orthopaedic Specialists, Inc., Minneapolis, Minnesota

William G. Boissonnault, M.S., P.T.
Clinical Instructor, Department of Physical Medicine and Rehabilitation, Program in Physical Therapy, University of Minnesota, Minneapolis, Minnesota; Assistant Professor, Institute of Graduate Physical Therapy, St. Augustine, Florida; Clinical Assistant Professor, Department of Rehabilitation Sciences, College of Allied Health Sciences, University of Tennessee–Memphis, Memphis, Tennessee; Partner and Therapist, Physical Therapy Orthopaedic Specialists, Inc., Minneapolis, Minnesota

Mark R. Bookhout, M.S., P.T.
Instructor, Office of Continuing Medical Education, Michigan State University College of Osteopathic Medicine, East Lansing, Michigan; President, Physical Therapy Orthopaedic Specialists, Inc., Minneapolis, Minnesota

Stephen D. Cain, B.A., B.S., Pharm. D.
Pharmacist, Boyton Health Service, University of Minnesota, Minneapolis, Minnesota

Paul H. Caldron, D.O., F.A.C.P., F.A.C.R.
Staff Rheumatologist, Arthritis Center, Ltd., Phoenix, Arizona

Jill Downing, M.D.
Instructor, Department of Preventive Medicine, Harvard Medical School; Assistant in Medicine, and Program Director, Cardiac Rehabilitation, Massachusetts General Hospital, Boston, Massachusetts

Jill A. Floberg, P.T.
Clinical Instructor, Curriculum in Physical Therapy, University of Washington School of Medicine, Seattle, Washington; Clinical Instructor, School of Occupational and Physical Therapy, University of Puget Sound, Tacoma, Washington; Clinical Instructor, School of Physical Therapy and Allied Health, Eastern Washington University, Cheney, Washington; President and Clinical Director, Olympia Physical Therapy Service, Inc., P.S., Olympia, Washington

Edward R. Isaacs, M.D., F.A.A.N.
Non-Geographic Faculty, Assistant Professor, Department of Neurology, Virginia Commonwealth University Medical College of Virginia School of Medicine, Richmond, Virginia; Instructor, Office of Continuing Medical Education, Michigan State University College of Osteopathic Medicine, East Lansing, Michigan

Steven C. Janos, M.S., P.T.
Adjunct Assistant Professor, Department of Physical Therapy, Programs in Physical Therapy, Northwestern University Medical School, Chicago, Illinois; Physical Therapy Orthopaedic Specialists, Inc., Minneapolis, Minnesota

Robert D. Karl, Jr., M.D.
Clinical Associate Professor, School of Occupational and Physical Therapy, University of Puget Sound, Tacoma, Washington; Clinical Associate Professor, Department of Radiology, University of Washington School of Medicine, Seattle, Washington; Chief of Radiology, South Region, Group Health Cooperative of Puget Sound; Consultant in Radiology, Madigan Army Medical Center, Tacoma, Washington

Patricia M. King, M.A., P.T.
Assistant Professor, Department of Rehabilitation Sciences, University of Tennessee–Memphis, College of Allied Health Sciences, Memphis, Tennessee; Assistant Professor, Institute of Graduate Physical Therapy, St. Augustine, Florida

Michael B. Koopmeiners, M.D.
Assistant Professor, Department of Family Practice and Community Health, University of Minnesota Medical School—Minneapolis, Minneapolis, Minnesota

Frank W. Ling, M.D.
Associate Professor and Director, Division of Gynecology, Department of Obstetrics and Gynecology, University of Tennessee, Memphis, College of Medicine, Memphis, Tennessee

Diane Madlon-Kay, M.D.
Physician, Department of Family Medicine, St. Paul-Ramsey Medical Center, St. Paul, Minnesota

Dudley M. McLinn, M.D., P.A.
Specialists in Internal Medicine, P.A., Abbott Northwestern Hospital, Minneapolis, Minnesota

Kevin McMahon, M.D., F.A.A.O.S., I.A.C.S.
Potomac Valley Orthopaedic Associates, Montgomery General Hospital, Olney, Maryland

Theresa Hoskins Michel, M.S., P.T., C.C.S.
Assistant Professor, Graduate Program in Physical Therapy, Massachusetts General Hospital Institute of Health Professions; Cardiopulmonary Clinical Specialist, Department of Cardiopulmonary Physical Therapy, Massachusetts General Hospital, Boston, Massachusetts

Craig A. Myers, P.T.
Staff Physical Therapist, Department of Obstetrics and Gynecology, and Medical Student, University of Tennessee–Memphis, College of Medicine, Memphis, Tennessee

Terry Randall, P.T., O.C.S., A.T.C.
Institute of Health Professions, Massachusetts General Hospital, Boston, Massachusetts

Michael Ryan, M.D., F.A.C.P.
Adjunct Professor, Department of Health, Physical Education, and Recreation, Northern Arizona University; Medical Director, Cardiopulmonary Rehabilitation Program, Phase I, Flagstaff Medical Center, Flagstaff, Arizona

Foreword

Heraclitus, the Greek philospher, stated, "There is nothing permanent except change." The profession of physical therapy exemplifies this bit of ancient wisdom. Since the beginning of the profession in 1921 in response to the needs of injured World War I veterans, physical therapists have developed from mere technicians who followed the prescriptions of physicians into increasingly autonomous professionals with a distinct body of knowledge and specialized diagnostic procedures.

This change is illustrated by comparing the Physical Therapy Code of Ethics in 1935 with the latest edition in 1981. In the earlier version, the professional scope of physical therapists was severely limited by the statement, "Diagnosing and stating the prognosis of the case and prescribing treatment shall be entirely the responsibility of the physician. Any assumption of this responsibility by one of our members shall be considered unethical." In the 1981 edition, the only restriction relating to providing services is in the clause, "Physical therapists [will] comply with the laws and regulations governing the practice of physical therapy." The updated laws have allowed physical therapists increasing autonomy in all areas relating to the provision of physical therapy services, while still clearly leaving the area of differential diagnosis to physicians.

Examination in Physical Therapy Practice acknowledges that medical care is a partnership among providers. All but one chapter is written by a physician and either co-authored by or written with input from a physical therapist, in order to take advantage of both perspectives. This is what makes this book unique. I have never read a text that so thoroughly merges the minds of physicians and physical therapists. In this book, both disciplines work as equal partners in the process of healing the patient.

This long overdue text is an effort to give physical therapists the knowledge necessary to make them full partners in the differential diagnostic process. Physical therapists are educated thoroughly in the area of treating problems with the musculoskeletal system, but our education is understandably lacking in the area of differential diagnosis. By contrast, in medical school physicians often spend little time learning about physical therapy treatment and a great deal of time on differential diagnosis. Therefore, physicians and physical therapists must work in concert to fill the gaps in one another's expertise. This book is an effort to expand the awareness of physical therapists so that we may be informed partners in the diagnostic process.

Differential diagnosis is defined by *Dorland's Illustrated Medical Dictionary* as "the determination of which one of several diseases may be producing the symptoms." Differential diagnosis of the neuromusculoskeletal system is a complex process, particularly for the many physicians who specialize in the diagnosis of systemic disease. These physicians will typically conduct a clinical examination, collecting signs and symptoms to develop an impression or a hierarchical problem list, based on the results of certain differential tests and measurements, they may decide to send the patient for physical therapy treatment. It is my experience that these physicians do not expect the physical therapist to assist them in gathering data or developing a clinical impression. Although we may be asked to evaluate and treat a patient while the physician is developing his or her diagnostic impression or problem list, we are not asked to provide information regarding our findings or the patient's responses that would facilitate the differential diagnostic process. It is my contention that we need to provide important qualitative and quantitative information that can assist the physician in completing the differential diagnosis. The physical therapist must be accountable for accurate, timely communication with the physician, and must be sensitive to the physician's role and responsibilities. The issue of legal accountability is critical; physical therapists must be able to substantiate their findings and conclusions on a sound, scientific basis.

Theories of medical treatment are separated into two broad categories: those that are focused on pathology and those that are focused on signs, symptoms, and the patient. Before Hippocrates, the Cnidian school of medicine rested on the notion that for every illness there existed one specific cause and one specific treatment. Modern medicine, or at least one aspect of it, is very Cnidian in its approach: for every infection there is a specific antibiotic for treatment; for every injury there is a specific routine of exercises. One can view this Cnidian approach as a pathology-focused treatment in which the medical practitioner focuses on the diagnosis that the patient's condition has been given, and offers whatever the standard treatment is for this diagnosis. The problem with the pathology-focused or single-cause, single-treatment approach is that it fails to appreciate the broader picture of the disorder. This approach also ignores the fact that the physical body that houses the ailment also houses an emotional and intellectual being—the human patient.

An injury invariably affects a patient intellectually and emotionally as well as physically, and an essential aspect of effective treatment is that the whole person must be acknowledged and ministered to in order for treatment to progress optimally. In short, the foundation of treatment should rest on the signs, symptoms, and patient-focused treatment model of medicine, the roots of which can be traced to Hippocrates. In this approach, the practioner looks at the total wellness of the patient and focuses on strengthening the body's defenses against illness or injury, as well as treating the signs and symptoms with a foreign agent or set of physical treatments. Treatment is a living process. It is growth. Knowledge can guide but not totally direct treatment. The patient and his or her response guide treatment in the final analysis. Therefore the successful physical therapist must have a broad background of knowledge to determine when things fit and when they do not.

In the signs, symptoms, and patient-focused model of treatment, when patients are referred to physical therapists by physicians, we first perform an evaluation to diagnose the movement dysfunction and to assess the functional profile. As treatment is provided, the therapist carefully monitors the patient's response and communicates with the physician about the patient's progress. When we are approached directly by the patient, we must be aware of the origin of the complaint; if it resides in a system other than the musculoskeletal system, it will require a diagnosis from a physician. We also must be aware of whether the musculoskeletal complaint requires diagnostic tests, measures, and treatment other than what can be provided by the physical therapist.

Pathology is not a fixed set of signs and symptoms. It is a living, changing condition. The position of the physical therapist as a member of the health care team is unique. The nature of treatment allows the therapist to spend more time with the patient than almost any other practitioner. Therefore, the change in pathology can be carefully monitored by the therapist. As a result, more detailed knowledge about pathology in other body systems can assist the therapist in evaluating situations in which changes indicate other factors that need to be addressed by the physician. The knowledge of medical diagnostics helps the therapist to make better-informed decisions. Only time can tell what effect this expanding knowledge will have on health care. If it helps us to better function as members of the medical team, then I feel that it will advance the cause. However, if we use this knowledge to become more independent of other practioners in the treatment of patients, then I feel it is detrimental to both the profession and the patients.

In our society, it is more acceptable to acknowledge a physical problem than it is to attribute emotional stress as a precursor or cause of disease. Physical therapists are in an ideal position to question and listen to a patient to help uncover emotional concomitants to the presenting physical problem. This information may be communicated to the physician by the patient only if he or she acknowledges its relevance. Therefore the physical therapist must inform the physician of a patient's emotional stress, especially in situations where lack of progress suggests that the stress may be of a magnitude requiring intervention by a psychologist or psychiatrist.

Too often the question of why a physical therapist should know more about medical diagnosis rests on arguments surrounding the issue of direct access. However, there is a far broader issue that concerns the therapist's accountability for the wellness of the patient. Since the physical therapist spends more time with the patient and is in a position to question the patient more often than the physician, the therapist is in an ideal position to assist in the often difficult process of differential diagnosis. Physicians do not often consider physical therapists resources to them in this process. Therapists need a broader view of pathology in order to communicate with physicians at a more appropriate level. By filling a major gap in the literature that is available to physical therapists, this text meets that need.

Peter I. Edgelow, M.A., P.T.
Faculty, Physical Therapy Residency Program
in Advanced Orthopedic Manual Therapy,
Kaiser Permanente Medical Center,
Hayward, California

Preface

Since state chapters of the American Physical Therapy Association have made the commitment to support patient direct access to physical therapy, concern has been raised about the safety and well-being of patients who have not been seen by a physician prior to being treated by a physical therapist. The fear expressed is that a patient suffering with a serious medical condition (e.g., cancer) that goes undetected by the physical therapist will receive months of inappropriate treatment. This delay in the medical diagnostic process and subsequent medical treatment could have a profound effect on the patient's prognosis. Concern over the possible development of this clinical scenario is shared by all practicing therapists.

The argument that physical therapists do not have the knowledge and skills necessary for diagnosing medical illnesses and therefore put patients at risk is only half true. Although physical therapy academic programs do not provide the training necessary for therapists to diagnose specific illnesses and diseases, the lack of these diagnostic skills should not imply that physical therapists are jeopardizing the well being of their patients. Therapists are highly educated in the assessment and treatment of the many elements related to movement dysfunction, but if the scope of our training was solely limited to that arena, patients would truly be at risk and our responsibilities as members of the health care team would not be fully met.

For the well-being of the patient, therapists should have the knowledge and clinical tools to medically screen patients for the presence of conditions that require the expertise of a physician; this is an absolute complement to the skills required for the assessment and treatment of movement dysfunction. This general medical screening implies ruling out the involvement of a body system (such as the gastrointestinal or cardiovascular systems) rather than ruling out specific diseases (such as pericarditis, osteomyelitis, or prostate cancer). If the therapist suspects pathologic involvement of a body system, referral of the patient to a physician is indicated for either formulation of a specific diagnosis of the medical condition, or ruling out of such a condition.

Written for the clinician and student, *Examination in Physical Therapy Practice* provides information to help ensure that patients are given appropriate physical therapy treatment. The primary objective of the book is to supply the information necessary to screen the various body systems. Chapter 1 gives the foundation of this screening, reviewing examination and treatment principles for ruling out the presence of pathologic conditions. Since it contains information that will help the therapist decide exactly which body systems to screen, it is highly recommended that this chapter be read prior to reading any other component of the text. Chapters 2 through 11 provide detailed information about screening the various specific body systems. An overview of anatomy and physiology, relevant to the screening procedures or to understanding the pathological processes discussed, is presented. In addition, symptoms and signs suggestive of the presence of systemic disease are described. Certain specific disease entities are reviewed in each chapter, but the list of diseases covered is not an all-inclusive list. The emphasis is on the diseases therapists are more likely to encounter clinically. Chapter 12, "Clinical Pharmacology for the Physical Therapist," discusses the effect that groups of medications can have on a patient's presentation during the evaluation or on the patient's response to seemingly appropriate treatment. Prescription and over-the-counter medications are so widely used by patients that therapists need to be aware of how the medications can affect the outcome of the physical therapy care. Chapter 13, "Radiologic Assessment of the Musculoskeletal System," covers material that should facilitate the understanding of medical literature, as well as communication with physicians. In addition, information is included in the final two chapters that should enhance the therapist's understanding of certain disease processes. Finally, the appendices include a glossary of terms to facilitate the understanding of medical terminology used throughout this book, and a review of systems summary which can be used as a quick reference source.

Besides providing the information necessary to screen the various body systems for the presence of disease, the other important objective of this book is to enhance the level of professional communication between therapists and physicians. The purposes of the medical screening examination are to detect the presence of conditions that may require the expertise of a health professional other than a physical therapist, and to recognize the pre-existing medical conditions that may affect the outcome of seemingly appropriate physical therapy care. If suspicion is raised regarding the status of a body system, referral of the patient to a physician should occur. The information provided in this book should allow the therapist to communicate a specific list of clincial findings to the physician regarding the purpose of the referral.

The intent of this book is not to allow the physical therapist to become more autonomous within the health care system, but to help ensure that patients receive the appropriate medical care. Instead of isolating therapists from physicians, screening for the presence of disease entities in a professional manner should only enhance and facilitate communication between physical therapists and physicians. In this spirit of collaboration between the two professions, most of the chapters in this book are co-authored by a therapist and a physician, and the chapters that are solely authored by a physician were written with significant input from physical therapists. This cooperative effort should ensure that the information covered is accurate and appropriate, and relevant to physical therapy practice.

William G. Boissonnault, M.S., P.T.

Acknowledgments

I would like to acknowledge the physical therapy staff of Physical Therapy Orthopaedic Specialists, Inc. (PTOSI), Minneapolis, for their dedication to providing the highest quality of patient care and for helping to create a work environment that is stimulating, challenging, and conducive to professional growth. Special thanks go to Mark Bookhout and Don Darling, co-founders of PTOSI, for their patience and support throughout the undertaking of this project.

Acknowledgments also go to Bette Ann Harris, Carl DeRosa, Peter I. Edgelow, and Corinne Ellingham for their encouragement and assistance in generating a prospective list of contributing authors. I would like to thank Marg Saeger (PTOSI) for her endless patience and timeliness regarding the preparation of portions of this book. I am also indebted to Media Services, Abbott Northwestern Hospital, Minneapolis, for their outstanding work on illustrations, tables, and photographs.

Finally, I would like to express my admiration for the contributing authors who invested their valuable time and energy in this project. I learned a great deal through my written and verbal communications with them, and the challenge of creating this book would not have been met without their efforts. In this group, I include Peter I. Edgelow, whose enthusiasm and insight were invaluable in the planning and completion of this project.

Contents

Appendix

1

Screening for Medical Disease: Physical Therapy Assessment and Treatment Principles

WILLIAM G. BOISSONNAULT, M.S., P.T.
STEVEN C. JANOS, M.S., P.T.

The Challenge of Patient Examination

If there is something you have not studied,
or, having studied it you are unable to do it,
do not file it away; if there is a question
that you have not asked or to which
you have been unable to find the answer,
do not consider the matter closed;
if you have not thought of a problem,
or, having thought of it,
you have not resolved it,
do not think the matter settled;
if you have tried to make a distinction
but have not made it clear,
do not sink into contentment;
if there is a principle which
you have been able to put into practice,
do not let up.
If one man gets there with one try,
try ten times.
If another succeeds with a hundred tries,
make a thousand.

Proceeding in this manner, even one
who is a bit slow will find the light,
even a weak man will find energy.*

Numerous challenges face the clinician responsible for patient management. The ultimate challenge is the development of a comprehensive treatment program designed to meet the patient's individual needs. Phys-

*From Kei-Hua, E: Kung-Fu Meditations and Chinese Proverbial Wisdom. Farout Press, Thor Publishing Co., Ventura, CA

ical therapists are well trained to treat patients conservatively who present with mechanical musculoskeletal system dysfunction. For the purposes of this book, mechanical musculoskeletal dysfunction is defined as impaired or altered function of skeletal, arthrodial, and myofascial structures resulting from either trauma or abnormal postures.[1] To help develop the appropriate treatment program, the therapist relies on the examination process to identify the anatomic source(s) of the patient's symptoms, to determine the stage of wound healing of the lesion (acute, subacute, or chronic condition), and to identify dysfunction of the neuromusculoskeletal system that may be directly or indirectly influencing the patient's complaints. Inherent in the attempt to identify the source of a patient's symptoms is ruling out certain structures that could be responsible for the complaints. This process should include screening structures such as visceral organs for disease that, if present and responsible for symptoms, would not respond to physical therapy management. In addition, screening the musculoskeletal system for the presence of diseases such as cancer or infections that, if present, would require immediate medical intervention, is also necessary. In order for the therapist to answer the question "Does this patient present with a condition that will respond to physical therapy treatment?" the patient must be screened for the presence of medical diseases. Answering this question must be one of the primary goals of the therapist's examination process.

1

Differentiating between mechanical musculoskeletal dysfunction and pathologic conditions as the source of a patient's symptoms can be extremely difficult. Pathologic conditions such as gastric ulcers, prostate cancer, kidney infection, and pathologic fracture secondary to a metastatic tumor may be manifested primarily as a mechanical musculoskeletal dysfunction (e.g., joint hypomobility, abnormal muscle tonus), with the sole symptom possibly pelvic, thoracic, or cervical pain. Most patients with medical disease are prompted to consult a physician because of the overt nature of the medical symptoms, but patients with certain chronic visceral diseases and serious conditions, such as cancer, may not experience the expected medical symptoms.. These patients may arrive at the physical therapy clinic with a diagnosis of thoracic outlet syndrome, mechanical low back pain syndrome, or cervical strain. The physical therapist must be aware of the symptoms and signs suggestive of medical disease that are responsible for symptoms and must have a working knowledge of the disease entities most likely to be primarily manifested as pain complaints. This knowledge will facilitate the process of referral of the patient to the appropriate physician for medical examination and subsequent diagnosis.

Ruling out pathologic conditions as responsible for all or a portion of a patient's complaints is not the only reason a therapist should screen for medical disease. Assuming that a patient's symptoms are arising from mechanical dysfunction, a medical condition may be present that will influence the outcome of the treatment deemed appropriate by the evaluation findings. For example, certain cardiovascular or endocrine system disorders may have an impact on the wound-healing process of the lesion, delaying or preventing the expected changes from occurring. Certain psychological disorders may prevent a patient from responding as expected to physical therapy procedures seemingly appropriate based on the physical examination. In addition, the presence of certain medical conditions may influence the choice of treatment intervention. For example, a metabolic bone disease such as osteoporosis may influence the type of passive stretching exercise the therapist will use or the position in which the stretching is carried out to increase range of motion (ROM). Patients often arrive at the physical therapy clinic already having been diagnosed as having a med-

ical condition. In these cases, the therapist must ask the appropriate questions regarding the patient's past and current medical history, to obtain this information. In other cases, symptoms have not progressed to the point where they have been brought to the physician's attention. The physical therapist carrying out a detailed evaluation may pick up enough clues to lead to suspicion of the presence of a medical condition. Referral of the patient to a physician would then be appropriate either to rule out the presence of a medical disease or to formulate the specific diagnosis.

The purposes of this chapter are to

1. Review evaluation principles that will assist the therapist in the differentiation of mechanical musculoskeletal dysfunction versus disease entities as the source of a patient's complaints—a process that will include a detailed review of the subjective and objective examination findings that could be considered clinical red flags regarding the presence of medical disease
2. Discuss examination findings that will aide the therapist in determining the presence of medical conditions that may have an impact on the patient's response to therapeutic intervention but that are not necessarily involved in the patient's symptomatic presentation
3. Present an examination scheme that incorporates the specific questions and physical examination techniques that a therapist can use to assist in the process of ruling out the presence of medical conditions
4. Review the principles of how a patient does or does not respond to treatment that may raise suspicion regarding the etiology of the patient's complaints and the appropriateness of continued physical therapy

EXAMINATION PRINCIPLES

Subjective and objective examination findings that may suggest the presence of medical disease are discussed in the following sections. Figure 1-1 is a schematic representation of how components of the subjective and objective examination can help guide the therapist

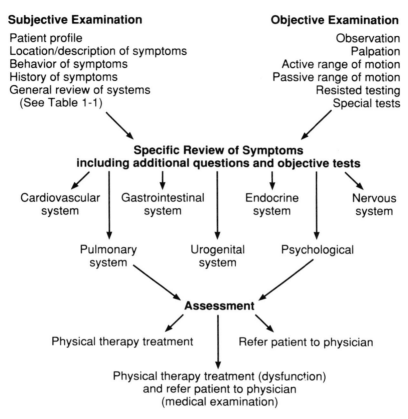

Fig. 1-1. Components of a physical therapy evaluation that may provide the clinical information that leads to referring the patient to a physician.

toward either implementing physical therapy treatment or referring a patient to a physician for a medical consult, or both, if some of the symptoms are believed to be related to mechanical dysfunction and others possibly to disease. No single question or examination procedure definitively rules out or confirms the presence of a pathologic disorder, but certain symptoms and signs, if noted, should raise suspicion in the therapist's mind of the presence of such conditions. This section presents specific questions designed to screen a patient's general health and the various organ systems for disease. Also discussed is the interpretation of specific patient responses to questions that may direct the therapist to ask additional questions or implement specific objective tests to provide more information regarding the patient's health status. Objec-

tive examination techniques that specifically assess the status of nonmusculoskeletal system structures are described. Finally, interpretation of objective examination findings suggestive of the presence of a condition that may not be amenable to physical therapy care is presented.

Subjective Examination

Performing a complete and thorough subjective examination in a timely fashion can be difficult. A history that is carried out in an organized and effective fashion can greatly facilitate the decision-making process in determining how to structure and organize the objective examination, differentiating between mechanical dysfunction and pathologic origins of symptoms, and developing an effective treatment regimen.

The subjective examination can be broken down into four parts: location and description of symptoms, symptom behavior, history, and review of systems. The location and description of symptoms will usually provide the therapist with the reason the patient has come to the clinic—that is, the patient's chief complaint. Symptom behavior refers to changes in symptoms over a 24-hour period. This information will reflect the severity (symptoms affecting function) and irritability (how easily the symptoms are provoked and then subsequently alleviated) of the patient's condition. Also, if multiple symptoms are present, this information will help determine whether the symptoms are related to a single lesion. The history of the patient's condition includes a chronologic description of the symptoms, including onset of symptoms, symptom change since onset, and treatment received for the condition. Review of systems provides additional information regarding the patient's status that may have a significant impact on the outcome of the physical therapy program. It includes a review of the visceral organ systems, emotional status, personal and family medical history, and occupation.

The following section focuses on the information obtained in the subjective examination that should raise suspicion in the therapist's mind regarding the presence of a medical condition that would not respond to physical therapy management or that would have an impact on the outcome of physical therapy treatment. The categories of information to be described include a patient profile, location and description of symptoms, symptom behavior, onset of symptoms (history), the patient's current and past medical history and family medical history.

General Patient Profile

During the subjective examination, the therapist should record general patient information. This information would include the patient's age, sex, race, and occupation. Certain disease entities are more common within specific age groups. For example, prostate cancer is more common in men over the age of 50[2], and the onset of ankylosing spondylitis often occurs between the ages of 15 and 35.[3] The incidence of certain disease processes is much higher in one sex than in the other. For example, ankylosing spondylitis appears predominantly in males,[3] while breast cancer appears predominantly in females. Bladder cancer is much more common in men.[4] Migraine headaches[5] and rheumatoid arthritis[6] are of higher incidence in women than in men. Race may also predispose certain groups to a higher incidence of specific diseases. An example would be sickle cell disease, which is more prevalent in the black population.[7] There is a higher incidence of cancers of the skin such as basal and squamous cell carcinoma and melanoma in the white population.[8] Finally, a patient's occupation may facilitate the development of certain disease process. Exposure to extremes of hot or cold temperatures; to industrial toxins, such as lead, arsenic, and asbestos; or to extreme levels of mental or emotional pressures may contribute to the patient's clinical presentation.[5] For example, air pollutants such as coal or flour dust and fibrous substances such as asbestos can contribute to lung disease.

When appropriate, age, sex, race and occupation are noted as they relate to specific disease entities described in the remaining chapters of this book. This information can be easily gathered by the physical therapist during the examination process and may provide valuable clues regarding the presence of a suspicious condition.

Location and Description of Symptoms

The patient's chief complaint provides important initial information for the clinician. Documenting the chief complaint includes noting the location of the symptom and how the patient describes the symptoms. This information can be effectively illustrated with the use of a body diagram. Once the chief complaint has been described by the patient, the therapist should screen the remainder of the body for the presence of other symptoms. For example, let us say the patient's chief complaint is a deep, dull, aching sensation in the central low lumbar spine and right buttock, the therapist should then follow with the specific questions: Do you have any symptoms in the pelvic region, lower extremities, middle or upper back, abdominal region, chest, upper extremities, neck and head, or facial areas? Affirmative answers can then be documented on the body diagram, while asymptomatic regions can be noted with a symbol such as a check mark (Fig. 1-2). Patients may be so preoccupied with their low back pain that they forget to inform the physician that they also are experiencing headaches or right shoulder pain. Patients may not volunteer to the therapist that they have abdominal or facial pain. Their rationale may be "Why does my therapist need to know if my stomach hurts when I am here because of my low back pain?" Yet these "other symptoms" may be related to the low back pain, possibly the result of a mechanical musculoskeletal dysfunction condition or could be related to a disease process that is affecting a number of body parts simultaneously. Even if these "other symptoms" are not directly related to the low back pain complaints, the presence of the dysfunction or disease process responsible for the symptoms may interfere with the patient's progress during physical therapy for the low back pain. Appropriate treatment, including medical care by a physician, may enhance the therapist's chances of helping the patient. Assuming that these "other symptoms" and their etiology have nothing to do with the low back pain, but considering that they could be the result of a medical condition, the therapist has the responsibility to recommend that the patient see a physician for medical examination. The therapist should periodically repeat the process of screening the patient for location of symptoms. New symptoms may develop while the patient is under the care of the therapist, and it may be weeks or months before the patient is scheduled to see the physician. These new symptoms could be representative of the development of a pathologic condition. Again, the patient may not volunteer that these symptoms have appeared, under the misapprehension that they have nothing to do with what the patient is being treated for by the physical therapist.

Clinically, location of symptoms can be misleading regarding the anatomic source of the symptoms. For example, visceral structures can be the source of local chest and abdominal pain and have the potential to refer pain to other regions of the body. The nociceptors innervating viscera are located in the loose connective tissue walls of the structure and in the walls of the local blood vessels investing the visceral struc-

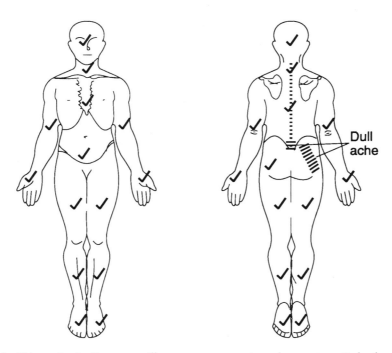

Fig. 1-2. Using a body diagram to illustrate symptomatic and asymptomatic body regions.

ture. Adequate chemical or mechanical stimulation will activate the nociceptive systems of a viscus. The result can be the perception of local pain and/or cortical misinterpretation of this sensory input (referred pain). It should not be assumed, however, that visceral structures are solely responsible for complaints such as abdominal pain. Simons and Travell[9] demonstrated that numerous muscles can be the source of abdominal pain. Other musculoskeletal structures, such as ligaments and facet joints, can also refer pain to the abdomen.[10,11] But at this point in the patient examination—investigating the chief complaint—the therapist must consider all possible sources of abdominal pain, including visceral structures. The organ systems to be screened with the presence of upper abdominal pain include the cardiovascular, pulmonary, gastrointestinal, and urogenital systems and the spleen, a component of the hematologic system. If lower abdominal pain is present, the cardiovascular, gastrointestinal, and urogenital systems should be screened. (See the corresponding chapter for each of the organ systems for a checklist of items to be used to help screen the various organ systems for the presence of disease.)

Once the nociceptive system of a visceral structure has been activated, the presence of the phenomenon of referred pain is possible. Referred pain is defined as pain experienced in tissues that are not the site of tissue damage and whose afferent or efferent neurons are not involved in the physiologic process of pain perception.[12] A diseased viscus may be manifested solely as back, buttock, or neck pain, while local abdominal symptoms or other complaints related to medical illness remain absent (Fig. 1-3). Therefore, a patient describing symptoms in the trunk (excluding the abdomen) or head and neck region could direct the therapist to screen the various organ systems for the presence of disease. If head or neck symptoms are present, the endocrine, nervous, cardiovascular, pulmonary, and gastrointestinal systems should all be screened. If shoulder symptoms (including the scapular and clavicular regions) are present, the cardiovascular, pulmonary, and gastrointestinal systems should be screened. All these systems should also be screened in the presence of upper and middle thoracic complaints. All these systems (with the exception of the pulmonary system), as well as the urogenital system, should be screened in the presence of lumbar or

pelvic complaints. Again, the other chapters of the book contain information that can be used to help screen these various organ systems. Determining which organ systems or disease entities should be screened for during a patient examination presents a difficult clinical decision. The location of the patient's symptoms is a key factor to consider when faced with this decision.

Investigating the chief complaint also includes the interpretation of the terms the patient uses when describing symptoms. Certain descriptors may be indicators of the presence of disease. Visceral pain has generally been described as ranging from sharp, severe, localized pain to poorly localized dull and vague sensations. The problem is that these same descriptors are also used by patients when describing symptoms for mechanical musculoskeletal dysfunction conditions. Therefore, the clinician is helped little by the presence of these particular complaints regarding the origin of symptoms. Other descriptors used by patients can be helpful, however. Sensations of cramping, colicky pain have been attributed to spasm of the smooth muscle wall of hollow viscus. The intensity of the cramping sensation varies as the smooth muscle wall rhythmically contracts and relaxes. This contraction-relaxation cycle may last up to a few minutes. Gastroenteritis, constipation, menstruation, gallbladder disease, and ureteral obstruction have all been implicated in the cramping pain experienced in the abdomen or referred to the back.[13] Complaints of a throbbing, cramping, or aching type of pain could be suggestive of cardiovascular system involvement. Symptom descriptors such as pressure, tightness, or heaviness in the thoracic, cervical, facial, or upper extremities as well as complaints of restless legs, weakness, and the sensation of pins and needles should also prompt screening of the cardiovascular system. Weakness, poor balance, numbness, and pins-and-needles sensation should also direct the therapist to clear the patient for nervous system involvement.

At times, patients have difficulty in pinpointing the location of their symptoms and in describing exactly what their symptoms feel like. Therapists must do all they can to facilitate this information-gathering process of important clues that may raise suspicion of a disease entity. The next important category of information in

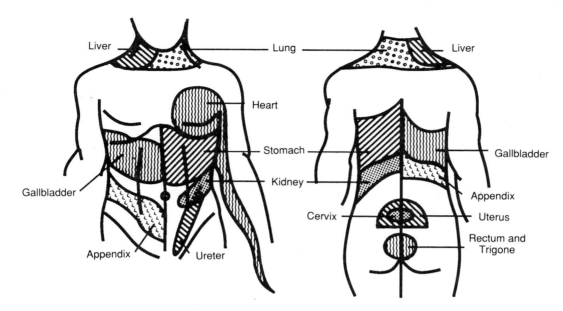

Fig. 1-3. Possible pain-referral patterns of visceral structures.

the subjective examination (behavior of symptoms) is closely related to the chief complaints.

Symptom Behavior

Symptom behavior is described as a change in the location, intensity, and/or quality (e.g., pins-and-needle sensation progressing to numbness) of the patient's complaints as related to activity, cessation of activity (i.e., rest), and assumption of specific body positions.[14] A common descriptor of pain from a visceral structure is a diffuse poorly localized dull sensation. Kellgren[10,15] and Inman and Saunders[16] also described a similar pain sensation that results from irritation of deep ligamentous and musculature structures of the spine. Therefore, the chief complaint may provide minimal insight regarding whether the source of the patient's pain is a visceral or a musculoskeletal structure.

Questions regarding the behavior of the patient's complaints may help the therapist considerably with this differentiation, when faced with this clinical problem. Classically, a change in the location and/or intensity of the symptoms from mechanical musculoskeletal dys-

function can be associated with either an alteration in body posture or specific activities. Therefore, if the patient's complaints do not vary with movement or rest, the therapist should be suspicious of a pathologic disorder as the cause of the symptoms. Often patients state that their symptoms are constant, but further questioning indicates that the intensity of the complaint does vary during a 24-hour period. If the symptoms are most severe at night, for example, the patient wakes at 2:00 AM with severe low back pain, the therapist should again be suspicious of the etiology of the symptoms. This is because, in most mechanical musculoskeletal dysfunction conditions, symptoms should be less severe when at rest. Patients with pain from dysfunction may wake up during the night stiff, sore, or with exacerbation of their chief complaint, but in most cases the symptoms are most severe with activity or assumption of a weight-bearing posture.

The therapist must be aware that the presence of symptoms that vary with movement or change in posture does not rule out the possibility of disease. For example, if a pathologic fracture secondary to a metastatic lesion is responsible for the patient's hip pain, certain activities such as standing and walking may increase the intensity of the pain significantly, while positions such as supine or side lying may not eliminate the pain but could decrease the intensity of the symptoms. Another example is occlusive arterial disease. A classic symptom is intermittent claudication, often marked by pain in the buttocks, thighs, or calves, associated with physical activity and relieved with rest. In both examples, other information obtained during the history and the objective examination will provide clues raising suspicion of the possible presence of a disease process despite symptom behavior findings that are classically representative of a mechanical dysfunction condition.

The behavior of symptoms from the visceral organs will vary depending on the function of the structure. Therefore, a patient report of intermittent symptoms does not rule out the possibility of the presence of disease. If the patient's central, mid-thoracic spine pain was the result of a duodenal ulcer, gastrointestinal system activity may alter the pain complaints. For example, the pain from the ulcer may begin a couple of hours after eating and then be relieved when the patient eats. Careful questioning related to the change of symptoms experienced over a 24-hour period may reveal important information patients would not normally have volunteered, as they may not have made the connection between their symptoms and gastrointestinal system function.

Each symptom noted when documenting a patient's complaints should be fully investigated regarding its behavior. This includes noting whether the symptoms are constant or intermittently present. If intermittent, what is the change in symptoms related to activities over a 24-hour period? If multiple symptom locations are noted, as in the patient with low back, buttock, and calf pain, the therapist should not assume that one lesion is responsible for the symptoms in all three locations. The low back and buttock pain may be a result of mechanical musculoskeletal dysfunction at L5–S1, while the calf pain may be due to peripheral vascular disease. The physical therapist must pay careful attention to the behavior of each symptom, to avoid being fooled, ultimately preventing

delay in providing appropriate medical care to the patient.

Symptom Onset

The mechanism of the onset of symptoms may also provide clues regarding the possible presence of a disease entity. The classic case involves symptoms related to a mechanical musculoskeletal dysfunction thought to be the result of a traumatic accident or incident or of an event marked by repetitive microtrauma or sustained postural strains. These events may include lifting an object, falling, or taking an extended car ride or plane trip, or the patient may report awakening with shoulder or low back pain after a day of heavy yard work. The therapist should be aware of a pathologic lesion if the onset of the patient's complaints is truly insidious, if new symptoms occur insidiously during the course of treatment, or if resolved symptoms return during the course of treatment for no apparent mechanical reason. Often patients cannot relate the onset of their symptoms to a particular accident or incident. Careful questioning by the therapist regarding the activities the patient engaged in before the initial perception of symptoms often pinpoints the problem. For example, the patient may have had a change in activity level, such as beginning to run after not running for 6 months; being promoted to an administrative position on the job, involving sitting for 8 hours a day; or beginning gardening and doing yard work after a winter of relative inactivity.

If the patient relates the onset of symptoms to a specific incident, such as lifting an object, the physical therapy should not rule out the prospect of a disease process as responsible for the complaints. For example, in the presence of a bony neoplastic lesion, a lifting or bending activity may sufficiently load the weakened structure as to produce a fracture and pain. The symptoms may not be severe enough to present as a medical emergency, and the patient could arrive at the physical therapy clinic with complaints of low back or hip pain. Another example could be a child with no previous history of knee pain who falls and hurts her knee. Persistent knee pain precipitates a visit to the clinic. It is possible that a previously asymptomatic and undiagnosed tumor could now be responsible for the inordinate duration of the pain, considering the degree of trauma. It is hoped that other examination findings besides the onset of symptoms or lack of response to treatment will make evident the possible presence of a pathologic condition and subsequent referral to a physician.

Review of Systems

Review of a patient's current and past medical history can provide valuable insight regarding the possible presence of a .medical condition, including psychological conditions, which may have a direct impact on a patient's initial symptomatic picture, or which may have an impact on how a patient responds to physical therapy care. This information can be grouped into three categories: (1) the patient's current health status, (2) the patient's health status just before the onset of symptoms, and (3) the patient's past medical history beyond the chronologic timeframe of the symptomatic condition.

Evaluating the patient's general health during the initial evaluation may provide information that will direct the therapist to screen specific or multiple organ systems. Figure 1-4 presents a checklist of items that review the patient's general health and that provide initial information for each of the organ systems. Positive patient responses to any of the items should direct the therapist to ask additional questions and/or perform objective tests that will provide more information regarding the patient's condition.

The first item on the checklist, *fever/chills/sweats* is associated with common ailments, such as "the flu," but these complaints are also associated with the presence of occult infections and cancer. *Unexplained weight change*, especially weight loss, is a potential symptom of a variety of ailments, including gastrointestinal disorders (e.g., ulcers or cancer), diabetes mellitus, hyperthyroidism, adrenal insufficiency, common infections and malignancies, and depression.[17] If the patient has noted weight loss, questions should follow regarding a change in diet or activity level that might explain it. The complaint of *malaise, fatigue, or loss of energy* is not an uncommon complaint offered by many patients, especially those with a long history of symptoms. This nonspecific complaint can be a result of a number of different disease entities, including depression, infections (e.g., hepatitis or tuberculosis), hypothyroidism, diabetes mellitus, anemia, cancer, nutritional deficits, and rheumatoid arthritis.[18] Certain medications may also produce malaise as a side effect.

Nausea and vomiting are most directly related to involvement of the gastrointestinal system. These complaints also may denote either pregnancy or cancer or may be a side effect of certain medications. Complaints of *numbness or weakness* should direct the therapist to investigate the status of the nervous system. *Syncope*, the sudden but temporary loss of consciousness, is a condition associated with inadequate blood flow to the brain. Patients may also describe dizziness and lightheadedness. These symptoms may be associated with side effects of medications for cardiovascular system diseases (e.g., blood pressure problems) or may be a result of hypoglycemia in a diabetic patient. The significance of *night pain* is described under Symptom Behavior. This complaint may indicate the presence of serious pathology such as cancer. Complaints of *dyspnea* or shortness of breath could be an indicator of cardiovascular or pulmonary system disease. If this complaint is present, additional questions and objective tests should follow for further assessment of the status of these two systems. In addition, *a history of smoking* significantly increases the risk of the development of diseases in these two systems, as well as other organ systems. Complaints of *dysuria, urinary frequency changes, and sexual dysfunction* should direct the therapist to specific screening of the urogenital system. Questioning a patient regarding *alcohol and drug usage* can be difficult and awkward for the therapist. (See Ch. 11 for suggestions regarding the investigation of a history of substance abuse.) Also, noting which *medications* the patient is taking can be helpful. We recommend the *Drug Use Education Tips* published by the American Academy of Family Physicians, Kansas City, Missouri, as a resource for information on the most commonly used medications. Noting specific medications and familiarity with potential side effects may explain some of the patient's complaints, including malaise, lightheadedness, or constipation. Asking patients why they are taking certain

Review of systems: General health			
Item	Yes	No	Comments
1. Fever/chills/sweats	_____	_____	_____
2. Unexplained weight change	_____	_____	_____
3. Malaise	_____	_____	_____
4. Nausea/vomiting	_____	_____	_____
5. Bowel dysfunction	_____	_____	_____
6. Numbness	_____	_____	_____
7. Weakness	_____	_____	_____
8. Syncope	_____	_____	_____
9. Dizziness/lightheadedness	_____	_____	_____
10. Night pain	_____	_____	_____
11. Dyspnea	_____	_____	_____
12. Dysuria	_____	_____	_____
13. Urinary frequency changes	_____	_____	_____
14. Sexual dysfunction	_____	_____	_____
15. History of smoking	_____	_____	_____
16. History of substance abuse	_____	_____	_____
17. Medications	_____	_____	_____
18. History of illness	_____	_____	_____
19. History of surgery	_____	_____	_____
20. Family medical history	_____	_____	_____

Fig. 1-4. Checklist designed to review the patient's general health status, as part of the subjective examination process. (Modified from Boissonnault and Bass,[24] with permission.)

medications may also reveal the presence of a medical condition the patient might not otherwise have volunteered.

Questions regarding the patient's *medical history* are important to include in this screening process. This includes inquiring whether the patient is currently being treated by another health care professional for a medical condition. The therapist should present a specific list of disorders to the patient: "Are you being treated for heart or vascular problems, stomach ailments, cancer, infections, psychological disorders, or pelvic or groin problems?" This approach can be very useful, as many patients forget about a particular condition, do not volunteer information they perceive as unimportant, or do not volunteer sensitive information, such as having cancer or being treated for a psychological condition. This checklist should include questions about the patient's surgical history. The patient's *family medical history* will provide important screening information. All patients being evaluated for any problem should be screened in this manner.

Questions related to the patient's health status just before the onset of symptoms can also provide valuable information, especially if the mechanism of the onset of symptoms is unclear or vague. The same questions designed to investigate the patient's current general health status can be used. Treatment for a medical condition just before, or simultaneous to, the onset of symptoms could be significant. For example, the presence of an infectious process before the onset of symptoms could have produced infection elsewhere in the body. Patients who had a bladder infection, but who thought they had recovered from it, may have developed a kidney infection, manifested primarily as low back pain. Osteomyelitis, a condition that may result in a deep, dull, central low back pain complaint, may be precipitated by other infectious diseases, including urinary tract infections. Certain cardiovascular conditions have a history of recurrence or progressing to a point where new symptoms develop. Therefore, a history of treatment for cardiovascular problems should lead the therapist to screen the cardiovascular system during the examination. Questions regarding the medications the patient had taken just before the onset of symptoms are also important. For example, taking nonsteroidal anti-inflammatory drugs (NSAIDs) can lead to the development of gastrointestinal disorders, such as a gastric ulcer. The symptoms from the ulcer may be masked while the patient is taking the medication but become noticeable once the patient stops taking the pills. The most overt symptoms related to the ulcer may be mid-thoracic pain, with the patient ending up at the physical therapy clinic for treatment.

Questions regarding the patient's medical history beyond the scope of the current symptomatic picture should provide medical information extending back to the patient's childhood. Again, it is important to question the patient regarding treatment of any medical conditions. Questions regarding surgery the patient may have undergone, and for what reasons, may also provide information regarding the presence of medical conditions with a pattern of recurrence. For example, a patient with a history of cancer who presents with complaints of pain and who has not been seen by a physician before the physical therapy evaluation should be referred to a physician, regardless of how mechanical the condition might appear to be. Once the patient has been cleared medically by the physician, physical therapy can proceed.

Investigating a patient's current and past medical history is an important component of the subjective examination process for any patient. These questions will help provide the therapist with information regarding the presence of medical conditions that may not be responsible for symptoms but could have an impact on how well the patient tolerates or responds to therapeutic intervention. These medical conditions may be directly related to the patient's complaints. Therefore, the patient's report of treatment for certain medical conditions may direct the therapist to more detailed screening of the visceral organ system.

Questions related to the health status of the patient's parents and siblings can provide important information. Certain disease entities, such as rheumatoid arthritis, diabetes, cardiovascular disorders, kidney disease, and cancer, have familial tendencies.[17] Therefore, this list of items should be presented to the patient. If family members are deceased, the physical therapist should inquire as to the cause of death and significant illness they were treated for before their death. In the following chapters, the disease entities most commonly encountered by physical therapists with significant familial tendencies are discussed in detail.

Summary

A complete subjective examination can provide helpful insight as to the presence of conditions that could interfere with a patient's response to what may be perceived as appropriate physical therapy. The preceding sections emphasized the subjective examination components related to ruling out the presence of disease that could be responsible for symptoms and to detecting the presence of disease entities that could interfere with a patient's appropriate progress while receiving treatment by a physical therapist. The history findings can also guide the therapist regarding when to implement special objective examination procedures for the purpose of gathering additional information regarding the patient's health status.

Objective Examination

Many of the objective tests used to provide information regarding the presence of disease fall outside the realm of the physical therapy profession. Examples of these tests include urinalysis, blood tests, and radiologic testing. Nevertheless, physical therapists can obtain important information if they have the knowledge and skills to implement test procedures such as assessment of blood pressure and arterial pulses and can carry out a thorough neurologic evaluation. In addition, having the knowledge to interpret the clinical findings from tests that do fall within the realm of the physical therapy profession, such as observation, palpation, and active, passive, and resisted testing, will provide invaluable clues regarding the nature of the lesion. The objective findings most suggestive of the presence of a pathologic disorder are emphasized in this section.

Detailed information related to the more general tests (i.e., observation and palpation) is provided in this chapter. It is often the information obtained during the history and observation and palpation components of the objective examination that directs the therapist to a more detailed review of the organ systems. An important aspect of the observation and palpation test-

ing is skin assessment, which is covered exclusively in this chapter. The other "special" tests of the objective examination, including assessment of pulses and blood pressure, percussion, and auscultation, are mentioned but are described in detail in the appropriate chapters.

One of the crucial factors to be considered by the physical therapist is related to provocation of symptoms. Alteration of symptoms from mechanical musculoskeletal dysfunction should be related to a change in the patient's posture or movement. Therefore, when symptoms cannot be reproduced, increased, or decreased by palpation, active or passive movement techniques, resisted tests, neurologic tests, or special tests, the therapist should be suspicious of a functional (psychological) or pathologic condition. Changes in symptoms during the physical examination do not absolutely rule out the presence of pathologic disorders. For example, infection of the intervertebral disc may cause severe low back pain that may vary in intensity with movement and changes in posture. A pathologic fracture of a vertebral body secondary to metastatic lesion may also result in similar findings. In these cases, other findings from both the history and physical examination, such as insignificant relief of symptoms when the patient is at rest, should help steer the therapist toward the appropriate conclusion regarding the source of the patient's symptoms. While therapists should be concerned if they fail to alter a patient's symptomatic presentation, there are times when mechanical dysfunction is still the primary lesion. The condition may not be irritable, taking considerable activity on the patient's part to provoke the symptoms, and the therapist cannot clinically stress the tissue sufficiently to bring on the complaints. The therapist may also not have stressed the appropriate region during the examination process. For example, a patient with lower-extremity symptoms resulting from a thoracic spine lesion may have been diagnosed as having mechanical low back pain syndrome. Screening the lumbar spine, pelvis, and lower extremities alone would not have demonstrated the source of the symptoms. Despite the above scenarios, if the therapist is confident that the appropriate body regions have been screened and the symptoms have not been altered, suspicion should be raised regarding the source of the symptoms.

Additional test procedures that can provide important information for the therapist can be grouped under the general categories of observation, palpation, percussion, auscultation, and neurologic examination.

Observation

Observation can provide important information regarding the possible presence of disease processes. A key item to include in the examination scheme is the assessment of skin condition. This assessment includes not only the skin itself but the hair and nails as well. Most abnormalities are benign entities, but certain skin lesions are suggestive of serious pathology, including melanoma and basal cell carcinoma. Characteristics of these serious lesions include variation in color within the noted area or structure, an irregular perimeter or border, a raised and irregular surface, a firm to hard consistency, and ulceration or crusting of the lesion. If the therapist notes a lesion or area of skin presenting with any combination of the above characteristics during the postural assessment or during a detailed regional examination, the patient should be asked whether the physician has noted this "spot" on the skin. Questioning the patient regarding noting a change in size, shape, or color of this area would also be appropriate. If the patient states that the physician is not aware of the area of skin involved, a recommendation that a visit to the physician would be advisable should be made in an unalarming fashion. It would then be appropriate for the therapist to telephone the physician regarding why the patient is being sent for examination. There are numerous skin lesions that may be observed by the therapist that are not life threatening but that do require medical examination and subsequent treatment. These conditions include psoriasis, herpes zoster, and scleroderma. Psoriasis may be marked by reddened patches of skin, accompanied by erythematous plaques and silvery scales. These lesions are more commonly observed on the elbows, knees, scalp, and intergluteal cleft. Herpes zoster (shingles) may be manifested as reddened areas of the skin within a dermatomal distribution. Vesicles may be found within the reddened area, and intense burning and tenderness may accompany the skin

changes. Scleroderma is a rheumatic disease characterized by a hardening of the skin. The patient may note a tightening sensation of the skin, especially of the hands and face. The skin lines may be absent, and skin mobility could be significantly restricted influencing ROM.[8]

Assessment of skin color can also be easily carried out during the postural or regional examination. Cyanosis, a dark bluish coloration of skin, including nails and/or the mucous membranes secondary to poor oxygenation of the blood, can be a sign of advanced lung disease or cardiovascular system involvement. Centrally, the lips, buccal mucosa, or tongue are usually the best structures to assess for the presence of cyanosis, whereas the skin and nails of the upper and lower extremities are the best areas for peripheral assessment. Jaundice, the yellowish coloration of structures, including the skin, tongue, and lips, can be representative of a liver disease or a blood disorder. The scleras of the eyes may also show the color change associated with jaundice. Pallor or paleness of skin can be suggestive of cardiovascular system disorders, including arterial insufficiency and anemia. Abnormal redness may also be indicative of the presence of a disease process. Skin marked by the presence of red streaks can be suggestive of the presence of an infectious process.[17]

Assessment of skin condition also includes observation of body hair and nails. Hair loss of distal extremity parts, such as hands and forearms or feet and lower legs, can be indicative of a peripheral vascular disease. More general hair loss may also be associated with anemia and hypopituitarism, while increased hair patterns can be seen in Cushing's disease and with certain cancers, such as of the adrenals and gonads. Deformities of the nails can also be markers of disease. Clubbing of the nails can be indicative of pulmonary system disease including lung cancer. Clubbing of the nails is described as the angle between the fingernail and nail base exceeding 180 degrees, with the nail base being swollen and soft.[17] Transverse sulci running perpendicular to the longitudinal axis of the nail (Beau's lines) may accompany anemia, malnutrition, and the acute stage of infectious diseases. Pitting of the nails have been associated with psoriasis, diabetes, and peripheral vascular disease. Nails that are spoon shaped (concave) can be associated with anemia, chronic infection, malnutrition, and Raynaud's disease.[18]

Palpation

Palpation is another important component of the objective examination that can indicate signs of the presence of disease. Palpation can be used for skin temperature, lymph nodes, vascular pulses, and abnormal soft tissue or bony masses. Besides observation, assessment of the skin and associated structures includes palpation for skin temperature. General decreased skin temperature is one sign of hypothyroidism, while general increased skin temperature is one sign of hyperthyroidism.[17] Localized increased temperature is associated with the presence of an inflammatory process but, if the tissue temperature is very warm to hot, an infectious process must also be considered.

Palpable lymph nodes may suggest the presence of infection or neoplasm. Although palpable lymph nodes are not generally found in healthy people, lymph nodes of up to 1 cm are considered normal. The presence of palpable lymph nodes that seem to be fixed or immovable from underlying tissues should raise concern. Normal lymph nodes should not be tender to touch, but nodes that are not tender are not necessarily normal. Lymph nodes to which malignancy has spread are usually not tender.[8] Areas that should be palpated for lymph nodes include the submandibular, supraclavicular, anterior and posterior cervical regions, and the axilla. Another important region of the lower quarter to be palpated is the femoral triangle, especially around the inguinal ligament. Generally lymph nodes are also found in close proximity to all the major peripheral joints, including the elbow, wrist, knee, and ankles.

Palpation of peripheral arterial pulses may reveal important information regarding the status of the cardiovascular system. An absent or diminished pulse suggests vascular obstruction that may be related to the patient's complaints. Lower-extremity pulses to be assessed include the femoral artery in the femoral triangle, the popliteal artery, and the dorsal pedis and posterior tibial arteries. In the upper extremity, the brachial artery in the cubital fossa and the radial and ulnar arteries at the wrist should be assessed. Central pulses that can be palpated include the aorta and iliac arteries. The carotid artery can be used, but the therapist must consider that even light pressure on the vessel may stimulate the carotid pressure receptors, resulting in a drop in the heart rate. (See Ch. 2, for the parameters of a normal versus abnormal pulse.)

When assessing the abdomen, and especially before doing soft tissue mobilization techniques for the abdominal region, the therapist should palpate for the presence of an aortic aneurysm. Most aortic aneurysms occur caudal to the renal arteries and produce a pulsation that is more prominent and distinct within a confined region than in a normal aorta. A palpable pulse greater than 2 to 3 inches wide should raise suspicion of the presence of aneurysm.

Palpation for the presence of abnormal soft tissue and bony masses is an ongoing process during the examination. The clinician must have in-depth knowledge of normal anatomy to be able to detect abnormalities. Many therapists lack familiarity of the normal anatomy of the abdomen, yet the abdomen is an area that often needs manual treatment, to improve extensibility of scar tissue, to treat trigger points in the abdominal muscle wall or iliopsoas muscle groups, and to decrease tone in musculature accessible through the abdominal wall, including the abdominals, respiratory diaphragm, and iliopsoas groups. (See Ch. 4, for a detailed description of normal abdominal anatomy.)

Percussion

Applying a vibratory force to bone tissue may provide information regarding the presence of a disease state or fracture. In the spine, the spinous processes is percussed with a reflex hammer or with fingertips with the patient in a forward-flexed posture. The presence of infection or tumor may be marked by provocation of either severe pain and tenderness or a deep, dull, throbbing pain that does not decrease in intensity immediately after completion of the technique. (See Ch. 9, for more information regarding the use of percussion as an examination procedure.)

Percussing other body regions, such as the thorax and abdomen, can also give important information regarding the health and location of soft tissue structures. Percussing over solid organs, such as the liver or spleen, should produce a decreased resonance or dullness to the sound. Assuming that there are no abnormal masses in the abdomen, percussing over most of the abdominal cavity will usually produce a tympanic sound (low-pitched, drumlike noise). Exceptions may occur if percussing over the suprapubic region when the bladder or uterus are distended. Normal fluid and fecal material may also produce a duller sound. Physical therapists can use percussion to locate structures such as the liver or spleen and take the appropriate precautions when doing deep soft tissue mobilization techniques in the upper abdominal region. (See Ch. 4 for further information regarding assessment of the abdomen.)

Auscultation

Listening for body sounds to help assess the status of an organ system is a common evaluation tool used by therapists working in a hospital setting. In certain situations in an outpatient setting, auscultation may provide valuable information to the therapist regarding a patient's health status. (See Chs. 2 and 3 for more detailed guidelines regarding the use of ausculation and interpretation of ausculatory findings.)

Neurologic Examination

This section provides an overview of neurologic examination principles with emphasis on reflex, sensory, and motor testing. (See Ch. 8 for a detailed description of assessment of the neurocranium and other components of the central and peripheral nervous system.)

An argument could be made for performing a neurologic examination on all patients, to obtain a baseline of normal regarding the status of their nervous system. There are times, however, when inadequate time to complete the initial evaluation prevents the therapist from including the neurological examination in the initial visit, or the patient's complaints might not warrant including the neurologic examination within the initial assessment scheme. A neurologic examination should be carried out during the initial evaluation for any patient who describes such symptoms

as radicular pain (pain that follows the path of a nerve), weakness, numbness, and/or paresthesias. Some patients may note that they have been dropping objects, stubbing their toes, or tripping over their feet, indicating possible weakness. Others may describe a hand that feels heavy or dead or as though it is falling asleep or hypersensitivity or irritability of the skin, indicating possible sensory changes. Any of the above complaints should direct the therapist to carry out a neurologic examination during the initial assessment. If positive neurologic signs are detected during the evaluation, retesting the status of the nervous system should be a part of each subsequent visit (before and after treatment) to closely monitor the patient's status. This should be done even if the patient reports significant reduction in pain complaints or possibly being pain free. It is possible in this situation that the compression on the nerve has progressed to complete occlusion. The patient's perception is that the problem has subsided, because of the reduction in pain, but in fact the condition has worsened. Progressive worsening of neurologic signs should be brought to the physician's attention immediately.

The three most commonly used components of the neurologic examination are reflex, sensory, and motor testing. Appendices 1-1 and 1-2 list specific tests that can be performed in weight-bearing (standing, sitting) and non-weight-bearing positions (prone, supine). To provide more valid and reliable information, the tests should be performed with the patient positioned in a consistent fashion. For example, if during a lower-quarter screening examination a portion of the neurologic assessment is done with the patient sitting and the remainder with the patient supine, inconsistent or false-negative findings may occur because of the change in pressure exerted on the nerve or the change in the degree of stretch placed on the nerve as the lumbar spine assumes a different position. False-negative findings may occur, however, even if all the tests are done with the patient remaining in a single position. Patients with a lumbar spinal nerve root compression secondary to lateral foraminal stenosis may be sitting with the lumbar spine in a kyphotic posture or may be supporting the trunk weight on their hands (propping themselves up, unweighting the lumbar spine). These positions may sufficiently relieve the compressive forces on the nerve so all the neurologic tests are negative. Another example would be a patient with cervical radiculopathy. The test results may be altered or influenced by inconsistencies in the patient's head and neck posture. While sitting, the patient may be watching the therapist perform the different tests, placing the neck in a variety of forward-bent, side-bent, and rotated positions. This altered head and neck posture would again alter the environment of the nerve root. The therapist must closely monitor the patient's trunk, head, and neck position while carrying out neurologic assessment. Consistent spine positioning and considering weight-bearing versus non-weight-bearing postures can greatly enhance the gathering of this important clinical information.

Testing for the status of deep tendon reflexes can be carried out for selected upper- and lower-extremity muscles and selected facial and trunk musculature. The reflex response can be graded using a 0 to 4 scale. A 2+ grade represents a normal response, a 0+ represents an absent response, while 1+ represents a diminished response. A 3+ grade indicates a brisk response and a 4+ grade indicates a very brisk response. Grieve[12] recommends repetitive testing, tapping the tendon up to six times in order to detect the possible presence of a fading reflex response indicating a developing nerve root lesion.

When assessing the abdominal reflexes, instead of tapping, the skin is stroked with the end of the reflex hammer. Each of the four abdominal quadrants (see Fig. 4-2) is gently stroked, noting movement of the umbilicus. If the reflex is intact, the umbilicus will move toward the stimulus. The upper abdominal quadrants represent the T7–T10 segments, while the lower abdominal quadrants represent the T10–L1 segments.[20]

The most commonly used sensory tests are light touch and pin prick. The clinician notes hyperesthesia, hypoesthesia, numbness, and or paresthesia as indicators of involvement of the sensory component of the nervous system. Careful comparison of left versus right corresponding body parts can help the therapist detect these sensory changes. If the patient notes a difference in the quality of pinprick or light touch stimulus (i.e., "I don't feel as much on the left side"), the therapist can then compare different regions within the same extremity to help determine whether the left side is hypoesthetic or if the right side is hyperesthetic. The location of the sensory changes will help the therapist differentiate between a peripheral nerve lesion and a spinal nerve root lesion. (See Figs. 8-4 and 8-5 for the sensory fields—dermatome versus peripheral nerve supply.)

Testing the motor component (myotome) of the nervous system consists of assessing strength of a selected muscle or muscle group that primarily represents a single neurologic segment of the spinal cord. The process of strength assessment usually begins with observation of active ROM of the joint the muscle crosses, against gravity. Active ROM, gravity eliminated, can be implemented if indicated. Assuming the patient can move the joint against gravity, either an isometric contraction against manual resistance or applied resistance throughout the active ROM can then be incorporated into the testing process. A 0 to 5 grading scale can be used to document the test findings. A 0 grade indicates no contraction noted, 1 indicates a flicker/trace of contraction, 2 indicates active movement with gravity eliminated, 3 implies that active movement can occur against gravity, 4 indicates active movement against gravity plus against manual resistance, while a grade 5 indicates normal strength with manual resistance applied.[21]

Applying these test procedures should allow the clinician to detect many of the patient's neurologic motor deficits, but to avoid false-negative findings the therapist should also incorporate repeated contractions or sustained isometric contractions of the muscle or muscle group. Cailliet[22] states that minor compromise of a nerve may be manifested by muscle fatigue rather than by frank weakness. The sign, fatiguability, is more likely to be present in the early stages of nerve root compromise. Detecting muscle fatigue could easily be missed if the myotome test consisted only of a "break" strength test. Even using sustained manual isometric contraction for large, powerful muscles such as quadriceps or the gastrocnemius/soleus may not reveal the muscle fatigue. Cailliet recommends using repetitive unilateral heel raising to assess the gastroc soleus group as a more delicate method of testing for minor impairment of the S1 nerve. Repetitive unilateral standing deep knee bends could be used for assessing the quadricep muscle group. Careful monitoring of the patient's posture while performing these movements would be extremely important. For the smaller muscle groups (e.g., anterior tibialis, extensor hallucis longus, and biceps), a sustained isometric contraction should be sufficient to screen the upper-and lower-extremity myotomes adequately for the onset of fatigue.[22]

If weakness is noted, the therapist must consider other sources of the deficit besides spinal nerve root involvement. A peripheral nerve lesion or a local muscle condition may also produce the weakness discovered. For example, if the patient presents with shoulder abduction weakness (C5–C6, axillary nerve), the therapist must consider: Does the lesion lie in the C5–C6 nerve roots, in the axillary nerve, or in the shoulder abductor muscle (supraspinatous will be considered)? Other C5–C6 muscles (elbow flexors, musculocutaneous nerve) that are not innervated by the axillary nerve can be tested. If the elbow flexors are also weak, a spinal nerve root lesion as the source of the weakness is supported. If the elbow flexors are strong, an axillary nerve lesion or structural muscle weakness may be responsible for the abduction weakness. A local supraspinatous muscle lesion would be marked by clinical findings, such as absence of other neurologic signs and observable or palpable changes in the muscle. Appendices 1-1 and 1-2 list the upper- and lower-extremity muscles and their central and peripheral innervations, which can be used for these testing purposes. In addition, correlation of other neurologic signs, such as location of sensory changes and deep tendon reflex findings, may help with this differentiation.

Monitoring the status of a patient's nervous system is an important responsibility of the physical therapist. Progressive worsening of neurologic signs warrants an immediate phone call to the physician. Immediate medical intervention may be necessary to prevent irreversible damage to the nerve tissue.

Summary

Incorporating the above principles and items of the subjective and objective examination into the evaluation scheme should not add inordinate time to the patient's initial visit. To keep the examination time ef-

ficient, the therapist must develop a well-organized subjective and objective examination format that begins with questions and techniques aimed at providing general information regarding the patient's status. The information obtained during the subjective examination will help the therapist decide (1) which body region(s) to assess objectively; (2) which specific examination techniques to use or omit; (3) the sequence of objective testing, including patient positioning; and (4) the degree of aggressiveness of the various techniques. The subjective examination will also provide valuable information regarding the origin of symptoms, mechanical versus pathologic. Starting the objective examination with an upper- or lower-quarter screening examination can also save the therapist valuable time. These general clearing tests help direct the therapist to examine specific body regions in detail and determine areas of mechanical dysfunction that are directly or indirectly related to the patient's symptoms. In addition, tests are included that help screen the patient for the presence of medical disease. Figure 1-5 presents a general examination scheme; Appendices 1-1 and 1-2 detail the components of suggested upper- and lower-quarter screening examinations.

Owing to time constraints, normally only one of the two screening examinations will be performed during the initial evaluation. Generally, the location and description of symptoms from the history will determine which quadrant examination will be used. Structuring these examinations by position is usually physically easier for the patient and more time efficient for the therapist. The sequence of positioning suggested is standing, sitting, supine, and then prone, although the acuteness of the patient's condition and behavior of the symptoms could alter this sequence. Specific approaches to carrying out and interpreting the tests designed to screen the patient for medical conditions (see Appendices 1-1 and 1-2) are described throughout this book. Numerous textbooks are available that describe other tests designed to screen for mechanical dysfunction.

Upon completion of the examination, the therapist may have more questions than answers regarding the source of the patient's symptoms or, in fact, may be confident that the patient has presented with a condition for which physical therapy is appropriate. It may

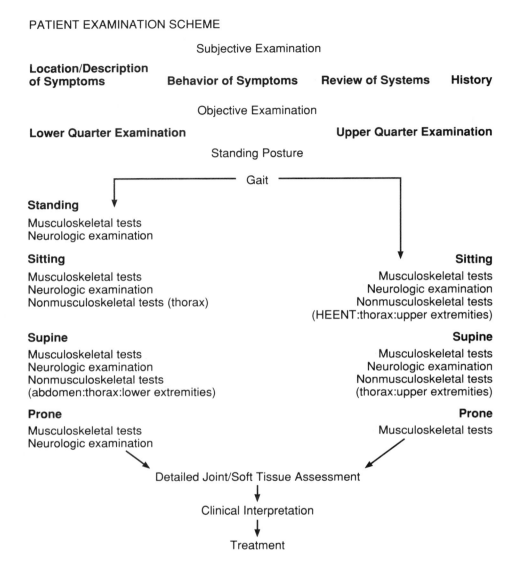

Fig. 1-5. General patient examination scheme leading to detailed assessment of specific body regions.

not be until noting how the patient responds to treatment that the therapist begins to question the underlying condition responsible for the symptoms or to be suspicious of the development of another pathologic process. Constant reassessment of the patient's status is an essential component of the ongoing examination process. The following section describes the principles related to reassessment, once treatment has been initiated.

Response to Treatment

Once the therapist has gathered information from the subjective and objective examination, analysis and interpretation of findings follows. A problem list is generated from the examination. This is then followed by devising a hypothesis as to what the underlying pathologic process may be giving rise to the patient's signs and symptoms and what possibly precipitated their onset. Relative to diagnosis and treatment of mechanical dysfunction, Maitland[23] refers to the term *assessment* in two ways. The first meaning includes interpreting the history of the patient's disorder and the symptoms and signs, so that a diagnosis can be made; determining the stage in the natural history of the disorder; and the psychological effect the disorder is having on the patient, taking into account such factors as ethnic background, home, and job situation. The second meaning refers to determining the effect the treatment has had, by checking the patient's symptoms and signs after each application of every technique. This assessment is used to prove the value of the technique used at that particular stage of the disorder.

From this information, goals and a prognosis are developed for the patient's treatment program. Prognosis is very important in guiding the therapist. The therapist should have expectations as to how the patient should respond to treatment, both subjectively and objectively. Any deviation from these expectations should raise a question as to why the patient is not responding appropriately. A treatment plan is then generated to address the patient's problems in the most comprehensive yet efficient manner. This plan should consist of at least three elements, including diagnostic, therapeutic, and educational components.

Take the case of a young patient, in excellent general health, who twists her ankle and suffers an apparent grade II sprain of the anterior talofibular and calcaneal fibular ligaments. She has no additional injuries and no prior history of ankle dysfunction and is seen the day of the injury. One would expect a relatively quick, continuous, and probable full functional recovery with physical therapy intervention. If it turns out that, with appropriate treatment, swelling, pain, and dysfunction do not dissipate as quickly as expected, one might consider the possibility of a more extensive sprain and/or fracture; if not already done, radiographs would need to be taken. A second patient in her mid-30s, is deconditioned and overweight and has a chronically unstable lateral ankle. If she suffers a recurrent sprain, one would expect slower progress and a longer treatment course and the possibility of some permanent loss of function of the ankle in the future, with a much

higher probability for recurrence of symptoms without proper treatment.

Many times, signs and symptoms that were first seen on initial examination change with subsequent visits. This may be true if (1) treatment affects the patient in an adverse way, (2) an additional event influences the patient during the treatment course, and (3) the patient has an active pathologic process that becomes worse during the treatment time.

During the course of treatment, the physical therapist must continue to correlate subjective and objective information. At times, function may improve before symptoms, or vice versa, and it may be left to the therapist to determine whether this is the normal course for the diagnosed problem(s).

It is not uncommon for a patient to have more than one complaint and, equally, to have more than one condition responsible for the complaints. This can be ascertained by analyzing the description and behavior of symptoms from the history and the objective clinical signs obtained during the evaluation. Patients may have both musculoskeletal and nonmusculoskeletal symptoms simultaneously, making assessment of differential diagnosis more difficult. A number of patient cases are described to illustrate the above points.

CASE STUDIES

Case 1

A patient saw her internist with primary complaint of left-sided frontal headaches, as well as left-sided neck and shoulder symptoms. Her physician did a physical examination, ordered a computed tomography (CT) scan, and a benign meningioma was found. Subsequent surgery alleviated the problem. Several months later, the headaches were gone, but the left-sided neck and shoulder symptoms persisted. The patient was referred to an orthopaedic surgeon and subsequently to physical therapy and clinical signs of a grade II strain of the left supraspinatous were found. Subsequent treatment alleviated the symptoms.

Case 2

A therapist asked a colleague from the same clinical facility, on an informal basis, to treat her lower back, which was painful as of late. Symptoms were local central pain, not accompanied by neurologic signs or symptoms or by radicular symptoms, but with some decrease in active ROM of trunk, with pain provoked during these movements. The symptomatic therapist was treated twice with heat and passive mobilization exercise. After the second treatment, ROM had markedly improved; however, subjectively there was not a concurrent improvement in pain; in fact, the symptoms were now more constant and intense in nature. At that time, the treating therapist began a more thorough review of the history and review of systems and found she had had surgery several years earlier for pancreatic cancer. The patient offered that she had regular physical examinations and a recent CT scan 1 month before that was negative. She was advised to return to her physician, who ordered repeat scans that revealed metastatic lesions in the abdomen and anterior lumbar spine. Although secondary to abnormal circumstances regarding the abbreviated initial examination, it was the incongruous change in signs versus symptoms that stimulated the treating therapist to perform a more thorough examination and to refer this patient back to the physician.

Case 3

A 54-year-old woman was referred by a physician who reported a diagnosis of C4–C5 nerve root impingement secondary to an osteophyte in the right intervertebral foramen. She had insidious onset of 1-month duration of intermittent right posterolateral cervical aching with intermittent radiation of the aching to the right side of her head, "through the head" to the right eye (Fig. 1-6). Behavior of symptoms revealed that looking over the right shoulder increased the cervical pain. The patient also noted gross loss of motion in all directions. The primary complaint was that of increased pain and headaches with lying, especially at night before sleep. The pain also woke her two to three times each night. The patient relieved her symptoms temporarily with deep pressure in the right occipital area and with massage and heat.

Review of systems revealed that the patient is currently undergoing chemotherapy for inoperable breast cancer. There are active metastases in her lungs. A bone scan and CT scan of the cervical region were performed 2 weeks before physical therapy examination, and these were unremarkable. The patient had undergone a mastectomy on the right 1 year ago, after which she claimed complete return to function of the right upper extremity without complaint of symptoms. She complained concurrently of some shortness of breath, depression, and nausea but had experienced these since starting chemotherapy. She denied dizziness, syncope, or changes in vision.

Objective Examination

Active ROM of the shoulders into abduction and flexion was 140 degrees bilaterally without pain. Active cervical ROM revealed that chin to chest caused minimal ache in the neck, extension 45 degrees with increase in strain in the mid-cervical area, side bending right 20 degrees with an increase in right-sided neck pain with radiation into the head, and side bending left 40 degrees and pain free. Left rotation 70 degrees produced a slight increase in right-sided neck symptoms, and right rotation 10 degrees produced a marked increase in neck symptoms with radiation to the head. General passive ROM essentially showed the same pattern of restriction of movement and provocation of symptoms as active ROM.

Passive accessory intervertebral movement testing of the cervical spine demonstrated hypomobility throughout the upper cervical region, but without reproduction of symptoms. Passive physiologic intervertebral movement testing also revealed a decrease in mobility throughout the cervical region, especially with a decrease in right passive rotation of C1, which when tested appeared to diminish the patient's symptoms. There was minimal tenderness to palpation in the cervical spine, especially in the upper cervical area, with some spasm noted here bilaterally. Radiologic findings were reported as moderate cervical spondylosis.

The therapist's assessment of this time was (1) primary dysfunction at C1–C2 into right rotation as most limited, but both directions restricted; (2) pain severe relative to her functional level (the patient was slightly

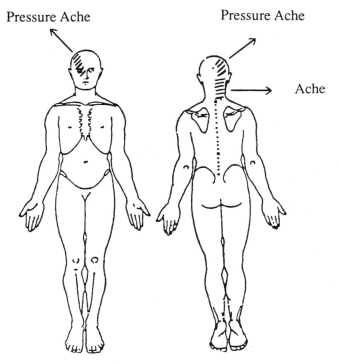

Pressure Ache   Pressure Ache

Ache

Fig. 1-6. Symptom location for a 54-year-old woman. Intermittent ache, right posterolateral cervical region, and pressure-like ache in the right side of cranium.

hysterical using many descriptors, such as "miserable" and "incredible," to describe her pain); and (3) her medical history is positive for cancer, but this apparently has been ruled out recently. A trial of manual therapy to improve rotation right at C1–C2 was initiated. The patient did not appear irritable to this movement and was thought to tolerate treatment well. Given that symptoms are decreased with this technique, the patient should show short-term improvement.

Treatment and Response

On day 1, manual therapy to increase right rotation resulted in a slight decrease in symptoms and a 5-degree increase in right rotation. On day 2, the patient reported a significant decrease in headaches since her first visit, especially immediately after treatment. ROM and right rotation were worse at this time; treatment continued with heat and manual treatment to C1, which afforded the patient some relief and slight increase in right rotation.

On day 3, pain was now intense and sleeping very difficult. The patient was now hysterical. She came to the clinic 4 hours before her appointment time crying. On reassessment she was noted to be in a right side bent and left rotated head posture, more so than previously. Some relief of symptoms was afforded simply by assuming a supine position. Manual treatment techniques gradually allowed her to increase her right rotation and extension, but after sitting or standing after treatment, her pain and antalgic cervical posture returned within several minutes. Subsequently, the patient's physician was called and her response to treatment was explained. She was referred back to her physician for reexamination. She was then referred to an orthopaedic surgeon and sent for magnetic resonance imaging (MRI) to the upper cervical spine. Approximately 5 days later, the patient called with information concerning the diagnosis as metastatic disease to the right C2 vertebra with extension into the right epidural space and right C2–C3 neural foramen (Figs.1-7 and 1-8).

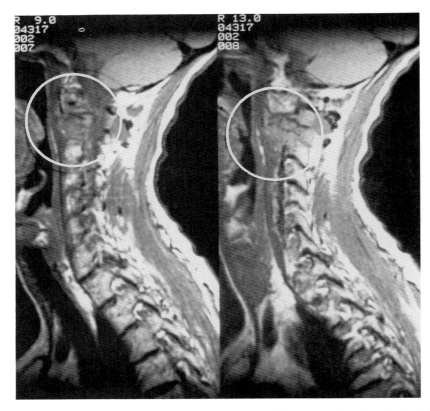

Fig. 1-7. Sagittal view, magnetic resonance imaging. The metastatic lesion is circled.

Case 4

A 29-year-old flight attendant was referred with a diagnosis of supraspinatus strain and bursitis of the left shoulder. She presented with complaints of left-sided anterolateral shoulder pain and of an occasional sharp but more often burning sensation with occasional grinding and snapping into the shoulder; she also had left-sided cervical spine stiffness, left interscapular aching, and tightness. She had a history of occasional symptoms in the right shoulder in the same location. The patient related that her left shoulder was irritated by overhead movements after several repetitions, especially lifting overhead, lifting her flight bag during work, and lying on her left side. She obtained relief with medications, heating pad, how shower, and deep massage. Medication included ibuprofen several times a day.

Review of systems revealed little; she was in good health. A history of endometriosis 1 year earlier in 1989 was noted. Previous surgeries included thyroid surgery 10 years earlier secondary to Graves' disease. The patient stated that she was right handed. The patient believed that her mother was diagnosed as having rheumatoid arthritis.

History

Two years earlier, while pulling a garment bag from the overhead compartment in an airplane, she had felt a quick jolt of pain in the left shoulder; she felt a pop, and her arm dropped down to her side. The pain was eased immediately afterward but again was painful later that night, primarily at the top of the shoulder. She later saw a physician for this problem and, over the course of a year, had radiographs taken and several subsequent injections into the left subacromial bursa.

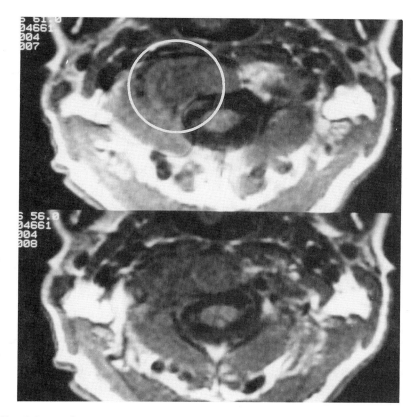

Fig. 1-8. Axial view, magnetic resonance imaging. The metastatic lesion is circled.

This afforded minimal relief of symptoms for a short period of time. Upon objective examination, palpation demonstrated tenderness and some thickening of the subdeltoid bursa, more so on her left. Active elevation was slightly hypermobile at the shoulders bilaterally, with pain on the left from 150 degrees until the end of ROM. Internal rotation was slightly limited with slight pain at the end range. Passive physiologic movement demonstrated a similar pattern of movement and pain complaints. Muscle testing revealed 4/5 strength and complaint of pain with resisted abduction and external rotation of the left shoulder.

The patient demonstrated an apparent subdeltoid bursitis/strain of the rotator cuff on the left with generalized hypermobility of both glenohumeral joints, postural dysfunction through the upper quarter facilitating anterior positioning of the humeral head bilaterally secondary to decreased muscle tone, and protraction of the shoulders, generalized weakness in the shoulder girdles bilaterally, and localized stiffness in the cervical and thoracic spine. She had no other complaints or problems of the joints of the upper or lower extremities at that time.

Treatment and Response

The initial treatment course consisted of ultrasound, massage, and passive mobilization exercise followed by resistive exercise/home program for the shoulder girdles. Over the next several visits, she responded very well to treatment with decreased pain, increased ROM, and increased strength of the left shoulder girdle. She continued to work full-time as a flight attendant during her physical therapy treatment course. There were several episodes of exacerbation of symptoms during this time, but each episode was directly related to increased physical exertion of the upper

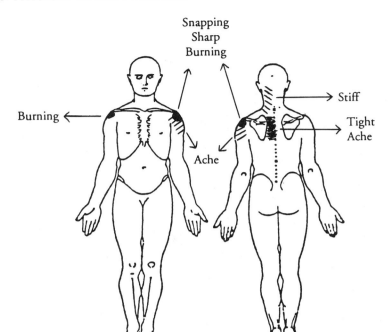

Fig. 1-9. Symptomatic complaints at the initial visit.

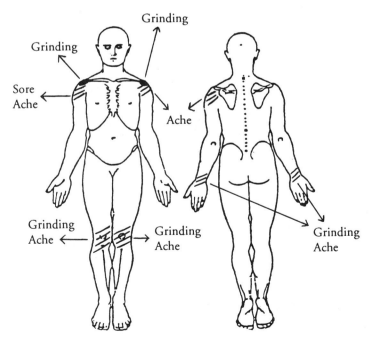

Fig. 1-10. Symptomatic complaints several months after the initial evaluation.

extremities while at work. Overall she continued to improve. The patient was seen for several months, for a total of 12 visits. Several of these sessions emphasized an exercise training class for strengthening of the shoulder girdles, head, neck, and upper extremities. She returned to physical therapy for reassessment and for manual treatment after a 2-week layoff. At this time she had increased complaints of generalized soreness and achiness in several of her joints, including increased pain in both shoulders (Figs. 1-9 and 1-10). On objective examination, she was noted to have an increase in synovial thickening, swelling, and pain upon palpation of both glenohumeral joints and associated bursae, with decreased abduction and increased crepitation of the shoulders bilaterally.

Secondary to exacerbation of left shoulder symptoms, onset of right shoulder symptoms similar to the left, and multiple other joint complaints (wrists and knees), the patient was asked to seek consultation from a rheumatologist. It was approximately 1 month before she could see this physician, at which time she returned for physical therapy and stated that she had been diagnosed as having systemic lupus erythematosus.

Case 5*

History

The patient was a 47-year-old highway maintenance workerwas referred to the clinic with a diagnosis of mechanical low back pain syndrome. His chief complaints were constant sharp pain across the lumbosacral junction accompanied by a numb feeling in both buttocks and intermittent numbness in the right anterior thigh. He also complained of intermittent cramping and throbbing pain in the calves bilaterally (Fig. 1-11). The low back and buttocks symptoms were aggravated by sitting for more than 30 to 45 minutes and standing in one place for more than 5 to 10 minutes and by transitional movements such as sit to stand. The intensity of these symptoms decreased by assuming a recumbent position or by constantly changing positions. The right anterior thigh and calf symptoms were specifically provoked by walking a distance of 3

to 4 blocks. The symptoms were then relieved by sitting for short periods of time. The patient described his low back condition as originating in 1978 when reaching out of the cab of his truck to pull a rope; he had felt a sharp tug in the low lumbar region. He had had constant low back and buttock symptoms since the incident, despite receiving four to five separate series of physical therapy sessions. The calf symptoms began in 1985 during the patient's involvement in a fitness program, with just the left calf symptomatic. This problem was diagnosed as a vascular condition and was subsequently treated by angioplasty. The patient felt partial relief of the left calf pain after the procedure but had noted an increased left calf pain and insidious onset of right calf pain during the past year.

The patient's medical history included undergoing three left knee surgeries and bilateral elbow surgery. He suffered a myocardial infarction in 1986. He had a 26-year history of smoking 1 to 2 packs of cigarettes per day. His family medical history showed that his mother had died of a cardiac condition at age 62 and his father of a myocardial infarction at age 58. Radiologic tests of the lumbar spine revealed degenerative facet joint disease from L3 to S1.

Objective Examination

Observation demonstrated a decreased lumbar lordosis and slight lateral shift of the trunk to the right. There appeared to be hair loss of the lower legs and feet. Slight increase in paraspinal muscle tone was noted from L4–S1 bilaterally with palpation. Also, weak dorsalis pedis and posterior tibial artery pulses were noted bilaterally. These low lumbar and buttock symptoms were provoked with active forward and backward bending in standing. All active movements were moderately restricted. Sharp local low back pain was provoked with passive stress on the L5–S1 segment. Significant hypomobility was noted at L5–S1 and at the thoracolumbar junction. The calf and right anterior thigh symptoms were not provoked with active movements or passive overpressures of the trunk and joints of the lower extremities. When the patient was asked to ambulate, these symptoms were provoked by the time he had walked 100 to 150 feet. Sitting down quickly relieved the thigh and calf symptoms. The low

* From Boissonnault and Bass,[25] with permission.

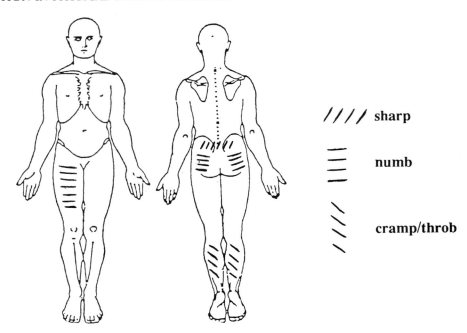

//// sharp

≡ numb

⟋⟋ cramp/throb

Fig. 1-11. Symptom location for a 47-year-old man. Constant lumbosacral junction and buttock complaints with intermittent right thigh and calf complaints. (From Boissonnault and Bass,[25] with permission.)

back and buttock symptoms did not change during the ambulation or subsequent sitting. The patient was then asked to ride a stationary bike; within 1 to 2 minutes, the right thigh and calf symptoms returned. Shortly after the patient stopped pedaling, the symptoms disappeared. Again, as with the ambulation, the low back and buttock symptoms did not change with the bike riding.

Assessment and Outcome

The presentation of multiple symptomatic areas is especially challenging when trying to determine the origin of symptoms. Is a local lesion responsible for each symptomatic area? Is one lesion responsible for all the symptoms? Answering these questions requires a detailed history regarding the behavior and chronologic history of each of the symptoms described by the patient. Also, a careful screening of the appropriate body regions with palpation, active and passive movements, resisted testing, and special tests can provide valuable information regarding the source of the various symptoms.

It was apparent, after the evaluation, that this patient's low back and buttock symptoms were related and that

the right anterior thigh and bilateral calf 'symptoms were related as well. The evaluation findings also suggested that the lumbar and buttock symptoms were the result of mechanical musculoskeletal system dysfunction, while the right thigh and calf symptoms might be related to peripheral vascular system disorder. The lumbar and buttock symptoms were consistently aggravated by sitting, standing, and transitional movements and alleviated by assuming a recumbent position. There was a common precipitating incident for the lumbar and buttock complaints.

Both symptoms were provoked with active movements of the trunk and passive stress on the L5–S1 segment. The anterior thigh and calf symptoms presented with a different behavior pattern; they were only provoked with a specific amount of activity, walking, or biking, then subsequently relieved with sitting. This is the classic pattern of clinical findings associated with intermittent vascular claudication. This finding led to the detailed question regarding the cardiovascular system. These questions revealed the 26-year history of smoking, the myocardial infarction in 1986, past treatment for peripheral vascular disease, and the significant family history of cardiovascular system disease. In addition, careful assessment of the lower-extremity pulses and observation of skin condition had revealed additional signs suggesting possible involvement of the cardiovascular system causing a portion of this patient's complaints.

All this information was communicated to the referring physician. Further medical testing was carried out revealing the presence of significant peripheral vascular disease. While these medical tests and subsequent treatments were being implemented, the patient received physical therapy for the dysfunction related to the lumbar and buttock complaints.

SUMMARY

This chapter emphasizes the information obtained during the subjective and objective examination that would direct the therapist to a more detailed screening of the various organ systems. A general health screening list was presented that could easily be incorporated into the subjective examination. These items should be screened in all patients. An upper- and lower-quarter screening examination scheme were also presented. This examination format illustrates how tests that screen for the presence of mechanical dysfunction and medical disease can be clinically integrated.

The information provided is not intended to prepare the therapist to make a medical diagnosis and suggest medical treatment. Rather it is to assist the therapist in screening for the presence of medical disease and to be able to communicate with the physician as to why the patient is being referred. To demonstrate the application of this information, a final patient case history follows.

REFERENCES

1. 1990 Yearbook and Directory of Osteopathic Physicians. 1981 Ed. p. 675. American Osteopathic Association, Chicago, 1990
2. Rous SN: The Prostate Book. WW Norton, New York, 1988
3. D'Ambrosia RD: Musculoskeletal Disorders, Regional Examination and Differential Diagnosis. 2nd Ed. JB Lippincott, Philadelphia, 1986
4. Schrier RW, Gottschalk CW (eds): Diseases of the Kidney. Vol. 1. 4th Ed. Little, Brown, Boston, 1988
5. Seidel HM, Ball JW, Dains JE, Benedict GW: Mosby's Guide to Physical Examination. CV Mosby, St. Louis, 1987
6. Kelley WN, Harris ED Jr, Ruddy S, Sledge CB: Textbook of Rheumatology. Vol. 1. 3rd Ed. WB Saunders, Philadelphia, 1989
7. Kelly WN, Harris ED Jr, Ruddy S, Sledge CB: Textbook of Rheumatology. Vol. 2. 3rd Ed. WB Saunders, Philadelphia, 1989
8. Schwartz MH: Textbook of Physical Diagnosis, History, and Examination. WB Saunders, Philadelphia, 1989
9. Simons DG, Travell JG: Myofascial origins of low back pain. 2. Torso muscles. Postgrad Med 73:66, 1983
10. Kellgren JH: On the distribution of pain arising from deep somatic structures with charts of segmental pain areas. Clin Sci 4:35, 1939
11. McCall IW, Park WM, O'Brien JP: Induced pain referral from posterior lumbar elements in normal subjects. Spine 4:441, 1979
12. Grieve GP: Common Vertebral Joint Problems. Churchill Livingstone, Edinburgh, 1981
13. Raj PP: Prognostic and therapeutic local anesthetic block. p. 908. In Cousins MJ, Bridenbaugh PO (eds): Neural Blockade in Clinical Anesthesia and Management of Pain. 2nd Ed. JB Lippincott, Philadelphia, 1988
14. Maitland GD: Vertebral Manipulation. 5th Ed. Buttersworth, London, 1986
15. Kellgren JH: Observations of referred pain arising from muscle. Clin Sci 3–4:175, 1938
16. Inman VT, Saunders JB: Referred pain from skeletal structures. J Neuro Ment Dis 99:660, 1944
17. Bates B: A Guide to Physical Examination and History Taking. 4th Ed. JB Lippincott, Philadelphia, 1987
18. Malasanos L, Barkauskas V, Stoltensberg-Allen K: Health Assessment. 4th Ed. Mosby, St. Louis, 1990
19. Zohn DA, Mennell J: Musculoskeletal Pain, Diagnosis, and Physical Treatment. Little, Brown, Boston, 1976
20. Hoppenfeld S: Physical Examination of the Spine and Extremities. Appleton and Lange, E. Norwalk, CT, 1976
21. Devinsky O, Feldmann E: Examination of the Cranial and Peripheral Nerves. Churchill Livingstone, New York, 1988
22. Cailliet R: Low Back Pain Syndrome. 2nd Ed. FA Davis, Philadelphia, 1968
23. Maitland GD: Peripheral Manipulation. 2nd Ed. Buttersworth, London, 1977
24. Boissonnault B, Bass C: Pathological origins of trunk and neck pain: part I—abdominal and visceral disorders. JOSPT 12(5):213, 1990
25. Boissonnault B, Bass C: Pathological origins of trunk and neck pain: part II—disorders of the cardiovascular and pulmonary systems. JOSPT 12(5):208, 1990

Appendix 1-1

Objective Examination: Upper-Quarter Screening Examination

Standing
1. Posture
2. Gait

Sitting
3. General survey (and vital signs); skin (lips, nails, hair, lesions)

4. Head
   A. Eyes
      i. Observation
      ii. Acuity
      iii. Peripheral vision (optic II)
      iv. Pupillary reaction (oculomotor III)
      v. Near reaction (oculomotor III)
      vi. Extraoccular movements (oculomotor III, trochlear IV, abducens VI)
      vii. Corneal reflex (trigeminal V and facial VII)
   B. Ears
      i. Observation
      ii. Palpation
      iii. Acuity (vestibular-cochlear VIII)
         a. Weber lateralization (bone conduction)
         b. Rhine test (air versus bone conduction)
      iv. Equilibrium (vestibular-cochlear VIII)
   C. Nose
      i. Observation
      ii. Nasal breathing
      iii. Palpation
      iv. Sinuses (frontal and maxillary)
      v. Smell (olfactory I)
   D. Mouth/throat/pharynx
      i. Gums
      ii. Teeth
      iii. Roof of mouth
      iv. Tongue (hypoglossal XII motor; facial VII sensory)
      v. Gag reflex and rise of soft palate/uvula (glossopharyngeal and vagus, IX and X)

5. Neck
   A. Observation
   B. Inspection
   C. Soft tissue palpation (muscle)
   D. Lymph nodes (suboccipital, pre- and postauricular, tonsillar, cervical, supraclavicular)
   E. Salivary glands (parotid, submandibular)
   F. Carotid pulses
   G. Thyroid gland
   H. Trachea

6. Upper extremities
   A. Observation
   B. Skin
   C. Pulses (brachial, radial)
   D. Lymph nodes (epitrochlear)
   E. Muscle tone
   F. Bony contour

7. Thorax
   A. Observation
   B. Breathing effort, rate, rhythm, depth
   C. Type of respiration
   D. Palpation of axillary (lymph nodes)
   E. Auscultation, palpation, and percussion of posterior and upper thorax

8. Temporomandibular joint
   A. Open and close (observe and palpate)
   B. Jaw reflex (trigeminal V)

9. Cervical spine
   A. Vertical compression and distraction
   B. Active motions (with overpressures)
      i. Flexion
      ii. Rotation (check vertebral artery)
      iii. Sidebending
      iv. Backward bending
   C. Resisted motions
      i. Forward bend (C1, C2, C3 and spinal accessory XI)
      ii. Backward bend (C1–C8 and spinal accessory XI)
      iii. Sidebend (C2, C3, and spinal accessory XI)
      iv. Rotation
10. Scapula
    A. Active elevation, protraction, retraction, depression
    B. Resisted elevation (spinal accessory XI)
11. Shoulder/elbow/wrist/hand
    A. Active motions
    B. Passive motions (with overpressure)
12. Neurologic
    A. Resisted myotomes (function and provocation)
       i. Shoulder abduction C5–C6 (axillary n.)
       ii. Elbow flexion C5–C6 (musculocutaneous n.)
       iii. Elbow extension C7 (radial n.)
       iv. Wrist extension C6 (radial and ulnar n.)
       v. Thumb extension C8 (radial n.)
       vi. Finger abduction/adduction T1 (radial and median n.)
    B. Reflexes
       i. Deep tendon reflexes
          a. Biceps C5–C6
          b. Brachioradialis (pronator) C6
          c. Triceps C7
       ii. Pathologic (Hoffman's)
    C. Cutaneous sensation (trigeminal V, C2–T6/T8)

Supine
13. Palpation, auscultation, and percussion (chest and upper abdomen)

Prone
14. Additional specific palpation

Appendix 1-2

Objective Examination: Lower-Quarter Screening Examination

Standing
1. Observation (posture and gait)

2. Inspection

3. Palpation

4. "Squat" clearing

5. Vertical "quick" compression (heel bounce)

6. Active trunk motions (with over-pressure)
   A. Forward bend (plus PSIS)
   B. Right and left side bend
   C. Backward bend
   D. Rotation

7. Resisted testing (myotomes)
   A. Heel raise (S1, S2)
   B. Toe raise (L4, L5)

Sitting
8. Observation (posture/respirations)

9. Palpation (auscultation and percussion) of posterior thorax

10. Vertical trunk compression/distraction

11. Trunk rotation (with overpressure)

12. Trunk forward bend (PSIS, if positive in standing)

13. Neurologic testing (trunk weight-bearing)
    A. Sensory dermatomes (T7–S2)
    B. Resisted myotomes
       i.   Hip flexion L1, L2, L3 (femoral nerve)
       ii. Hip adduction L1, L2, L3 (obturator nerve)
       iii. Knee extension L2, L3, L4 (femoral nerve)
       iv. Anterior tibialis L4 (deep peroneal nerve)
       v.   Extensor hallucis longus L5 (deep peroneal nerve)
       vi. Ankle eversion L5, S1, S2 (superficial peroneal nerve)
       vii. Knee flexion L5, S1, S2 (sciatic nerve—tibial)
       viii. Plantar flexion S1, S2 (tibial nerve)
       ix. Trunk flexion/extension/side bend/rotation (thoracic and lumbar segments)
    C. Deep tendon reflexes
       i.   Knee jerk L2, L3, L4
       ii. Hamstring L5
       iii. Ankle jerk S1, S2

Supine
14. Neck flexion (dural tension)

15. Palpation/auscultation/percussion; anterior lower thorax

16. Palpation/percussion of the abdomen and pelvis
    A. Liver
    B. Stomach
    C. Spleen
    D. Kidneys
    E. Colon (ascending and descending)
    F. Bladder
    G. Prostate/uterus
    H. Ovaries
    I. Inguinal area and nodes

17. Pulses
    A. Aorta

B. Renal arteries
C. Iliac arteries
D. Femoral arteries
E. Popliteal arteries
F. Posterior tibial/dorsalis pedis arteries

18. Sacroiliac gap testing

19. Observation/palpation soft tissues/ bony contour of lower extremities

20. Hip active/passive ROM (with overpressure)
    A. Flexion (clear knee first)
    B. Internal rotation
    C. External rotation

21. Knee active/passive ROM (with overpressure)
    A. Flexion
    B. Extension

22. Ankle foot ankle/passive ROM (with overpressure)
    A. Dorsiflexion
    B. Plantar flexion
    C. Inversion
    D. Eversion

23. Toes (active/passive range of motion with overpressure)

24. *Neurologic testing (non-weight-bearing)
    A. Straight leg raise (with and without ankle dorsiflexion and neck flexion)
    B. Sensory/dermatomes T7–S2 (S3–S5)
    C. Reflexes
        i. Superficial abdominal reflex T7–L1
        ii. Cremasteric L1, L2
        iii. Plantar response (Babinski)

Prone

25. Observation/palpation posterior trunk and lower extremities

26. Hip extension active/passive ROM

27. Knee flexion

28. Femoral nerve stretch test

29. Neurologic
    A. Sensory/dermatomes S1–S2 (S3, S4, S5)
    B. Superficial (anal) reflex (S3, S4, S5)

---

* Should repeat any other neurologic test, i.e. DTRs, myotomal, sensory testing that may have been positive in weight-bearing position.

2

Screening for Cardiovascular System Disease

THERESA HOSKINS MICHEL, M.S., P.T., C.C.S.
JILL DOWNING, M.D.

Physical therapists have always had an important role in the evaluation and treatment of peripheral vascular diseases and, for at least the past decade, have expanded their efforts in cardiac rehabilitation. Some of the earliest writings by physical therapists describe tests available for the evaluation of the peripheral vascular system, as well as walking programs designed for the treatment of indolent ulcers and intermittent claudication.[1,2]

Today, the practice of physical therapy extends to all body systems and to nearly all disease entities. The cardiovascular system continues to require the expertise of physical therapists versed in this system and should be considered by any physical therapist who is screening particular signs or symptoms involving chest, neck, face, and the upper or lower extremities. This chapter describes disease entities that may give rise to such signs or symptoms. Information is provided on medical screening procedures and physical therapy evaluation techniques used to assess the cardiovascular system.

It is often difficult to differentiate the sources of local peripheral edema, jaw pain, or tingling in the fingers, any of which may have a cardiovascular origin. In the absence of a specific diagnosis, the physical therapist must decide when these complaints need to be referred to a physician for a differential diagnosis. The evaluation procedures described in this chapter will help the physical therapist provide vital information to the physician. By screening a patient's left shoulder pain and ruling out angina pectoris, the physical therapist can proceed to evaluate other potential sources of the complaint without imposing undue restrictions on the patient's activity.

There is not always a clear-cut differentiation between cardiovascular causes of symptoms and musculoskeletal system dysfunction. Many complaints of pain in the upper or lower extremities are extremely confusing to the patient and the health professional, even after a thorough medical screen. The physical therapist's ability to provide pertinent information about these complaints can prove invaluable. In the event that cardiovascular disease is present, the physical therapist needs to recognize the implications this presents for treatment precautions. For example, heart disease may impose limits on the intensity and type of physical activity that are safe for the patient. Wound healing will be impaired in the patient with vascular compromise.

This chapter provides an overview of the anatomy and physiology of the heart and peripheral vasculature. The general symptoms and signs of cardiovascular diseases are described, and the screening procedures available to the physical therapist are presented. Objective tests used for the medical screening of these symptoms or signs are listed with parameters for normal or abnormal, such as blood pressure, pulse palpation, and electrocardiography (ECG). Finally, specific common cardiovascular diseases are presented, including the pathophysiology, histology, and usual findings of diagnostic medical tests.

CARDIOVASCULAR ANATOMY AND HISTOLOGY

The cardiovascular system is a massive network of three types of blood vessels connected to a pump, the heart. Efferent flow of oxygenated blood is carried in arteries of progressively diminishing caliber. Veins convey blood back to the heart. The interface between these two types of vessels in many parts of the body is the third type of vessel, the capillary. Another network of vessels is the lymphatics, which carry a tissue fluid known as lymph away from peripheral circulation and toward the heart, ultimately draining into the venous system through the thoracic duct. The main transport function of the lymphatics is to remove fluid and large diameter molecules from the systemic circulation. The heart itself is somewhat pyramidal in shape and is encased in a double-layered sac known as the pericardium. It is located within the middle mediastinum and is divided into four chambers: the right and left atria and right and left ventricles. Three external surfaces can be identified: the sternocostal, or anterior; the diaphragmatic, or inferior; and the base, or posterior surfaces. In addition, the distalmost tip of the left ventricle defines the apex. Directed down, forward, and to the left, it is at the fifth left intercostal space, $3\frac{1}{2}$ inches (9 cm from the midline (Fig. 2-1).

Unoxygenated or venous blood returns to the heart through the inferior vena cava, passing into the right

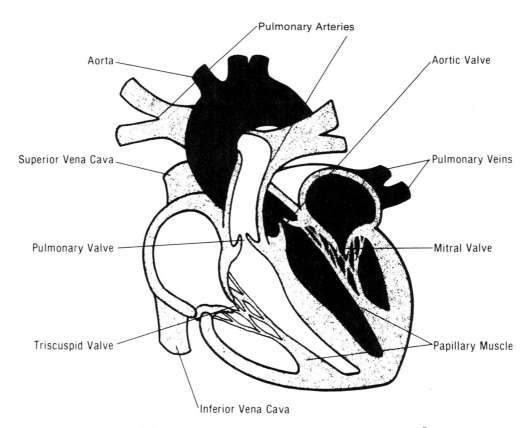

Fig. 2-1. Cross section of the heart and great vessels. (From Cohen and Michel,[7] with permission.)

atrium. It then flows into the right ventricle, pulmonary artery, and pulmonary vascular bed, where carbon dioxide and oxygen are diffused. Freshly oxygenated blood returns to the heart through the pulmonary veins into the left atrium and left ventricle. Blood is ejected into the aorta for systemic distribution. The flow of blood out of each chamber is regulated by the presence of a heart valve. The tricuspid valve is located between the right atrium and right ventricle, the pulmonic valve between the right ventricle and pulmonary artery, the mitral valve between the left atrium and left ventricle, and the aortic valve between the left ventricle and aorta (Fig. 2-1). The heart itself is composed of three layers of tissue. The thick cardiac muscle, the myocardium, is covered externally with serous pericardium called the epicardium and internally with a layer of endothelium, the endocardium.

The heartbeat originates in a specialized system of cardiac muscle cells that generate and conduct electrical impulses. Known as the conducting system of the heart, this system provides for the synchronized contraction of cardiac muscle and a cardiac output that meets the body's metabolic needs. Structurally it is composed of the sinus node, the atrioventricular (AV) node, the AV bundle with its right and left branches, and the subendocardial plexus of Purkinje fibers (Fig. 2-2). The heart is nourished by an arterial supply provided by the right and left main coronary arteries, which arise from the aorta directly above the aortic valve (Fig. 2-3). The number and configuration of branches that arise from these two vessels vary considerably from one individual to the next. In most cases, however, the right coronary artery travels anteriorly and inferiorly along the right side of the heart, perfusing the right atrium, the right ventricle, portions of the left ventricle, and the sinus and AV nodes. The left main coronary artery usually gives rise to the left anterior descending and circumflex branches and perfuses the entire left ventricle and most of the left atrium. Cardiac innervation is by both the sympathetic and parasympathetic fibers of the autonomic nervous system. Sympathetic fibers arise from the cervical and upper thoracic portions of the sympathetic trunks and from the parasympathetic supply from the vagus nerves.

The flow of oxygenated blood to the peripheral tissues is carried by arteries. Regardless of their diameter, all arteries consist of three microscopic layers: the intima, media, and adventitia. From inside out, the intima is thin and forms the interface between the vessel and the circulating blood. It is composed of the endothelium, a basement membrane, and an elastin membrane. The media is formed by layers of smooth muscle cells and an elastic membrane. Finally, the adven-

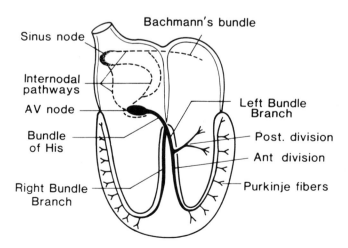

Fig. 2-2. Diagrammatic representation of the conducting system of the heart. (From Albarran-Sotelo et al.,[18] with permission.)

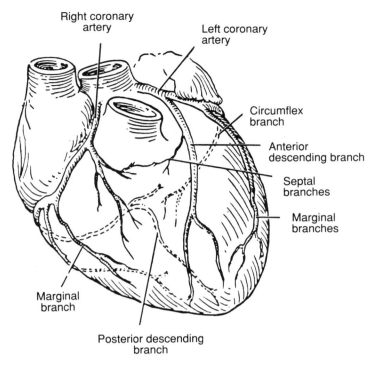

Fig. 2-3. Coronary arteries, showing the arterial supply to the surface of the heart. (From Ross,[8] with permission.)

titia of the artery appears with its collagenous support structure through which pass blood vessels, lymphatics, and nerves to the artery itself (Fig. 2-4). At the level of the arteriole, blood passes to the capillary, where it equilibrates with the interstitial fluid. Capillaries drain through venules to veins. While the same microscopic layers are present in veins, they contain little smooth muscle tissue in the media. Vein walls are therefore, thin, and easily distended. In the veins of the extremities, a series of bicuspid valves are present, preventing the retrograde flow of venous blood back toward the tissues.

Cardiovascular Physiology

The cardiovascular system transports substances absorbed from the gastrointestinal tract and oxygen from the lungs to the tissues and returns the products of metabolism to the kidneys and carbon dioxide to the lungs. It has a role in controlling body temperature and distributes hormones and other substances im-

portant to cell function. The functions of the cardiovascular system and the influences on it can best be appreciated by looking separately at the heart and the circulation.

The Heartbeat

The heartbeat consists of an orderly sequence of events involving contraction of the atria, known as atrial systole, followed by contraction of the ventricles, ventricular systole. This is followed by diastole, during which all four chambers are relaxed. The heartbeat originates in the specialized myocardial cells of the cardiac conduction system. Because of faster rates of discharge, the sinus node has the role of cardiac pacemaker. The electrical impulses it generates spread across the atrial myocardium, through the AV node, and into the ventricles. The ventricles are depolarized in an "inside-outside" fashion, stimulating the endocardium, myocardium, and finally the epicardium. An inherent property of all excited muscle cells is the

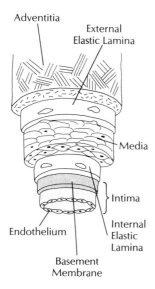

Fig. 2-4. Cellular architecture of the artery. (Modified from Stein et al.,[19] with permission.)

ization, plateau, and slow repolarization phases. When electrodes are placed on the skin, the action potential that is recorded extracellularly resembles the PQRST pattern of the ECG (Fig. 2-5). More correctly, it is the sum of all myocardial action potentials for any one heartbeat. When detected from certain body surface locations, the ECG stands as a record of the electrical behavior of the heart during the cardiac cycle. The P wave is generated at the time of atrial depolarization, the QRS by ventricular depolarization, and the ST segment and T wave by ventricular repolarization. The size and shape of any one PQRST complex vary with the placement of the electrodes, or leads, used to record it.

Mechanical Events of the Cardiac Cycle

Once activated, myocardial contraction begins shortly thereafter. Contraction of the atria, known as atrial systole, begins after inscription of the P wave on the ECG. Ventricular contraction or ventricular systole begins near the end of the R wave and ends just after the T wave. With all chambers relaxed in late diastole, the tricuspid and mitral valves that partition the atria and ventricles are open, and the pulmonary and aortic

ability to produce an action potential that is transmitted along its membrane. The electrical event that occurs is a result of chemical changes resulting from ion fluxes across the muscle cell membrane. A transmembrane action potential is composed of rapid depolar-

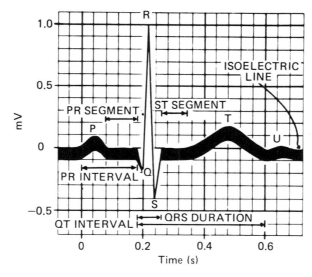

Fig. 2-5. PQRST pattern of the electrocardiogram. (From Ganong,[9] with permission.)

valves are closed. Blood is able to flow throughout the heart, filling the four chambers. While 70 percent of left ventricular filling occurs now, the remainder is accomplished during the next phase, atrial systole. With the onset of the next phase, ventricular systole, the tricuspid and mitral valves close. The ventricular muscle mass contracts very little, but intracavity pressures rise sharply. This period of ventricular systole is referred to as isovolumic contraction. It will last approximately 0.05 seconds, until pressure in the right ventricle exceeds pulmonary artery pressure (10 mmHg) and left ventricular pressure exceeds aortic pressure (80 mmHg), and the respective pulmonary and aortic valves open (Fig. 2-6). Ventricular ejection occurs with peak left ventricular pressure reaching 120 mmHg and peak right ventricular pressure 25 mmHg. The amount of blood ejected by each ventricle per stroke is 70 to 90 ml, approximately 65 percent of total volume of blood present in the left ventricle at the time of systolic contraction. It is this value of 65 percent that is referred to as the left ventricular ejection fraction.

Contraction of the heart muscle forces blood out into the aorta in a pulsatile fashion. As this pressure wave travels along arterial walls, the walls expand. This expansion is palpable as the pulse. The rate at which this pressure wave travels is dependent on the characteristics of the vessel in which it is traveling and is faster than the velocity of blood flow. For example, there is a 0.1-second delay between peak left ventricular systolic ejection and palpation of the radial pulse at the wrist. Various characteristics of a pulse can be described. The most obvious—strength of pulse—is determined by the pulse pressure, and not the mean pressure. While the pulse is generated by the arterial pressure wave and is palpated over an artery, it can be transmitted to the great veins of the neck, producing three characteristic waves in the jugular venous pulse: the a, c, and v waves. These waves reflect, respectively, atrial systole, bulging of the tricuspid valve into the atria during isovolumic contraction, and the rise in atrial pressure before the tricuspid valve opens in diastole.

A series of vibratory sounds, known as heart sounds, are set up with each cardiac cycle. Two heart sound produced by the normal heart are S1, the first heart sound, caused by closure of the tricuspid and mitral valves at the start of ventricular systole; and S2, the second heart sound, which arises when the aortic and pulmonary valves close. While both sounds are a mix of vibrations caused by different events of the cardiac cycle, two components of S2 can be discerned by the trained human ear. The first, known as A2, is due to closure of the aortic valve. The second, P2, stems from pulmonic valve closure. A third heart sound (S3) and a fourth heart sound (S4) can occur during diastole in both normal and abnormal states. Other sounds, not necessarily abnormal, which are generated in various parts of the vascular system by turbulent flow, include murmurs, bruits, clicks, rubs, hums, and souffles. Murmurs can be a cause for concern, as they may reflect disease in one or more heart valves. Murmurs are sounds made up of many frequencies. The characteristics of a particular murmur depend on the velocity of blood flow, the morphology of the valvular orifice, and the resonating properties of the surrounding structures. A valve can malfunction in two ways. Normal forward flow of blood can be hindered by a narrowed valve, a condition known as stenosis. A valve that fails to close adequately and that leaks blood back into the chamber from which it just came is called incompetent or insufficient. This condition is referred to as regurgitation of the valve. Appropriate location of the stethoscope on the chest wall (Fig. 2-7) can determine which valve is producing the murmur. Whether the lesion is stenotic or insufficient can be decided by correlating the timing of the murmur (whether in diastole or systole) with knowledge of the mechanical events of the cardiac cycle. Blood normally flows through the aortic and pulmonary valves in systole. A murmur in systole will be caused by a stenotic lesion and a murmur in diastole by a regurgitant flow. Because the normal flow of blood through the mitral and tricuspid valves is in diastole, the reverse is true. A murmur arising from either of these valves in systole is caused by regurgitation, and stenosis of the valve will be heard in diastole.

Cardiac Output

The pumping function of the heart is regulated by a number of different mechanisms that match the output of the heart to tissue perfusion needs over a large range of physiologic demands. Cardiac output is the amount of blood moved per minute by the heart from the great veins into the aorta. It is also referred to as minute volume, defined as the product of stroke volume and heart rate. Because the size of the individual

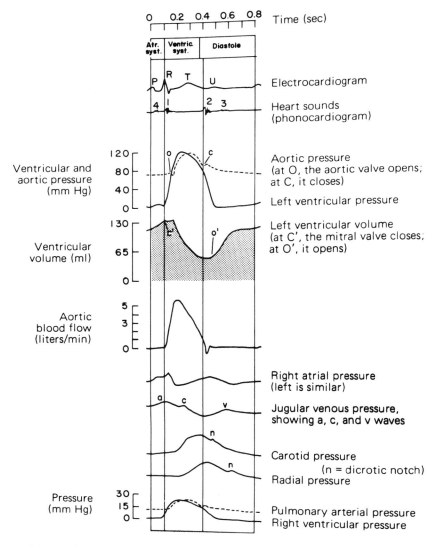

Fig. 2-6. Events of the cardiac cycle. (From Cohen and Michel[7] as adapted from Ganong,[10] with permission.)

determines the perfusion needs, cardiac output is frequently expressed as a function of body surface area. The cardiac index is the cardiac output in liters per minute divided by the body surface area in square meters.

$$CI = \frac{CO \text{ L/min}}{BSA \text{ m}_2}$$

Cardiac output can range from 20 to 30 percent below normal resting supine values, as with assumption of the upright position from a supine value, to 700 to 800 percent above resting levels with extreme effort. The two major clinical measurements of cardiac output use either the Fick principle or the indicator dilution technique; cold saline is the indicator and thermodilution the specific technique. This measurement is accomplished by injecting saline into the right atrium through one port of a Swan-Ganz catheter. Temperature change is registered at a thermistor in the pulmonary artery at the balloon tip of the catheter.

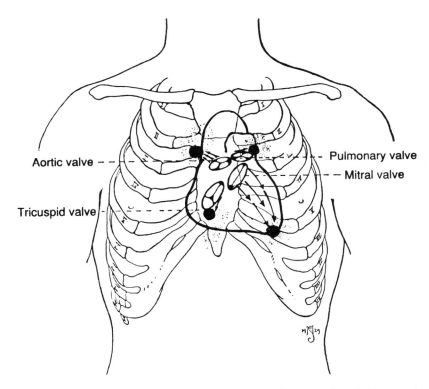

Fig. 2-7. Anatomic location of heart valves and of areas in which sounds are best heard. (From Delp and Manning,[11] with permission.)

Regulatory mechanisms can work on either or both components of the cardiac output equation: heart rate or stroke volume. Heart rate is controlled primarily by autonomic nervous system input. Sympathetic stimulation causes an increase in heart rate and parasympathetic stimulation decreases it. Stroke volume is also influenced by neural stimulation, with sympathetic afferents giving greater strength to muscle fiber contraction at any given length and parasympathetics having the opposite effect. The effect of the release of catecholamines by sympathetic stimulation on heart rate is referred to as chronotropic action. Their effect on the strength of myocardial contraction is known as inotropic action. An inherent property of the myocardial muscle mass, independent of innervation, to regulate stroke volume stems from the generation of tension within the fiber at any given cardiac muscle fiber length. Classic physiologic studies of this length-ten-

sion relationship for the isolated muscle strip plot sarcomere length against isometric tension. This force of contraction is dependent on preload, the initial load on the muscle prior to contraction, and afterload, the tension at which the load is lifted. In the individual patient, preload translates into the degree to which heart muscle is stretched before contraction and afterload, the resistance against which blood is expelled. When preload is thought of more generally as venous return and afterload as peripheral resistance or impedance, it becomes clear that these variables can be manipulated therapeutically to affect myocardial fiber shortening, stroke volume, and cardiac output. Other regulatory mechanisms of cardiac output that work more slowly, effecting change by determining extracellular volume and secondly blood volume, are the renin-angiotensin system and centrally mediated release of antidiuretic hormone, or vasopressin.

Blood Pressure

Whereas cardiac output is the amount of blood ejected from the heart throughout a complete cardiac cycle, actual tissue perfusion over a broad spectrum of physiologic demands is determined by the arterial (or blood) pressure. The highest pressure point of the pulse wave is the systolic pressure and the lowest pressure, at the end of diastole, is the diastolic pressure. The difference between systolic and diastolic pressure is the pulse pressure. Mean pressure is the average pressure during the cardiac cycle. It is not an arithmetic average, but rather a geometric mean, that can be approximated with the following formula (Fig. 2-8):

Mean pressure
    = diastolic pressure plus $\frac{1}{3}$ pulse pressure

Multiple cardiovascular regulatory mechanisms for controlling blood pressure have evolved. These adjustments include both local and systemic mechanisms that (1) affect the diameter of arterioles and other resistance vessels, (2) increase or decrease blood storage in the venous system, and (3) vary the rate and stroke volume of the heart. The autonomic nervous system has a major regulatory role, involving sensory input from peripheral baroreceptors and from chemoreceptors located in the walls of the heart. In the major blood vessels, it is relayed to a sort of cardiovascular center in the medulla. Although not a true center in the anatomic sense, investigation of the function of the medulla can pinpoint areas that, when stimulated, result in vasoconstriction or vasodilation of various vascular beds. Also contributing to pressure control at the individual organ or vascular bed are metabolic end products and other vasodilatory peptides that affect vascular smooth muscle tone, as well as the inherent response of resistance vessels to varying degrees of stretch.

Oxygen Consumption of the Heart

Unlike skeletal muscle, which requires glucose or glycogen for metabolism, cardiac muscle can take advantage of a number of energy sources, including esterified and nonesterified fatty acids, lactate, ketone bodies, and amino acids. All metabolic pathways are aerobic, however, requiring oxygen for adenosine triphosphate (ATP) regeneration. Oxygen consumption of the heart is determined by heart rate, intramyocardial wall tension, and contractility of the myocardium. Measurements of wall tension and contractility are not readily available clinically. An excellent correlation exists, however, between myocardial oxygen consumption and the rate pressure product or double product obtained by multiplying heart rate and systolic blood pressure measured at any given workload.

SIGNS AND SYMPTOMS OF CARDIOVASCULAR DISEASE

Every organ in the human body relies on the anatomic integrity and physiologic effectiveness of the cardiovascular system for tissue nutrition. Impairments in this system can cause symptoms anywhere throughout

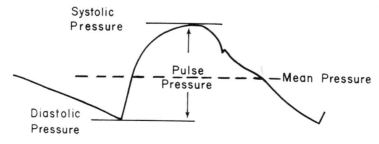

Fig. 2-8. Schematic arterial pressure pulse-labeled to show pressure values usually measured. (From Little,[12] with permission.)

the body. Some of these symptoms can be very clear-cut sequelae of cardiovascular disease, such as intermittent claudication. Many symptoms are confusing, such as fatigue, and are likely to be presented to a physical therapist. The physical therapist should be familiar with those symptoms that are likely to implicate the cardiovascular system: pain, irregular heartbeat (palpitations), lightheadedness, syncope, fatigue, dyspnea, and cough.

Pain

Pain that is cardiac in origin is referred to as *angina pectoris*. This condition is defined as an imbalance of myocardial oxygen supply and oxygen demand, arising when the available blood supply is inadequate to meet the metabolic requirement of cardiac muscle. Angina pectoris is a symptom of myocardial ischemia. Typical angina occurs substernally, with a referral pattern to the left shoulder and along the inside of the left arm in the usual ulnar distribution. Atypical angina may occur in the face, jaw, teeth, either or both shoulders, and down either or both arms. Angina is usually described as a pressure and not necessarily as a pain. It may be accompanied by nausea, vomiting, epigastric distress with burping, or none of these. Because of these associated symptoms, it may easily be mistaken for indigestion. Often patients will remember sensations of numbness or tingling in their left hand associated with angina. These, too, are often misleading for patients who do not know they have coronary artery disease (CAD).

To aid in making a differential diagnosis for the source of thoracic pain, the following rules of thumb are presented. Thoracic pain that worsens with inspiration, is sharp and improves with a change in position, is usually pericarditis, not angina. A sharp stabbing pain that occurs with a deep breath, described as a knife in a local area, is probably pleurisy. Myocarditis and endocarditis do not necessarily produce chest pain, but a chest tightness with breathlessness may easily be confused with angina. There is often low-grade fever and malaise, as well as arthralgias accompanying cardiac infections or inflammations. The pain associated with aortic aneurysm is usually a hot sensation, throbbing in nature, and increasing in intensity with increased physical activity. A dissecting aortic aneurysm presents as a pain, sudden in onset, a searing heat, often located in the patient's back, and accompanied by a rapid decrease in blood pressure. Pain that is burning, limited in area over the cutaneous distribution of a nerve, and accompanied by swollen local lymph nodes may indicate herpes zoster, especially if it is brought on by recent stress or in an immunocompromised patient. Skin vesicles eventually appear.

Angina can occur from etiologies other than coronary artery disease or coronary vasospasm. Aortic stenosis and outflow tract obstruction caused by hypertrophy of the septum known as idiopathic hypertrophic subaortic stenosis (IHSS), can result in inadequate blood flow into the coronary circulation during diastole. Chest pain on exertion accompanied by breathlessness can be a symptom of inadequate blood flow, rather than coronary vessel disease. Another clinical entity that sometimes causes chest pain attributable to blood flow dysfunction is mitral valve prolapse.

Typical angina is described in the following terms:

Onset: exertional, or under conditions of stress
Location: substernal with left shoulder and arm radiation
Quality: pressure, tightness that may not be perceived as pain
Intensity: ranging from pressure or tightness to severe crushing sensation
Duration: usually longer than 1 minute but less than 10 minutes
Relief: stopping exercise, sublingual nitroglycerin
Associated symptoms: breathlessness, diaphoresis; sometimes nausea and vomiting when severe

Atypical angina usually refers to angina that is nonexertional. It can occur as a pain, tightness, or tingling located in the jaw, in the neck, or in the back, radiating down either or both arms, or as something quite unique to the patient.

Myocardial ischemia may be "silent," and not at all perceived as pain. Anginal equivalents can occur such as diaphoresis, dyspnea, or fatigue. If a patient has had angina in the past, the medical history should mention the specific anginal pattern with clear descriptors. In

High suspicion of myocardial ischemia:

1. *Chest pain brought on by exertion, cold air, drag on cigarette, and after a heavy meal:* This pain is often accompanied by dyspnea, diaphoresis, and nausea.
2. *Angina:* Stable angina has a regular, consistent, predictable onset, location, relief, and duration. Unstable angina is characterized by increasing frequency; onset is now earlier, more easily induced, and spreading or radiating in location; it requires more sublingual nitroglycerin and takes longer to obtain relief.
3. *Prinzmetal or variant angina:* Rest angina occurs during sleep and is unrelated to exertion, from vasospasm of coronary arteries. It may be associated with high anxiety.
4. *Chest pain brought on by exertion, accompanied by dyspnea, wide pulse pressure (SBP versus DBP):* Besides CAD, chest pain may relate to left ventricular hypertrophy or other syndromes of ventricular strain. Check the ECG for left ventricular hypertrophy, seen as an increased QRS voltage with secondary changes in T-wave amplitude and ST segment. Check the echocardiogram for aortic stenosis, mitral valve prolapse, and IHSS.

addition, the presence of CAD should be documented by tests and by an analysis of the risk factors for this disease.

Leg Pain

Leg pain is a very nonspecific symptom that can be very localized, quite general, and variable under different conditions. Causes of leg pain can be vascular, such as phlebitis, vasculitis, or ischemia, as in intermittent claudication or anterior compartment syndrome. Other causes of leg pain may be secondary to musculoskeletal disorders, as in arthritis. Leg pain may be neural in origin, as in sciatica or in neuropathy of diabetes mellitus, or may be due to soft tissue con-

ditions, such as cellulitis. Muscle imbalance or weakness as occurs with shin splints can produce leg pain that may be confused with anterior compartment syndrome or pain associated with stress fractures. Descriptors of pain, location of discomfort, and associated findings may be the most critical aspects of the differential diagnosis. Localized edema of both ankles may be present with venous stasis ulcers. Skin discoloration (blue to black with gangrene, brown to purple with venous stasis) and presence of hair loss and trophic changes of skin will lead to the conclusion of arterial or venous insufficiency. Peripheral neuropathies and sympathetic neuropathies can produce trophic changes and pain as well. The physical therapist looks for long scars along the course of a vein as evidence of previous revascularization surgery, such as a saphenous vein for coronary artery bypass graft (CABG).

Pain with acute swelling in the anterior tibial compartment is associated with cramping, increases with walking or running, and stops with rest. It occurs secondary to increased capillary permeability or hematoma within tight connective tissue in the shin area. Calf pain with slow walking that develops into a cramp unless walking is discontinued is symptomatic of calf muscle ischemia caused by peripheral vascular disease. The former is usually found in young athletes and is known as anterior compartment syndrome.[3] A case study is provided by Cohen and Michel.[4] By contrast, the patient with intermittent claudication is usually older; has a duller ache that may occur in the buttock, thigh, calf, or all of the above; and comes on with walking, intensifies if walking continues, and disappears with rest.

Other forms of leg pain relating to vascular insufficiency include gangrenous lesions yielding very intense, constant localized pain associated with blackened lesions in the skin, most often of the toes or heel. Venous stasis ulcers produce a raw, throbbing, constant, nauseating pain in an ulcerated area, usually surrounded by brownish discolored skin, and local edema. Pain over a localized distribution, associated with a red, hot area, and swelling may be a symptom of thrombophlebitis. This occurs most commonly in patients who have been bedridden or immobilized for a long period.

Physical Therapy Evaluation of Leg Pain

Fingertip palpation of peripheral pulses is one of the most important procedures to employ. The femoral pulse is found in the groin, medial to the inguinal ligament. The popliteal pulse is behind the knee joint in the popliteal fossa. The tibial pulse is posterior to the medial malleolus, and the pedal pulse is found on the mid-dorsum of the foot. If a pulsatile mass is palpated anywhere in the body, such as in the abdomen or groin, it needs to be checked urgently, as it may be an aneurysm.

Another significant evaluation is that of reactivity of the arterial system. The reactive hyperemia test is the use of gravity to drain the limb of a significant volume of blood and the rapidity with which the arterial system can compensate for this blood redistribution. To perform this test, the patient is supine, and the lower limb being tested is elevated over the patient's head level, approximately 45 degrees of hip flexion. The leg is kept in this position for 1 to 3 minutes, or until the color of the foot, ankle, and lower leg is quite blanched. With a stopwatch, the examiner times how long it takes for the skin to turn pink as soon as the limb is brought to the dangling position while the patient is sitting. Normally, this time is less than 1 second. Anything above 1.5 seconds represents some degree of arterial insufficiency. This test takes an eye sensitive to color change. Another similar test, perhaps a little more risky for the seriously impaired patient with arterial insufficiency, measures reactive hyperemia to cold water immersion. Instead of gravity, the use of cold water immersion will produce blanched or mottled skin, which can be rewarmed with rapid immersion in warm water, and the time to return to pink skin is taken as the test of arterial insufficiency. Again, normal reaction time is less than 1 second.

To determine the pressure of the systolic pulse wave in a peripheral vessel, a sphygmomanometer cuff is inflated above the site of the suspected lesion. The Doppler probe is placed along the vessel being studied. As the pressure is slowly released, flow is first detected at the point of systolic pressure. When the sphygmomanometer is applied at serial points along the limb, a gradient in pressure between any two measurement sites will localize the segment in which arterial obstruction is significant. This test may be performed by a physical therapist or may be done in a vascular diagnostic laboratory. Skin temperature can be a useful measure, and a temperature map can help assess areas in which arterial supply is inadequate. Thermography provides the same measurement but is a much higher, more sensitive technology. It is also more expensive.

High suspicion of vascular cause of leg pain:

1. Gangrene anywhere on the peripheral body part indicates arterial insufficiency.
2. Nonhealing ulceration on the peripheral body part indicates a vascular problem—either arterial insufficiency or venous stasis.
3. Ischemic pain with activity of muscle involved in the activity is the result of arterial insufficiency. Intermittent claudication is the peripheral example, in which onset occurs with walking; pain is in the calf muscle, in the hamstring muscle group, or in the gluteal group. Testing for reactive hyperemia will result in delayed skin coloration. Doppler tests, especially under low-level exercise conditions, help pinpoint location, and identify severity of stenoses.

Irregular Heartbeat

By definition, irregularities of heart rhythm (palpitations) are abnormal but may be quite benign or dangerous to the patient. Some patients may not perceive them at all, while others may find them quite bothersome. The physical therapist must distinguish between irregularities that are not hemodynamically compromising and those that need immediate medical attention. In general, atrial arrhythmias, or extra beats originating in the atria but not from the sinus node, are of the benign variety. However, a new onset may be significant hemodynamically, especially if the ventricular response rate goes above 160, at which rate diastolic filling time may be sufficiently reduced to undermine the cardiac output. There is also a much increased risk of clot formation with atrial arrhythmias leading to the potential risk of thrombus or embolus. Ventricular arrhythmias are more likely to lead to serious hemodynamic compromise. In addition, a primary conduction defect can lead to a rhythm disturbance, which can be quite serious. First-degree AV block appears as a prolongation of the PR interval and represents a slowing of conduction through the atria. This block does not challenge the patient hemodynamically. Second-degree AV block appears in two forms: type I (or Wenckebach), and type II. Both types occur when some impulses are conducted from atria to ventricles, while other impulses are blocked. Wenckebach AV block almost always occurs at the AV node and is often due to increased parasympathetic tone or to drug effect. It is usually transient and does not compromise the patient. Progressive prolongation of the PR interval indicates decreasing conduction velocity, until finally an impulse is completely blocked. Only a single impulse is blocked, and the cycle is repeated. Type II AV block occurs when the block is below the level of the AV node in the bundle of His, generally the result of an organic lesion. Thus, it is associated with a deterioration to third-degree or complete heart block. In type II second-degree AV block, the PR interval does not lengthen before a dropped beat. The block may be intermittent, or the conduction ratio may vary. If it is a constant conduction ratio, the palpable pulse is regular. Third-degree AV block indicates complete absence of conduction between atria and ventricles. P waves occur at their own rate and rhythm; QRS complexes appear at a different (slower) rate and rhythm without any relationship to each other. The block is usually below the AV node, thereby carrying a poor prognosis. In this case, the QRS rate is the ventricular escape rhythm, with its inherent firing rate of less than 40 per minute. There may be periods of asystole in this case. Figure 2-9 presents an overall view of the major arrhythmias.

Physical Therapy Evaluation of Irregular Heartbeat

Since not all patients have symptoms associated with their irregular heartbeat, the physical therapist's pulse palpation may demonstrate the first sign of this problem. Any pulse point will reflect the irregularity. The first step is to define the nature of the irregularity, then determine the amount of hemodynamic dysfunction caused by the arrhythmia. The vital signs should be taken. Heart rate must be counted for a full minute to determine the total number of fully perfused beats. The heart rhythm, taken peripherally, may be described as regular, regularly irregular, or irregularly irregular. When an irregular pulse is found, an apical auscultation simultaneously performed with a peripheral palpation will help elucidate the significance. The presence of the S1 or S2 (*lubb-dupp*) heart sound during a peripheral pause in pulse is noted. If there is no palpable pulsation, even when a normal heart sound is heard, there is no perfusion with the beat. The frequency and regularity of the pause in palpated pulse should be noted to help assess its severity. Blood pressure may be difficult to perform accurately during an irregular heartbeat, since the systolic reading depends on the normal Karotkoff sound, which will be absent during the pause of a premature contraction. The absence of a timely beat may be misread as the diastolic pressure rather than as a pause, since it may appear as cessation of sound.

Lightheadedness

Lightheadedness is a common experience. There are many causes, some simple and easily removed, such as hyperventilation, others complex and associated with severe compromise. For this reason, it is critical to ascertain whether there are any associated symptoms accompanying the experience of lightheadedness. The most frequent etiologies are ventricular ectopic activity, hypotension, hyperventilation, hypoglycemia, and cerebral ischemia.

A person who feels lightheaded may appear pale, and may also be diaphoretic, but may in most respects be reasonably normal in appearance. If a patient loses consciousness, there is more cause for alarm (see under Syncope). Patients experiencing a transient ischemic attack (TIA) may also have slurred speech, loss of motor control on one side or a portion of their body, or incoordination of motion.

The medical history should help the physical therapist determine any previous history of any of the above.

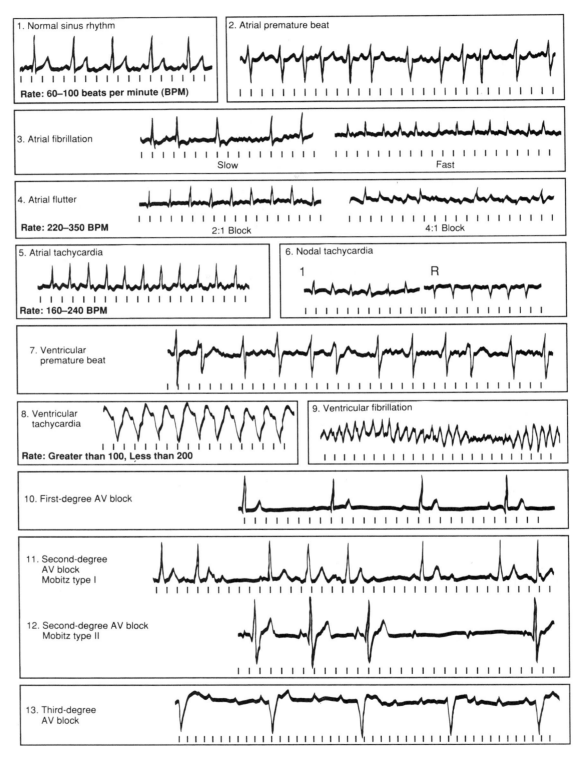

Fig. 2-9. Patterns of the major arrhythmias.

The physical therapist should be especially on the alert for mention of diabetes mellitis (hypoglycemic reaction to insulin); TIAs (cerebral ischemia); and any sign of arrhythmias, such as ventricular ectopic activity

---

Physical Therapy Evaluation of Lightheadedness

Rule out cardiac cause

1. Check the ECG for ventricular arrhythmia. If not seen, VEA is less likely to be the cause. The best monitor for VEA is the Holter monitor for a continuous ECG over 12 or 24 hours.
2. Look for ECG signs of ischemia (i.e., ST segment depression or elevation). Since myocardial ischemia results in some dysfunction, there may be hypotension with resulting lightheadedness. If ST segments are isoelectric, there is probably no myocardial ischemia as a cause of lightheadedness. However, the presence of chest pain with or without ST-segment change with lightheadedness must be further worked up for myocardial ischemia.
3. Take the blood pressure. If hypertensive, or normotensive, hypotension is not the cause. In the case of orthostasis, hypotension occurs only in response to position change (i.e., from the supine to upright position), causing lightheadedness.
4. Check heart rate. If not less than 60 beats per minute (bpm), bradycardia is not the cause.
5. Check respiratory rate. If elevated, the probable cause is not cardiac but respiratory.
6. Check blood sugar. If low, and accompanied by diaphoresis, pallor, and fatigue, the probable cause is hypoglycemia.
7. Check motor coordination. If not incoordinated or hemiparetic, and speech is normal, the cause is probably not cerebral ischemia, although there certainly can be less straightforward presentations of cerebral ischemia.

High suspicion of cardiac cause:

1. *Skipped beats on pulse taking:* Check the ECG for VEA, paroxysmal atrial tachycardia (PAT), bradycardia, and heart block.
2. *Hypotension:* A low systolic reading suggests hemodynamic compromise. A low pulse pressure (narrow margin between systolic and diastolic reading) and not necessarily hypotension per se also suggests cardiac problem.
3. *Chest pain:* Chest pain may also be present with or without ST-segment depression on ECG.

(VEA). If this symptom has occurred frequently, the chart may have a description of what provokes it. For example, orthostatic intolerance produces lightheadedness with postural change from recumbancy to the upright position. There may also be an indication of how long this symptom lasts, how frequently it appears, what relieves it, and whether it leads to loss of consciousness. Hyperventilation is often a result of anxiety and may become chronic. If chronic, lightheadedness may be a persistent experience, accompanied by tingling of the fingers, numbness, and an increase in respiratory rate. Sustained VEA will result in hypotension and may represent a serious dysfunction of the myocardium. However, many people experience transient VEA, which is well tolerated. VEA can occur from caffeine ingestion, with lightheadedness resulting from lack of perfusion to the brain. Hypotension with change of position may be transient, may be associated with prolonged bed rest or recent surgery, or may represent congestive heart failure and a seriously failing left ventricle. It is therefore important to look at the patient's chart for concurrent diagnoses, such as diabetes, sustained VEA, and TIAs. Some antihypertensive or antiarrhythmic drugs produce lightheadedness when the dose is being adjusted in some patients, as blood pressure may become more labile, or a cardiac rhythm may be stimulated by the altered dose. Examples of these types of such drugs are methyldopa and quinidine sulfate.

Syncope

Syncope, or loss of consciousness, is generally caused by cardiovascular problems. It is not always serious, however. It can range from nothing more than vasovagal syncope, with a spontaneous rapid recovery, to ventricular fibrillation or cardiac standstill, prompting immediate emergency intervention to prevent death.

A medical history for a patient who has experienced loss of consciousness in the past should include a description of the conditions that provoked this state, as well as the probable cause. Vasovagal syncope can be triggered by fear, pain, the sight of blood, hunger, and fatigue and is most frequently encountered in persons in a high anxiety state. Commonly, premonitory signs or symptoms provide a warning, including pallor, yawning, sighing, hyperventilation, epigastric discomfort, nausea, and/or blurred vision. In the case of loss of consciousness caused by orthostatic hypotension, the blood pressure will fall precipitously when the

---

Physical Therapy Evaluation of Syncope

High suspicion of cardiac cause:

1. Check for the presence of ventricular ectopic activity on the ECG.
2. Check supine and standing blood pressure for orthostatic intolerance as a cause of loss of consciousness.
3. Check blood pressure of both arms and legs for the presence of electromechanical dissociation of the myocardium.
4. To assess the likelihood of cardiac arrest, if the patient is status post anterior myocardial infarction, there is a higher incidence of aneurysm. Check using echocardiogram for evidence of aneurysm. Consider the possibility of rupture. Also, if the patient is status post posterior myocardial infarction, there is a higher likelihood of mitral regurgitation attributable to papillary muscle involvement. There may be rapid fulminating pulmonary edema.

---

patient moves from a supine to standing position and is preceded by lightheadedness when the person is upright. There is also a compensatory tachycardia, which would not be present during vasovagal syncope. Hypoglycemia in diabetes mellitus may result in loss of consciousness, especially during exercise. A seizure is typically characterized by muscle jerking, breath-holding, and choking sounds, and the patient may lose consciousness. Grand mal seizures generally abate spontaneously after 3 to 4 minutes and are characterized by lip or tongue biting and by incontinence of the bowel and bladder. The seizures are followed by a state of mental confusion. Most other causes of loss of consciousness are life-threatening or could become so, such as ventricular ectopy (ventricular fibrillation or tachycardia), asystole, pulmonary embolus, aortic stenosis, and IHSS. Carotid sinus hypersensitivity could produce loss of consciousness when a patient wearing a high collar turns the head, which causes spontaneous stimulation of the carotid sinus. Other examples of types of syncope include micturition syncope, Stokes-Adams attacks (i.e., transient asystole or ventricular fibrillation in the presence of atrioventricular block) sinus arrest, hyperventilation syncope, and cough syncope. Exertional syncope has been found in patients with aortic stenosis, IHSS, pulmonary hypertension, asystole, and ventricular tachycardia.

Fatigue

Fatigue is defined as the loss or lack of energy with which to perform a necessary activity. Sources of fatigue at very low-level exertion may be neurologic, muscular, metabolic, cardiac, or pulmonary. A medical history is an important reference for sorting out the cause of fatigue in any given patient. However, fatigue is rarely the single presenting symptom reported on the patient's medical chart. Most tests are not specific for fatigue, but the combination of many test results may elucidate the cause of fatigue and whether it is pathologic.

If the patient's history indicates that fatigue is a major complaint, an interview should provide descriptors. Fatigue may be general whole-body fatigue, or it may be quite localized. It may be accompanied by other

<hr>

Physical Therapy Evaluation of Fatigue

High suspicion of cardiac cause:

1. Look for signs of falling blood pressure, which occurs in cardiac tamponade, congestive heart failure (CHF), and inotropic incompetence. In CHF, check for appearance of rales in both lung bases, using the diaphragm of the stethoscope, and check for a gallop rhythm using the bell of stethoscope over the apex with the patient in a left side-lying position (see Auscultation, under Physical Examination). In cardiac tamponade, look for dyspnea, weakness, malaise, chest pain, anorexia, and weight loss with diaphoresis.
2. Check for hypotension with tachycardia or with severe bradycardia.
3. Check the patient for pallor.
4. Check pulses and ECG for frequent VEA.
5. Look for test results on ETT, echocardiography, or magnetic resonance imaging (MRI) to indicate the presence of CAD, aortic valve dysfunction, cardiomyopathy, or myocarditis.

<hr>

associated symptoms, such as pain in a muscle (or cramp) or chest pain (or dyspnea). Normal causes of fatigue, related to high levels of energy output, include local muscle glycogen depletion (after very prolonged high level effort), lactate accumulation in muscle and blood (at relatively high levels of exertion), poor motivation or loss of motivation, calcium ion depletion (prolonged use of a muscle), and dehydration (on hot days after long periods of exercise). In addition, some pathologic conditions that contribute to early fatigability include a low cardiac output state, such as CAD, aortic valve dysfunction, cardiomyopathy, and myocarditis. Anemia can cause extreme fatigue. Hypothyroidism results in lethargy and a general loss of energy. Hyperthyroidism may also lead to chronic exhaustion. Psychiatric disorders, especially depression, are usually associated with chronic fatigue. Conditions resulting in hypoxia also result in fatigue and other associated symptoms of increased respiratory rate, dyspnea, and lightheadedness. These conditions include respiratory failure, acute pulmonary embolus, and arteriovenous shunt of the heart or lungs. Finally, hyperglycemia such as may occur in a diabetic patient with an insulin deficiency will result in extreme fatigability. General metabolic derangements and systemic illnesses that create fatigue include some cancers, chronic renal failure, and chronic liver failure.

Dyspnea

Breathlessness, or dyspnea, is a common experience whenever we engage in fairly strenuous exercise. It is accompanied by a respiratory rate usually over 40 breaths per minute, and can be extremely frightening if extreme. The fear of suffocation accounts for associated symptoms and behaviors. Breathlessness can be an acute problem, such as occurs in the choking victim, or can be chronic, under conditions of low-level exertion in severe chronic obstructive pulmonary disease (COPD), or at rest, in CHF. There may be several causes for dyspnea. The increase in metabolic demand for oxygen provides a chemical stimulus to increase respiration, which may lead to the patient's perception of breathlessness. It may actually be caused by the inappropriate length-tension relationship of the diaphragm muscle when the muscle length is too short, as in high exercise demand, or when the muscle length is too overstretched, as in COPD patients, to meet the tension requirement of a particular activity. In left ventricular congestive failure, caused by a failing pump, fluid is retained in the left atrium, which backs up much like a clogged drain, in the pulmonary circulation. The fluid leaks out into the alveoli, blocking the exchange of gases and creating the demand for better oxygenation, or better ventilation. The impossible demand, unable to be met by the inadequate supply, produces dyspnea.

The medical history will enlighten the physical therapist about the likely etiology of breathlessness. What is the smoking history of the patient? The pack-year history, or the number of years times the number of packs of cigarettes smoked per day, should be available from a history. The higher the pack-year exposure to

Physical Therapy Evaluation of Dyspnea

High suspicion of cardiac cause:

1. If the blood pressure (BP) is low, heart rate (HR) is high, rhythm of ECG shows premature atrial contractions (PACs), respiratory rate is high, oxygen saturation is normal, and temperature is normal, it is likely to relate to CHF.
2. A low blood pressure with fatigue, dyspnea, anorexia, weight loss, and malaise may indicate cardiac tamponade.
3. An echocardiogram may show mitral stenosis.
4. Pulmonary embolism will produce abrupt onset of dyspnea, which may be very severe, and should correlate with a drop in oxygen saturation by pulse oximetry.
5. Chronic pericarditis will produce tachycardia with dyspnea and may flare up acutely with sharp chest pain.
6. Check for cyanosis of nail beds and lips as an indication of tissue hypoxia.
7. Check whether the patient has secretions chronically, or suddenly, with acute onset of pulmonary edema.

smoking, the more damage to the tissue. Environmental exposure to damaging substances can also be a cause of breathlessness. Air pollutants may include chemical substances, fibrous particulate substances (e.g., asbestos), and dust from occupations working with substances (e.g., coal dust and flour dust), which can all contribute to long-term lung disease. The result is chronic breathlessness because of the loss of available lung tissue for gas exchange.

Cardiac causes of dyspnea include coronary insufficiency, mitral valve disease, myocardial dysfunction, and constrictive pericarditis. Breathlessness may occur under different conditions, and it may help to delineate which condition is pertinent to each patient. Dyspnea on exertion (DOE) is one condition common to both cardiac and pulmonary disease. Many patients have some elements of both diseases (attributable to many common etiologies, such as smoking). In DOE, breathlessness is brought on by activity. In severe DOE, activities are curtailed when they induce the unpleasant sensation of dyspnea. Thus begins the spiral of deconditioning, which produces a lower anaerobic threshold, and an earlier onset of DOE. Thus, dyspnea induces more deconditioning, which exacerbates the symptom of breathlessness.

Another condition is paroxysmal noctural dyspnea (PND), in which a patient awakens from prolonged sleep with dyspnea. Its frequent occurrence implies CHF. Chronic pulmonary edema or cor pulmonale is worsened by a long period of recumbency and by consequent shifts in hydrostatic fluid. Orthopnea is the final condition, in which the supine position is not tolerated; propping several pillows below the head can relieve dyspnea.

Findings from the maximum stress test with gas analysis can illuminate the various etiologies of dyspnea. If deconditioning is the primary cause, expected findings will be early dyspnea, a low maximal oxygen consumption ($\dot{V}O_2$), and a low anaerobic threshold. If the patient has congestive heart failure, made worse by exercise, there will be a low, nonresponsive cardiac output, reflected in the systolic blood pressure by a flat or dropping measurement with increasing exercise. In addition, there will be early onset of anaerobic metabolism and a rapid rise in heart rate. The third heart sound may become audible during exercise. When the peripheral circulation is the limiting factor to a patient's exercise tolerance, dyspnea may occur early in the test because of earlier anaerobic metabolism in the local ischemic muscle bed. There will be a low maximal $\dot{V}O_2$, and low anaerobic threshold, and very likely, local muscle pain in an area of active contraction.[5]

Cough

Cough occurs as a protective reflex to expel foreign matter from the large airways, thus avoiding obstruction of the airways. In general, a cough should not be suppressed, but when it becomes chronic, ineffective, and irritating, cough suppression is sometimes a goal.

Physical Therapy Evaluation of Cough

High suspicion of cardiac cause:

1. Chest radiography showing cardiomegaly, a boot-shaped heart, and Kerley B lines points to a cardiac etiology.
2. Sputum that is pink and frothy, with no evidence of infection (bacteria or viral, which produces purulent sputum), gives a cardiac diagnosis.
3. An echocardiogram that shows myocardial wall hypokinesis, akinesis, dyskinesis, or mitral valve dysfunction, and an ejection fraction of less than 40 percent implicates cardiac disease.
4. Adventitious breath sounds, such as rales and rhonchi, may implicate either pulmonary or cardiac problems, or both but, in the presence of a gallop rhythm heart sound, certainly suggest myocardial dysfunction.

The therapeutic goal, however, is most likely to enhance cough effectiveness.

Most causes of cough involve infectious, neoplastic, or allergic disorders of the lungs and tracheobronchial structures. Cardiovascular diagnoses that contribute to the symptom of cough include left ventricular failure with pulmonary edema, pulmonary venous hypertension, pulmonary infarction, and expanding aortic aneurysm that compresses the tracheobronchial tree. In some patients, a premature ventricular beat can cause a cough.

A medical history should describe whether myocardial damage or mitral stenosis in the past may account for CHF before this episode or new-onset CHF. If pulmonary edema has occurred, there is usually a description of the sputum produced, which is frothy and pink, and the cough will be bubbling, loose, and rattling. Cough caused by pulmonary venous hypertension secondary to mitral stenosis or chronic CHF tends to be dry, irritating, and nocturnal.

HISTORY

One of the most important means to obtain information is the patient interview. Key questions about each symptom listed in Table 2-1 as well as questions about the patient's medical history, and family history, can be very instructive in ascertaining the likelihood that a given symptom is cardiovascular in origin. The interview can also indicate the significance or severity of symptoms.

Table 2-1. Key Questions for Cardiovascular Symptoms

Angina
Description of chest pain
  Where is it?
  When does it occur?
  How long does it last?
  What gives relief?

Sweating
  Do you sweat with chest pain?
  Do you ever sweat without exercise? (cold sweat)
  If so, when?

Palpitations
  When do these occur?
  How do they affect you? (e.g., scared, dizzy, weak.)
  How do you get rid of them?

Breathlessness
  What brings on breathlessness: (activity, sleep, certain positions)
  What gives relief? (pursed-lips breathing, sitting upright, leaning forward with support, rest)

Lightheadedness/Loss of consciousness
  Have you ever felt dizzy or blacked out?
  If so, how often?
  If so, what brings it on?
  If so, how do you get relief?

Fatigue
  How is your energy level in general?
  How well do you sleep at night?

Cardiac risk factors
  Have you ever been told that you have high blood pressure?
  Do you now, or have you ever, smoked? Cigarettes? Other? How long, and how many?
  Have you ever had your blood cholesterol checked? Do you know the level? Do you know what it should be?
  Do you have diabetes?
  What is your best body weight? Are you over, under, or OK now?
  What activities do you do regularly?
  Has anyone in your immediate family ever had a heart attack?
    Has anyone had chest pain or cardiac surgery?
  Have you ever had a heart attack, chest pain, or cardiac surgery?

Patient's Past and Current Medical History

Many signs and symptoms of the cardiovascular system stem from atherosclerotic disease. Questions about risk factors for CAD are therefore important. If a patient has been a smoker, any exposure to nicotine, however remote, should raise a high suspicion for cardiopulmonary signs and symptoms. Additional questions about the other key cardiac risk factors (i.e., hypertension and cholesterol or diet habits) can provide valuable insight into the probability that the patient has CAD or peripheral vascular disease (PVD). The physical therapist should ask about the patient's own knowledge of CAD and whether the patient has ever had a heart attack, angina, a problem with heart rhythm, or been told that he or she has high blood pressure.

Family Medical History

CAD and often PVD have a strong family history. Thus, a patient who is a reasonable historian should know whether parents and/or siblings experienced similar signs or symptoms or carried the diagnosis. Questions designed to uncloak this information can be very enlightening, since a positive response gives a much higher suspicion for cardiovascular disease.

PHYSICAL EXAMINATION

Observation

The observer's eye, when fully opened to postural, color, skin, or other changes that occur with cardiovascular disease, can be decisive in assessing the presence and extent of a disease process. The most obvious example is in PVD. Skin color changes and skin texture can define arterial or venous insufficiency. Arterial problems result in blue to black skin lesions in regions of smooth, hairless skin. Venous problems produce brown or purple areas of discoloration, often extending much farther than areas of arterial lesions, with roughened skin texture. Edema of both ankles occurs

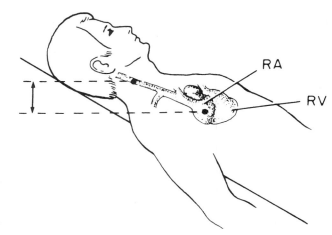

Fig. 2-10. Examination of jugular venous pulse and estimation of venous pressure. RA, right atrium; RV, right ventricle. (From Sokolow and McIlroy,[13] with permission.)

with venous stasis, which tends to be relatively painless.

In CHF, edema of both ankles can occur when right ventricular failure is involved. This edema is not associated with discoloration, is painless, and is usually associated with rapid weight gain (4 to 5 pounds over 2 to 3 days), jugular venous distention (JVD), and ascites. JVD is determined by placing the patient supine in a 45-degree head-up position and measuring the number of centimeters up from the right atrium that the distention of the jugular vein appears in the neck (Fig. 2-10).

Left ventricular failure results in breathlessness, which can be quite acute. In the situation of acute pulmonary edema, the patient appears to be starved for air. The patient will be gasping, often leaning forward on both arms to fix the shoulder girdle, which facilitates the accessory muscles of breathing. This appearance is identical to that of the person with primary lung disease who is air hungry. A cough may be present that will be productive of frothy pink sputum. In chronic CHF, the cough may be productive of white bubbling sputum and accompanied by a wheeze.

In the case of a cardiac or pulmonary shunt, in which

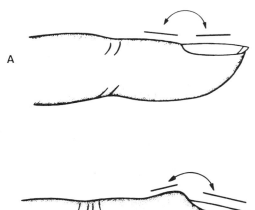

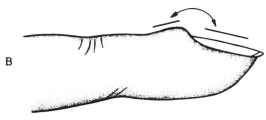

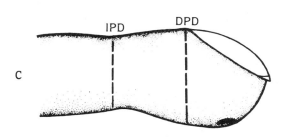

Fig. 2-11. **(A)** Normal digit configuration. **(B)** Mild digital clubbing with increased hyponychial angle. **(C)** Severe digital clubbing. Depth of finger at base (DPD) is greater than depth of interpharyngeal joint (IPD) with clubbing. (From Wilkins et al.,[14] with permission.)

blood bypasses the pulmonary alveoli and arrives insufficently oxygenated in the periphery, chronic tissue hypoxemia is the result. Fingernail and toenail clubbing can be observed. There is an alteration in the angle between the nail bed and the skin, an angle normally close to 180 degrees. In the presence of clubbing, this angle is increased to 200 degrees or more[6] (Fig. 2-11).

Patients with heart disease may experience angina in a variety of ways. They may appear anxious but otherwise show no obvious signs of cardiac embarrassment.

When patients are pale, diaphoretic, cyanotic, or weak, there is usually hemodynamic compromise with a poor cardiac output. For the patient who has irregular heartbeats or palpitations, the physical appearance provides important clues about the hemodynamic significance of their arrhythmia. A compromised patient will appear pale, even ashen, may be diaphoretic, and may have cyanotic lips and nail beds.

Palpation

Palpation is a very useful technique for differentiating chest pain syndromes. Chest wall pain may be elicited by finger probing over trigger points, by applying pressure over joint structures (especially costochondral junctions), or by applying pressure with the heel of the hand at the sternocostal joints. Angina will not be elicited by palpation techniques.

Pulse counting is usually done by palpation. Usual sites for determining a patient's heart rate is the radial pulse or the brachial pulse. The carotid pulse is not recommended, as the slightest pressure over the carotid pressure receptors can result in a vagal response with a drop in heart rate, which will alter the response being monitored. In some thin patients, an apical pulsation can be palpated by placing the hand over the cardiac apex position at the fifth intercostal space to feel for the point of maximal impulse sensation. This is a very effective point in children.

For the patient experiencing a cardiac arrhythmia, palpation by the physical therapist may provide the first evidence of the source of the problem. What the physical therapist feels should help a physician or someone trained in arrhythmia detection to recognize it and initiate appropriate treatment. A pulse pattern should be described as follows:

Is the rate regular or irregular? (Count for a full minute if necessary.)
If the ECG is observed, are there P waves?
Are P-to-P wave and R-to-R intervals regular or irregular?
Is there a P wave before each ventricular complex?
Are the P waves and QRS complexes identical and normal in configuration?

What is the hemodynamic significance of the arrhythmia?

The systolic blood pressure should be taken and the patient's appearance noted.

The peripheral pulses are palpated primarily to determine the presence or absence of a pulse. Absence of a palpable pulse indicates poor vascular supply, requiring follow-up evaluation procedures, such as Doppler flow evaluation, to determine the severity of the problem. Primary sites for palpation include the carotid pulse, both sides, radial and brachial pulses (femoral, popliteal, and tibial). A carotid pulse will be absent or distant in patients who have carotid stenosis. This leads to symptoms of lightheadedness, loss of consciousness, and strokelike symptoms of slurred speech, sagging facial muscles on one side, and weakness on one side of the body. TIAs, by definition, are reversed, leaving no sequelae, but should be considered as serious warning signs of vascular disease.

Patients who lack a tibial pulse in one or both feet (dorsum) should have their popliteal pulses checked, as well as the femoral pulses, to determine if these too are absent. Thus, the presence of a palpable pulse should mean that blood supply is adequate; when the pulse disappears to palpation, there may be vascular insufficiency.

Palpation can also be useful in early detection of an aneurysm. When a throbbing mass is palpable along an artery, the presence of an aneurysm should be suspected, and immediate referral to a physician for a diagnostic evaluation is indicated.

Palpable peripheral edema occurs from both cardiac disease and peripheral vascular or lymphatic disease of various etiologies. General edema is readily observable in the patient who has widespread CHF. Right ventricular failure causes increased systemic venous pressure as a result of failure of the pump to push fluid forward into the pulmonary circulation. Elevated jugular venous pressure, ascites, bilateral pitting edema of ankles, feet, and even knees may be present. The more severe case is ultimately characterized by anasarca.

Lymphedema is an abnormal accumulation of lymph in the extremities that occurs with infections of the lymphatics, with trauma to lymph channels (e.g., in burns and radiation), with allergic reactions, and with tumors obstructing a channel. The form this edema takes is localized edema, which can lead to extensive fluid accumulation from the level of the obstruction to all distal parts. Body parts thus affected feel pulpy and appear quite bloated.

Local edema may result from any loss of fluid balance between the interstitial and vascular compartments in any segment of the body. Hydrostatic pressure, inside blood vessels, develops as a result of gravity, the force of systolic ejection, and total blood volume. When one or more of these forces prevail over the tissue tension and oncotic pressures, tending to push fluid inward into vessels, edema can result. It may remain local to an area of dependency, characterized by insufficient fluid supply. This fluid accumulation can be palpated but may be less obvious than central or lymphatic sources of edema. It will feel boggy but sometimes will resist pitting.

It is difficult to assess a patient's vascular status accurately by palpating skin temperatures. The only useful evaluation is to compare the temperature of bilateral extremities by palpation and to note any obvious difference. Skin temperature should be accurately measured with a skin thermometer or thermistor, which will enable the therapist to draw a temperature map of limbs. This map can help assess the areas in which arterial supply is inadequate, as the skin distal to a vascular lesion will be significantly cooler than the proximal skin. Localized distribution of hot, red skin, often accompanied by swelling, may be thrombophlebitis. This condition occurs most commonly in patients who have been bedridden or immobilized for a long period and does not correlate with other vascular diseases.

Thermography is a high-technology application of the principle of making a temperature map of a body area. The result is a beautiful color representation of temperature differences, which can yield valuable information about sites that are cooler than expected. It is difficult to use for diagnosis or treatment planning, as there is no baseline color map with which to judge the severity or significance of the findings. Furthermore, the results are not quantifiable.

Auscultation

In order to gain insight into the source of a symptom that may be cardiovascular, or pulmonary, both breath sounds and heart sounds should be auscultated. The patient who is experiencing chest pain may avoid taking a deep breath for fear of worsening the sensation. Muscular splinting may reduce air movement at the bases of both lungs. Patients who are extremely anxious may breathe shallowly or may hyperventilate. Typically, patients with central nervous system (CNS) depression breathe very shallowly. Inspiratory rales will be heard bilaterally in the presence of pulmonary edema. In patients who have chronic CHF, a wheeze may develop if their failure is worsening; rales (crackles) should be audible as well.

Heart sounds normally occur as four distinct sounds: two very prominent high-frequency sounds, the *lubb-dupp* or S1 and S2, and two low-pitched less obvious sounds, heard most distinctly in pediatric populations because of the lack of subcutaneous tissue, and in adult patients who have exaggerated S3 and S4 heart sounds resulting from disease states. Both the S3 and S4 heart sounds are diastolic filling sounds generated by the influx of blood from atria to ventricles during diastole. In patients with CAD who have ventricles with decreased contractility caused by a scar from a myocardial infarction or by ischemia, the decrease in ventricular compliance results in greater volume of blood entering and even greater sloshing of blood as it enters the chambers. These factors amplify the filling sounds. The S3 heart sound occurs shortly after S2, or after semilunar valve closure. When this sound is auscultated, it most likely indicates a large area of noncompliant ventricular muscle, and the entering blood is unable to be accommodated by a stretchy, elastic wall. Patients with an S3 heart sound are typically in heart failure and will require medical attention to compensate for their failure. The S4 heart sound occurs at the end of diastole, when the last bit of blood enters the ventricles from an atrial "kick" as both atria contract. An area of scar or poor wall motion in the ventricles will magnify the S4 heart sound. It does not indicate

CHF per se. However, the presence of both an S3 and S4 heart sound is described as a gallop rhythm and represents a critical condition of CHF.

Auscultation of heart sounds requires skill, which can only be acquired with practice. However, this skill may be one of the most critical for the patient who has known CHF compensated by medication. This patient needs to perform exercise and may be pushed over the edge by exercise, into decompensation.

To auscultate for S3 and S4 heart sounds, the patient is placed in the left lateral decubitus position, to increase the volume of blood returning to the heart. The bell of the stethoscope is used on the xiphoid, lower left sternal border and listened to during inspiration. The bell of the stethoscope is placed on the apical space over the 5th intercostal space left of the sternal border. The physical therapist listens for S3, S4 on expiration. The sounds may be heard immediately after the "dupp" of "lubb-dupp" (S3) and immediately preceding the "lubb" for S4. The following is a useful mnemonic for each:

"Ken-tuck-key"
S1   S2   S3

"Ten-nes-see"
S4   S1   S2

Blood Pressure

A clinical measure of blood pressure is one of the most useful simple measures available for assessing cardiac status and patient response to treatment, position change, exercise, and anxiety. The systolic blood pressure represents the product of the cardiac output and the total peripheral resistance. As such, it is an index of myocardial contractility. Unfortunately, there is a high degree of error in the measurement as compared with that taken with an arterial line (anywhere from 5 to 20 mmHg difference), even by experienced clinicians. For therapists who are unaccustomed to auscultation techniques and to the sounds produced in the circulatory system known as Karotkoff sounds, this technique may be quite inaccurate and not at all helpful.

When the systolic reading is high, there may be a high

cardiac output (as during exercise), or a high degree of peripheral resistance, as in anxiety states or under conditions of stress, or both. Conversely, a low systolic reading implies low cardiac contractility, although this is not necessarily low. There may be a low cardiac output, a low degree of total peripheral resistance, or both. The patient who fails to show an "adaptive" blood pressure response to exercise and who has a flat or falling systolic reading with exercise probably has an inadequate cardiac output, may have a failing ventricle with loss of contractility, and may also have inappropriate peripheral vasodilation.

The product of the systolic blood pressure and the heart rate during exercise at any point is an index of myocardial work. Thus, a patient who has known cardiac disease and who performs exercise should always have both systolic blood pressure and heart rate monitored to determine the degree of work the heart is placed under. If the patient experiences angina with exercise, the rate pressure product will always be the same at the threshold for angina. This stands to reason, since myocardial ischemia occurs when there is an imbalance between myocardial supply of oxygen and the demand for oxygen. The supply is determined by the amount of blood flow allowed through coronary stenoses, and the demand is the work of the heart. Since the heart functions as a pump, it is intuitively easy to see why it pumps harder when it must work faster (increased heart rate) and when it must increase the power of its contraction (increased contractility, or systolic blood pressure).

Systolic readings during exercise may become very high at maximal levels, and the upper limits of safety are a matter of controversy and not at all standard. Younger subjects can easily tolerate high readings of 220 mmHg, whereas older people may not, even if they have no disease. There is no agreement about setting upper limits for specific age groups, and there must be a high degree of individualization. Common sense dictates that the person with an aortic aneurysm should have a low upper limit for systolic blood pressure, perhaps 170 mmHg. Many elderly subjects may be subject to aortic disease without clinical manifestations and should therefore be held to an upper limit of perhaps 190 mmHg. However, the patient with hypertension has accommodated to much higher pressures over time and should show excessively high systolic responses to exercise.

Diastolic blood pressure should not be higher than 90 mmHg but can drop to zero by auscultation in certain exercising subjects. For people with resting diastolic readings above 90 mmHg, significant hypertension is present that should be reported to the patient's doctor, if it is an uncommon finding for this patient. Some patients, however, have labile pressures with a diastolic reading that may be as high as 105 from time to time. This is usually well tolerated and is often left untreated. The significance of the higher diastolic reading is that the myocardium at rest is still facing a high fluid pressure, which implies that there may be a loss of contractility or onset of failure.

The difference between the systolic and the diastolic blood pressure is called the pulse pressure. This difference should not narrow with exercise, or it is a grave sign of pending cardiac failure. Clearly, if the cardiac output is falling with a resultant drop in systolic pressure, and the amount of pressure in diastole is rising with fluid backup and loss of contractility, the pulse pressure is narrowing. This becomes an important indicator for eventual distress.

All patients who have known heart disease, and any who exhibit signs or symptoms of heart disease, should have their blood pressure measured. Blood pressure should be measured at rest and with the patient in supine, sitting, and standing positions, to determine orthostatic adjustment before exercise, and certainly during and after exercise.

ELECTROCARDIOGRAM

The ECG is the surface recording of the electrical activity of the heart. It tells nothing about the mechanical, contractile function of the heart or about its effectiveness as a pump. However, the ECG does shed light on two overall aspects of myocardial function: the excitability of cardiac tissue, and the nutritional status of regions of the heart. When 12 leads are monitored, representing the standard measurement of electrical activity, the nutritional status of all the different aspects, from base to apex, from anterior to posterior, and from lateral to inferior, can be assessed. When ischemia is present, the sensitive segment on the ECG is the region representing ventricular repolarization, known as the ST segment. When injury and/or necrosis is present, the same segment will register a different change. Ischemia depresses the ST segment; injury elevates it. The particular lead(s) where these signs are found indicate(s) the location of injury, without specifying an anatomic distribution.

Hyperexcitable states of the myocardium include extra beats generated from irritable foci; hypoexcitability may be seen as conduction pathway delays or blocks. For this parameter, any lead will show the same information, although some may be easier to see than others. Thus, a rhythm-strip ECG is a single lead tracing over a period of time in order to track the relative excitability of the tissue. On a single-lead rhythm strip, taken at rest, consecutive beats should be checked for regular intervals of P-QRS-T, which do not vary from beat to beat. In heart block or sinus arrest, segments of this normal waveform may be prolonged, missing, or dissociated, thereby creating pauses in the palpated pulse. Premature beats can readily be found as those appearing early, and therefore too close to the previous beat for the normal R-to-R interval. The configuration of these premature beats is critical. If they resemble the normal beat, but occur early, and have a P wave before the QRS complex, they are usually atrial or junctional, whereas if they have a wide, quite different configuration from the normal beat, and have no P wave before the QRS, they are ventricular. If there is more than one premature beat, they may all be the same in configuration, or there may be more than one type, or multiform. Uniform beats originate from a single ectopic focus; multiform beats originate from several ectopic foci.

The significance of an irregular heartbeat can be determined from a functional evaluation. The physical therapist can choose one or more pertinent activities for the patient to perform while being monitored with a rhythm-strip ECG. In addition, vital signs will help determine the hemodynamic status of the patient during the activity. Since activity increases myocardial work, this may induce an irregular heartbeat, especially in cases in which myocardial dysfunction or hy-

Observations that the physical therapist should make during activity on the patient who has a rhythm-strip ECG recording include the following list of 11 items:

1. Describe heartbeat in terms of rate and rhythm, whether premature or not.
2. Describe P waves, PR and QRS intervals, and morphology. If ventricular in configuration, what is the frequency of the premature beat? If it is less than 6 per minute, this is probably well tolerated. If it is greater than 6 per minute, check vital signs for evidence of hemodynamic intolerance.
3. Describe signs and symptoms of hemodynamic compromise.
4. Note what provoked the arrhythmia.
5. Note what caused any change in it.
6. Check the relationship of P waves to QRS complexes. If P waves appear at their own rhythm, unrelated to QRS complexes, the patient may have third-degree heart block, which will not be tolerated well for long. Some cases of atrial to ventricular dissociation are tolerated without any problem.
7. If P waves occasionally trigger QRS complexes in a normal sequence, but at other times are not followed by QRS complex, the patient may have second-degree heart block and that could deteriorate into third-degree heart block.
8. PVCs are more serious if they occur frequently, are multiform, and/or if they occur early (R on T) because they are more likely to deteriorate into ventricular tachycardia.
9. Ventricular tachycardia, seen as couplets or triplets of PVCs or as salvos of several more PVCs, may deteriorate into ventricular fibrillation and become life-threatening or may not promote adequate peripheral perfusion, resulting in hemodynamic compromise.
10. Ventricular fibrillation calls for immediate electrical countershock as an emergency measure. Cardiopulmonary resuscitation (CPR) should be initiated and a "code" called.
11. Sinus arrest results in no pulse and a flat-line ECG, calling for immediate emergency care. CPR should be initiated and a "code" called.

poxia are responsible for the arrhythmia. Some arrhythmias occur at rest or at low levels of activity and are abolished with higher energy requirements, because of the overriding influence of the sinus node when exercise demands induce sympathetic stimulation to that node. Many arrhythmias will not be influenced by activity, but activity will be tolerated less well than rest. This is due to the inadequate hemodynamic response available to support activity requirements under conditions of myocardial arrhythmias.

Some additional problems with cardiac rhythm can arise. These include severe sinus bradycardia, which may result in serious hemodynamic compromise and require emergency measures but yield no irregularity of pulse. Severe sinus tachycardia may not be well tolerated by some patients because of the severe anxiety associated with the sensation of flutter in their chests and because of inadequate diastolic filling time. Medical treatment may be necessary, although usually not on an urgent basis.

CARDIOVASCULAR PATHOPHYSIOLOGY

The seven most frequently encountered cardiovascular disease states seen in patient populations from an industrialized society are coronary artery disease (CAD), arrhythmias, heart failure, hypertension, valvular heart disease and endocarditis, pericardial disease, and aortic and vascular tree disease.

Coronary Artery Disease

Whether presenting as chronic angina pectoris, unstable angina with or without myocardial infarction (MI), sudden death, or congestive ischemic cardiomyopathy, the underlying pathologic lesion will be a unifying one in most cases (i.e., atherosclerosis of the coronary arteries). Atherosclerosis involves a progressive thickening and hardening of the medium-sized and large muscular arteries, usually the coronary, carotid, basilar, vertebral, aortic, and iliac vessels. Epidemiologic efforts have identified two sets of risk factors that predispose to the development of atherosclerosis. The first set are considered nonmodifiable

and include a family history of CAD before the age of 60, as well as being male. Modifiable risk factors, the second set, include a history of hypertension or diabetes mellitus; hyperlipoproteinemia involving an elevation in the low-density lipoprotein (LDL) fraction and/or depression of the high-density lipoprotein (HDL) cholesterol fraction; recent tobacco abuse; obesity; sedentary life-style; and an ill-defined psychological profile characterized by high levels of stress, hostility, and isolation.

Controversy continues to surround the step-by-step explanation of atherosclerotic vascular injury. One increasingly accepted view is that proposed by Valentin Fuster and his investigative group. Initial change is thought to occur as early as age 3 years with the development of the fatty streak, a slightly raised lesion in which limited numbers of smooth muscle cells and lipid containing macrophages invade the endothelium or inner lining of the blood vessel wall. In the genetically predisposed person or one with known risk factors, these lesions may mature, becoming fibrotic and increasing shear stress from blood flow, hyperlipidemia, hypertension, immune injury, or cigarette smoking, endothelial lining cells are lost and platelets deposited, initiating fibrous intimal hyperplasia. If exposed to elevated levels of circulating lipids, lesions progress to atherosclerotic plaques with further accumulation of lipid-laden macrophages, migration of smooth muscle cells, and collagen synthesis. With further maturation of the lesion, elevated cholesterol concentration within the lipid fraction results in cholesterol crystal formation in the older, deeper layers.

Once platelets deposit or adhere to the vessel wall, a series of molecular processes occur, resulting in platelet aggregation and thrombus formation. Presumably the gradual narrowing of coronary flow can cause the chronic pattern of exertionally related angina pectoris. Rupture or fissure of a plaque causes a sudden change in lesion shape, triggering the cascade of events that leads to intraluminal thrombosis, resulting in unstable angina (Fig. 2-12). Whether a person goes on to suffer an MI will depend on the degree and duration of inadequate coronary blood flow. Sudden ischemic death can result, too, in this setting of prolonged coronary

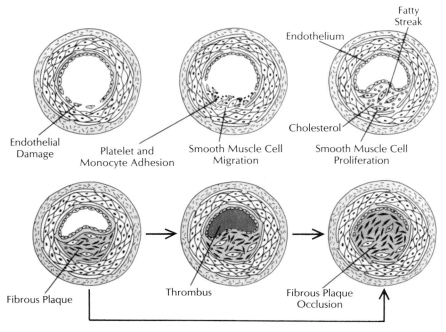

Fig. 2-12. Proposed cellular changes involved in plaque formation, thrombosis, and vascular occlusion. (Modified from Stein et al.,[19] with permission.)

insufficiency, in which fatal ventricular arrhythmias are triggered.

Patients with atherosclerotic CAD can present with (1) a chronic pattern of effort- or stress-related chest pain known as angina pectoris; (2) chest pain that is new, increasing in intensity or frequency, occurring at lower workloads or requiring more sublingual nitroglycerin for relief, called unstable angina; (3) chest pain and other constitutional symptoms associated with MI; or (4) death. Indeed, of the roughly 1.5 million people in the United States who suffer an MI annually, 540,000 (36 percent) will die—350,000 of those before medical attention can be obtained.[2] While patients typically present in middle or advanced age, coronary atherosclerosis progresses over decades. Autopsies of young adults killed in military combat or accidentally frequently demonstrate evidence of coronary atherosclerosis. Both sexes are susceptible, with incidence rates of disease for women increasing and surpassing those of men once into the postmenopausal years.

Several tests and studies are frequently done to evalu-

ate patients suspected of having, or known to have CAD. A resting ECG is normal up to 50 percent of the time in those with chronic stable angina. Evidence of previous injury may be seen in the form of Q waves in a particular distribution. The most common findings are nonspecific ST-segment and T-wave abnormalities. If the patient is unstable, transient depression or elevation of the ST segment often associated with T-wave inversions is seen. Recording of an ECG during and after some type of stressful intervention, such as exercise, is valuable in assessing cardiovascular reserve and the possible degree of hemodynamic compromise. Exercise tolerance tests are often performed in the group of patients. A definitive diagnosis of CAD requires highlighting of the coronary blood vessels with radiocontrast in a procedure known as coronary angiography. This technique is part of cardiac catheterization, with left ventriculography also performed at this time. By injecting radiocontrast into the left ventricle, an estimation of cardiac performance and evidence of any prior injury can be obtained. Noninvasive evaluations of left ventricular performance can be obtained by cardiac ultrasound (echocardiography) and radionuclide angiography with a first-pass radionuclide angiogram and the gated blood pool study.

Exercise Tolerance Test

Patients with suspected CAD, whether the symptom of chest pain is present or not, will most likely be evaluated in a cardiology stress-testing laboratory. Although diagnosis is an important goal of the exercise tolerance test (ETT), other very significant items of information can be derived. These include definition of a dose-response relationship between exertion and cardiovascular adaptation, establishment of an optimal prescription for exercise, identification of a patient's limitations to exercise, induction of arrhythmias, and assessment of efficacy of a recent addition to one's antianginal regimen or recent procedure. A variety of protocols exist using either a treadmill or a cycle ergometer. The advantages of using a standardized protocol are many. A patient's response can be compared with that of a larger pool of similar subjects. Also, a baseline can be established in the patient's dose response, which can be compared with a future ETT after an intervention, after a period of time has elapsed, or upon the appearance of a new sign or symptom. Exercise is carefully titrated in increasing doses. This is why a consistent protocol with known energy requirements must be used, so that the cardiac responses to each "dose" or exercise level may be identified. Cardiac responses monitored include heart rate, blood pressure, and ECG changes. The ECG provides information about the status of myocardial perfusion (ST segment) and the rhythm. Arrhythmias arise when the myocardium is hypoxic, with metabolic abnormalities, or because of inherent conduction problems. Blood pressure monitoring gives important information about the hemodynamic responsiveness of the heart under exercise conditions. Systolic readings may be abnormally high or low, may drop when they should be rising, or may be normal, all of which can help determine the significance of the chest pain. When a standard Bruce treadmill protocol is used, the normal systolic rise is 12 mmHg per stage. With cycle ergometry, the blood pressure rise should be higher than with treadmill testing because of the muscular activity in the arms contributing to stabilizing the torso.

In the case of chest pain, the ETT can be used to determine the symptom threshold, in terms of either the workload at which chest pain arises or the heart rate and/or blood pressure at which chest pain appears. The product of heart rate and systolic blood pressure at the point that angina occurs can be used clinically as the rate-pressure product (RPP) at angina threshold. This index correlates highly with actual measurement of myocardial oxygen consumption, providing a handy clinical tool for the indirect measure of myocardial work. The equation that no longer balances supply with demand demonstrates an RPP at which angina occurs and supply is inadequate. This relationship is relatively fixed until one of several things happen: the disease progresses and the RPP is lower at a given angina threshold; a therapy such as β-blockade is instituted that affects heart rate and blood pressure even at angina threshold; or an exercise training program is successfully undertaken that can raise the RPP where angina is experienced or eliminates the experience of angina, even up to maximal exercise.

In using the ETT results to establish an exercise prescription, the anginal threshold heart rate is taken as the symptom-limited maximal heart rate, and not the true physiologic maximum. A percentage of this symptom-limited maximum heart rate is then used as a target heart rate for training. Frequently, 10 bpm less than symptomatic maximum is chosen for a target. American College of Sports Medicine guidelines recommend 70 to 85 percent of the symptom-limited maximum heart rate level or use of the Karvonen equation:

Target heart rate

$$= (HR_{max} - HR_{rest}) \times 0.7 + HR_{rest}$$

The ETT results may show that a patient who experiences chest pain has no ischemic ST-segment change. The question arises as to whether the chest pain is actually not of cardiac origin or is a false-negative ECG finding. The test may demonstrate no chest pain but a positive ST-segment change. Is this silent ischemia or a false-positive ECG finding? When a test is negative for both chest pain and ischemic ST-segment change, is the patient actually free of hemodynamically significant CAD, or was the exercise level attained inadequate to produce diagnostic information? To clarify such situations, current practice is to perform a diagnostic ETT with myocardial imaging techniques using thallium in order to observe myocardial perfusion.

The physical therapist may be in a position to need such information in a patient for whom a standard stress test is unavailable or not possible. It is quite reasonable to perform a standardized exercise at initial low levels with gradually increasing increments of effort with appropriate patient monitoring without calling it a formal stress test. If an appropriate activity can be identified that can be performed under relatively controlled conditions (e.g., 6-minute walk test, one flight of stairs, or wheelchair propulsion over an identified distance), the method of performance must be documented to make it repeatable, and the same parameters must be monitored in order to develop the dose-response relationship.

Arrhythmias

Rhythm disturbances involve an abnormality in the generation and/or propagation of the heartbeat. This can occur as an isolated situation or may be related to other underlying problems of the cardiovascular system. Its presence may be unknown to the patient, may cause troublesome symptoms resulting in no blood pressure abnormalities, or may lead to sudden death. Separate from this general discussion of the pathophysiology of arrhythmias is the earlier discussion on recognition of specific arrhythmias.

Cardiac arrhythmias are thought to arise as a result of one of two possible mechanisms. The first involves a disturbance in automaticity, the inherent property of the conduction system to generate a heartbeat. If the rate of the normal cardiac pacemaker is too fast or too slow, this is referred to as sinus tachycardia or sinus bradycardia. Other parts of the conduction system (i.e., the AV nodal junction), as well as the atrial and ventricular myocardium, are capable of impulse generation. These can be single beats arising early, known as premature ventricular or atrial beats (also contractions, complexes, and depolarizations), or accelerated junctional beats. Sustained rhythms of more than three beats in duration include the atrial, supraventricular, and ventricular tachycardias.

The second mechanism for arrhythmia generation results from a disturbance in conductivity, the appropriate distribution of a normal heartbeat throughout the myocardium. The conduction abnormality can result from AV block. As such, it is classified as first-, second-, or third-degree block.

First-degree AV block: The site of conduction delay is nearly always in the AV node. Recognition is made by prolongation of the PR interval on the 12-lead ECG.

Second-degree AV block: This abnormality is divided into Mobitz type I, in which delay is within the AV node, and Mobitz type II, with delay occurring below the AV node in the His-Purkinje system.

Third-degree AV block: Also referred to as complete heart block in which conduction of the heartbeat from atria to ventricles is completely blocked, the actual site of the block is in the bundle-branch system.

Further disturbances in conduction can give rise to the phenomenon known as re-entry. In re-entry, an impulse that would normally reach a branch point and travel at equal rates of speed down both branches on toward the ventricle, is slowed in one branch and blocked in the other. The impulse will be delayed in reaching its destination down one branch. Because the block experienced by the impulse in the other branch was unidirectional, the stage is set for the delayed impulse to now go backward up the unidirectionally blocked branch, re-entering the system as an ectopic or abnormal beat. This mechanism is seen with such cardiovascular diseases as CAD and cardiomyopathy. It too can give rise to isolated or sustained premature beats or rhythms.

Also seen in conduction disturbances is the phenomenon of bypass tract conduction or pre-excitation. In this condition, depolarization of the ventricular myocardium occurs earlier than expected because conduction is occurring by way of an anomalous pathway or bypass tract that conducts much more quickly than the normal conduction system. Wolff-Parkinson-White syndrome is an example of this phenomenon. It is characterized on the ECG by a short PR interval and frequently with a δ wave preceding each QRS complex, lending a widened, bizarre appearance. Clinically, these patients will present with palpitations or lightheadedness resulting from a variety of tachyarrhythmias that can develop.

The 12-lead ECG and rhythm strip are the most important tools for diagnosing these disorders. A Holter monitor is often ordered to diagnose rhythms or conduction abnormalities that may be transient and not present at the time an ECG is obtained; to quantify frequency of a problem; or to determine possible arrhythmic precipitants of a symptom complex. The Holter monitor continuously scans and records two chest leads over a 24-hour period.

A recently developed technique, known as signal-averaged ECG, is used to identify patients at risk of future malignant arrhythmias, as is the case in postinfarction patients or in patients with a cardiomyopathy. With this technique, low-amplitude electrical activity occurring in the late phase of the QRS complex is amplified and averaged in a computer-assisted process. These late potentials are the presumed substrate for re-entrant ventricular arrhythmias. If a patient has been discovered to have serious arrhythmias that will require drug therapy, or if a serious arrhythmia is suspected but cannot be documented, electrophysiologic studies (EPS) may be pursued. These invasive studies require the placement of one or more intracardiac catheters to record and stimulate portions of the heart that are electrically silent on the body surface ECG (e.g., sinus node, right or left atrium, His bundle, right bundle branch, left bundle branch, and specific sites within the right or left ventricle).

Heart Failure

Defined broadly, heart failure is the condition in which the heart is unable to supply all body tissues adequately with oxygenated blood. Heart failure can occur even though the heart muscle is normal, as in situations in which venous return to the heart is impaired (e.g., constrictive pericarditis or restrictive cardiomyopathy). Most cases result from the actual inability of the myocardium to contract sufficiently. This condition is generally produced by cumulative ischemic injury, as seen with ischemic cardiomyopathy. It can also result from any of the following: chronic alcohol exposure, the peripartal state, Adriamycin toxicity, diabetes, sarcoidosis, Chagas' disease, or amyloidosis.

Patients with heart failure will present with congestive symptoms, the particular pattern of which can help in defining the failure as left sided, right sided, or biventricular. A distinction is made between chronic and acute heart failure. A chronic condition is present and unchanged for a minimum of 3 months, and an acute situation is manifested within minutes to hours, usually in association with myocardial ischemia or infarction. The acute presentation is often referred to as pulmonary edema.

Hemodynamically, abnormalities include decreased cardiac output and elevated ventricular filling pressures. Hypoperfusion, as a result of a drop in cardiac output, can lead to confusion, weakness, and cold and clammy extremities. Elevated left ventricular filling pressures, clinically measured as mean left atrial pressure or left ventricular end-diastolic pressure, cause pulmonary venous congestion, leading to exertional dyspnea, nonproductive and nocturnal cough, orthopnea, and paroxysmal nocturnal dyspnea. Elevated filling pressures of the right heart, measured by use of a central venous pressure (CVP) catheter, are associated with systemic venous congestion manifested by pedal edema, abdominal discomfort and/or distention, and anorexia.

A major component in the clinical presentation of these hemodynamic abnormalities is the compensatory attempts made by the body. While initially helpful, these efforts invariably become counterproductive. The sympathetic nervous system and the renin-angiotensin system are stimulated, leading to increased heart rate, increased filling pressure, and increased contractility. In addition, myocardial hypertrophy occurs. When carried to the extreme, increased arterial vascular tone results in increased peripheral resistance and afterload on the already failing left ventricle. Venoconstriction shifts blood volume into the central circulation, worsening congestive symptoms. Finally, filling pressures past an optimal point simply add to congestion.

Once heart failure becomes even moderate in extent, the patient will be easily fatigued with minimal effort, will often require multiple daily medication, and will have a host of cardiac management problems. Whether the CHF patient is being examined de novo, having the efficacy of a new drug assessed, or being seen for follow-up management, left ventricular function must be evaluated. The most accurate and thorough determination of left ventricular performance is invasively at cardiac catheterization when pressure, flow, and volume can be measured and dimensions calculated. Noninvasive measures can be done with echocardiography and radionuclide angiography. Increasingly, structured exercise protocols are being added to these assessments of left ventricular performance for better definition of the functional response to interventions and overall prognosis.

Hypertension

Arbitrarily defined as a blood pressure above 140/90 mmHg, hypertension affects 20 percent of adult Americans. Of those, 90 percent have no identifiable secondary cause of the hypertension and are said to suffer from essential or primary hypertension. The remaining 10 percent have treatable or reversible causes of hypertension, such as renal parenchymal disease, renovascular disease, primary aldosteronism, Cushing's syndrome, pheochromocytoma, coarctation of the aorta, or hyperparathyroidism. Although largely asymptomatic, left untreated, hypertension will shorten life by 10 to 20 years, primarily because of acceleration of atherosclerosis, but also by leading to stroke, heart failure, peripheral vascular disease, renal insufficiency, and retinopathy.

Blood pressure is determined primarily by cardiac output and peripheral resistance. The multifaceted, regulatory networks that control cardiac output, fluid status within and outside the vascular bed, and vascular caliber and responsiveness all must respond to the increased pressure load of hypertension. Many observations have been made about hypertension, but the underlying cause has not yet been identified. Two main mechanistic theories prevail: (1) an increased level of cardiac function results from overstimulation by the sympathetic nervous system, and (2) primary retention of salt and water by the kidneys may lead to elevated blood pressure levels. Heredity obviously has a role to play in many instances of essential hypertension. Another contributing factor is the person's environment, including percentage body weight above ideal, alcohol intake, salt intake, smoking history, and possible oral contraceptive use.

The diagnosis of hypertension can be made during the physical examination, requiring no more than a stethoscope and sphygmomanometer. Because most hypertension by far is classified as essential hypertension, the standard evaluation initially includes only a few simple laboratory tests of blood and urine, to determine severity of cardiovascular disease, possible causes of hypertension, overall cardiovascular risk, and baseline values for judging therapeutic efficacy. These include hemoglobin and hematocrit values; complete urinalysis; serum postassium, calcium, creatinine, and uric acid; and plasma lipid profile (total cholesterol, LDL and HDL cholesterols, and triglycerides) and plasma glucose.

Valvular Heart Disease and Endocarditis

The four heart valves can develop abnormalities either obstructing the forward flow of blood (stenosis) or allowing blood to leak backward into the preceding chamber (regurgitation). Involvement of either the mitral or aortic valve is more common and more debilitating than right-sided lesions.

Mitral Stenosis

Mitral stenosis is almost always a result of rheumatic fever. There is always a delay of many years between the acute fever and the development of symptoms. Rheumatic fever distorts the valve apparatus in a number of ways, all of which result in fusion of the valves. A normal valve opening or orifice is 4 to 6 cm². A reduction to 2 cm² is considered mild and to 1 cm² critical. At this level of stenosis, a pressure gradient between left atrium and left ventricle develops. This increase in pressure is transmitted backward, in turn raising the pulmonary venous and capillary pressures. This results in exertional dyspnea. Further clinical compromise is dictated by the degree of increased pulmonary vascular resistance and lowered cardiac output.

Women have a higher incidence of mitral stenosis. Typically, the patient with mitral stenosis will present with dyspnea, largely the result of reduced compliance of the lungs. Other complications of this lesion include infective endocarditis, hemoptysis, chest pain of unclear etiology, and thromboembolism. Often atrial fibrillation will develop. Once patients become moderately symptomatic, medical management becomes more difficult, and invasive procedures are entertained. In certain situations, mitral valvuloplasty is a consideration. Operative approaches that are available for rheumatic mitral stenosis include closed mitral commissurotomy (reopening of the valve leaflets by splitting along the fused commissures), open commissurotomy with the aid of cardiopulmonary bypass, and mitral valve replacement.

Mitral Regurgitation

Abnormalities of any portion of the mitral valve apparatus can result in incompetence. Leaflet involvement is seen most commonly in chronic rheumatic heart disease. The mitral annulus, a portion of the fibroskeleton of the heart that is the attachment point of the leaflet base, can become dilated or calcified, resulting in regurgitation, especially in the elderly. Abnormalities of the chordae tendineae, either congenital or a consequence of infective endocarditis, trauma, rheumatic fever, or myxomatous degeneration, can result in problems, often acutely and without warning. Finally, the papillary muscle, which completes the connection between leaflet and chordae to the ventricular wall, can rupture, usually as a result of ischemia. Pathophysiologically, the left atrium receives a significant portion of the blood flow in systole, which would normally have been ejected into the aorta. There is also overloading and eventual dilatation of the left ventricle as the left atrium chronically discharges its excessive blood volume into it during diastole. Whether the patient presents with fatigue and exhaustion from a low-output state or with pulmonary edema and right-sided failure depends on the chronicity of the lesion.

Because of the multiple etiologies resulting in mitral regurgitation, the natural history of the disease is quite variable and appears to be dependent on both the regurgitant volumes as well as on the underlying etiology. Acute pulmonary edema, hemoptysis, and systemic embolization are less likely to occur than in mitral stenosis. If symptoms do develop, the presenting picture is that of CHF. Medical management is focused on afterload reduction. Once surgery is decided on, options include annuloplasty (repair or support of the existing valve structure) or valve replacement.

The mitral valve prolapse syndrome involves a common cardiac valvular abnormality that can include mitral regurgitation. For most people with this diagnosis, it remains an echocardiographic finding with no resultant symptoms, functional implications, or effect on future outcomes. In a few cases, symptoms can include palpitations, chest discomfort, and, when mitral regurgitation is severe, symptoms of heart failure. Etiology of the chest discomfort is postulated to involve increased papillary muscle tension and left ventricular wall motion abnormalities. The clinical course can be complicated by arrhythmias, endocarditis, progressive mitral regurgitation requiring valve replacement, and cerebral embolization.

Aortic Stenosis

Valvular aortic stenosis is usually either congenital or degenerative in origin. In most cases, nodular calcium deposits on the valve cusps prevent normal opening during systole. With obstruction to left ventricular output, a pressure gradient develops between the left ventricle and the aorta. Output is maintained by hypertrophy of the left ventricle. Patients with aortic stenosis can remain symptom free until late in the course of the disease, when the heart can no longer meet the oxygen demands of the massively hypertrophied left ventricle.

The natural history of patients with aortic stenosis is characterized by a long latent period. Despite increasing obstruction of the aortic valve and myocardial hypertrophy, the patient is asymptomatic. Typically, symptoms develop in the sixth decade of life, which include angina, syncope, and dyspnea. By the time symptoms appear, the prognosis is poor, and only with invasive intervention is there any hope of interrupting the projected 2- to 5-year survival. Angina experienced by the patient with aortic stenosis is attributed to the increased oxygen demands of the hypertrophic myocardium as well as diminished oxygen supply caused by compression of the coronary vessels. CAD can coexist and can also contribute to symptoms.

The ECG will demonstrate left ventricular hypertrophy in most patients, seen as a marked increase in voltage of the QRS complex. Chest radiography commonly demonstrates post-stenotic dilatation of the ascending aorta. If the aortic stenosis is severe, calcification of the valve is almost always present in the adult patient. The most sensitive and specific noninvasive test is the echocardiogram. With its various modes of inquiry, it can define abnormal valvular shape and restricted leaflet motion, measure blood flow through the valve, measure the pressure gradient across the valve, and calculate valve area. When surgery is contemplated, cardiac catheterization is usually performed to assess pressure gradients and valve area, using catheter measurements, as well as to evaluate for coronary atherosclerosis. Aortic valve replacement is the definitive procedure for critical aortic stenosis. Valvuloplasty of the aortic valve is generally reserved for patients considered too frail to withstand surgery.

Aortic Regurgitation

Aortic regurgitation can result either from valve leaflet abnormalities (e.g., rheumatic fever or infective endocarditis) or from abnormalities of the aorta (e.g., Marfan's syndrome, syphilis, or rheumatoid arthritis). In a patient with chronic regurgitation of blood, the left ventricle compensates by dilating. Symptoms arise when the heart fails to achieve an effective forward cardiac output. When acute, the left ventricle is unable to compensate by dilating; left ventricular failure quickly occurs as the ventricle is unable to meet the burden of acute, severe volume overload.

Chronic aortic regurgitation is characterized by a latency period during which the left ventricle is slowly dilating; the patient is asymptomatic until late in the course of the disease, once left ventricular dysfunction has developed. These symptoms include exertional dyspnea, orthopnea, and paroxysmal nocturnal dyspnea. The left ventricle tolerates acute, severe regurgitation poorly; the patient with acute regurgitation usually presents with sudden cardiovascular collapse (i.e., weakness, severe dyspnea, and hypotension).

Electrocardiographic findings of aortic regurgitation are relatively subtle. The chest radiographic findings are dependent on the duration and severity of regurgitation as well as left ventricular function. In chronic aortic regurgitation, marked enlargement of the cardiac silhouette and dilation of the ascending aorta are common findings. The echocardiogram demonstrates

abnormal valve function, the effects of regurgitation on surrounding structures, changes in left ventricular size and function, and turbulent regurgitant flow across the aortic valve in diastole. Severe aortic regurgitation is an indication for surgical replacement of the valve.

Infective Endocarditis

Heart valve leaflets are derived from endocardium. When they become infected, the condition is referred to as endocarditis. A large variety of bacteria can infect the heart valves, as can yeast and fungi. In general, normal valves in a healthy person do not become infected. An abnormal, damaged or prosthetic valve is much more vulnerable to infection. The likelihood of infections is increased by other systemic illnesses, burns, placement of inert material (e.g., a catheter line or pacemaker wire near or through the valves), and intravenous drug abuse. Once infected, vegetations develop on the leaflets. These vegetations can embolize to other parts of the body; rupture the surrounding structures, leading to valvular lesions; produce a persistent bacteremia; or develop into an immunologic disorder.

Patients with endocarditis can present with symptoms of only a few days' duration, yet be critically ill. This condition is referred to as acute bacterial endocarditis. Conversely, chronic illness with symptoms of fatigue, weight loss, low-grade fever, and arthralgia is the picture of subacute bacterial endocarditis. The diagnosis is made when multiple blood cultures demonstrate the offending organism. Echocardiography can demonstrate valvular and myocardial function and the presence of valvular vegetations. Patients are treated with organism-specific intravenous antibiotics for extended periods.

Pericardial Disease

The double-layered tissue lining the heart can become inflamed and accumulate fluid, known as an effusion, between the two layers. The usual presentation is that of chest pain, a pericardial friction rub, and typical ECG abnormalities. The numerous causes of this inflammation include viral infection, bacterial infection, uremia, trauma, postpericardiotomy syndrome, neoplasia, and postinfarction syndrome. Effusions usually resolve spontaneously, but some can become chronic. In the event of scarring of either the parietal or visceral pericardium, constrictive pericarditis develops, interfering with cardiac filling. The patient presents with exertional dyspnea, abdominal swelling, fatigability, and edema. Cardiac tamponade arises when the accumulation of fluid around the heart is hemodynamically compromising. Typically urgent in nature, cardiac tamponade often requires hemodynamic support and periocardiocentesis.

Aortic and Vascular Tree Diseases

The aorta can be afflicted by any of four entities. Aneurysms or widening of the aorta can arise. If all three layers of this large artery are involved, it is a true aneurysm. If the intima and media are disrupted and it is only the adventitial layer with a perivascular clot expanding outward, it is referred to as a false aneurysm. Most aneurysms are caused by atherosclerosis, but trauma, infections, or genetically weakened media, known as cystic medial necrosis, can have the same result. Dissection of the aorta can occur in which the intima is disrupted. Blood enters between the vessel layers, separating them further. A weakened medial layer predisposes to this predicament, as seen with cystic medial necrosis, Marfan's syndrome, chronic hypertension, pregnancy, coarctation of the aorta, or a bicuspid aortic valve. A third entity is occlusive disease of the aorta caused by atherosclerosis. As in the coronary vascular bed, there is plaque formation, rupture, hemorrhage, and thrombus formation. Fourth, aortitis, or inflammation of the aorta, can also occur. Syphilis is the best known etiology, although other infectious and noninfectious agents have been identified.

Aneurysms of the aorta in the abdominal region are generally asymptomatic, picked up incidentally on a routine physical examination. Aneurysms can cause a sense of fullness or a continuous, gnawing pain in the low back. Expansion of the aneurysm produces sudden, severe pain in the same low back or lower abdominal region. Actual rupture links excruciating pain with hypotension and shock. A physical examination is limited, in that it can reveal an enlarged, pulsatile mass at best. Diagnoses and definition of the aneurysm

are accomplished with a variety of procedures, which may include plain films of the chest and abdomen, ultrasound, computed tomography (CT) scanning, and angiography. Because aneurysms will continue to expand and lead to rupture if left alone, elective surgery is recommended once aneurysms reach a certain diameter. Whether elective or emergent, surgery involves resection of the aneurysm and insertion of a prosthetic vascular graft.

In an older patient population the effects of atherosclerosis involving the vascular system are seen more distally. Patients typically present with intermittent claudication. As the blood supply to the lower extremity is further impaired, pain can be present at rest, and ulcers or gangrene of the toes and distal foot develop. The more distal vasculature can also be acutely occluded or interrupted by embolism, thrombosis, or injury.

The symptoms, findings on physical examination, and testing procedures are discussed earlier in this chapter. Older patients may have symptoms for many years; efforts are aimed at modifying risk factors, such as cessation of smoking, weight loss, and exercise training. If pain becomes intolerable even without exertion, tissue appears threatened by insufficient blood supply, or testing suggests critical occlusive disease, patients may undergo percutaneous angioplasty by means of fluoroscopically guided catheters or surgery for either vascular repair or bypass graft placement.

SUMMARY

This chapter discusses the anatomy, physiology, and pathophysiology of the cardiovascular system as it applies to patients seen by health care providers in daily practice. The clinical entities identified are discussed according to the symptoms presented to the physical therapist. By building on this information with the appropriate physical evaluation and diagnostic testing, the therapist can develop a practical approach to data collection, understanding, and management of the patient with cardiovascular disease.

PATIENT CASE HISTORY 1

History

The patient was a 42-year-old social worker who came to the clinic with a diagnosis of mechanical low back pain syndrome. Her chief complaint was a constant dull ache in the central lower thoracic and upper lumbar regions. Sitting and standing for more than a couple of minutes would increase the intensity of the aching. Assuming a supine or side-lying position for 20 to 30 minutes would decrease the intensity of the ache to its usual level of discomfort. The aching was least intense early in the morning but increased progressively through the remainder of the day. Although the ache made falling asleep difficult, once asleep, the patient was not awakened by pain. The symptoms began 18 months before the physical therapy evaluation. The patient described the aching as beginning 4 to 5 days after she had cleaned her closet. She underwent physical therapy for 6 weeks, receiving ultrasound, hot packs, transcutaneous electrical nerve stimulation (TENS), and electrical stimulation. The patient had received no relief of symptoms. She also described an intermittent deep throbbing pain in the same general area. The onset of this symptom was associated with increased exertion, such as climbing stairs or walking uphill. She could obtain relief by stopping and sitting or by leaning forward with her upper body supported by a car, railing, or tree. She noted shortness of breath when the throbbing sensation was present. These symptoms began insidiously 12 months before the evaluation. She had not seen a physician specifically for these symptoms.

The patient also described an intermittent sharp pain in the right lumbosacral junction region. This symptom was associated with a few repetitions of bending or lifting. Stopping the activity usually eliminated the pain within minutes. This symptom dated back to the L4–L5, L5–S1 lumbar fusion operation she had undergone in 1983.

The patient's medical history included a lumbar decompression surgery L4–L5, L5–S1 in 1980 and subsequent decompression and lumbar fusion of L4–L5, L5–S1 in 1983. Her surgical history also included a hysterectomy. Outside of being treated for colitis in 1983, the patient stated that her general medical history was negative. She also denied any history of smoking. The only medication she was taking was cyclobenzaprine (Flexeril). The only significant family medical history item she offered was that her father had died from a cerebrovascular accident.

Physical Examination

In a standing position, the patient presented with a decreased low lumbar lordosis and a markedly increased lordosis in the mid-lumbar region. A slightly increased mid-thoracic kyphosis was also noted. Slight increase in muscle tone was noted in the left and right paraspinals from T10 to L3. Trunk active range of motion (ROM) in standing demonstrated provocation of the sharp right lumbosacral junction pain with one repetition of backward bending. There was a marked increase in the mid-lumbar spine lordosis, as if she were hinging at that region during the movement. A sharp stretching sensation was provoked in the right middle and lower lumbar spine region extending to the right iliac crest with side bending to the left and forward bending. She experienced immediate relief from this discomfort when returning to the upright posture.

The neurologic examination was negative; peripheral pulses were symmetric and perceived to be normal. Muscle length testing demonstrated moderate tightness of hamstrings and hip flexors, as well as weakness in the abdominals and hip extensors. There was no palpatory tenderness at the interspinous spaces of the thoracic or lumbar spine, but central pressures (passive accessory vertebral motion testing) at T4, T8, and T12 provoked significant local tenderness, accompanied by segmental hypomobility. Central pressures at L3 increased the intensity of the patient's chief complaint, deep aching. Right unilateral pressure at the L5–S1 segment provoked sharp pain at the lumbosacral junction. Passive intervertebral physiologic motion testing of the spine demonstrated hypermobility at the L3–L4 and L2–L3 segments in backward and forward bending. With the patient positioned supine, abdominal palpation was carried out. Significant tenderness was provoked with palpation along the linea alba, approximately 2 to 3 inches above the umbilicus. Palpating the lateral extent of the aorta, the arterial pulse indicated a localized, enlarged, pulsatile mass, approximately 3 inches above the umbilicus. After maintaining slight to moderate pressure over this tender site for 20 to 30 seconds, the patient noted the deep throbbing pain in the lower thoracic and upper lumbar region. This was the same sensation she experienced when walking up flights of stairs or uphill. The throbbing sensation receded quickly when the palpatory pressure was released. At this point, the patient was again questioned regarding her past medical history, especially noting any cardiovascular system involvement. She denied any significant history initially but then remembered going to the emergency department because of severe palpitations 5 months before this clinical visit. She stated that her pulse rate had been 200 bpm, but nothing was found medically; by the next day, the symptoms had passed and had not occurred since. She was again asked about family medical history related to cardiovascular system conditions. This time she offered that three of her grandparents had died of MI and that her brother had been diagnosed as having a mitral valve prolapse condition.

Assessment and Outcome

The patient had come to Minneapolis from another state to see the physician who had done the lumbar fusion surgery. Possible surgery to the L3–L4 segment was to be considered for the thoracolumbar junction symptoms (aching). The patient was referred to the physical therapist for consultation regarding the appropriateness of physical therapy treatment for her current complaints. She was scheduled to have a discogram at the L3–L4 and L2–L3 segments the day after the physical therapy consultation. She was then to see the physician.

On the basis of the clinical examination, it was apparent that the sharp pain in the right lumbosacral junction and the dull ache at the thoracolumbar junction region were related to dysfunction of the musculoskeletal system. Provocation and alleviation of these symptoms were related to specific movements or postures. Also, both symptoms were provoked during the initial evaluation with passive segmental testing (central pressures at L3 and right unilateral pressures at L5–S1). However, the third complaint, deep throbbing pain, immediately raised suspicion. A throbbing sensation is not a description generally used by patients who present with mechanical dysfunction conditions. Throbbing or pulsating sensations are often associated with involvement of components of the cardiovascular system. A symptomatic aortic aneurysm could cause this type of pain complaint anywhere in the thoracic spine (usually midline), the chest, or abdominal regions. Because of the anatomic location of the aorta, numerous other structures may be impinged on by the aneurysm, causing a multitude of seemingly unrelated symptoms. These structures include spinal nerves, the esophagus, and the bronchi. The fact that the throbbing pain was brought on by physical exertion, such as stair and hill climbing, and was then relieved by cessation of the activity also suggests possible cardiovascular system involvement. Even though the throbbing pain and the dull ache were located in the same body region, the behavior of the symptoms was very different. The dull ache was provoked by sitting or standing for more than a few minutes, while physical exertion was what provoked the throbbing sensation. Physical examination findings also suggested two different lesions responsible for the different symptoms at the thoracolumbar junction. Passive intervertebral segmental testing provoked the aching at the L3 level, and abdominal palpation provoked the throbbing pain in the same area. The fact that the patient had a significant family medical history for cardiovascular system pathology also added weight to the concern regarding the origin of the throbbing complaints.

At completion of the initial evaluation, the patient was asked to remain in the clinic while the referring physician was contacted. The above information was communicated with emphasis on the factors that raised concern regarding the origin of the throbbing pain at the thoracolumbar junction. The discogram was put on hold and tests were run to check for the presence of an aortic aneurysm. A large aneurysm was found, and the patient returned home for medical consultation. She was also referred to a physical therapist at home for treatment of the dysfunction related to the complaints associated with the L5–S1 and L3–L4 segments.

Abdominal palpation played an important role in the decision to contact the physician regarding this patient's status. The abdomen is an important area to be assessed by the physical therapist. Multiple musculoskeletal system structures are located in the abdominal cavity (e.g., anterior lumbar spine, psoas major, and abdominal muscles) that, when dysfunctional, could affect the patient's symptoms and response to treatment. A number of other structures, including the visceri, may affect the clinical picture as well. Screening this region may prevent a delay in the patient receiving important medical treatment. (See Ch. 4 for a detailed description of abdominal anatomy and how to screen this region; Chs. 5 and 6 also present relevant information.)

PATIENT CASE HISTORY 2

History

The patient was a 66-year-old retired man who came to the clinic with a diagnosis of right sacroiliac joint pain. His chief complaint was intermittent aching in the right buttock and right calf. Walking was the only activity that provoked his symptoms. He would be pain free when ambulation was initiated, but consistently after walking 10 to 15 minutes the aching in the right buttock and calf would begin. If the patient continued to walk, the intensity of the pain increased tremendously; if he sat down, he would be pain free within minutes. The patient also described the sensation of restless legs periodically after he had been in bed for a short period. Walking short distances would relieve this discomfort. The patient's chief complaint and symptom behavior pattern were consistent from early morning to bedtime.

These symptoms began insidiously 16 months before the initial evaluation. During the past 16 months, the patient had received two 4-week sessions of physical therapy consisting of lower-extremity stretching and strengthening exercises, ultrasound to the right buttock and sacroiliac joint, hot packs to the lumbar and buttock regions, and prone press-up exercises. Outside of feeling a little looser, the patient's symptoms did not change. He received cortisone injections to the right sacroiliac joint and to trigger points in the gluteus medius, with only slight, temporary decrease in the intensity of the symptoms.

The patient's medical history included lumbar decompression surgery for a herniated nucleus pulposis at L5–S1 in 1963. He stated that the only residual effect was low lumbar stiffness. He had also suffered a heart attack in 1981 and received a pacemaker. The patient has smoked one pack of cigarettes daily for the past 50 years. He denied any bowel or bladder dysfunction. Special tests over the past 16 months included radiographs that he recounted as indicating loss of disc space height at L5–S1 and possible right lateral stenosis at L5–S1.

Physical Examination

In the standing position, slight atrophy of the right gluteals, thigh, and calf was noted. A reduced lumbar lordotic curve and increased midthoracic kyphosis were present. There was no provocation of symptoms with active movement of the trunk in standing or with overpressure, including the quadrant positions. Backward bending and right side bending ROM was significantly reduced in the low lumbar spine. Right hip internal rotation and the combined motion of hip flexion and adduction were moderately reduced compared with the left hip. Neurologic evaluation and sacroiliac joint and hip provocation tests were negative. Muscle length tests demonstrated bilateral lower-extremity tightness of the hip flexors, external rotators, and adductors, with the right side being tighter than the left. Manual muscle testing showed weakness of the right hip extensors and abductors. Muscle palpation produced numerous tender areas with increased muscle tone of the right gluteals and hip external rotators. There was no palpatory tenderness over the posterior sacroiliac joint ligaments or at the interspinous spaces of the lumbar and thoracic spine. Joint mobility testing demonstrated hypomobility at the right hip joint, right sacral base, L5, and thoracolumbar junction. There were no palpable differences between the lower-extremity pulses.

Because of an inability to provoke the patient's symptoms, I instructed that he walk until the symptoms were severe, just before the second physical therapy visit. Although I was unable to aggravate the patient's symptoms by stressing the thoracic and lumbar spine, sacroiliac and hip joints, and corresponding soft tissue structures, I found greater difficulty in palpating the right lower-extremity pulses compared with the left. This had not been the case during the initial evaluation, when the patient was asymptomatic.

Assessment and Outcome

The referring physician was contacted after the second physical therapy visit. He was informed of the several factors suggesting a vascular occlusive disease, as a possible source of the patient's symptoms: intermittent claudication, weaker right lower-extremity pulses after ambulation, and a history of smoking and heart attack. Of equal concern was the inability to provoke symptoms with palpation and active and passive testing. Because of the presence of significant right hip, sacral, and lumbar dysfunction, as well as muscle imbalances that might be related to the symptoms, it was agreed that physical therapy was to continue for 2 or 3 weeks including the initiation of a lower extremity conditioning exercise on a stationary bicycle. Depending on the patient's response to treatment, a decision would then be made regarding any additional medical tests to be carried out. The patient was seen twice a week, receiving joint mobilization for the right hip, right sacral base, and hypomobile segments of the lumbar and thoracic spine. In addition, soft tissue mobilization and muscle-stretching exercises and strengthening exercises were carried out for the involved areas. Objectively the patient improved; backward bending and right side bending ROM improved significantly, as did right hip joint mobility. Despite these improvements, the patient's tolerance for walking only slightly improved as the behavior of the right buttock and calf symptoms changed little. The patient was sent back to the physician for additional tests, which indicated significant occlusion of the right iliac artery. Subsequent treatment of the occlusion completely eliminated the patient's symptoms.

This patient presented with many of the important findings discussed in Chapter 1 (i.e., the possible presence of pathology, including insidious onset of symptoms, an inability to provoke symptoms by stressing the structures of the musculoskeletal system, and the lack of subjective improvement despite significant objective improvement). In addition, numerous symptoms and signs suggested a vascular condition, including intermittent claudication symptoms, the complaint of restless legs, a long history of smoking, a previous heart attack, and decreased pulses after long enough ambulating to provoke symptoms. Sufficient dysfunction was present in the lower quarter, however, to raise suspicion of a mechanical origin of the symptoms of musculoskeletal dysfunction as well. At times the significance of musculoskeletal system dysfunction related to the patient's complaints presents a difficult clinical situation. Careful and frequent reassessment of symptoms and signs after treatment help the clinician decide whether the patient should be assessed medically to rule out the presence of pathology. Communication with the physician regarding clinical findings that have raised suspicion in the therapist's mind is then essential to ensure the proper course of treatment for the patient. In this patient's case, months of symptoms and unnecessary treatments might have been avoided had a more complete and concise evaluation been made initially. Fortunately for this patient, his condition was treated successfully. For other pathologies, such as cancer, a few months can make a difference in the prognosis for recovery.

REFERENCES

1. Wise CS: Physical medicine in disease of peripheral circulation. JAPTA 30:499, 1950
2. Stillwell DM: Bisgaard treatment for static edema and its sequelae in the lower extremity. Arch Phys Med Rehabil 37:693, 1956
3. Mubarak SJ, Hargens AR: Compartment Syndromes and Volkmann's Contractures. Saunders' Monographs in Clinical Orthopedics. Vol. 3. WB Saunders, Philadelphia, 1981
4. Cohen M, Michel TH: Cardiopulmonary Symptoms in Physical Therapy Practice. Churchill Livingstone, New York, 1988
5. Kanarek DJ, Hand RW: The response of cardiac and pulmonary disease to exercise testing. Clin Chest Med 5:181, 1984
6. Wilkins RL, Sheldon RL, Krider SJ: Clinical Assessment in Respiratory Care. CV Mosby, Princeton, NJ, 1985
7. Cohen M, Michel TH: Overview of the cardiac system. p. 15. In Cohen M, Michel TH (eds): Cardiopulmonary Symptoms in Physical Therapy Practice. Churchill Livingstone, New York, 1988
8. Ross G (ed): Essentials of Human Physiology. Year Book Medical Publishers, Chicago, 1978
9. Ganong WF: The heartbeat and electrical activity of the heart. p. 445. In Review of Medical Physiology. 13th Ed. Appleton & Lange, E. Norwalk, CT, 1987
10. Ganong W: Review of Medical Physiology. 8th Ed. Lange Medical Publications, Los Altos, CA, 1977
11. Delp M, Manning R: Major Physical Diagnosis. 8th Ed. WB Saunders, Philadelphia, 1979
12. Little RC: Physiology of the Heart and Circulation. 4th Ed. Year Book Medical Publishers, Chicago, 1978
13. Sokolow M, McIlroy M: Clinical Cardiology. Lange Medical Publications, Los Altos, CA, 1981
14. Wilkins RL, Sheldon RL, Jones-Krider S: Clinical Assessment in Respiratory Care. 2nd Ed. CV Mosby, St. Louis, 1990
15. American Heart Association: Textbook of Advanced Cardiac Life Support. p. 2. American Heart Association, Dallas, 1987
16. American College of Sports Medicine: Guidelines for Exercise Testing and Prescription. p. 67. Lea & Febiger, Philadelphia, 1986
17. Braunwald E: Valvular heart disease. p. 1123. In Braunwald E (ed): Heart Disease. A Textbook of Cardiovascular Medicine. 1st edition. WB Saunders, Philadelphia, 1980
18. Albarran-Sotelo R, Atkins JM, Bloom RS: Arrhythmias. p. 48. In: Textbook of Cardiac Life Support. American Heart Association National Center, Dallas, 1987
19. Stein B, Israel D, Cohen M, Fuster, V: Ischemia and infarction III: pathogenesis of coronary occlusion. p. 87. Hosp Pract [off] 23(4):87, 1988

SUGGESTED READINGS

Braunwald E (ed): Heart Disease. A Textbook of Cardiovascular Medicine. WB Saunders, Philadelphia, 1980

Cohen M, Michel TH: Cardiopulmonary Symptoms in Physical Therapy Practice. Churchill Livingstone, New York, 1988

DeGowin E, DeGowin R: Bedside Diagnostic Examination. 4th Ed. Macmillan, New York, 1981

Delp M, Manning R: Major's Physical Diagnosis. 8th Ed. WB Saunders, Philadelphia, 1975

Eagle KA, Haber E, DeSanctis RW, Austen WG (eds): The Practice of Cardiology. 2nd Ed. Little, Brown, Boston, 1989

Tilkian SM, Conover MD, Tilkian AG: Clinical Implications of Laboratory tests. 4th Ed. CV Mosby, Washington, DC, 1987

3

Screening for Pulmonary System Disease

DAVID ARNALL, Ph.D., P.T.
MICHAEL RYAN, M.D.

The physical therapist is recognized as a valued member of the health care team, providing care for patients with lung disease in both an outpatient and inpatient setting.[1-3] As the role of physical therapy continues to grow with the pulmonary patient population, accurate assessment of ventilatory muscle strength and oxygen-carbon dioxide exchange capacity becomes increasingly important. As home health care becomes more prevalent in the face of diagnosis-related groupings (DRGs), the role of physical therapists in the outpatient care of pulmonary patients will increase. Therapists interested in orthopaedics or sports medicine cannot reasonably expect to function clinically without knowing something about baseline measurements of both ventilatory and respiratory function.[4-7] With so many patients, young and old, having respiratory disease, physical therapists will need the assessment and treatment tools necessary to address the respiratory problems, as well as the orthopaedic conditions.

To help prepare the therapist for screening and assessing the pulmonary system, this chapter presents an overview of pulmonary anatomy relevant to the assessment tools of auscultation and percussion. The assessment and interpretation of breath and vocal sounds are presented in great detail. Pertinent evaluation information obtained through chart review, history taking, and physical examination is related to specific pulmonary disease entities. The disease entities discussed in this chapter are those that physical therapists are most likely to encounter in the clinical set-

ting. Because of the serious nature of many of the pulmonary system illnesses, it is not as likely that the physical therapist or patient would be fooled by trunk or neck pain masking underlying pulmonary pathology as compared with other organ systems. There are numerous pulmonary conditions upon which the physical therapist can have a significant impact, however, and these are discussed in detail.

PULMONARY ANATOMY

Anatomy and physiology are the foundations upon which all evaluation and treatment is built. When auscultating the patient's chest wall, the physical therapist must have a clear understanding of the external chest wall markings that overlie the lung, as well as the relationship of the external landmarks to internal pulmonary anatomy. The anatomy briefly reviewed here will help the clinician begin auscultating the lungs with a more secure feeling that the placement of the stethoscope has some meaning with reference to the underlying lobes and bronchopulmonary segments.

The left and right lungs are grossly divided into regional lobes demarcated by the presence of fissures that penetrate deep into the lung fields frankly dividing the lung into upper, middle, and lower lobes on the right and upper and lower lobes on the left lung. The left lung does not have a middle lobe (Figs. 3-1 and 3-2).

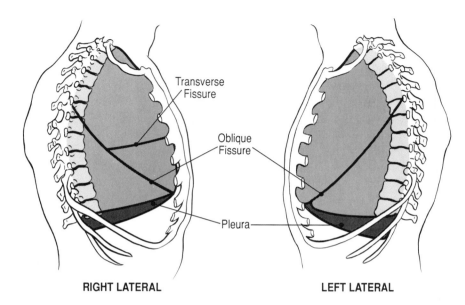

Fig. 3-1. Lateral views of the lobes, fissures, and pleura of the lungs in relationship to elements of the bony thorax.

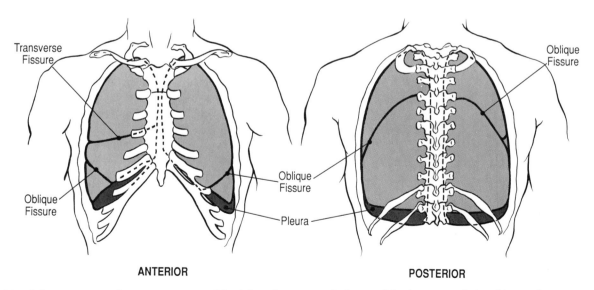

Fig. 3-2. Anterior and posterior views of the lobes, fissures, and pleura of the lungs in relationship to elements of the bony thorax.

The lobes of the right lung are separated by two large pulmonary fissures: (1) the horizontal or transverse fissure, and (2) the oblique fissure. The horizontal or transverse fissure divides the right upper lobe from the right middle lobe. The oblique fissure divides the right middle lobe from the right lower lobe. The upper and lower lobes of the left lung are separated by the presence of the oblique fissure.

The major lobes of the left and right lungs are further divided into bronchopulmonary segments that are not immediately seen in the cadaver because there are no anatomic fissures dividing the major lobes into the smaller bronchopulmonary segments. Rather, the bronchopulmonary segmental divisions of the lobes and their corresponding names are determined by the names of the segmental bronchi that serve these areas of the lung. The various bronchopulmonary segments of each major lobe are listed in Table 3-1.

When the physical therapist learns the external surface anatomic landmarks overlying specific bronchopulmonary segments, auscultation of the patient's lung fields becomes meaningful. Figures 3-3 and 3-4 outline pictorially the thoracic cage bony structure and the surface markings overlying the bronchopulmonary segments. From these drawings, it is easy to determine which major lobe, and often which bronchopulmonary segment, is being auscultated. It will be useful to refer to Figures 3-3 and 3-4 while reading the descriptions of the bronchopulmonary segments. The following discussion describes placement of the stethoscope on the chest wall to listen to specific regions of the lung.

Right Lung

Upper Lobe

The right upper lobe is composed of three bronchopulmonary segments: apical, posterior, and anterior.

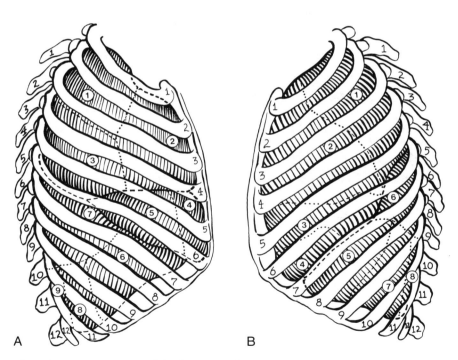

Fig. 3-3. Bronchopulmonary segments of the lungs in relationship to elements of the bony thorax. **(A) Right lung.** *Right upper lobe:* 1, apical segment; 2, anterior segment; 3, posterior segment. *Middle lobe:* 4, medial segment; 5, lateral segment. *Right lower lobe:* 6, anterior basilar segment; 7, superior segment; 8, lateral basilar segment; 9, posterior basilar segment; *, medial basilar segment not shown. **(B) Left lung.** *Left upper lobe:* 1, apico posterior segment; 2, anterior segment; 3, superior lingula; 4, inferior lingula. *Left lower lobe:* 5, anterior basilar segment; 6, superior segment; 7, lateral basilar segment; 8, posterior basilar segment.

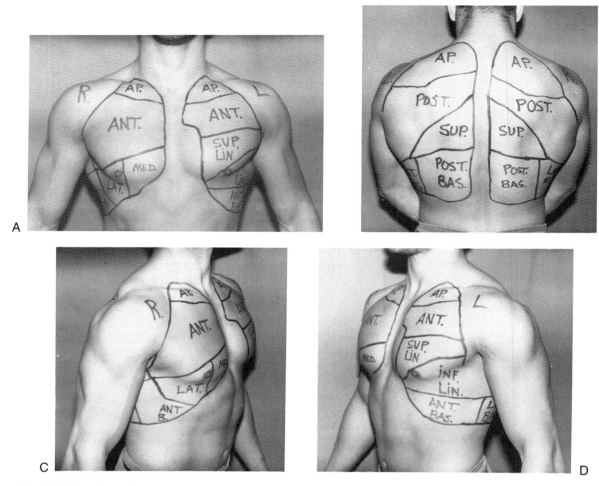

Fig. 3-4. Bronchiopulmonary segments of the lungs in relationship to surface anatomy. **(A)** Anterior view. **(B)** Posterior view. **(C)** Right lateral view. **(D)** Left lateral view. (AP, apical segment; ANT, anterior segment; MED, medial segment; LAT, lateral segment; SUP LIN, superior lingula, left lung; INF LIN, inferior lingula, left lung; ANT BAS, anterior basilar, left lung; POST, posterior segment; SUP, superior segment; POST BAS, posterior basilar.)

Apical Segment

The apical bronchopulmonary segment is not as often auscultated because it is not as frequently involved in disease pathologies as other segments. The apical segment of the right upper lobe can be auscultated by placing the diaphragm of the stethoscope over the upper trapezius muscle just above and behind the clavicle. This segment can be auscultated at this point be-

cause the tip of the apical segment peaks out over the clavicle. In the adult, the vesicular breath sound or the bronchovesicular breath sound are the normal breath sounds heard in this segment. When the vesicular breath sound is heard, the inspiratory to expiratory (I:E) ratio is usually $1:\frac{1}{4}$, meaning that normally the expiratory phase is only one-fourth the duration of the inspiratory phase. It is also common, during the vesicular breath sound, not to hear the expiratory phase

Table 3-1. Bronchopulmonary Segments of Each Lobe of the Right and Left Lung

Right lung
    Upper lobe
        Apical segment
        Anterior segment
        Posterior segment
    Middle lobe
        Medial segment
        Lateral segment
    Lower lobe
        Anterior basilar segment
        Superior segment
        Medial basilar segment
        Posterior basilar segment
        Lateral basilar segment

Left lung
    Upper lobe
        Apicoposterior segment
        Anterior segment
        Superior lingular segment[a]
        Inferior lingular segment[a]
    Lower lobe
        Anterior basilar segment
        Superior segment
        Posterior basilar segment
        Lateral basilar segment

[a] The lingular segments are part of the upper lobes of the left lung but are anatomically analogous to the medial and lateral segments of the right middle lobe.

at all. Therefore, in a normal vesicular breath sound, the expiratory phase will be abbreviated or completely absent as compared with the inspiratory phase.

If the bronchovesicular breath sound is heard, the clinician will usually hear the vesicular portion of this breath sound during the inspiratory phase of the respiratory cycle, while the more tubular, high-pitched bronchial portion of this breath sound is heard during exhalation. The I:E ratio is usually close to 1:1, meaning that inspiration is heard as long as expiration. In teens and children, the normal breath sound is usually the bronchovesicular breath sound. The differences in the breath sounds in teens and children compared with adults is probably due to maturational factors.

Posterior Segment

The posterior segment of the right upper lobe can be auscultated if the diaphragm of the stethoscope is placed over the lower trapezius just below the spine of the scapula. The medial border for this lobe is the thoracovertebral border of the spine (some anatomists call this region the paraspinous gutter), while the lateral border is located approximately between the 3rd and 6th ribs along the mid-axillary line. The inferior border of this bronchopulmonary segment is along the 6th rib as it approaches the spinous process of T5. The inferior border of the posterior segment of the right upper lobe is also demarcated by the oblique fissure. The superior border is just anterior to, and at the same level as, the spine of the scapula, which lies immediately to the right of the dorsal spinous process of T3. The vesicular breath sound is most commonly the normal breath sound heard in this segment in the adult. The I:E ratio for this breath sound is normally 1:0 or 1:$\frac{1}{4}$.

However, it is also normal to hear the bronchovesicular breath sound with the softer, breathy vesicular sound heard in the inspiratory phase and the harsher more tubular, hollow, and high-pitched bronchial sound heard during expiration. The I:E ratios are usually 1:1 for the bronchovesicular breath sound. Teens and children will very often demonstrate the bronchovesicular breath sound in this bronchopulmonary segment.

Anterior Segment

The anterior segment of the right upper lobe can be easily auscultated because the surface area for auscultation is so extensive. The anterior segment can be auscultated at its inferior border above or on the level of the 4th rib, lateral to the sternocostal margin at its medial border, just below the clavicle at its superior border with the lateral border extending to just posterior to the mid-axillary line. The normal breath sound is a vesicular breath sound in the adult. The I:E ratios for this breath sound is usually 1:0 or 1:$\frac{1}{4}$. In some adults, a bronchovesicular breath sound can be heard immediately over the sternocostal border and immediately below the clavicle. In children below the age of 12 to 14 years, the bronchovesicular breath sound predominates throughout the lung field of the anterior segment.

Middle Lobe

The right middle lobe consists of two bronchopulmonary segments: medial and lateral.

Medial and Lateral Segments

The medial bronchopulmonary segment is medial and anterior to the lateral segment. Unless the clinician is experienced, it can be difficult to know which segment is being auscultated. These two relatively small segments can be auscultated over the wedge-shaped area shown in Figure 3-2. This area is between the 4th and the 6th ribs anteriorly, which encompasses the nipple of the right chest wall. (The nipple is a good landmark only in young boys, in girls before pubescence, and in men who do not have substantial upper body fat reserves that mimic breast tissue. In other sex and age groups, the nipple often has too much inferior displacement, making it an unreliable external thoracic wall landmark.) Moving laterally and posteriorly along the fifth rib, the wedge-shaped area narrows and terminates just posterior to the mid-axillary line. If the stethoscope is placed on the anterior surface of the chest wall between the 4th and 6th ribs on or medial to the nipple and lateral to the sternum (Fig. 3-3), the chances are fairly good that the medial segment is being auscultated. If the stethoscope is placed lateral to this area, the lateral segment is probably being auscultated (Fig. 3-3). The normal breath sound heard in the healthy adult is always the vesicular breath sound for both the medial and lateral segments of the right middle lobe. In children and young teens, the bronchovesicular breath sound is often heard.

Often the most posterolateral area of the right middle lobe can be identified by following the 6th rib along its posterior and oblique upward direction toward the mid-axillary line. When coming to the point on the chest that marks the junction of the transverse and oblique fissures (slightly posterior to the mid-axillary line) and crossing over that point, one will often hear a change in the breath sounds going from a higher-pitched to a lower-pitched vesicular breath sound. The subtle change in pitch is an indication that one has crossed over from the middle lobe to the lower lobe in the vicinity of the superior segment of the lower lobes.

Lower Lobe

The lower lobe of the right lung consists of the five segments: anterior basilar, lateral basilar, posterior basilar, superior, and medial basilar.

Anterior Basilar Segment

The anterior basilar segment of the right lower lobe can be auscultated by placing the diaphragm of the stethoscope on the anterior chest wall on its superior border at the 6th rib and as far down as its inferior border at the 10th rib 2 to 3 inches above the costal margin. The stethoscope can be moved laterally within this lobe as far as the mid-axillary line. The medial limit for this segment is along the mid-clavicular line. The normal breath sound that is heard in the basilar segments is always the vesicular breath sound in the adult, with an $I:E$ ratio of $1:0$ or $1:\frac{1}{4}$. The bronchovesicular breath sound may still be heard in children and in young teens.

Lateral Basilar Segment

The lateral basilar segment of the right lower lobe is lateral to the anterior basilar segment. It occupies an area below the 8th rib on the lateral surface of the chest wall and 2 to 3 inches posterior to the mid-axillary line. In the adult, the normal breath sound heard in this basilar segment is always the vesicular breath sound, with an $I:E$ ratio of $1:0$ or $1:\frac{1}{4}$. The bronchovesicular breath sound may still be heard in children and in young teens.

Posterior Basilar Segment

The posterior basilar segment of the right lower lobe occupies a space on the posterior surface of the thoracic wall between the vertebral column at its medial border and the lateral basilar segment at its lateral border. The superior border of this segment is located below the dorsal spinous process of T9 vertebra, with the inferior border located at the dorsal spinous process of T11 vertebra. The normal breath sound in the healthy adult is always the vesicular breath sound, with an $I:E$ ratio of $1:0$ or $1:\frac{1}{4}$. The bronchovesicular breath sound will often be heard in children under the age of 12 to 14 years.

Superior Segment

The superior segment of the right lower lobe is located on the posterior wall of the thorax below the oblique fissure, which runs generally along the 6th rib. The inferior border of the superior segment curves posteriorly from the mid-axillary line to the dorsal spinous process of the ninth thoracic vertebra. The medial border for this segment is the vertebral column between the dorsal spinous processes of T5–T9 with the lateral border being the oblique fissures that angles obliquely downward along the 6th rib. The normal breath sound that is always heard in this segment of the lung in healthy adults is the vesicular breath sound, with an I:E ratio of 1:0 to 1:¼. The bronchovesicular breath sound will often be heard in children under the age of 12 to 14 years.

Medial Basilar Segment

The medial basilar segment cannot be auscultated because it is located medial to the anterior basilar segment juxtapositioned to the heart. It has no thoracic surface area exposure from which to be auscultated.

Left Lung

Upper Lobe

The left upper lobe is divided into four segments: apicoposterior, anterior, superior lingular, and inferior lingular.

Apicoposterior Segment

The apicoposterior segment of the left upper lobe is positioned in the thoracic cage similar to that of the right apical and posterior bronchopulmonary segments. The landmarks for auscultation are very similar. The normal breath sounds heard in these segments may be vesicular to bronchovesicular, depending on the cellularity and age of the patient. The vesicular breath sound is a breathy, muffled, whispy, low-pitched sound that usually has an I:E ratio of 1:0 or 1:¼. If the bronchovesicular breath sound is heard, the vesicular portion of the breath sound is heard during the inspiratory cycle, while the bronchial portion is heard during exhalation. The I:E ratio for the bronchovesicular breath sound is usually 1:1.

Anterior Segment

The anterior segment of the left upper lobe has virtually the same location as the anterior segment of the right lung. The normal breath sound typically heard in a healthy adult will be the vesicular breath sound, although the bronchovesicular breath sound is a common variant when auscultating near the sternoclavicular, sternocostal, and clavicular borders. In young teens and children, the bronchovesicular breath sound is heard as the normal breath sound.

Superior and Inferior Lingular Segments

The superior and inferior lingular segments occupy roughly the same space as the medial and lateral segments of the right middle lobe. The left lung does not have a middle lobe. However, the analogous structures in the left lung are the superior and inferior lingular segments. In the adult, the normal breath sound heard in these segments is always the vesicular breath sound. The bronchovesicular breath sound can often be heard in young teens and children.

Lower Lobe

The lower lobe of the left lung is composed of five segments: anterior basilar, superior, posterior basilar, and lateral basilar.

Anterior Basilar Segment

The anterior basilar segment of the left lung has an anatomic distribution similar to that of the analogous segment on the right side. The normal breath sound that is always heard in the adult is the vesicular breath sound. The bronchovesicular breath sound can often be heard in young teens and children.

Superior segment

The superior segment of the left lower lobe is positioned in the thoracic cage in an area analogous to the same segment on the right side. The normal breath sound heard in this segment is always the vesicular breath sound in the adult. The bronchovesicular breath sound can often be heard in young teens and children.

Posterior Basilar Segment

The posterior basilar segment of the left lower lobe is located at its superior border just below the spinous process of T9 along the vertebral column extending inferiorly to about the dorsal spinous process of T11. It extends laterally out to a point on the posterolateral thoracic wall roughly analogous to a line dropped vertically between the surgical neck of the scapula and the glenoid fossa of the scapula. The vertebral column is its medial border, and the lateral basilar segment its lateral border. The normal breath sound heard in the healthy adult is always the vesicular breath sound. The bronchovesicular breath sound is often heard in young teens and children.

Lateral Basilar Segment

The lateral basilar segment of the left lower lobe is located analogously to the right lateral basilar segment. The normal breath sound heard in healthy adults is always the vesicular breath sound. The bronchovesicular breathy sound may be heard in young teens and in children.

PHYSICAL ASSESSMENT OF PULMONARY STATUS: AUSCULTATION

Stethoscope as an Evaluation Tool

The physical therapist should understand how to perform a chest assessment using a stethoscope. This basic tool in the pulmonary evaluation is of immense help in understanding the patient's pulmonary condition. The following discussion presents a brief overview of how to auscultate or listen to the chest using a stethoscope. The clinician should understand quite clearly that practice under the tutelage of an experienced auscultator is invaluable. However, it is hoped that the rudimentary information presented here will stimulate the reader to become a knowledgeable auscultator.

The stethoscope is a diagnostic tool that has been used for well over 150 years to determine the condition of certain organs. Laennec, a French physician, was an early proponent for using the stethoscope to auscultate, or listen to the lungs. Laennec's stethoscope was a simple tube, considerably different from the stethoscopes of modern medicine. The modern stethoscope is divided into three major components (Fig. 3-5): the head (or chestpiece, which includes the bell and the diaphragm), tubing, and ear pieces.

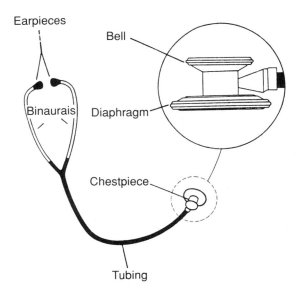

Fig. 3-5. Components of the stethoscope.

Head or Chestpiece

The modern stethoscope is most often duosonic. This means that there is a bell on one side and a diaphragm on the other. Stethoscopes are still made that are unisonic (i.e., having a diaphragm only). The bell transmits low-frequency tones at the expense of the high-frequency tones. It is therefore very useful for listening to rhonchi, or wheezes, in the central airways of the lung or for a heart murmur, such as the murmur that frequently appears in patients with mitral valve stenosis. The diaphragm facilitates tone transmission of high-frequency tones at the expense of low-frequency tones. The diaphragm is therefore useful for hearing bronchial breath sounds and bronchovesicular breath sounds.

Tubing

The tubing of the stethoscope is usually thick walled and flexible, with the inner bore diameter the size of the earpieces. Double tubing is superior to a single tube stethoscope because of the enhanced transmission of sound. The length of the tubing connecting the head and the earpieces should be 8 to 16 inches. The shorter the tubing, the better the transmission of the sound waves. The tubing has to be long enough, however, for the clinician to use comfortably during a chest examination.

Earpieces

Earpieces should be chosen that fit into the ears comfortably and exclude as much extraneous room noise as possible. Many nurses, respiratory therapists, physicians, and physical therapists choose soft rubber earpieces instead of the hard plastic earpieces that frequently come with the stethoscopes. The soft rubber earpieces not only conform more easily to the ear channel but also block some of the room noise more efficiently than do the plastic earpieces.

What Can Be Heard with the Stethoscope?

Vocal and Breath Sounds

While listening with the stethoscope placed on the chest wall, the sounds produced by the passage of air in and out of the lung during respiration will be heard. These sounds are created by the turbulence and vibration of air passing in and out of the lung through the various generations of the bronchopulmonary tree. Some of the sounds that a clinician will encounter are normal breath sounds heard in patients with healthy lungs. These sounds will be made by air passing in and out of clear unobstructed bronchial passages. Other sounds, known as adventitious breath sounds, are abnormal and are typically created by having air pass through bronchial passages obstructed by mucus. The ease with which these sounds or vibrations are transmitted depends on the elasticity (or compliance) of the tissue, the mass (or volume) of the transmitting medium, and the density of the transmitting medium. For example, the alveoli, or air sacs, surrounding all the bronchial structures dampen the transmission of sound. In a healthy lung, this has the effect of damping the higher-frequency sounds in favor of the lower-frequency sounds. Therefore, what is heard over the lateral and posterior-inferior chest walls is a muffled, breathy sound. In areas of the chest wall in which there is a smaller number of alveoli, such as near the trachea and over the costosternal border, the sounds are of higher frequency and tend to

be tubular, harsh, and somewhat metallic in quality, much like hearing air blowing through a tube.

Transmission of Vocal or Voice Sounds

During the standard chest assessment, the clinician listens to the chest wall with a stethoscope, while the patient utters a word such as "ninety-nine" or a long vowel sound, such as the letter "E" or "A." The quality of the spoken or whispered word, whether clearly understood or so muffled as to be unintelligible through the stethoscope should be noted. Two types of vocal or voice sounds can be heard: normal vocal sounds and abnormal vocal sounds.

Normal Vocal Sounds. As air passes over the vocal cords, vibrations are produced in the larynx, and sound is created. The sound waves are transmitted through the respiratory tract, through the chest in all directions, to the thoracic wall. The vocal sounds are loudest near the trachea and the major bronchi because there is less lung tissue to muffle the sound transmission. Words spoken while auscultating in the area of the trachea or costosternal borders will be "fuzzy" but intelligible. Vocal sounds heard during auscultation in the more distant areas of the lung field (e.g., the posterior basilar segments) are less intense and much more muffled. Indeed, in a normal lung, the syllables of the words cannot be understood at all. The clinician hears what sounds somewhat like talking with a mouth full of food. No one can understand what has been mumbled—only that something has been said.

Abnormal Vocal Sounds. There are several abnormal vocal sounds to be aware of that are common in patients with consolidation disorders (e.g., pneumonia, atelectasis). Consolidation is a process in which the lung becomes less compliant (flexible and extensible) because of the presence of larger than normal amounts of fluid collecting in the interstitial spaces and in the bronchial passages. Bronchophony, whispered pectoriloquy, and egophony are examples of abnormal vocal sounds heard over an area of consolidation in the lung.

Bronchophony. Bronchophony is an abnormal vocal sound in which the transmission of the spoken word is increased both in intensity and in clarity. During the examination, the clinician will ask the patient to utter a specific word or a letter, such as "ninety-nine" or "EEEEE." If the patient has a bronchophony, the clinician will be able to hear through the stethoscope the word or enunciated long vowel sound. The clarity of the word or vowel phonation will be related to how well developed the consolidation has become, as well as to the size of the consolidated area. To some degree, it will be clear enough to actually understand the exact words or vowel sound. The presence of bronchophony is a sign that sound is being transmitted through a more solid lung (i.e., there is not as much spongy air space to muffle the transmission of the sound wave).

At this juncture, it would be wise to insert a cautionary note. When practicing listening to the lung fields with the stethoscope, it is important to remember that certain lung fields have normal sounds (typical sounds) that are associated with their anatomy and location. For instance, the upper lobes are juxtapositioned to the trachea and transmit voice sounds rather well. There simply is not a great deal of parenchymal and alveolar tissue in the upper lobes to muffle the sound waves transmitted from the larynx to the chest wall. In addition, there is a great deal of cartilaginous and bony anatomy as well as the substantial cartilaginous ring structure of the upper airways, all of which permit sound waves to be effectively transmitted to the thoracic wall. It may appear to the beginning auscultator listening to the thoracic wall around the trachea, the costosternal borders, or the thoracovertebral borders that the subject has a bronchophony, when this is not the case, simply because the sounds are so easily transmitted in the upper lobes next to the trachea and mainstem bronchi. However, in all other lung fields, the vocal sounds will be unintelligible in a clear lung. If the phonated word or vowel sounds can be heard in these areas (the right middle lobe, left lingula, bilateral basilar segments), it can be strongly suspected that the area is consolidated.

Whispered Pectoriloquy.   During whispering, the vocal cords do not oscillate, since there is no turbulent airflow through the trachea, glottis, and larynx. In a normal lung, the whispered voice is not heard at all or, at best, only faintly and indistinctly. No syllables can be distinguished throughout the entire chest, except perhaps very faintly around the sternum and the trachea in the upper lobe areas of the lung, where the bony anatomy transmits the sound.

To test for a whispered pectoriloquy, the patient is asked to whisper the number series "1-2-3-4." If a whispered sound can be heard that is definitely and clearly recognizable, the patient has a whispered pectoriloquy. The patient must whisper very quietly (no phonated words), if this test for consolidation is to be of value. Whispered pectoriloquy is never a normal sound and always indicates consolidation of the lung field in the area being auscultated.

Egophony.   The word *egophony* comes from the Greek "voice of the goat." Egophony refers to the nasal or bleating quality of speech transmitted through consolidated lung tissue. The uttered word will frequently sound much like that produced when children playfully talk with their noses pinched, having a very nasal, whinning, or bleating character. Egophony is a modified form of bronchophony, in which there is not only an increase in the clarity of the spoken voice, but a change in the character of the sound as well. When the patient phonates the long vowel sound of the letter "EEEEE," the auscultator hears the long vowel sound "AAAAA." With egophony, when sound waves pass through the consolidated lung tissue, the sound is transmutated, producing the phenomenon known as E-to-A egophony. The precise mechanism for this abnormal vocal sound is not clearly understood but is no doubt related to the way in which sound waves are transmitted through a fluid-filled or obstructed lung field.

Transmission of Breath Sounds

Normal Breath Sounds.   There are four basic types of normal breath sounds: tracheal, bronchial, vesicular, and bronchovesicular. Each of these breath sounds is normal when heard through the stethoscope in the appropriate anatomic region of the lung. However, hearing the tracheal, bronchial, and bronchovesicular breaths sounds in regions of the lung in which they are not usually transmitted is considered an abnormal finding.

Tracheal Breath Sounds.   Tracheal breath sounds are only heard over the trachea below the larynx. Since this breath sound is located only over the trachea, and not in the lung fields, the tracheal breath sound is usually not auscultated. However, it is important to know the character of a tracheal breath sound because the bronchial breath sound is quite similar. In fact, medical professionals who listen to the lungs on a daily basis consider the tracheal and bronchial breath sound almost identical but merely located in different areas on the chest wall.

The tracheal breath sound is heard through the stethoscope as a high-pitched loud, tubular, hollow, raspy, metallic sound. It has been likened to wind rushing through a hollow tube. On auscultation, both the inspiratory and expiratory phases of the ventilatory cycle are clearly heard. The I:E ratio is almost always equal in length; occasionally the expiratory phase is slightly longer (i.e., I:E ratio = 1:1 or 1:1$\frac{1}{2}$). Usually there is a pause between the expiratory and inspiratory phases. The expiratory phase is coarser or louder than the inspiratory phase. It can be represented diagrammatically as follows:

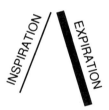

Bronchial Breath Sounds.   Bronchial breath sounds are normally heard over the upper lobes of the lungs close to the sternum along the anterior midline of the thorax at the jugular notch of the manubrium, as well as directly over the manubrium. They are also heard along the sternocostal margins of the sternum. On auscultation, they are tubular and metallic in quality, high-pitched, and resonant. Like the tracheal breath sound, the bronchial breath sound is much like hearing air blown through a hollow tube.

Bronchial breath sounds differ from tracheal breath sounds in that the bronchial breath sound is not as loud as the tracheal breath sound. Bronchial breath sounds are not as loud because there is more soft and bony tissue muffling the sound transmitted to the sternal chest wall from the trachea and the mainstem bronchi than on the neck anterior to the trachea.

A bronchial breath sound heard on or next to the sternum is considered a normal breath sound. Bronchial breath sounds have a louder and longer expiratory phase (I:E ratio = 1:$\frac{1}{4}$ to 1:$\frac{1}{2}$). There is usually a characteristic pause between inspiration and expiration, but on occasions this pause may be absent. A normal bronchial breath sound can be represented diagrammatically as follows:

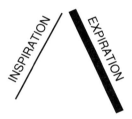

However, if the bronchial breath sound is heard in any other area of the lung, such as in the lingula, the right middle lobes, or the bilateral lower lobes, it is considered an abnormal sound of serious import. It is then an indication of enhanced sound transmission caused by fluid filling the lungs, of atelectasis, or of a compressed consolidated lung.

Vesicular Breath Sounds.   Vesicular breath sounds are normally heard over the entire anterior, lateral, and posterior chest walls, excluding the areas described under Bronchial Breath Sounds (Fig. 3-6).

Vesicular breath sounds are a muffled low-pitched sound as compared with bronchial or tracheal breath sounds. It has often been said that vesicular breath sounds are like wind rustling through the leaves of a tree. Vesicular breath sounds are so muffled as compared with the other breath sounds that they sound like respirations in the next room through a house wall.

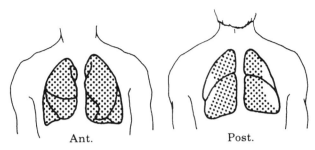

Fig. 3-6. Dots signify where vesicular breath sounds are normally heard. Anterior (ANT) and posterior (POST) views of the trunk.

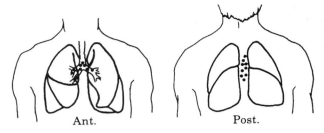

Fig. 3-7. Dots signify where bronchovesicular breath sounds are normally heard. Anterior (ANT) and posterior (POST) views of the trunk.

Inspiration will be higher in pitch, louder, and the more dominant audible respiratory phase with inspiration being three times longer than expiration (I:E ratio = 3:1). Therefore, expiration will be much shorter and much more faint. There is usually no pause between the longer inspiratory and shorter expiratory phases. Often the expiration phase is completely absent (I:E ratio = 1:0). A normal diagram below:

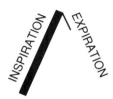

Unlike the bronchial breath sound, which is considered an abnormal breath sound when heard in an atypical area of the lung, the vesicular breath sound is not considered abnormal solely on the basis of geographic placement. Rather, the vesicular breath sound may be viewed as abnormal when it is diminished in normal intensity or is distantly heard in its expansive lung field distribution. This occurs when the lung tissue is no longer being adequately ventilated, producing a faint or a distant breath sound. Distant vesicular breath sounds are commonly heard in patients who are in the early stages of pneumonia, in patients who are experiencing the onset of atelectasis, and in patients with chronic obstructive pulmonary disease (COPD). An abnormal vesicular breath sound will often have a pause between the inspiratory and expiratory phases, giving it the character of a bronchial breath sound.

Bronchovesicular Breath Sounds.   As the name implies,

the bronchovesicular breath sound is a combination of vesicular and bronchial breath sounds. The pitch in inspiration and expiration is the same. There is usually a short pause between inspiration and expiration. Expiration is as long as inspiration (I:E ratio = 1:1). These sounds are heard on the anterior chest wall over the sternum at the angle of Louis and along the lower costosternal borders of the sternum, as well as the interscapular region between T3 and T6 (Fig. 3-7). The bronchovesicular breath sound is the predominant and normal breath sound in children under the age of 13 years. It is represented diagrammatically as follows:

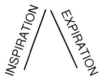

However, when the bronchovesicular breath sound is heard in an area of the lung that normally has vesicular breath sounds, it is considered abnormal. The vesicular sound may be heard more on inspiration and the bronchial breath sound component more during exhalation when the bronchovesicular breath sound is heard in an abnormal location. Bronchovesicular breath sounds designate partial consolidation in the lungs typically seen with the buildup of secretions or in atelectasis, or in a combination of both.

Diminished Breath Sounds.   These are often called decreased breath sounds. They designate an interference with the conduction of breath sounds and will therefore be decreased or absent. Decreased breath sounds indicate decreased airflow to a particular region of the lung.

The causes of diminished breath sounds are as follows:

1. Fluid in the pleural space: hemothorax (blood); inflammatory pleural effusion
2. Air in the pleural space: pneumothorax
3. Thickening pleura caused by fibrosis: effusion, empyema·
4. COPD, caused by decreased air velocity and sound conduction as a result of overinflation of the lung
5. Bronchial obstruction: plugged lumen
6. Hypoventilation of the lung caused by pleurisy or splinting produced by a thoracic incision

In all but the first example, decreased breath sounds are a result of an interposed liquid medium as well as a definite decrease in ventilation of the underlying lung.

Adventitious Sounds

Adventitious sounds are not heard normally over any anatomic region of the chest. Adventitious sounds are not like the breath sounds previously discussed. Adventitious sounds are superimposed on top of the breath sound. They indicate air passing through obstructed regions of the lung. The most common adventitious sounds are rales, rhonchi, and stridor.

Rales

Râle is a French word meaning "rattle." This term was in common use during late eighteenth century and early nineteenth century Europe and was synonymous with impending death. Its usage today is no longer associated with the impending death of the patient. It is now a word that implies alveolar obstruction or collapse. Since rales is a word of European origin, its meaning in modern American English over the past several decades has become obscured. Clinicians have recently sought a more descriptive word that accurately describes the quality of the adventitious sound. The recent change in medical nomenclature for rales is *crackles*. In truth, both terms are still used and appear with frequency on the medical chart. The terms

in this section are presented side by side in an effort to ease the transition to the "new age" term.

Rales, or crackles, are popping sounds heard through the stethoscope during the inspiratory phase of ventilation. They sound like popcorn popping or like the crackles or popping of wood burning in a fireplace. Because the crackles can be heard separately and clearly one from another, they are sometimes called discontinuous sounds. Rales, or crackles, result from the passage of air through mucous secretions in the distal regions of the bronchopulmonary tree, that is, the last two to three generations of the lung. In fact, the crackle, or popping, sound occurs from the reinflation of the air sacs or alveoli of the lung during inspiration, which were collapsed because of fluid filling or mucous obstruction. The reinflation or the sudden reopening of the alveoli is believed to account for the popping that is heard—somewhat analogous to the popping sound of an opening parachute.

The sound of a rale will vary according to the size of the chamber involved and the character of the exudate responsible for the collapse. Rales, or crackles, may be wet or dry, depending on the amount of the moisture in the lung. Also, rales can be classified as fine, medium, or coarse in character.

Fine rales (crackles). Moisture is found deep in the terminal areas of the tracheobronchial tree. They have a fine crackling sound. These sounds indicate inflammation or congestion involving the alveoli. They can be heard at any stage during inspiration but are commonly heard at the beginning of inspiration. They look very much like this:

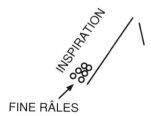

FINE RÂLES

Medium rales (crackles). Medium rales sound heavier or louder than fine rales. They can be heard at any stage of inspiration but are commonly heard halfway through the inspiratory phase. They tend to be the result of air passing through mucus in the acinus and tend to reflect a more tenacious exudate in the distal airway. They look like this:

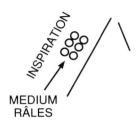

MEDIUM
RÂLES

Coarse rales (crackles).   Coarse rales are a sign of heavy involvement of the distal airway, as the exudate is very wet and tenacious. They frequently appear early in the inspiratory phase and are a sign of serious pulmonary involvement. They look like this:

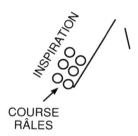

COURSE
RÂLES

Rhonchi

Rhonchi have been given a new name, as has the term rales, that more accurately describes the sound. The newer term cohabitating in the medical records with the older term of rhonchi is *wheeze*. Rhonchi, or wheezes, are continuous in their sound, unlike rales, which are discrete and singularly crackly. Rhonchi, or wheezes, are continuous "snoring" or rumbling-type sounds that can be heard throughout inspiration and expiration. Rhonchi, or wheezes, are sounds produced by the passage of air through the trachea, the bronchi, and bronchioles, which have been narrowed or nearly closed by disease and mucous plugging. Rhonchi, or wheezes, represent an obstructive event in the central airways. They can often be cleared by coughing and suctioning, whereas rales are not cleared in this manner.

Stridor

Stridor is a particularly loud musical sound that is most prominent during inspiration. It can be heard at a distance from the patient, without the use of a stetho-scope. Stridor is produced when the patient is experiencing laryngeal or tracheal obstruction. Stridor is the sound heard in children with croupe. It is that high-pitched, raspy, throaty, wheezy, or crowing sound that is so indicative of the child's respiratory distress. Although stridor is usually heard during inspiration, it can be heard during inspiration and expiration as the airway becomes increasingly obstructed. The larynx or the trachea can be increasingly obstructed by the growth of laryngeal tumors, by a worsening tracheal stenosis, or when some object has been inhaled or aspirated into the upper airway of the lung. When particularly severe, stridor is associated with gasping respiration and the use of accessory respiratory muscles in an attempt to increase airflow.

Pleural Friction Rub

The visceral and parietal pleural surfaces glide over each other without difficulty because the surfaces are smooth and glistening. The thin fluid layer between these pleural coverings acts to lubricate the surfaces and allows them to slip past each other noiselessly and effortlessly during the respiratory phases of breathing. When these surfaces become inflamed, they can become rough and self-adherent, creating a pleural friction rub.

A pleural friction rub is a continuous sound that is usually heard at the middle to end of the inspiratory phase, and perhaps at the beginning of the expiratory phase. Pleural friction rubs have a characteristic squeaking, grating, creaking, or clicking sound. A tell-tale sign of the presence of a pleural friction rub is the cessation of breathing at the point that the patient feels pain during breathing. Patients will splint or momentarily hold their breath because of the pain they feel as the roughened and inflamed pleural surfaces stick together. Rubs are most commonly heard over the posterolateral and anterolateral chest well and on the posterior chest wall. Pleural friction rubs can be caused by pleurisy, pneumonia, and thoracic surgery.

Helpful Hints for the New Auscultator

New auscultators should practice in a quiet room. In the hospital intensive care unit, the background noise can be so intense as to make it almost impossible for the new auscultator to hear anything meaningful in the thoracic cavity. It is useful to practice on healthy subjects first, in a quiet place, to learn the normal breath sounds and where they are located. It would be wise to practice on scores of people and to evaluate the different regions of the lung methodically, in order to learn what normal breath sounds are like. In review, the tracheal breath sound is normally heard only over the trachea. The bronchial breath sound is normally heard only over the sternum, along the sternocostal border, and in some patients along the thoracovertebral border from T1 to T6. A bronchial breath sound heard anywhere else is considered abnormal and portends the presence of lung disease. The vesicular breath sound is normally heard over the remaining portions of the chest wall. The clinician has to remember that certain sounds are normal when found in the right place in the lung. However, that same sound located in a region of the lung field in which it is not normally heard is a sign of pathology. The clinician must become very familiar with the lung sounds heard in their normal anatomic location. This will be essential when a real pathology is present and altered lung sounds are heard.

For proper evaluation of the gradations of sounds heard through the stethoscope, the clinician should move the stethoscope in an orderly pattern from side to side, that is, move from the right basilar segments to the left basilar segments or from the anterior segment of the right upper lobe to the left anterior segment of the left upper lobe. Essentially, the auscultator listens to one full inspiratory and expiratory cycle on the right and then repeats this on the left. In so doing, one can compare right side to left side and can detect differences in amplitude and pitch between the right and left lung fields.

The new auscultator may initially encounter some real problems in filtering out local extraneous noise. Local extraneous noise in this case has reference to the noises transmitted through the stethoscope that originate from either the patient or the clinician. Extraneous local noises might include the following:

1. The creaks and cracks of the auscultator's own phalangeal joints are easily mistaken for chest sounds; they are transmitted to the ears while the stethoscope is handled and as the diaphragm is firmly pressed on the patient's chest. New auscultators have been known to report that the patient has rales or crackles, when in fact all the clinician really heard was local extraneous noise from the digits holding the stethoscope.
2. When listening to the chest wall of a hairy male subject, the sound of hair scratching across the diaphragm is often mistaken for fine rales. Once the source of this local noise is identified, the auscultator can learn to ignore the sound or can try dampening the area with some water to make the hair lie close to the chest wall.
3. Local extraneous noise may come from clothing rubbing on the stethoscope. Many times in older patients with rheumatoid arthritis, the crepitant noise from arthritic joints can interfere with listening to the chest wall. Speech as well as bowel sounds can also provide considerable interference with the sounds of a patient's lungs, especially in patients who are on bed rest.

Practice makes perfect, and that adage is certainly true for anyone interested in becoming good at chest auscultation. The idea is to start out slow and listen to normal healthy lungs first. Some very fine tapes and book publications discuss in great detail how to listen to the chest when conducting a pulmonary assessment.

ASSESSMENT OF THE PULMONARY PATIENT

Chart Review

The physical therapist should have a thorough understanding of the patient's past medical history. Knowledge of the patient's medical background can help in forming a meaningful rehabilitation plan and in making realistic goals to meet the rehabilitation needs of the patient.

Medical History

If the medical chart is accessible, the medical history should be thoroughly reviewed. Is there something about the medical history that will give some background to understand the patient's current medical problems? For instance, does this patient's current hospital visit represent a repeat admission for the same problem, or is this admission completely unrelated to the acute or chronic respiratory problems? For example:

1. Is an emphysemic patient being admitted for removal of plates and screws from an open-reduction internal fixation (ORIF) performed several months or years ago? If this is the case, the patient's emphysema is a secondary problem and will have to be managed while the patient is in physical therapy for gait training and muscle strengthening. It may well be necessary to address the respiratory problem first before thinking of doing anything else with the patient's musculoskeletal system.
   or
2. Is the patient being readmitted because of a recurrent infection in a total hip prosthesis? It may well be accompanied by a secondary pneumonia resulting from the older sedentary patient's inactivity or bed rest. Once the infection is under control, the therapist may well be asked to see this patient for muscle strengthening, range-of-motion (ROM) exercises, and increasing out-of-bed activities, such as gait or bicycle exercises. However, the lung condition will be the major acute obstacle for the patient's need to increase physical activity leading to recovery.

It is clear that as America ages, more and more of our patients will have multiple system impairments. In the future, it may well be the exception, rather than the rule, that we will be seeing a patient for a single problem.

Psychosocial History

The physical therapist should know the patient's psychosocial history. This information will be readily available in the medical chart. However, if the chart does not contain this information or is not available for review, the patient's psychosocial history may be obtained from the patient, the family, or relatives. Psychosocial information may be extremely helpful to the therapist in understanding the patient's attitudes toward members of the rehabilitation team, motivations or lack of motivations for recovery, interactions with family members. The complexities of a patient's emotions and feelings are best understood within this setting of knowledge. All too often, the success or the failure of a patient's rehabilitation program rests on the level of trust, support, and love that the patient feels in the family. The behavior of a patient reflects the nuances of familial interaction.

Some of the information gleaned by the therapist may include the age of the patient and the patient's marital status. Marital status can be an important piece of background information to be used to enhance the patient's desire to participate in the rehabilitation process. It may also explain why the patient is not participating in the rehabilitation program. For example, the patient may have no one to "go home to" as discharge from the hospital grows nearer. Some patients who feel lonely and who do not have a loved one to return home to may feel there is no reason to live anymore. They may have no incentive to participate actively in their own rehabilitation and may well refuse to take responsibility for their own recovery.

Radiographic Results

It is important to read the radiographic reports. These reports will be very useful in demonstrating what part of the lung field is involved in the disease process. The radiographic report will indicate whether the patient has a panlobar (diffuse) problem or a discrete lobar involvement. In many instances, the radiologist will have access to old films and will state in the report how the most recent radiograph compares with older radiographs. These comments will be helpful because they will give some idea of whether the patient is improving, has remained the same, or is deteriorating with time. Radiographic reports will tell the therapist whether the disease process is acute or chronic. All this information will help the therapist plan reasonable rehabilitation goals.

Pulmonary Function Test

The chart should be reviewed to see whether pulmonary function studies have been completed. These tests measure the patient's lung volumes and capacities. They are very useful because they are a measure of the patient's ability to ventilate and exchange two critical gases—oxygen and carbon dioxide—in and out of the lung.

Pulmonary function tests are particularly useful in the diagnosis of chronic obstructive pulmonary disease (COPD), such as asthma, emphysema, chronic bronchitis, and bronchiectasis. In suspected COPD, the patient will have a classic reduced ability to exhale air forcibly from the lungs. Therefore, critical volume measurements of the patient's ability to expire air forcibly from the lungs will be reduced; that is, forced expiratory volume in 1 second (FEV_1), forced expiratory volume in 3 seconds (FEV_3), and forced vital capacity (FVC) will all be smaller than in patients with normal lung function.

Pulmonary function tests are also useful but less diagnostic in patients suspected of having restrictive lung disease. Restrictive lung diseases such as adult respiratory distress syndrome (ARDS), infant respiratory distress syndrome (IRDS), sarcoidosis, and any number of pulmonary fibrosis syndromes all make the lung less flexible or compliant. The lung affected with a restrictive disease is a stiffer lung. Expansion and contraction of the bronchopulmonary tree are much more difficult, and the volume of air that can be brought in and out of the lungs is reduced. Also, a number of medical conditions restrict normal expansion and contraction of the lung, such as flail chest, a thoracic cage affected by ankylosing spondylitis, rib fractures, as well as blunt chest trauma, in which case patients refuse to deep breathe because they are splinting against the pain that deep inspiration might cause. These conditions affect the normal mechanics of breathing. Patients with these medical problems will have pulmonary function tests that may display a normal FEV_1 but a smaller than normal FVC.

If the patient has had a pulmonary function study, the report will describe the results in terms of obstructive or restrictive lung disease. These reports, coupled with the information on the radiographic report, as well as the blood gas report, are very helpful in describing the patient's pulmonary disease state.

It will be very helpful to find out whether serial pulmonary function tests (PFTs) are available. These tests will show whether the patient's pulmonary status has changed over the past few months or years.

Blood Gases

The therapist should read the blood gas reports. They will show whether the patient has adequate gas diffusion. Blood gas reports have a wealth of information describing the acid-base balance of the patient. Some of the information to be aware of is the partial pressure of oxygen (PaO_2), partial pressure of carbon dioxide ($PaCO_2$), pH, and bicarbonate ion concentration in the blood.

Normal blood gas readings are described as partial pressures of a specific gas (oxygen and carbon dioxide) and are given the units of millimeters of mercury pressure (mmHg). The normal values for oxygen are 90 to 100 mmHg and for carbon dioxide 35 to 45 mmHg. If the patient has a partial pressure of oxygen (PaO_2) of less than 80 mmHg, severe CNS effects will be noted because the CNS does not function well when the patient is hypoxic. If the partial pressure for carbon dioxide ($PaCO_2$) rises above 60 mmHg, the patient will likely be in respiratory distress because of the retention of carbon dioxide, a condition known as hypercapnia.

The normal pH of the blood is 7.35 to 7.45. For a number of reasons, the pH level of the blood can be altered. If the pH falls lower than 7.35, the patient is said to be acidotic. Acidosis is usually caused by failure to ventilate the lungs adequately. The exchange of oxygen and carbon dioxide across the alveolar-capillary interface is reduced, and the blood begins to collect ever-increasing amounts of carbon dioxide because of continued cellular metabolism. As more and more carbon dioxide collects in the blood, the pH of the blood begins to fall, pushing the patient further and further into acidosis. The reasons for acidosis are legion. Each year millions of patients experience respiratory acidosis because of COPD, drug overdose, or airway obstruction.

Chronic Obstructive Pulmonary Disease

Patients who smoke constitute the largest class who experience chronic acidosis. People with emphysema and chronic bronchitis experience increasing difficulty in exchanging oxygen and carbon dioxide over the years of their smoking lifetime. This is directly attributable to the constituents of the burning tobacco, which stimulate an inflammatory reaction in the lung tissue that causes fibrosis and scarring of the gas-exchange surfaces of the lung. The alveolar-capillary interface where oxygen and carbon dioxide are normally exchanged is so eroded by fibrosis as to impede the exchange of oxygen and carbon dioxide. The smoker becomes increasingly short of breath because of poor gas-exchange mechanics. These patients will have slightly lower Pao_2 values and higher $Paco_2$ values on the blood gas report. Patients with COPD will often be seen with Pao_2 values within the range of 80 to 90 mmHg and $Paco_2$ values within the range of 50 to 60 mmHg. As the destruction of the gas-exchange surfaces continues through continued tobacco abuse, the patient will experience increasingly severe respiratory difficulties. Death by respiratory failure can eventually be the end result if the smoking behavior cannot be stopped.

Drug Overdose

Drug overdose patients will be acidotic as a result of severe CNS and respiratory center depression. The poor blood gas values in these patients are a direct result of the failure of the respiratory system to stimulate adequate ventilation of the lungs. The poor respiratory mechanics must be corrected immediately, to avoid irreparable damage to the CNS.

Airway Obstruction

Airway obstruction is another common reason that patients may experience acute blood-gas derangements. Objects or mucous secretions may be obstructing the tracheobronchial tree, resulting in inadequate ventilation.

Laboratory Reports

The therapist should read the laboratory reports for bacteriology, for sputum cultures, for hematology, and for urinalysis. Some common blood laboratory values to be familiar with the following:

Platelets	200,000–400,000/mm³
Red blood cells	5,000,000–6,000,000/ml
White blood cells	4,500–10,800/ml

Hemoglobin		
	Females	13–14 g/dl
	Males	15–16 g/dl
Hematocrit		
	Females	34–46%
	Males	40–52%

Work History

What is the work history of the patient? Is the patient retired, or is it likely that the patient will return to work? How happy was the patient with his or her job before the present illness? How anxious is the patient to return to the workplace? Is the patient involved in a worker's compensation dispute subsequent to an injury on the job? Is a lawsuit pending in the courts during the course of rehabilitation? The answers to many of these questions may influence the patient's desire to participate actively in rehabilitation.

Discharge Planning

Will the patient return home immediately after discharge, or will there be the need for a short stay at an extended-care facility? Is there a likelihood of home discharge and the need for some health services in the home? Will treatment be continued on an outpatient basis? The excitement of getting out of the hospital is sometimes dampened by the need to go to an extended-care facility. The patient's zeal for rehabilitation can be affected by what type of discharge is expected. The therapist can help the patient see the benefits of an extended-care facility. The time spent in helping patients cope with discharge can go a long way in helping them work hard for rehabilitation, making the therapist's job much easier. Depression concerning the illness frequently encumbers that patient's speedy progress in rehabilitation, but when it is complicated by depression about discharge to an extended-care facility, the therapist can find it very difficult to motivate the patient to work hard for recovery.

History

The therapist should interview the patient or the patient's family for the relevant history concerning the illness for which the patient is being admitted. The following questions should be included:

1. What is the patient's smoking history? How long has the patient been a smoker? How much did the patient smoke per day?
2. What is or was the patient's occupation? Did the patient's job present an occupational risk to the patient's pulmonary health? If there was an occupational hazard, to what extent was that health hazard responsible for the present hospital admission?
3. Can the patient document a history of shortness of breath secondary to smoking, or does the patient think the shortness of breath started just before admission to the hospital?

The next step is to determine the patient's responses to activity. How is the patient able to tolerate mild to moderate activity? The following questions should be considered:

1. Can the patient get out of bed and walk unattended or is the patient restricted to bed rest?
2. Does the patient require oxygen supplementation during exercise? Is oxygen necessary even at rest? What are the oxygen saturation values for the patient at rest, during ROM exercises, and during ambulation? Oxygen saturation is determined by an oximeter and is useful in determining the oxygenation capacity of the patient.
3. Does the patient tolerate positional changes—can the patient lie flat in the bed during sleep or must the patient sit up in bed during their sleep hours? Many patients in respiratory distress cannot tolerate the supine or prone flat positions. These patients will often experience less shortness of breath when in the sitting position. While in the sitting position, the abdominal contents are being pulled on by gravity and pulled away from the diaphragm, permitting maximal downward excursion of the diaphragm. This position allows for a deeper inspiratory effort and therefore reduces the sensation of shortness of breath.

Physical Examination

Thoracic Function

The examination begins with manual evaluation of the chest wall. This aspect of the chest evaluation looks at the anatomic and mechanical movement of the thoracic wall. The following information should be included in the evaluation notes:

1. Can the patient take a deep breath or does the patient complain of being unable to take a deep breath? What is the cause of the patient's complaint of shortness of breath? Frequently patients with pneumonia or other diseases, such as asthma, bronchitis, or emphysema, will complain of shortness of breath. They will try to ventilate the entire lung by taking in deep breaths, but the complaint of shortness of breath persists. This problem is due either to fluid filling in the acinus (acinus is a term that refers to the basic respiratory unit of the lung consisting of the respiratory bronchioles, the alveolar duct, the alveolar sac, and the alveoli), or to obstruction of the conducting airways (trachea, mainstem bronchi, lobar bronchi, segmental bronchi, small bronchi) and the peripheral airways. Very often the patient who complains of shortness of breath will have evidence of this in the movement of the chest wall. The therapist should manually place the palmar surfaces of the hands firmly on the lateral chest wall. The patient should be asked to take a deep breath while the therapist feels the amount of excursion of both sides. Using the simple manual test, the therapist can often feel the loss of chest wall excursion on the side that is affected with disease. The therapist should note whether there is equal bilateral expansion of the chest wall. If there is less excursion on the right, that outcome should be noted.
2. Is there pain on deep breathing? Pain frequently accompanies pulmonary problems. Patients with pneumonia frequently experience pain in the region of the atelectasis and fluid infiltration of the lung. This pain is usually encountered on inspiration and can be so severe at times as to limit the depth of the inspiratory effort. The splinting and shallow breathing that result from chest wall pain only complicate the patient's recovery. Deep breathing and coughing are effective treatments for clearing secretions from the lung. Many times the therapist's greatest task in treating patients experiencing chest wall pain is to get them to produce an effective deep breath and cough.
3. Is there any use of the accessory respiratory muscles? Patients in respiratory distress will call upon

the accessory muscles of respiration (e.g., the sternocleidomastoids, the paraspinal muscles, and the shoulder girdle muscles). During inspiration, the neck, back, and shoulders should be observed to see whether the patient is activating the accessory muscles of breathing during inspiration. Cavitation of the thoracic wall—a depression of the thoracic wall between the ribs during inspiration—is a sign that the patient is experiencing respiratory distress. Cavitation is seen especially in children who are diagnosed with IRDS. In these infants, every inspiratory muscle is called into action in order to mount enough driving pressure to open up the collapsed or collapsing lung. The negative driving pressure exerted by the infant during the inspiratory maneuver is so great as to cause the intercostal spaces to be drawn inward below the surface level of the ribs, giving the appearance of indentations, or cavitations, between the ribs.

4. Does the patient suddenly halt inspiration and splint or exhibit a chest wall "catch"? This can be indicative of the presence of a pleural friction rub. Also, if there are simple rib fractures, sometimes a crepitus and a splinting occur when the bony ends of the fractured ribs cause chest wall pain.

5. What is the rate and depth of respiration?

Productive or Nonproductive Cough

1. Can the patient illicit a good, round double cough? Patients must be able to take in a deep breath and produce a deep double cough in order to clear the secretions from their lungs. Deep coughing mobilizes the secretions, while a shallow-in-the-throat cough does little but inflame the throat.

2. What is the quantity, color, and general consistency of the mucus that is coughed up? If the mucus is green, it is a sign that infection is probably present. If the mucus is frothy and pink or red, blood is most likely being coughed up with the mucus.

Breathing Patterns

1. Is there any paradoxical breathing? Paradoxical breathing is a pattern seen frequently in high paraplegics and in quadriplegics. Normally, the abdomen and the chest rise concomitantly during inspiration because, as the chest wall expands and rises, the contracting diaphragm pushes down against the abdominal contents, forcing the abdomen to rise as well. In patients who have lost innervation to the intercostal musculature (especially the external intercostals), the chest will not rise as much and may actually appear to fall during inspiration while the abdomen rises. Quadriplegic patients who only have a neurologically intact diaphragm through the phrenic nerve (C3, C4, C5) and who have lost all thoracic innervation will exhibit this type of paradoxical breathing.

2. Is expiration longer than inspiration? Patients who have COPD will very often breathe with pursed lips. Breathing through pursed lips will produce a longer expiration compared with a shorter inspiration. In effect, these patients are creating a backpressure in their lungs to prevent the small bronchi and the terminal bronchioles from collapsing during mid- to end-expiration. The backpressure that these patients deliver to their lungs is much like the positive end-expiratory pressure (PEEP) given to ventilator-bound patients to prevent collapse of the acinus. In both cases—the COPD patient and the ventilator patient—PEEP is designed to keep the terminal airways open as long as possible to ensure a longer oxygen-carbon dioxide exchange.

3. Can the patient speak while breathing, or are breaths interspersed between words in a labored gasping type of speech?

4. Is there any vocal fremitus? Vocal fremitus describes the vibratory or buzzy sensation the therapist will feel if the hands are placed on the patient's chest as the patient speaks. Usually the therapist will place the palmar or the hypothenar regions of the hands on the thoracic wall. As the patient speaks, the rattling of the chest wall will be evident and is due to the passage of air and sound through secretions. Vocal fremitus is often observed in patients with COPD and pneumonia.

5. What is the rate of breathing?

Finger Percussion

Finger percussion is useful in determining which areas of the thoracic wall should be auscultated. The technique involves placing the middle finger—the "anvil"—of the nondominant hand on the chest wall and sharply and quickly tapping it over the distal interphalangeal joint (DIP), using the middle finger of the dominant hand as the "hammer." When the hammer firmly raps the anvil, a resonant note is heard. For those who do not have the power to create a nice resonant note with the hammer finger, sometimes using a reflex hammer instead of the hammer finger produces a loud enough note to be easily heard.

The therapist will listen for variations over the chest wall in the transmitted sound, much like the technique used when auscultating the chest wall with a stethoscope. A side-to-side movement should be employed to compare the sounds heard over the right lung field with the sounds heard over the left lung field.

Normally the percussion note should be the same side to side, when moving over the thoracic wall. However, in areas of consolidation, there will be a reduced resonance or a dullness to the sound produced during finger percussion.

Auscultation

The therapist should first listen for normal breath sounds (bronchial and vesicular) in the areas of the lung field in which they normally appear. The therapist should also listen for adventitious sounds over the entire lung field, such as rales, rhonchi, stridor (inspiratory stridor), and pleural friction rub, as well as the

voice sounds, such as bronchophony, egophony, and whispered pectoriloquy.

When auscultating the lung fields, the therapist starts by listening to the anterior chest wall. The therapist listens to one side and then the other side in the same segment of the lungs. Listening to the same segment of one lung permits a comparison between the sound that was heard and the sound that will be generated in the same segment in the other lung. This side-to-side movement of the stethoscope enables the therapist to evaluate the amplitude of both lung fields and to determine whether abnormal breath sounds or adventitious sounds are present. After evaluating the anterior chest wall, the therapist moves to the lateral chest walls and the posterior chest wall in a similar side-to-side evaluation method.

DISEASES OF THE PULMONARY SYSTEM

The preceding discussion described the normal assessment process. The following discussion is designed to aid in assessing the patient whose respiratory function is already known to be abnormal. A practical approach to pulmonary assessment is presented, based on common techniques applicable to both the outpatient and the inpatient setting (Table 3-2). These techniques are used as the groundwork to evaluate baseline functional capacity and subsequent trending in regard to four broad categories of pulmonary disease.

Assessment of the Pulmonary Patient

Read the chart
Gather pertinent history from the patient about present condition
Elicit the health history
Determine the level of activity that the patient can sustain
Note whether the patient is dependent on oxygen supplementation
Perform a manual evaluation of chest mechanics
Evaluate the patient's breathing patterns
Determine whether the patient can cough and deep-breath to mobilize secretions
Perform finger percussion and auscultation of the thoracic wall

---

Table 3-2. Pulmonary Evaluation Techniques

Outpatient	Inpatient
History (including medications)	History (including medications)
Physical examination	Physical examination
Spirometry (FVC, FEV_1, PEFR, $\dot{V}_E$)	Spirometry (FVC, FEV_1, PEFR, V_T)
Maximum inspiratory or expiratory force	Maximum inspiratory or expiratory force; PEEP
Compliance (dynamic)	Compliance (static and dynamic)
	Arterial blood gases
Oximetry	Cardiac monitor, oximeter
ECG, chest radiography	Ventilation-perfusion calculated
Functional capacity ($\dot{V}_{O_{2max}}$)	shunt or V_D/V_T

The assessment techniques presented in Table 3-2 serve to contrast the normal setting with the abnormal condition, given the specific disease state. The emphasis is on outpatient assessment techniques, unless the patient's situation (e.g., intensive care unit for coma) renders the technique inadequate. In such circumstances, additional special techniques are suggested.[8]

Tests that should be readily available to, or performed by the physical therapist for completion of the assessment include simple spirometry, used to obtain a forced vital capacity (FVC) and a forced expiratory volume in 1 second (FEV_1); manometry to measure maximum inspiratory pressure or force; and ear or fingertip oximetry; the ECG and a chest radiograph should also be on hand for viewing by the therapist.

As with cardiac rehabilitation, the therapist must have an estimate of the patient's functional respiratory capacity (FRC). Several regression equations have been developed to measure the patient's FRC.[9] The following equation is standard:

$$VE_{max}(L/min) = 37.5 \times FEV_1 \tag{1}$$

The following measurement of functional capacity has the additional advantage of predicting maximum oxygen uptake:

$$VO_{2max}(ml/min) = 216.8 + 22.3(VE_{max}) \tag{2}$$

The therapist will find the following equation useful because it also measures the patient's ventilatory muscle strength as a baseline as well as for trending purposes:

$$VE_{max} = 21.34 \times FEV(L) + 6.28 \times PIFR_1(L/sec) \tag{3}$$

The tests given as well as the equations derived should be adequate to present the therapist with enough information to evaluate the patient accurately and to provide an exercise prescription for that patient. These equations and assessment techniques will be effective in all types of respiratory disease.

We will now consider four general categories of pulmonary disease with which the physical therapist will need to be familiar. Obstructive pulmonary disease is the most common disease category. It includes obstructive sleep apnea, asthma, chronic bronchitis, emphysema, bronchiectasis, and cystic fibrosis. Restrictive pulmonary disease includes obesity, the most common limitation to chest expansion; ventilatory muscle dysfunction (i.e., denervation of the muscles of respiration—the ventilatory pump); cervical cord injury; and diaphragmatic paralysis. This category also includes common disease entities that compress or infiltrate the alveoli, including pneumonia, interstitial lung disease, lung tumors, and diseases of the pleural space. Pulmonary vascular diseases include pulmonary heart disease, pulmonary thrombosis and embolism, and heart failure. Ventilatory regulation disorders include central hypoventilation (sleep apnea) and central hyperventilation.

Table 3-3. Types of Lung Disease

Clinical Type	Distinguishing Features
Obstructive: emphysema, asthma, bronchitis, bronchiectasis, obstructive sleep apnea	Obstruction to inspiratory and expiratory airflow ($\downarrow FEV_1/FVC$); increased residual volume
Restrictive: obesity, interstitial lung disease (ARDS), ventilatory muscle weakness, lung volume loss	Decrease in all lung volumes; no obstruction to airflow
Pulmonary vascular disease: pulmonary artery embolism, pulmonary heart disease, chronic heart failure	Normal lung volume; decreased functional alveolo-capillary membrane area for O_2-CO_2 exchange
Ventilatory regulation: hypoventilation (central sleep apnea); hyperventilation	slowed or accelerated respiratory rate; normal A-a O_2 difference

Obstructive Pulmonary Disease

Obstructive pulmonary disease is defined by increased residual volume and obstruction to airflow during both inspiration and expiration. Certain historical information must be obtained for an effective concentration of the therapist's treatment approach. Of primary importance is a history of (1) those irritants that worsen the patient's symptoms, such as smoking, pollen exposure, fumes, or particles that seem to cause acute respiratory difficulty and repeated lung infections, and (2) possible influence of that patient's workplace, such as coal mining, uranium mining, and working around cotton gins or silage. It seems self-evident that if the patient is unable to avoid the aggravating irritant, as smoking, the efforts of the therapist are unlikely to be effective.

The interview should document the presence of cough, particularly if it is persistent (more than 3 months of daily coughing per year) and whether it is accompanied by wheezing, as with asthma, or by sputum production. If the patient is producing more than 3 to 4 tablespoons of mucopurulent or purulent secretion each day, such production suggests that postural drainage and percussion (frappage) may be of benefit. The therapist should note the appearance of the sputum (clear, mucoid, purulent, or bloody). The presence of blood in the sputum should alert both the patient and the therapist to the possibility of a more serious illness than bronchitis, even though chronic bronchitis is probably the most common cause of hemoptysis.

The patient's functional capacity should be estimated. Questions that may be useful to ask include the distance the patient can walk continuously at any rate on the level and whether shortness of breath (dyspnea) is present at rest or only with activity. Does shortness of breath during the night force the patient to arise in order to obtain relief? This would suggest paroxysmal nocturnal dyspnea and orthopnea, two symptoms relating more to left ventricular heart failure rather to than lung disease per se. An estimate of the patient's nutritional status, if only to ask about weight loss, is well worthwhile.

Inspection should include an estimate of mucous membrane cyanosis, specifically of tongue and buccal membranes, bearing in mind that the patient must have at least 4 g of desaturated hemoglobin per 100 ml of blood to make cyanosis visible; notation of membrane pallor suggesting significant anemia is important. Respiratory rate and manner should be noted, since a prolonged expiratory phase, particularly in the presence of chronic cough and pursed-lip breathing, is good confirmatory evidence that the patient is suffering from significant obstructive pulmonary disease. Whether the patient is able to speak fairly long sentences before taking a breath is also a useful clue to the severity of obstructive lung trouble.

The patient's seated position, as if supporting the torso

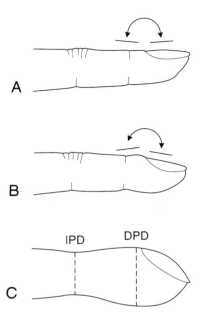

Fig. 3-8. Clubbing of the digits. **(A)** Normal digit configuration. **(B)** Mild digital clubbing with increased hyponychial angle. **(C)** Severe digital clubbing; depth of finger at base of nail (DPD) is greater than depth of interphalangeal joint (IPD). Abbreviations: DPD, distal phalangeal depth; IPD, interphalangeal depth. (From Wilkins et al.,[13] with permission.)

on extended arms, is a further clue to the presence of significant obstructive pulmonary disease. Another sign of obstructive disease is the chest appearing to be in continuous full inspiratory pause (i.e., barrel-shaped chest). Clubbing of the terminal phalanges is associated with chronic lung, heart, and liver disease (Fig. 3-8).

The severity of the clubbing is probably best related to the duration of the disease state as well as its severity. The presence of ochre-brown stains between the index and second finger of either the right or left hand characterizes the smoking of at least two packs of cigarettes per day.

Such evaluation of outpatient status must be expanded or varied in regard to the hospitalized patient, particularly the patient in the intensive or intermediate care unit.[8] Some information can be obtained from other personnel or from the patient's relatives. Under these circumstances, the therapist must rely on the observations noted earlier.

In addition, the therapist should note ventilator settings, if any are in use. Observation of the ventilator settings includes whether the patient is on spontaneous, assisted, or mandatory ventilation, as well as the tidal volume (V_T), respiratory rate, and fraction of inspired oxygen (FiO_2). The therapist should also note whether positive end-expiratory pressure (PEEP) or continuous positive airway pressure (CPAP) is being used. In general, PEEP will not be used in a patient with COPD, but the technique is used very effectively in other disease categories (see below).

If the hospitalized patient is breathing spontaneously, one should evaluate the patient for thoracoabdominal dyssynchrony, defined as a loss of the synchronized outward movement of the lower chest and upper abdomen during diaphragmatic contraction.[10] The chest will appear retracted as the epigastrium expands, and vice versa. This finding is of particular importance as an early indicator of ventilatory muscle fatigue, the cause of which must be corrected if physical therapy is to be beneficial.

To return to those techniques that are useful for both inpatient and outpatient evaluation, palpation and percussion of the patient's chest with obstructive pulmonary disease frequently reveal that the chest wall does not move when the patient takes a deep breath and that percussion of the lung bases will elicit no evidence of diaphragmatic motion, that is, the level of dullness between complete expiration and full inspiration. Percussion will also frequently indicate a hyperresonance of the chest, expected in a patient who has significant air trapping in emphysematous lung disease. The resonance felt by the percussed finger is a more sensitive indicator than the audible or auscultated note for detecting subtler changes of tissue density within the chest.

Palpation with the examining hand over the precordial area may indicate a right ventricular heave just left of the sternum or just beneath the xiphoid process. This finding is a reasonably good indicator of right ventricular hypertrophy or strain from pulmonary hypertension. Occasionally when the radial artery pulse or the apical cardiac impulse is palpated in the presence of COPD with pulmonary hypertension, the therapist will find that during inspiration, the radial pulse, systolic pressure, or apical impulse will be noticeably diminished ("paradoxical pulse").

Auscultation of the chest in any form of COPD is limited not only by the fact that even with the best stethoscope, one can hear no deeper than about 3 to 5 cm into the chest, but also by the decreased breath sounds related to airflow obstruction. In general, it will be found that the vesicular breath sounds are diminished during inspiration and the first portion of the expiratory phase and that adventitous sounds (e.g., rhonchi) will frequently be very prominent during the expiratory phase, especially during a forced expiration maneuver. A bronchospastic component occurs not only in the asthmatic, but also frequently in the COPD patient, such that expiratory wheezing will be present. By contrast, inspiratory wheezing usually suggests that there are multiple bronchiolar mucous plugs. The presence of inspiratory rhonchi, particularly in a patient with severe asthma, is a worrisome finding, since it is associated with recurrence of the asthma attack, the development of status asthmaticus (cessation of respiration), and death. This finding is sometimes difficult to separate from pneumonia, but in general the inspiratory rhonchi will be present throughout the lungs, rather than in an isolated lobe or lobes. The finding of coarse rhonchi and rales in an isolated area of lung, which clears with a deep breath or cough, objectively denotes an atelectasis of that segment of lung and suggests the need for more vigorous pulmonary therapy and evaluation for obstructing tissue.

A useful measurement of ventilatory muscle strength is maximum inspiratory pressure ($P_{i\ max}$) also known as maximum inspiratory force (MIF) or negative inspiratory force (NIF), which should be at a minimum minus 20 cm H_2O to produce adequate resting vital capacity. Maximum expiratory pressure ($P_{e\ max}$) can also be used.[7] A generated pressure of -40 to -60 cm H_2O is necessary to sustain the activities of daily living, including walking. This measurement should always be obtained in the outpatient setting. A similar measurement can be acquired in the inpatient setting, if the patient is responsive to command.[6–8]

The muscular power needed to provide a vital capacity (VC) of approximately 15 ml/kg (the capacity necessary for an adequate cough and respiratory reserve) is produced by a negative inspiratory force greater than -20 cm H_2O or more negative than -20 cm H_2O pressure in 20 seconds.[7] It should be noted that the normal negative inspiratory force (NIF) is in excess of -80 cm H_2O) with a range of -60 to -90 cm H_2O.[6] Other readily measured clinical evaluations of respiratory capacity include minute ventilation, which should be 6 to 10 L/min in an adult and is frequently used in correlation with the forced vital capacity already mentioned.[6]

Oximetry with either an ear probe or finger probe gives an adequate measurement of respiratory function, that is, oxygen exchange across the alveolar-capillary membrane both at rest and with activity, but does not reflect carbon dioxide exchange. Because of the simplicity and reproducibility of these tests, the maximum inspiratory pressure or maximum negative inspiratory force and oximetry should be repeated as a guide to the success or lack of success of therapeutic maneuvers.

A subcategory of upper airway obstructive disease is obstructive sleep apnea.[11] This entity is considered separately within the category of obstructive pulmonary disease for a number of reasons. First, this disease process, unlike most obstructive pulmonary disease, will respond readily to ventilatory muscle strengthening and weight loss. Second, obstructive sleep apnea is not a problem of intrathoracic airway obstruction, but rather of oropharyngeal upper airway obstruction secondary to decreased muscle tone. Third, obstructive sleep apnea overlaps with restrictive pulmonary disease because it is almost always seen in patients who are morbidly obese. It overlaps with central respiratory diseases because of the apparent insensitivity of the brain stem respiratory centers to hypoxemia or hypercapnia, or both.

The characteristic history obtained concerning these patients is that of overweight condition, daytime somnolence, morning headache, nocturnal snoring, and episodes of apnea, lasting more than 10 seconds and occurring more than five times within any given hour of sleep.

Inspection finds an overweight, thick, and short-necked patient, usually with a red face, who frequently will have a somewhat "froggy" voice, an increased respiratory rate when awake, and an irritable affect.[12] Palpation, percussion, and auscultation will rarely demonstrate anything of major importance other than poor thoracic expansion and decreased breath sounds. The forced vital capacity (FVC) and maximum minute volume (MMV) will generally indicate the classic decrease in lung volume measurements associated with restrictive defects. Oximetry during the patient's sleep will usually indicate significant hypoxemia (i.e., less than 88 percent oxyhemoglobin saturation). Hypercapnia may also occur. Observation of the patient's sleep pattern will demonstrate more than five episodes per hour of ventilatory muscle activity, but no air movement at the nose and mouth. The apneic episodes last more than 10 seconds each. Frequently such episodes will cease with a loud snort or cough and will be interspersed with loud snoring.[11] This disease process offers the physical therapist an excellent opportunity to attain real success with ventilatory muscle strengthening in association with a weight-loss program. CPAP will be necessary during the night for a period of weeks or months.

Restrictive Pulmonary Disease

Restrictive pulmonary disease is characterized by a decrease in all lung volumes. In contrast to obstructive pulmonary disease, the flow rates (FR), such as forced expiratory flow rate (FEFR), are normal or increased.[8] The diseases in this general category include (1) abnormalities of the thoracic cage, either congenital or acquired (multiple rib fractures); (2) respiratory muscle dysfunction, as with muscle weakness of any kind (e.g., medication effect, myasthenia gravis); and (3) diseases that invade the lung tissue (e.g., interstitial lung disease and pneumonia) or occupy the pleural space or lung parenchyma (e.g., tumors, pleural effusions, pneumothorax).

Restrictive pulmonary disease is less common than obstructive pulmonary disease but offers the physical therapist a good opportunity to improve the respiratory status of the patient with muscle and structural dysfunction. The basic concept that must be kept in mind in regard to restrictive pulmonary diseases is that the ventilatory muscles must generate a pressure great enough to overcome the recoil of the lung tissue. A measure of the ventilatory muscle strength required to increase the lung volume against the resistance of the lung tissue is called compliance (C).[6] A rough measure of dynamic compliance (C_{dyn}) can be obtained by measuring the vital capacity at the peak of the maximum inspiratory pressure ($P_{i\ max}$) (negative inspiratory force) that the patient can produce. The ratio of vital capacity (mm of air) to the maximum inspiratory pressure (negative inspiratory force; negative cm H_2O) gives a direct measurement of compliance, including the ventilatory muscle function:

$$C_{dyn} = \frac{VC}{P_{i\ max}}$$

This equation of vital capacity/maximum inspiratory pressure demonstrates that the more inspiratory pressure required to attain a given volume or a lesser lung volume obtained with a given maximum inspiratory pressure indicates decreased compliance. In order to obtain eupnea, the work of the ventilatory muscles must increase.

Abnormalities of the Thoracic Cage

The commonest disease state having to do with abnormalities of the thoracic cage is obesity. This morbid state restricts the expansion of the chest wall and restricts diaphragmatic function. This particular type of ventilatory disease has been termed obesity-hypoventilation syndrome. The history of these patients will frequently document an overweight condition for many years and a progressively sedentary life-style. Information from a family member may well indicate symptoms discussed concerning obstructive sleep apnea. Objective information frequently includes an elevated blood pressure (even with an oversized sphygmomanometer) and an elevated red blood count (secondary erythrocytosis) because of the hypoventilatory state and resultant hypoxemia. The chest circumference will not expand during inspiration to a significant degree when measured with a tape at the nipple line. Percussion of the chest will demonstrate inadequate descent of the diaphragm over the posterior portion of thoracic cage during inspiration. Auscultation will simply reflect decreased breath sounds and occasional basilar rhonchi.

Respiratory Muscle Dysfunction

Respiratory muscle dysfunction[7] includes generalized muscle weakness as from myasthenia gravis, Guillain-Barré syndrome, muscular dystrophy, metabolic disease states (e.g., severe potassium deficiency or phosphate deficiency), and specific antibiotic effects, particularly the commonly used aminoglycoside. Also included is cervical spinal cord damage with or without diaphragmatic paralysis. An important concept concerning this group of disease states is that diffuse neuromuscular weakness does not necessarily interrupt adequate ventilation and respiration unless the diaphragmatic function is also severely damaged.

The physical therapist's evaluation or assessment is of great help in this particular disease category. As always, the history is crucial to evaluation. Since these patients will almost always be hospitalized, and frequently will be in the intensive care unit, the history may have to be obtained from the chart and other people, rather than from the patient. A history of infectious disease will be of particular importance, not only for the possibility of a developing and perhaps correctable Guillain-Barré syndrome, but for sepsis with attendant aminoglycoside antibiotic use. Equally important is a history of metabolic disease states resulting in hypokalemia/hyperkalemia such as alcohol and diuretic use or acute renal failure, respectively. A history of cervical spine damage with the attendant possibility of intercostal muscle paralysis or diaphragmatic paralysis, including chest trauma with nonfunctional intercostal muscle and chest wall motion, will clarify the physical therapist's approach.

Objective findings must include observation of intercostal muscles and diaphragm contraction, especially the diaphragm. Palpation and inspection will demonstrate whether normal expansion of the lower rib cage and epigastric area occurs during inspiration. The therapist must be alert to the presence of the paradoxical inward motion of the lower thorax, as thoracoabdominal dyssynchrony would indicate that the diaphragmatic function is failing either from paralysis of the nerves innervating the diaphragm or from muscle weakness of any cause. Auscultation will generally indicate little or no air movement in the bases of the lungs. Decreased breath sounds in general correlate with the patient's inability to clear secretions from lung bases. The decreased ventilation in association with ventilation-perfusion mismatch at the same lung bases functions to weaken general muscle function, including the diaphragm. Negative inspiratory or positive expiratory force will be decreased, as will the forced vital capacity (FVC) and the forced expiratory volume (FEV_1) in 1 second.

If the physical therapist detects diaphragmatic failure, other members of the team should be notified, so that corrective action can be taken. From the therapist's point of view, the presence of true diaphragmatic failure requires repositioning of the nonventilated patient. The patient should be placed in the supine position, such that any diaphragmatic function present can be enhanced by moving the dome of the diaphragm cephalad with the passive motion of the abdominal viscera, giving the diaphragm a more efficient contractile effect. This positioning will be particularly effective in those quadriplegic patients who may have little intercostal muscle function but an intact diaphragm.

Bedside observations that the physical therapist will make are (1) a forced vital capacity and a maximum inspiratory pressure or similar to measure the lung volume produced and baseline ventilatory muscle strength, and (2) oximetry, which is useful because of the mentioned problem with ventilation-perfusion mismatching. in the lung bases. Auscultation is frequently useful for finding poorly cleared secretions in the form of rhonchi. Such findings should alert the therapist to two possibilities: (1) the ventilatory efforts are still inadequate, and (2) there is an impending atelectasis or pneumonia, or both.

Diseases that Invade the Lung Tissue or Occupy the Pleural Space or Lung Parenchyma

Another subcategory of restrictive disease includes disease states restricting lung volume, including intrapulmonary diseases of such diffuse types as pneumonia, interstitial pneumonitis, and adult respiratory distress syndrome (ARDS) or intrathoracic space-occupying lesions (most commonly pneumothorax or pleural effusions).

Once again, the history is basic to understanding the disease process with which the therapist is working, including a history of pneumonia, congestive heart failure, and multiple injury. This information will determine, to a large degree, what progress the therapist might expect to make. For example, very little will be accomplished by the therapist until a large pneumothorax or pleural effusion is evacuated, or a lung tumor (particularly endobronchial lesions and mass-effect lesions) can be either removed or relieved.

An example of this category of restrictive lung disease that is perhaps not so common, but that is devastating in its effects on the patient, carrying a high morbidity and mortality rate, is the ARDS.[12] This disease, with its profound hypoxemia due to severe alveolocapillary membrane block, as well as ventilation-perfusion abnormalities and worsening compliance, poses one of the most severe problems requiring the efforts of all members of the team, including the physical therapist, to obtain the best possible result.

The objective findings of this category are those of the given disease process. The space-occupying lesion frequently will produce dullness to percussion and absent breath sounds, particularly with pleural effusions, whereas a large pneumonia, particularly a multilobed variety, will produce dullness but increased breath sounds including "E" to "A" voice transmission change. Interstitial diseases including ARDS will produce the typical "Velcro" rales to auscultation, while the breath sounds are usually enhanced, not absent, and percussion usually indicates resonance. However, if a pneumothorax intervenes, as it frequently does during therapy for ARDS, the resonance remains the same or increases, whereas breath sounds will diminish, and there will be abrupt worsening in the patient's respiratory status.

Pulmonary Vascular Disease

In pulmonary vascular disease, the available alveolocapillary membrane for oxygen and carbon dioxide exchange is diminished. This general category can be considered a lung disease displaying changes in ventilation-perfusion secondary to other disease states. As the name implies, pulmonary vascular disease is usually accompanied by normal lung volume measurements, but the restriction in pulmonary function is in the arterial and capillary flow to segments or regions of lung tissue. Decreased perfusion results in a major ventilation-perfusion mismatch, with subsequent hypoxemia of the pulmonary venous blood. Usually a decrease in the carbon dioxide level of the blood occurs because of hyperventilation. Dead space ventilation increases above normal (normal is approximately 2 ml/kg of ideal body weight).[6] Since the hypoxemia increases the pulmonary vascoconstriction, a vicious circle develops, increasing ventilation-perfusion mismatch. The abnormalities noted above characteristically increase in severity with any exercise.

Other disease states most commonly associated with this particular situation include pulmonary heart disease secondary to any pathophysiology within the lung vascular bed, including vascular changes attending severe obstructive pulmonary disease or primary disease entities, such as lupus erythematosus, rheumatoid vasculitis, sarcoidosis, and interstitial lung disease of any type. Diseases primarily affecting the vascular bed include deep vein thrombosis with subsequent pulmonary embolism and pulmonary arteriolar obstruction. Over a period of time, left heart failure can cause a significant pulmonary vascular disease state, primarily by backpressure from an elevated left ventricular end-diastolic pressure. This permits transudation of serum into the interstitial portion of the lung, decreasing the diffusion of oxygen from the alveolar surface to the capillary bed.

The history is critical to this disease category. It will generally clarify the underlying or primary disease state (e.g., rheumatoid arthritis, sarcoidosis, lupus erythematosus) and gives some index of it's severity and current treatment. Acute symptoms are also of great importance; for example, dyspnea on exertion is an outstanding feature, as is a chronic nonproductive cough. Occasionally family members will note the development of cyanosis when the patient walks even a short distance. The patient rarely recognizes any fever, nor is one documented. However, profuse night sweats are common within this general category. A history of abrupt pleurisy is often obtained, not infrequently, from those patients with rheumatoid arthritis and lupus erythematosus, but commonly (about 20 to 30 percent of cases) abrupt pleuritic chest pain can be dated to the minute by a patient who has suffered a pulmonary embolism and infarction. Subsequent hemoptysis is characteristic.

If pulmonary thromboembolism is suspected, the examiner should seek a history of swollen painful legs (particularly with walking) or of pelvic heaviness or pain (particularly from patients who have recently traveled a long distance). The history should prompt observation of the lower extremities for increased girth, swelling, tenderness, and redness along the great veins of the lower extremity.

The physical findings in regard to this category include the physical manifestations of the underlying disease state. Such obvious findings as the malar rash of lupus erythematosus or the joint destruction of rheumatoid arthritis can be observed. Nonspecific cyanosis that occurs at rest, but particularly with exercise, is noted. The respiratory rate will generally be increased above normal. The patient with pleurisy is easily recognized by the guarding set of the trunk. Palpation may demonstrate a right ventricular heave or lift; if pulmonary hypertension has become chronic and significant, pulsus paradoxus will frequently be palpable. The patient will generally have a resonant chest, whereas auscultation may frequently show the same "Velcro" rales that we associate with any interstitial disease state. On occasion, the examiner will hear an evanescent pleural friction rub attending the pleuritic disease state, including pulmonary embolism and infarction.

Of particular interest in patients with superimposed right heart failure secondary to pulmonary hypertension and pulmonary vascular disease is the finding of fingernail and toenail bed clubbing or the finding of pretibial edema, suggesting decompensation of the right ventricle. These two findings will generally indicate a poor prognosis. Considerable care must be taken with these patients for any kind of rehabilitative therapy. The development of ischemic heart disease or of supraventricular arrhythmias (e.g., multifocal atrial tachycardia or atrial fibrillation) is very frequent in these patients.

Pulmonary function measurements will generally show a combination of obstructive and restrictive defects in those patients with interstitial lung disease. There will frequently be decreased compliance. As with other diseases, the maximum exercise ventilation will be diminished. This decrease in maximum ventilation should be correlated with oxygen consumption and measured in any of these disease categories in order to estimate the functional capacity at which physical therapy (e.g., by bike or treadmill walking) can be started.

Ventilatory Regulation Disorders

The characterization of a disordered ventilatory regulation[7,8] is defined by the limits of hypoventilation or hyperventilation. This category is generally a secondary disease state found in patients with other types of pulmonary disease that have already been considered. These patients seem to have a disordered central brain stem response either to elevated carbon dioxide or to lowered oxygen concentration, or both. If the brain stem is not the center of the disordered response, the peripheral chemoreceptors (e.g., in the carotid bodies) are at fault.

There are three general disease states included among the ventilatory regulatory disorders. First, there is central sleep apnea. This condition is usually related to previous damage to the brain stem by various insults, including blood vessel occlusion, injury, neoplasia (either benign or malignant), or infection (including viral). Central sleep apnea is occasionally idiopathic. A peculiar disease state is that of Ondine's curse. Such patients are noted to breathe normally when they are awake but fail to respire when asleep. Secondly, peripherally insensitive states to oxygen and/or carbon dioxide changes in the bloodstream include hypothyroidism in which the patient lacking adequate thyroid hormone is simply insensitive to oxygen and carbon dioxide fluctuations. These patients also have significant myxedematous accretions within the lung tissue. A common cause of death in the hypothyroid patient is hypothermia in coma. Another cause is pneumonia

to which the patient fails to mount a response. Finally, probably the commonest state of hypoventilation noted, usually suspected by the history, is that of hypoventilation associated with the intake of narcotic and sedative medications. This is particularly true in those with underlying chronic lung disease of any kind. While the history is important for these patients, necessary information is often lacking. Observation will indicate a hypoventilatory state with a slow or absent respiratory rate, despite a drop in oxygen saturation. If awake, the patient will be subject to confusion and hallucinatory disorientation.

To define this particular pattern of disease state, the therapist can measure the alveolar-arterial oxygen gradient, which should be normal in central or chemical hypoventilation, assuming normal lungs.[8] As a corollary to the normalcy of the A-a oxygen gradient, other lung volume measurements will generally be normal, although in the case of hypothyroidism a restrictive pattern will sometimes be noted.

In the case of hyperventilation in disorders of ventilatory regulation, it should be noted that hyperventilation, or the "hyperventilation syndrome," is certainly the most common of these states and seems to be largely a stress reaction to either psychological or physical stimuli. This particular central hyperventilation pattern should not be accepted, however, as the initial diagnosis, but rather should be a diagnosis of exclusion. Once again, there should be a demonstrably normal A-a oxygen gradient.

A number of medications or drugs will cause hyperventilation on the basis of either central or peripheral stimulation, although most of these act centrally. Most notable are the amphetamines and cocaine. The use of progesterone in the treatment of central sleep apnea and obesity-hypoventilation syndrome is also associated with hyperventilation. The hyperventilatory response to acidosis of any kind, whether lactic acidosis or a diabetic ketoacidosis, is an obvious example of chemical hyperventilation.

A careful history will describe the basis for the presence of these disease states. Objectively, a patient who has an increased respiratory rate above 18 per minute at rest, for example in the presence of Kussmaul breathing (deep rapid respiration) with either lactic acidosis or diabetic ketoacidosis, is particularly impressive. The appearance is that of a "driven" respiratory pattern. A peculiar fruity or acetone odor to the breath is a reasonably good tipoff to the presence of either ketoacidosis or early salicylate excess. Physical findings are rather minimal, although with diabetic ketoacidosis one will frequently note evidence of dehydration with dry mucous membranes, cracked lips, and decreased skin turgor. Lowered blood pressure is frequently present as well. The lungs will show no particular evidence of decreased chest expansion or dullness to percussion, unless some other process is present. Auscultation will generally detect clear breath sounds, unless such entities as aspiration have supervened. Generally speaking, lung functions will be normal, including the A-a oxygen gradient.

SUMMARY

This chapter presents a system for assessing the pulmonary system. The important evaluation techniques and tools were discussed and related to reviewing the patient's chart, taking a history, and performing a physical examination. Of the physical examination procedures discussed, auscultation is emphasized, including an overview of relevant anatomy. Identification and interpretation of normal and abnormal chest sounds are covered in detail. All the evaluation procedures and findings described will assist the therapist in developing an appropriate treatment program for the patient.

Numerous pathologic conditions are discussed throughout the chapter. Chronic pulmonary diseases are emphasized because of their relatively high incidence, their long-term debilitating effect on the patient, and the impact that physical therapists can have on the quality of life of these patients, if the appropriate treatment program is developed. The four general disease categories presented—chronic obstructive pulmonary disease, restrictive pulmonary disease, vascular diseases of the lungs, and disorders of ventilatory regulation—are roughly separated on the basis of basic physiologic measurements. The ability of the therapist to use the evaluative techniques described to separate the patient's disease state into one of the four categories will largely determine the most effective therapeutic approach.

REFERENCES

1. Hodgkin JD: Home care and pulmonary rehabilitation. p. 216. In Kacmarek RM, Stroller JK (eds): Current Respiratory Care. CV Mosby, St. Louis, 1988
2. Petty TL: Pulmonary rehabilitation: Why, who, when, what, how? J Respir Dis 2:200, 1990
3. American College of Sports Medicine: Guidelines for Exercise Testing and Prescription. 3rd Ed. Lea & Febiger, Philadelphia, 1986
4. Skinner JS: Exercise Testing and Exercise Prescription for Special Cases. Lea & Febiger, Philadelphia, 1987
5. Altose MA: The physiological basis of pulmonary function testing. Ciba Found Symp 31:21, 1979
6. Sharpiro BA, Harrison RA, Kacmarek RM, Cane RD: Clinical Application of Respiratory Care. 3rd Ed. Year Book Medical, Chicago, 1985
7. Bates DV: Respiratory Function and Disease. 3rd Ed. WB Saunders, Montreal, 1989
8. Luce JM, Tyler ML, Pierson DJ: Intensive Respiratory Care. WB Saunders, Philadelphia, 1984
9. Carter R, Linsenbardt S, Blevins W, et al: Exercise gas exchange in patients with moderately severe to severe chronic obstructive pulmonary disease. J Cardiopulm Rehabil 9:243, 1989
10. Carter R, Nicotra B: Recognition and management of respiratory muscle fatigue and chronic obstructive pulmonary disease (COPD). Int Med 9:171, 1988
11. Smith PL, Schwartz AR: Sleep disordered breathing in adults. Contemp Intern Med 1:72, 1990
12. Petty TL: Acute respiratory distress syndrome (ARDS). Dis Mon 36:9, 1990
13. Wilkins RL, Sheldon RL, Krider SJ: Clinical Assessment in Respiratory Care. 2nd Ed. CV Mosby, St. Louis, 1990

SUGGESTED READINGS

Cherniak RM, Cherniak L: Respiration in Health and Disease. 3rd Ed. WB Saunders, Philadelphia, 1983

Enright PL, Hyatt RE: Office Spirometry—A Practical Guide to the Selection and Use of Spirometers. Lea & Febiger, Philadelphia, 1987

Frownfelter DL: Chest Physical Therapy and Pulmonary Rehabilitation. 2nd Ed. Year Book Medical, Chicago, 1987

Irwin S, Tecklin JS: Cardiopulmonary Physical Therapy. 2nd Ed. CV Mosby, St. Louis, 1990

Lane EE, Walker JF: Clinical Arterial Blood Gas Analysis. CV Mosby, St. Louis, 1987

Morgan WKC, Seaton A: Occupational Lung Diseases. 2nd Ed. Keith C. Morgan and WB Saunders, Philadelphia, 1984

Murray JF: The Normal Lung—The Basis For Diagnosis and Treatment of Pulmonary Disease. 2nd Ed. WB Saunders, Philadelphia, 1986

4

Screening for Gastrointestinal System Disease

MICHAEL B. KOOPMEINERS, M.D.

The gastrointestinal (GI) system is responsible for providing the body with the essential nutrients for survival. The extraction of these essential nutrients from ingested food—digestion—begins in the mouth with the mechanical breakdown of food. As the bolus of food moves to the esophagus and progresses through the intestinal tract, chemical processes complete the digestive process. Undigestable food particles are stored in the sigmoid colon until they are eliminated through the rectum. The liver and pancreas, are also part of the GI system. These organs produce digestive enzymes and hormones to facilitate the breakdown of food particles.

Pathology of the GI system can lead to low back pain, leg pain, and thoracic spine complaints; less obviously, it can lead to shoulder pain. The physical therapist can identify markers of GI pathology. Once alerted to the possibility of visceral pathology, the physical therapist can provide appropriate consultation. Once it is established that the presenting complaints are secondary to biomechanical dysfunction rather than to visceral pathology, appropriate patient care can be initiated.

This chapter reviews the normal anatomy and physiology of the structures of the GI system. Figure 4-1 presents an anatomic overview of the GI system. It is not my intent to highlight all possible diseases of the GI system—only those conditions most likely to be encountered by the physical therapist are discussed. These conditions may mimic musculoskeletal system dysfunction or may have an impact on the type of physical therapy modality used.

ANATOMY AND PHYSIOLOGY OF THE GASTROINTESTINAL SYSTEM

The mouth provides an entrance to the GI system, as well as initiating digestion by the mechanical breakdown of ingested food material. The normal swallowing mechanisms, facilitated by cranial nerves X and XII, move the food bolus from the mouth to the esophagus. The esophagus is a hollow muscular tube that connects the mouth to the stomach. It runs in the chest cavity, lying in the midline in front of the vertebral column. High in the chest cavity, the esophagus runs behind the trachea; lower down, it runs behind the heart, with the descending aorta on its left. It attaches to the stomach just below the diaghram. The lower esophageal sphincter is a one-way valve that prevents stomach contents from regurgitating into the lower esophagus.

The upper esophagus is striated muscle under voluntary control. The lower esophagus and lower esophageal sphincter are smooth muscle under involuntary control mediated by the vagus, or 10th cranial nerve. The involuntary activity of the esophagus and of the intestinal tract is primary peristalsis, rhythmic progressive pulsatile contractions of the hollow viscus tube. The lower esophageal sphincter relaxes as a per-

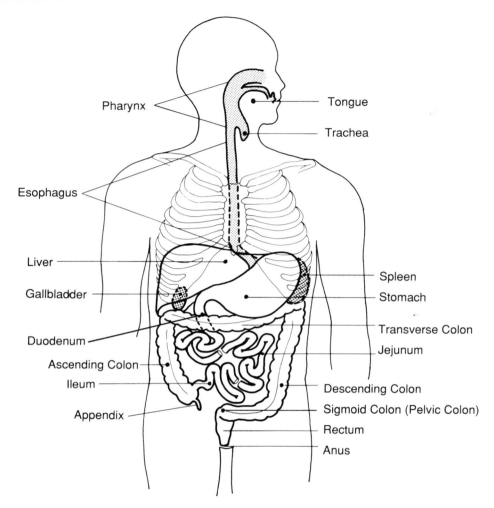

Fig. 4-1. Anatomic overview of the gastrointestinal system.

istalstic wave approaches so that food can enter the stomach.

Blood supply of the upper esophagus comes from the branches of the thoracic artery. Lower esophageal blood supply comes from the branches of the left gastric artery and inferior phrenic arteries. A plexus of veins drains the esophagus, forming multiple anastomosis with the portal venous system of the stomach. The esophagus has two main functions—transport of food and mechanical dispersion of food—the first step of digestion.

The stomach is a dilatation of intestinal tract separated

from the esophagus by the lower esophageal sphincter and from the first part of the small intestine by the pyloric valve. It is located in the mid-epigastric area of the abdomen immediately behind the transverse colon. It partially covers the pancreas, which is located deep in the abdominal cavity. Arterial blood supply comes from the celiac trunk off the aorta and from several branches off the splenic artery. The gastric veins enter the portal venous system. With obstructive liver pathology, such as cirrhosis, this venous system becomes engorged because of increased pressure necessary to "push" blood through the liver. This condition subsequently leads to esophageal varicose veins. The nerve supply is from the vagus nerve. A pacemaker in the proximal stomach initiates peristalsis for the upper intestinal tract.

Three mechanical functions of the stomach are identified: storage, mixing, and grinding. Outflow regulation of processed food particles to the small intestine is another important function. The rate of movement of the stomach contents to the small intestine must be balanced with the rate of pancreatic and biliary secretions, to permit efficient extraction of nutrients.

The stomach also has exocrine and endocrine functions. Exocrine functions (local secretion of chemicals) include secretion of acid, intrinsic factor, pepsin, mucus, and bicarbonate. All these ingredients are important for digestion. Although these secretions are normally very balanced, a mismatch of these secretions can lead to peptic ulcer disease.

Endocrine function is the secretion of hormones, which are chemicals produced in one part of the body that have an action in another part of the body. Specifically, the stomach produces various hormones that stimulate the pancreas, liver, and gallbladder to release their digestive enzymes into the duodenum.

The small intestine begins at the pyloric valve and ends with its connection to the large intestine in the right lower abdominal quadrant. It has three distinct parts: duodenum, jejunum, and ileum. The duodenum is the first 25 cm of the small intestine and lies in the right upper quadrant just below the liver. It is almost entirely retroperitoneal, surrounding the pancreas and lying on top of the ileopsoas muscle and moving across the vertebral column at the level of L4.

The duodenum receives the slurry from the stomach through the pyloric valve, as well as the fluids from the pancreas and liver through the common bile duct. This is the area of the small intestine that is susceptible to ulcers. The blood supply is from the inferior mesenteric artery and gastric artery and is drained by the portal veins. The vagus nerve through the celiac ganglion provides the nerve supply to the duodenum and to the rest of the small intestine. Pain in the small intestine is produced by distention or violent cramps. The function of the duodenum is to neutralize the acid in the food slurry delivered from the stomach, as well as mix the food slurry with the pancreatic and biliary secretions.

The jejunum makes up the bulk of the small intestine. This undulating hollow viscus tube in the abdominal cavity stretches for 2.4 m. It is attached by the omentum to the posterior aspect of the abdominal cavity over the vertebral column. The omentum is the conduit through which the blood supply, nerve supply, and lymphatic supply attach to the small intestine. The superior mesenteric artery and vein and the vagus splanchnic nerve provide the small intestine with the necessary blood and nervous functions. The jejunum is mainly concerned with absorption of nutrients, water, and electrolytes. It has a significant capacity for absorption, since its surface area is greater than that of double tennis court.

The ileum is the terminal 40 cm of the intestinal tract. It is located in the right lower abdominal quadrant and attaches to the colon through the ileocecal valve. The ileum provides the same functions as the jejunum, but it has a unique function of absorbing bile acids and intrinsic factor, recycling these chemicals in the body. Inability to reabsorb intrinsic factor causes a major disability in the form of vitamin B_{12} deficiency, which leads to pernicious anemia.

The large intestine (colon) stretches 1.5 m, beginning in the right lower abdominal quadrant, traverses the periphery of the abdominal cavity, and ends with attachment to the rectum in the posterior pelvis. The cecum located at the beginning of the colon is the blind-ended pouch to which the appendix is attached. The appendix and cecum are frequently retroperitoneal in the right iliac fossa, lying on top of the ileopsoas muscle. The ascending colon, on the right side of the abdominal cavity, is a retroperitoneal structure that lies on top of the quadratus lumborum, ileopsoas, and iliacus muscles. The transverse colon in the upper abdominal cavity runs over the stomach and the spleen, at the level of the umbilicus. The colon then turns caudally toward the rectum, becoming the descending colon, which, again, is retroperitoneal, lying on the psoas and quadratus lumborus muscles. The last part of the colon, or sigmoid colon, begins at the pelvic brim, crosses the sacrum, and curves and lies in the midline at the third sacral segment. The rectum lies in the mid-pelvis behind the prostate and bladder in males and behind the vagina in females.

The blood supply is from the superior mesenteric and inferior mesenteric artery. The portal vein drains the intestinal tract and goes through the liver before ultimately returning the blood to the central circulation via the inferior vena cava. The nerve supply is through the vagus nerve; the mid-colon contains an intrinsic pacemaker that controls the peristalsis activity of the mid- and lower colon. The function of the colon is to absorb water and electrolytes. The distal colon stores waste products in the form of feces. The rectosigmoid and anal canal have the function of expulsion of feces.

The liver is located in the right upper abdominal quadrant under the diaphragm, with its lower margins at the lower edge of the right rib cage. The gallbladder is located beneath the liver in the midclavicular line. A tight capsule surrounds the liver; stretching of this capsule causes the pain associated with liver pathology. The liver has two blood supplies: the hepatic artery makes up 10 percent of the blood flow and provides the necessary oxygen for the cells of the liver; and the portal vein makes up 90 percent of the blood flow coming into the liver. The portal vein carries recently absorbed nutrients from the stomach and intestine, as well as hormones secreted by the pancreas and GI tract, to the liver for processing.

The liver plays a major role in regulating the serum levels of solutes, such as fat, protein, and carbohydrate, needed by the muscles, brain, heart, and other organs to function adequately. Bile is produced in the liver and is instrumental in the absorption of lipids and lipid-soluable substances. The liver also has a role in drug metabolism, in the normal rate of production of red blood cells, and in vitamin K production, which is necessary for normal blood clotting.

Besides the plexus of arteries, veins, and lymphatics in the liver, there is another plexus of hollow collecting tubes, called the biliary tree. The biliary tree collects bile, the digestive enzyme produced in the liver, and transports it through the hepatic duct to the stomach. Branching off this hepatic duct and located beneath the liver is the gallbladder (Fig. 4-1). The gall-bladder is a storage sac that holds the bile until a bolus of food presents itself to the stomach. Hormone stimulation causes the gallbladder to contract and expel its contents into the hepatic duct, which ultimately empties into the duodenum. In addition to storing bile, the gallbladder concentrates bile by preferentially absorbing water. When it goes awry, this process contributes to the formation of gallstones.

The pancreas is another gland that is extremely important to normal functioning of the GI tract. It is located retroperitoneally, lying on top of the vertebral column, and extends to the left upper abdominal quadrant. It is surrounded anteriorly by the stomach, the duodenum on the right, the spleen on the left, and posteriorly by the vertebral column, kidney, aorta, and inferior vena cava. The pancreas secretes bicarbonate and digestive enzymes, the production of which is stimulated by eating. Bicarbonate is a major defense against gastric acid in the duodenum. Large acid production or too rapid delivery of the gastric acid to the duodenum will overwhelm the bicarbonate production of the pancreas and contribute to the formation of duodenal ulcers.

The pancreas has important endocrine functions. It secretes insulin and glugacon, as well as multiple other hormones necessary for normal regulation of glucose levels and several other substances in the bloodstream. The blood supply is extremely generous. The several major arteries going to the pancreas have generous anastomosis, but the nerve supply to the pancreas is relatively poor. As a result, the pain of cancer infiltration is minimal, making early detection of cancer of the pancreas extremely difficult.

Although the spleen is not part of the GI tract, it is intimately located in the left upper abdominal quadrant below the rib cage, surrounded by various organs of the GI system. It lies against the paraspinous muscles on the left side. The function of the spleen is to filter out foreign substances as well as old degenerating blood cells from the bloodstream.

The GI system is responsible for maintaining adequate levels of all the essential nutrients in the bloodstream to facilitate the normal activity of the organism. It does this through complicated mechanical and biochemical processes. Many of the organs that make up the GI system are located in close proximity to various "organs" of the musculoskeletal system. This association is not obviously appreciated at times, since the significant part of those relationships is hidden in the posterior aspect of the abdominal cavity. The importance of additional knowledge concerning the GI tract to the physical therapist becomes obvious when these relationships are appreciated.

DISEASES OF THE GASTROINTESTINAL SYSTEM

Visceral pathology of the GI system can present with symptoms easily confused with conditions of mechanical dysfunction. For example, right shoulder pain is a frequent complaint with liver or gallbladder pathology, and back pain can be associated with peptic ulcer or metastatic colon cancer. An awareness of GI conditions and the associated signs and symptoms that can present as mechanical dysfunction will enhance the physical therapist's skills to identify these conditions and direct the patient to seek consultation with a medical colleague.

Infectious Diseases of the Mouth and Throat

The most frequent category of diseases that affect the mouth and throat are infectious diseases. The presenting complaint for an infection of the throat may be neck pain associated with a reactive lymph node. If a swollen mass is found during the examination of the neck, the physical therapist should ask about sore throat, sore teeth, mouth sores, and so forth. If the swollen gland persists for 4 weeks, medical follow-up is warranted.

Esophageal Spasm

Esophageal spasm is a combination of esophageal colic and dysphagia of unknown cause. The spasm is exacerbated by hot or cold fluids, carbonated beverages, and exposure to stress. The resulting difficult swallowing, dysphagia, involves both liquids and solids.

The pain is colicky or crampy in nature, located substernally. It can radiate to the back, neck, jaw, or arms. The intensity is extremely variable, from minimal to severe symptoms. It may last for a few minutes to several hours. This condition may be confused with angina. A physical therapist may confuse this condition with disorders of the mid- and upper thoracic spine, left shoulder, and the anterior rib cage.

Acid Peptic Disorders of the Stomach and Duodenum

A common pathology of the stomach and the first part of the duodenum that the physical therapist will come across frequently is that of acid peptic disorders. This is a group of disorders with very similar pathologic processes, including reflex esophagitis, gastritis, gastric ulcer, duodenitis, and duodenal ulcer. The common pathologic process is that of damage to the mucosa. Simple irritation of the mucosa will lead to conditions such as gastritis, while an actual erosion through the mucosa is an ulcer, either gastric or duodenal, depending on its location. One or more organs can be involved simultaneously.

The precise mechanism of these conditions is unclear. It is not simply a condition of too much acid but an imbalance of the acid, pepsin, bicarbonate, and mucous production of the intestinal tract. Thirty-five percent of males and 25 percent of females are affected at any one time. However, only five to ten percent of the individuals are symptomatic. Seventy-five percent of affected individuals will have recurrent disease. Heavy smoking, heavy alcohol use, and use of nonsteroidal anti-inflammatory drugs (NSAIDs) increase the likelihood of this disease.

Acid peptic disorders present with a pain in the epigastric or right upper abdominal quadrant area of the stomach. The pain may radiate to the back; this is especially true of posterior penetrating ulcers of the stomach. It is frequently described as a gnawing episodic pain, worse at night or when the stomach is empty and usually improves with food intake. Some weight loss, nausea, vomiting, and anorexia may be associated with this condition. Black tarry stools or vomiting of blood signify bleeding, which is the major cause of death in these patients. Other major complications include perforation leading to acute abdominal pain and necessitating surgery, as well as gastric outlet obstruction.

Physical therapists should think of these conditions whenever they have patients with lower thoracic spine complaints and lower anterior rib cage and upper abdominal complaints. With the significant use of NSAIDs in the patient population seeking care from physical therapists, these conditions must also be monitored for in clients being treated for conditions other than thoracic spine/upper abdominal complaints.

Liver and Gallbladder Disorders

Hepatitis, inflammation of the liver, and cholecystitis, inflammation of the gallbladder, are conditions that can present with right upper abdominal quadrant pain, but also quite frequently present with right shoulder pain. The liver has multiple functions to perform. One is the production of bile acids, which are secreted and collected in the biliary duct system, coalescing into the hepatic duct and ultimately draining into the duodenum. The gallbladder is a small sac attached to the hepatic duct that stores the bile acids that are continually produced by the liver until they are needed, such as occurs after a meal. The gallbladder also concentrates the bile acids during the storage process by removing water. In so doing, precipitates will sometimes form in the bile acids, which will act as nideses for the formation of gallstones.

Gallstones

Gallstones vary in size from sand consistency up to stones several inches in diameter. The precise cause of the formation of these stones is unclear. Once formed, these stones can then irritate the lining of the gallbladder and/or occlude the outflow tract of the gallbladder, leading to inflammation and/or infection of the gallbladder. Ten to 20 percent of Americans have gallstones. The incidence increases with age. Obese females over 40 years of age have a significantly greater incidence of cholecystitis. Gallstones are frequently asymptomatic. Symptoms develop with occlusion of the outflow tract or inflammation of the gallbladder secondary to the gallstones. Pain is located in the right upper abdominal quadrant and may radiate to the back. Pain may also be referred to the scapula, right shoulder, or neck area. Pain is frequently abrupt in onset with a gradual defervescence of symptoms. Nausea, vomiting, and fever will occur with this condition—if not at the onset, certainly within hours of the onset. These patients will have tenderness, and occasionally a mass can be palpated in the right upper abdominal quadrant.

Cholecystitis and Hepatitis

While cholecystitis can occasionally confuse the physical therapist working with patients with right shoulder and right mid-back pain, hepatitis can do the same. Hepatitis is inflammation of the liver caused by several agents, such as the infectious agents of hepatitis A and B or a chemical agent of which alcohol is the most common. This disease may be entirely subclinical and unsuspected in an individual appearing relatively healthy, or it may be rapidly progressive and fatal. For the viral agents, the onset of symptoms is usually 2 to 14 days after exposure. Patients will be fatigued, anorexic, and nauseated, with occasional fever and emesis. Musculoskeletal complaints beside the right shoulder and right mid-back pain could include headache, myalgias, and arthralgias. Dark urine and light-colored stools are frequent observations made by patients with hepatitis. These patients will have tenderness in the right upper abdominal quadrant, and the liver will occasionally be palpable.

Viral hepatitis is an infectious disease and is potentially transmissible to the therapist. Type A is transmitted by the fecal-oral route. This is an important consideration when working with patients who are incontinent or disabled. Type B and type non-A, non-B (NANB) are transmitted by percutaneous, oral-oral, or venereal means. Needle sticks are a significant route of hepatitis B infection among hospital personnel.

Alcoholic hepatitis will present in an extremely similar manner but will also have associated with it the stigmata of chronic or acute alcohol use (see Ch. 11). Besides causing hepatitis, heavy alcohol use is a leading cause of pancreatitis, an inflammation of the pancreas. Pancreatitis can also be caused by gallstones or blunt abdominal trauma. In 20 percent of cases, no clear etiology is identified. Acute pancreatitis occurs in 20 of 100,000 patients. While this condition resolves spontaneously in many patients, chronic pancreatitis develops in 15 percent.

Pancreatitis

Pain is the dominant presenting complaint in patients with pancreatitis. There is a constant waxing and waning pain in the mid-epigastric and left upper abdominal quadrant area. One-half of patients will have pain radiating to the upper lumbar and lower thoracic area. The pain may also radiate retrosternally, to the right upper abdominal quadrant and left scapular and supraspinous area. These patients are very uncomfortable. Eating, alcohol intake, and vomiting will lead to exacerbation of the pain. On physical examination, they are frequently very tender in the mid-epigastric area and can also be tender in the lower thoracic, upper lumber spine area. These patients frequently have the associated stigmata of chronic alcohol use, gynecomastia (enlargement of the breast), jaundice, muscle wasting, abdominal bloating, and so forth.

Colon Disorders

Colon Cancer

Colon cancer has several characteristics that make it extremely important for the physical therapist to be aware of this condition. It is the most frequently diagnosed cancer in the United States. It is more prevalent in developed countries; the United States has one of the highest incidences in the world. Five to 6 percent of the population will develop colon cancer. The clinical importance lies in the frequency; also, early detection leads to substantial improvement in outcome. The physical therapist will encounter this disease either by local spread of the disease leading to local pathology that mimics complaints of mechanical dysfunction origin or by metastatic presentation of this lesion leading to complaints anywhere in the body, but more frequently in the thoracic spine and rib cage.

Risk factors for colon cancer are (1) age over 40 years; (2) prior history of inflammatory bowel disease, such as Crohn's disease, ulcerative colitis; (3) prior cancer of another organ; and (4) benign polyps of the colon.

Screening the stool for blood is advocated for any patient over 40 years of age. It is important to bear in mind, however, that this is a screening test and is not a definitive diagnostic procedure.

Patients with colon cancer may complain of gradually progressive constipation and/or a reduction in the stool caliber. New blood mixed in with the stools or old blood may also be a presenting complaint. Frequent nonspecific symptoms that are true of any cancer condition will also occur, such as weakness, malaise, anorexia, and weight loss. This cancer frequently metastasizes to the liver, lung, and bone. It is not uncommon for the diagnosis to be made by recognizing a metastatic lesion as opposed to the primary lesion in the colon. The physical therapist will find it extremely important to screen for this disease, especially in patients over 40 years of age.

Diverticulitis

Another relatively common colon disease process is that of diverticulitis. This local inflammation in the wall of the apex of the small outpouching of the colon is caused by trapped feces. It can occur anywhere in the colon but frequently presents in the descending or sigmoid colon in the left lower quadrant of the abdominal area. This, again, usually occurs in patients over 40 years of age and has no particular predilection for either sex. Constant left lower quadrant abdominal pain radiating to the low back, pelvis, or left leg are the complaints associated with this disease. Fever, if present, is usually low grade. Usually there is a change in the stooling pattern, becoming loose and watery or hard. Rarely is bleeding noted in this disease.

Enlargement of the Spleen

Enlargement of the spleen frequently presents with vague left upper abdominal quadrant pain, left flank pain, and mid-back pain. Two main causes of spleen enlargement are infectious mononucleosis and cancer. Both conditions occur in young individuals: mono, almost solely in individuals between 15 and 25 years of age; cancer, such as acute leukemia, and lymphomas, occurs in younger individuals more frequently, but can occur in any age. The most significant complication of spleen envolement is splenic rupture, which can lead to massive bleeding and occasional death. The therapist must be very aware of this fact when doing soft tissue work in the left upper abdominal quadrant on patients with suspected splenic enlargement. Additional symptoms besides pain that should make the therapist suspicious of pathology other than biomechanical are fatigue, malaise, weight loss, and lymph node enlargement.

One other condition may be encountered by the therapist, especially if their patient population includes a high percentage of blacks. Sickle cell disease, occurring almost exclusively in blacks, will most likely be diagnosed before seeing the therapist and can lead to chronic spleen enlargement.

Abdominal Hernia

An abdominal hernia is the protrusion of abdominal contents through an opening in the muscle walls that surround the abdominal cavity. Two common areas in which hernias occur are the inguinal area and the diaphragm. An enlargement of the normal opening for the esophagus in the diaphragm allows part of the stomach to protrude into the chest cavity. This common condition is called a hiatal hernia and leads to symptoms similar to those of esophageal spasm.

Hernias in the lower abdominal area are direct or indirect femoral hernias or inguinal hernias. The differences, although important to surgeons, are not necessary for the physical therapist to appreciate—only to realize the multiple terms used for hernia. The inguinal canal is the normal opening in the three layers of abdominal wall musculature that allows the spermatic cord and related vascular and nervous structures to traverse from the testicle in the scrotum in their intra-abdominal connections.

A small enlargement of the canal may permit a small protrusion and lead to subtle lower abdominal, hip, and anterior thigh pain. A larger opening and protrusion of intestine, while leading to similar pain complaints, will be less subtle to diagnose because of the presence of an obvious mass. The wide range of defects can make hernias difficult to diagnose even for

the astute surgeon. This condition should be thought of in patients presenting with lower abdominal wall complaints, as well as hip and anterior thigh complaints. Hernias will produce pain with contraction of the abdominal musculature. This may be intermittent; on one occasion, there may be trapping and pinching of abdominal contents in the hernia sac, and at other times, if no abdominal contents are present in the hernia sac, no complaints may be elicited from similar activity. If the onset of symptoms is sudden, the diagnosis is made easier. Frequently the onset is subtle, with gradually worsening symptoms over time as the opening enlarges with repeat minor injury.

Strangulation is the most serious complication of hernias. This occurs when the blood supply to the abdominal contents in the hernia sac is compromised by the pressure that builds in the canal. Ischemia causing pain is the clinical result of strangulation; left untreated, it can lead to bowel necrosis and bowel death. This not so subtle condition will be noted by progressively worsening pain, nausea, vomiting, and fever. If suspected, immediate physician referral is indicated.

Summary

Gastrointestinal pathology has multiple areas of symptomatic overlap, with conditions frequently cared for by physical therapists. Complaints can be as diverse as shoulder strap pain and local cervical pain, secondary to metastatic lesions from colon cancers, or low back pain from pancreatitis or hip pain from a hernia. The alert therapist along with collaborating medical care providers can ensure patients of high-quality appropriate medical care.

ABDOMINAL EVALUATION

A history of complaints that may be secondary to visceral pathology should prompt screening for GI pathology. The presenting complaints that should make a therapist suspicious of nonbiomechanical problems were reviewed above.

Directed questions of the patient about symptoms of

possible GI pathology is the next step in the evaluation. A series of items that can be noted by the therapist for his questioning process includes the following:

Hemoptysis
Nausea
Vomiting
Melena (black tarry stools)
Hematochezia (bright red blood in the stools)
Fatty food intolerance
Change in stool color
Constipation (hard to push out)
Diarrhea (frequent watery stool)
Change in urine color
Jaundice
Drug use
Sexual activity
Previous history of hepatitis
Previous history of a hernia

Each question is tied to one or more of the pathologies discussed above. Negative answers to all the questions may be enough reassurance that visceral pathology is unlikely. If the patient reports several of the symptoms, a screening evaluation of the abdomen would be the next step to take. Positive responses to all the questions, especially if there is an exaggerated quality to the answers, should raise the possibility of psychological problems (see Ch. 11).

Physical Therapy Evaluation of the Abdomen

A screening evaluation of the abdomen begins with inspection. Figure 4-1 shows the location of intra-abdominal contents in relationship to external landmarks. Figure 4-2 presents the common terminology for various abdominal regions. During inspection, the physical therapist looks for asymmetries in shape and size such as in the lower abdominal quadrant or the right upper abdominal quadrant possibly signifying hernia or gallbladder disease, respectively. Noting abdominal scars may remind the patient of surgery they had forgotten to mention during the subjective examination.

Auscultation/Percussion

Auscultation to screen for bruits is the next part of an evaluation. Particular attention should be paid to the mid-epigastric, right and left lower abdominal quadrants and to the femoral areas, since these are locations for aneurysms and obstructions of the blood vessels (see Ch. 2). Percussion, seemingly simple but time

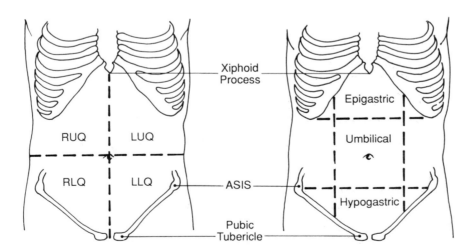

Fig. 4-2. Terminology used to delineate the regions of the abdomen. RUQ, right upper (abdominal) quadrant; LUQ, left upper (abdominal) quadrant; RLQ, right lower (abdominal) quadrant; LLQ, left lower (abdominal) quadrant.

consuming to master, is useful in evaluating liver and spleen size. Normal liver percusses to 4 to 5 inches in the midclavicular line (Fig. 4-3 and 4-4). A dullness in the quality of the noise in response to the percussion will signify a solid organ underneath the fingers; this is opposed to a more hollow-sounding resonance when hollow organs or cavities are percussed. This would help differentiate the location of the liver versus just percussing over lung tissue or the abdominal contents caudal to the liver. The spleen, found in the left upper abdominal quadrant, should be percussed over the rib cage at the caudal end of the anterior axillary line (Fig. 4-5). If the spleen is of normal size a hollowness should be noted during the percussion. If the spleen is sufficiently enlarged, a dullness may be noted during the procedure. To protect these structures, location of the liver and spleen should be noted before soft tissue mobilization techniques are performed in the upper abdominal areas. Percussion is one method to help delineate the boundaries of these two solid organs.

Palpation

Palpation in all four abdominal quadrants is the last part of the evaluation. Gastrointestinal system structures located in the right upper quadrant include the

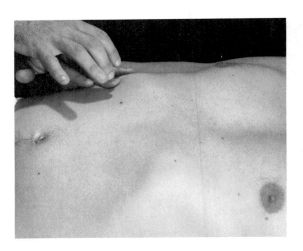

Fig. 4-4. Percussing for the caudal border of the liver in the midclavicular line.

liver, gallbladder, and components of the small and large intestine. A portion of the stomach, the tail of the pancreas, components of the small and large intestine, and the spleen all lie in the left upper quadrant. The right and left kidneys also lie far posterior in the respective upper quadrant. Components of the large in-

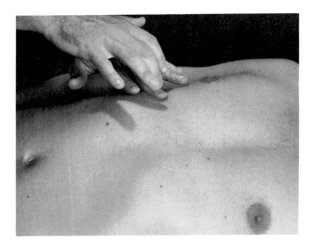

Fig. 4-3. Percussing for the cephalad edge of the liver in the midclavicular line.

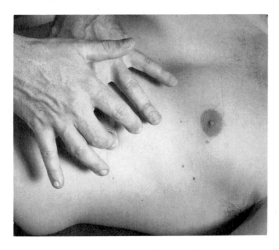

Fig. 4-5. Percussing for the spleen in the anterior axillary line.

estine, including the appendix, fill the right lower quadrant, while other components of the large intestine are located in the left lower quadrant. Masses associated with colon cancer or diverticulitis can be found anywhere in the abdomen but are more common in the left lower quadrant. Hernias will present as tender masses in the femoral triangle or groin area and can occur in both men and women. Midline masses that are pulsatile may signify the presence of an aneurysm and should be referred for immediate consultation if noted. Generally speaking, the therapist should have difficulty palpating the specific abdominal visceral organs if they are not diseased, because of the hollow soft nature of their structure. Exceptions may be solid organs, such as the liver, which may extend caudal to the rib cage, or fecal material, which may be palpable in the descending colon in the left lower quadrant.

Besides assessing for abdominal masses, tenderness and muscle guarding are other physical findings that may be elicited by palpation. A subset of tenderness that should raise concern is rebound tenderness. Rebound tenderness is when the pain experienced by the patient is worse with quick release of the palpatory pressure, as opposed to when the initial pressure was applied. If this sign is present, immediate referral to a physician should be made to rule out peritoneal irritation secondary to serious pathology, including abdominal bleeding. Abdominal muscle guarding or rigidity may occur in response to underlying visceral pathology. If noted, this self-protective reflex response should be correlated with other examination findings to help differentiate muscle guarding secondary to a local muscle injury, or to an injury to a deeper musculoskeletal system structure, from visceral pathology.

If the therapist finds a tender or painful area in the abdomen, the patient, in the supine position, can be asked to lift the head and neck off the table. As the abdominals tighten, the therapist again applies pressure to the painful area; if the pain is still present, the lesion probably lies in the superficial myofascial wall of the abdomen, as opposed to a deeper visceral structure. If, instead, tenderness and pain disappear when the abdominals tighten but return when palpated with the abdominals relaxed, a deep visceral structure could be the source of the discomfort. Correlation of these findings with other examination findings should again help the therapist determine the involvement of musculoskeletal system structures versus elements of the GI system.

Diagnosis

A definitive diagnosis is not the goal for a physical therapy screening evaluation of the abdominal area. The evaluation can give clues that visceral pathology may be present. When suspicion is aroused in the astute physical therapist, physician consultation is warranted to ensure nonvisceral causes of the patient's presenting complaints.

SUMMARY

Patients presenting to the physical therapist may have visceral pathology as the primary cause of their presenting complaint. Therapists need to be aware of this possibility and should have a plan to address it. To help with this, the anatomy and physiology of the GI system are reviewed; common conditions are outlined to increase the awareness of visceral pathologies that present, such as mechanical dysfunction conditions; and an evaluation process of directed questioning and physical evaluation is presented as a suggested approach to patients where visceral pathology is suspected. By incorporating these suggestions into their practice, the physical therapist will enhance the care given to patients who use their talents. For additional information regarding the GI system, the reader is directed to the Suggested Readings.

PATIENT CASE HISTORY 1
History

The patient was a 32-year-old unemployed laborer who came to the clinic with a diagnosis of grade I spondylolisthesis at L5–S1. He presented with a long history of episodic low back pain, with the episodes usually precipitated by a lifting injury. He had been seen by a physical therapist previously and was referred to the clinic for consultation and subsequent treatment. When questioned, he described his chief complaint as severe deep aching pain in the central mid-thoracic spine region. He acknowledged central low lumbar spine pain but nothing that compared with the intensity of the thoracic pain. The thoracic pain was intermittent but daily; when severe, the aching seemed to wrap around the rib cage bilaterally. The patient was unable to relate a movement or posture to provocation, aggravation, or alleviation of symptoms. He stated that the pain just seemed to come and go for no reason. He reported that these symptoms began 2 weeks ago, after the physical therapist had tried a new joint mobilization technique on this back. When questioned further, the patient revealed that the pain began in the evening, a few hours after the physical therapy visit. He had no previous history of thoracic pain.

The patient's general medical and surgical history were negative, and he was not taking any medication. He had no history of smoking, recent weight loss, fever, or chills.

Objective Examination

In standing, the patient presented with an increased mid-thoracic kyphotic curve and an increased low lumbar spine lordosis. Abnormal muscle tone was not detected in the thoracic spine. The thoracic symptoms were not provoked with active movements of the trunk, but backward bending was moderately restricted in the mid-thoracic spine. The thoracic symptoms were also not provoked with central and unilateral pressures for the thoracic spine, but stiffness was noted in T5–T10. The corresponding portion of the rib cage was also stiff.

Assessment and Outcomes

The thoracic symptoms failed to be provoked with palpation, active and passive tests, and vertical trunk compression and distraction. Because of the suspicious behavior of the symptoms (i.e.,

unrelated to movement or change in posture), the patient was further questioned. When asked about abdominal symptoms, the patient stated that he had been experiencing heartburn after meals but was not sure whether there was a correlation between the heartburn and thoracic symptoms. The heartburn episodes had only been present for the past 1 to 2 weeks. When questioned about medications, the patient again stated that he was not taking any. He had taken Motrin for a couple of months but had not taken any for 2 to 3 weeks.

After the initial visit, the referring physician was contacted regarding the thoracic symptoms that had begun since the last patient visit to the physician. The suspicious pattern of symptoms and signs was discussed with the physician: the presence of abdominal symptoms (heartburn) and mid-thoracic pain (a common pain referral area for gastrointestinal structures), an inability to provoke the symptoms during the examination, and a history of taking Motrin. (NSAIDs can cause GI ulcers but mask the ulcer symptoms while being taken.) The physician placed the patient on Tagamet and a bland diet. The thoracic symptoms were gone within 2 days and, according to the patient in a phone conversation, had not reappeared during the following 3-month period. The examination demonstrated numerous findings associated with the lumbar complaints. The mechanical musculoskeletal system dysfunctions related to these symptoms were subsequently treated.

PATIENT CASE HISTORY 2
History

The patient was a 51-year-old unemployed nurse and physical therapy aide who came to the clinic with a diagnosis of mechanical low back pain syndrome. Initially her chief complaint was constant central low lumbar aching. This aching was increased by sitting for more than 30 minutes, standing in one place more than 15 minutes, and by assuming a forward flexed posture for more than a few seconds. The symptoms were lessened by assuming a recumbent position and, when weight bearing, by constantly changing her posture. She also experienced intermittent sharp pain in the same location. The sharp pain primarily occurred with sit-to-stand movements after sitting for more than 30 to 45 minutes. She could fall asleep without difficulty but woke one to two times a night due to her low back pain. These symptoms began approximately 2 years prior to this evaluation and were precipitated by catching a patient who was falling. She experienced a significant increase in the low lumbar aching 7 months prior to the evaluation, following a long car trip.

The patient denied any other symptoms including numbness or pins and needles. She also denied any symptoms or signs suggesting bladder dysfunction. Surgical history included tonsillectomy, appendectomy, and hysterectomy, and she was being treated for migraine headaches. The medication she was taking included Midrin and Tylenol No. 3 (Tylenol with Codeine). A computed tomography (CT) scan had revealed a bulging disc at L4–L5.

Objective Examination

In standing, the patient presented with a slightly decreased low lumbar lordosis. Increased paraspinal muscle tone was noted in the low lumbar spine. Her chief complaint of aching was increased with one repetition of active trunk forward and backward bending, and left side bending and rotation. Right hip flexion to 95 degrees also increased the aching sensation. Central and right unilateral pressures (passive accessory vertebral motion testing) at L4 also intensified the aching sensation. Significant hypomobility was noted at the L5–S1 segment, left sacroiliac joint, and thoracolumbar junction. The neurologic examination was negative.

Assessment and Outcome

The patient was seen for eight treatment sessions with a goal to increase pain-free range of motion (ROM) so that she could tolerate an aggressive

exercise training program designed to prepare her for work as a physical therapy aide. She made excellent progress with the initial treatment and subsequent exercise program. She was no longer experiencing any sharp pain, and the central low lumbar ache was now intermittent. Her sitting and standing tolerance was much improved, and the low back pain no longer interrupted her sleep.

Approximately 1 month after the initiation of the exercise program, the patient began complaining of severe left lateral lumbar pain that spread out along the left iliac crest and into the left lower abdominal region. She returned to the original physical therapist for re-evaluation at that time. The patient described the symptom as an ache, but stated that she had never experienced the pain in these locations before (Fig. 4-6). The left mid- and lower lumbar pain was constant and increased if she sat for more than 30 minutes and with forward bending movements, especially those combined with left rotation. The aggravation or alleviation of the iliac crest and lower abdominal pain did not seem to be influenced by movement or assumption of various postures. The iliac crest and abdominal pain would come and go throughout the day and was severe enough to wake her at night. These new symptoms began 2 weeks prior to the re-evaluation, the day after Thanksgiving. She could not relate the onset of the symptoms to a particular traumatic incident or accident. When specifically questioned, in addition to these new symptoms, she revealed a recent onset of significant bowel dysfunction. The frequency of bowel movements had decreased, and she described a great deal of difficulty initiating a bowel movement. She denied ever having these problems previously.

During the objective re-assessment the left lumbar pain was increased with all active trunk movements in standing, but especially with forward and right side bending. Left unilateral pressures (passive accessory vertebral motion testing) on L4 and, to a lesser degree, on L3 significantly increased the left mid- and lower lumbar aching. The iliac crest and left lower abdominal ache were not provoked during the objective ex-

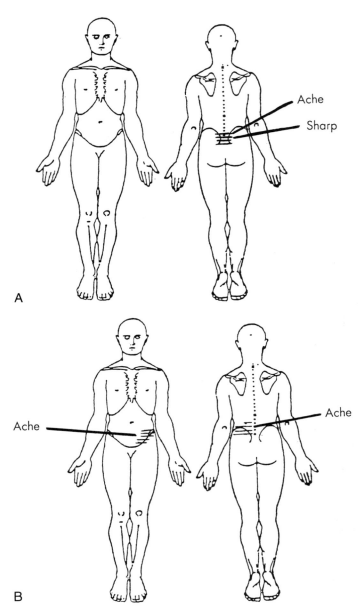

Fig. 4-6. (A) Chief complaint at the initial evaluation—constant central low lumbar aching and intermittent sharp central low lumbar pain. **(B)** Chief complaint at the re-evaluation—constant mid- and lower left lumbar aching and intermittent left iliac crest and lower abdominal aching.

amination, which included clearing tests for the thoracic, lumbar, sacroiliac joint, and hip joint regions. However, significant information was obtained with palpation of the abdomen.

With the patient in a supine position, severe muscle guarding was noted over the left mid- and lower abdominal regions. Generally, the lower abdominal area felt bloated compared to when it was assessed during the initial evaluation a number of weeks previously. Sharp local tenderness was provoked with palpation at points in the mid- and left lower abdominal areas. The tenderness was not present over the same points when the abdominal muscle wall was contracted (she was asked to curl up to tighten the abdominal wall).

Conclusion

At the time of the re-evaluation visit, the patient received treatment for the mechanical dysfunction that was felt to be related to the mid- and lower lumbar region pain. She was also instructed to see her family physician regarding the iliac crest and abdominal symptoms. The family physician was called by the physical therapist to discuss why the patient was referred; the following information was communicated: insidious onset of symptoms within a new location (especially the iliac crest and abdominal pain), the nonmechanical behavior of these symptoms (the iliac crest and abdominal symptoms did not seem to vary with movement or postural changes), the recent changes in bowel function, the inability to provoke the iliac crest and abdominal symptoms during the objective examination, the significant mid- and lower abdominal muscle guarding and local tenderness, and the bloated nature of the abdominal region.

The patient returned to the physical therapy clinic 4 days later stating that she had been diagnosed by her family practice physician as having irritable bowel syndrome, a motility disorder of the small intestine and large bowel. She had

been placed on a high fiber diet and began taking Metamucil. The iliac crest and abdominal pain quickly receded and had not been present 38 hours prior to her return to physical therapy. She also stated that she was not having difficulty with bowel movements any longer. Upon re-evaluation, palpation of the abdomen did not reveal the distention that was present previously, the abnormal muscle tone was not present, nor was local tenderness with palpation. The patient was once again treated for the mechanical dysfunction related to the left mid- and lower lumbar symptoms and subsequently returned to the group exercise class.

When the patient had returned for re-evaluation of the new symptoms, she was under the impression that this was a flare-up of her usual low back pain problem, despite the fact that the symptoms, especially the iliac crest and abdominal pain, were in a new location. Although she was aware of the changes in bowel movement pattern, she never considered contacting her physician regarding her symptoms because of the overriding nature of the increased low back pain. It was not until the specific location and behavior of the symptoms were discussed with the patient that she began to consider the possibility that these symptoms were not necessarily related to what she had originally been seen for. When initially asked about the presence of bowel dysfunction, she denied problems being present, but when given a specific list of bowel dysfunctions, she quickly noted the change in frequency of her bowel movements, as well as the difficulty in initiating them. Therapists should always include a list of specific examples of bowel dysfunction if a patient gives a negative initial response to the question, "Is bowel dysfunction present?" In this patient's case it was apparent after re-evaluation and response to treatment that the left mid- and lower lumbar symptoms were a result of local dysfunction, while the iliac crest and abdominal symptoms appeared to be related to a condition of the GI system. Fortunately, both conditions responded quickly to the appropriate treatment and the patient was able to resume the aggressive exercise program that had been initiated previously.

SUGGESTED READINGS

Braunwald E: Harrison's Principles of Internal Medicine. 11th Ed. McGraw-Hill, New York, 1989

Greenberger N: Gastrointestinal Disorder. A Pathophysiologic Approach. 3rd Ed. Year Book Medical Publishers, Chicago, 1986

Kelley WN (ed): Textbook of Internal Medicine. JB Lippincott, Philadelphia, 1987

Rubenstein E (ed): Scientific American Medicine. Scientific American, New York, 1990

Sleisenger M: Gastrointestinal Disease. Pathophysiology Diagnosis Management. 4th Ed. WB Saunders, Philadelphia, 1989

5

Screening for Male Urogenital System Disease

DUDLEY M. McLINN, M.D.
WILLIAM G. BOISSONNAULT, M.S., P.T.

The structures making up the male urogenital system include the kidneys, ureters, bladder, prostate gland, urethra, testicles, and epididymis. These structures are well known to cause both abdominal and low back pain. In addition, pre-existing conditions of the urogenital system, such as cancer or infections, may be associated with the development of disease processes in other areas of the body. It is, therefore, essential that the physical therapist have the clinical tools to screen patients for the presence of disease of the urogenital system. The purposes of this chapter are to provide:

1. A general review of the anatomy and function of the male urogenital system
2. An overview of the general symptoms and signs suggestive of urogenital system disease a physical therapist might expect to detect during the examination process
3. A more detailed analysis of the disease processes most likely to present primarily as pain syndromes and of prediagnosed conditions that could have an impact on the prognosis of physical therapy care

ANATOMY AND PHYSIOLOGY

The anatomic relationship of the urogenital system and of the abdomen, back, and peritoneum is shown in Figures 5-1 to 5-3. The kidneys and ureters exist bilaterally in the peritoneal cavity, separated from the gastrointestinal tract by the peritoneum. Normal kidneys can be difficult to palpate because of their anatomic location. Diseased kidneys could produce such symptoms as ileus or nausea because of the close proximity of the kidneys to structures of the gastrointestinal system. The ureters connect to the bladder, which is extraperitoneal, existing inferior to the peritoneal cavity. As the bladder fills, its borders extend cranially to where the structure may be palpable superior to the pubic symphysis. The prostate and seminal vesicles are located caudad to the bladder and are connected to the urethra. The prostate and seminal vesicles lie close to the bladder and rectum and, if pathologically enlarged (particularly the prostate), may encroach on these two structures impairing function (Fig. 5-4). The prostate is a chestnut-sized solid organ that can be easily palpated through the rectum. The testicles and epididymis lie in the scrotal sac and are connected to the vas deferens, which exits the scrotum through the inguinal canal. The vas deferens then empties into the urethra at its junction with the prostate gland. The vas deferens is also closely associated with the seminal vesicles at this junction. The testes are oval shaped and vary in size, with the left testicle commonly larger than the right. They are smooth and elastic in texture. The epididymis is posterior to, and distinguishable from, the testicles.

Neurologic control of the urogenital system originates in the brain stem and culminates in the sacral micturition center through the autonomic nervous system. Table 5-1 designates the spinal segmental innervation levels for the structures of the urogenital system. This

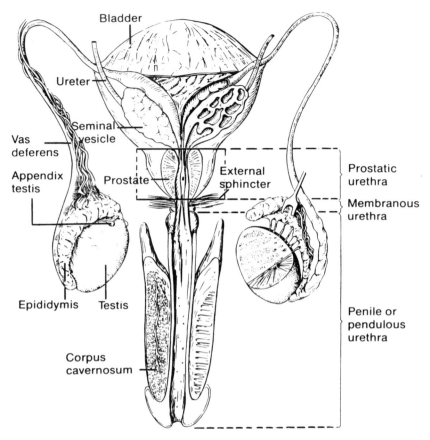

Fig. 5-1. Anatomic structures of the male urogenital system. (From Skögeland,[2] with permission.)

neurologic arrangement serves to stimulate or inhibit micturition through the two components of the autonomic nervous system. The cholinergic fibers stimulate micturition, whereas the sympathetic fibers inhibit micturition.

A primary function of the urogenital system is to act as a filter and drainage system for the body. An important function of the kidney is to regulate the body's extracellular fluid composition by filtering metabolic by-products in the blood, thereby maintaining the fluid and electrolyte balance. The kidney can regulate the body's extracellular fluid by altering the composition of plasma as it courses through the vascular network of the kidney. The altered plasma influences the interstitial fluid of the body and the intracellular fluid composition as it circulates. The blood enters the kid-

ney through a branch of the aorta, the renal artery (see Fig. 5-3). Ultimately the plasma brought into the kidney by the renal arteries filters through glomerular capillaries into the renal tubules.[1] As the filtrate passes through the renal tubules, its volume is reduced and its composition altered. The volume is reduced by the absorption of water and certain solutes, such as sodium, calcium, potassium, and phosphate, which are used by the body. The composition is further altered by the secretion of the solutes magnesium, hydrogen, and ammonia into the remaining filtrate. The resulting filtrate eventually forms the urine that enters the renal pelvis and exits the body through the urine drainage system made up of the ureters, bladder, and urethra.[2] The kidney also produces hormones, including angiotensin II, prostaglandins, and kinins, which are important mediators regarding the regulation of blood pressure. The release of angiotensin increases extra-

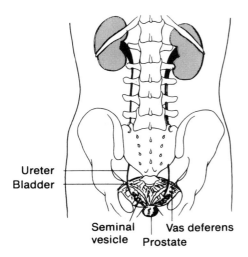

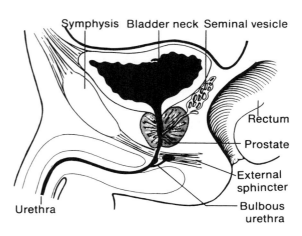

Fig. 5-2. Anatomic relationship of urogenital system structures and elements of the bony skeleton. (From Skögeland,[2] with permission.)

Fig. 5-4. Anatomic relationship of the prostate gland and the bladder, urethra, and rectum. (From Skögeland,[2] with permission.)

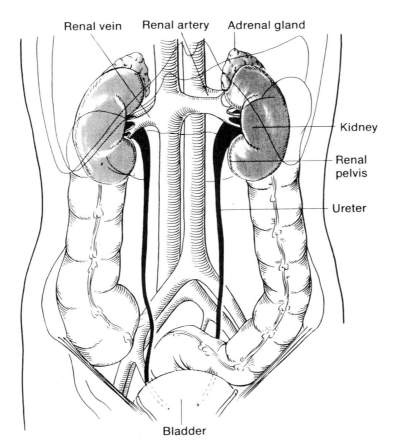

Fig. 5-3. Anatomic relationship of the kidneys and ureters and elements of the cardiovascular and gastrointestinal systems. (From Skögeland,[2] with permission.)

Table 5-1. Structures of the Male Urogenital System

Structure	Segmental Innervation	Possible Areas of Pain Referral
Kidney	T10–L1	Lumbar spine (ipsilateral) flank Upper abdominal
Ureter	T11–L2, S2–S4	Groin Upper/lower abdominal Suprapubic, scrotum Medial, proximal thigh Thoracolumbar
Urinary bladder	T11–L2, S2–S4	Sacral apex Suprapubic Thoracolumbar
Prostate gland	T11–L1, S2–S4	Sacral, low lumbar Testes Thoracolumbar
Testes	T10–T11	Lower abdominal Sacral

cellular fluid volume and elevates the blood pressure by enhancing sodium reabsorption within the kidney.[1] Through the production of the hormone erythropoietin, the kidney also helps regulates the synthesis of red blood cells. Therefore, if the kidneys are malfunctioning regarding hormone production, the patient may present with such conditions as hypertension and anemia. If the urine drainage system (the ureters, bladder, and urethra) is impaired, problems related to bladder distention and renal failure could develop.

The remaining structures of the male urogenital system include the testicles, epididymis, vas deferens, seminal vesicle, and prostate. The structures are involved in the important functions related to spermatogenesis, ejaculation, and male hormone production. Spermatozoa are formed within the testes and drain into the epididymis. Spermatozoa then pass into the vas deferens, which is continuous with the epididymis. Upon ejaculation, semen, including the spermatozoa, enters the urethra within the body of the prostate.[2] The testes also play an important role in male hormone production. The principal hormone produced within the testes, which is subsequently secreted, is testosterone. Luteinizing hormone (LH), released by the anterior lobe of the hypophysis (pituitary gland), stimulates the production of testosterone. Testosterone helps maintain the male secondary sex charac-

teristics, including hair distribution, body configuration, and genital size, by acting as a prehormone for a number of sex steroids, such as androgens and estrogens.[3] Testosterone also exerts an important growth-promoting affect. Malfunction of these structures of the urogenital system could lead to sexual dysfunction (e.g., infertility, pain with ejaculation, and impotency).

Knowledge of the anatomy and physiology of the urogenital system can facilitate the therapist's understanding of the symptoms and signs of pathologic conditions that present in the clinical setting. This information should assist the therapist in formulating questions to be added to the history and should help in the interpretation of information volunteered by the patient regarding the function of this organ system. In addition, knowledge of anatomy will help the therapist differentiate these structures from musculoskeletal system structures during the objective examination and subsequent treatment. The remainder of this chapter focuses on the clinical presentation of diseases of the male urogenital system.

SIGNS AND SYMPTOMS OF DISEASE

History

The physical therapist must rely on the history for most of the information regarding screening this system for medical disease. Few physical therapy objective tests or measures provide data related to the function of the urogenital system as opposed to systems such as the cardiovascular or pulmonary. Therefore, questions regarding pain complaints, bladder function, and sexual function are crucial in screening patients for disease of the urogenital system. The medical tests commonly used to assess the health of the urogenital system include urinalysis, diagnostic ultrasound, radiology, and semen analysis.

The location, description, and behavior of symptoms are all important factors to be considered during the history. The PQRST method is commonly used by physicians to organize the history-taking process:

P   Factors that provoke or palliate the pain.
Q   Quality of pain, that is, sharp, dull, burning, wave-like (colicky), or stabbing
R   Region and radiation of the pain
S   Severity of the pain (usually graded mild, moderate, or severe)
T   Timing as it relates to other events in daily living such as eating or sleeping (includes documenting whether the symptoms are constant or intermittent)

Urogenital system disease can result in abdominal, back, flank, or buttock pain. These symptoms may be described as a dull ache, burning sensation, or wave-like or colicky pain, depending on which structure is involved and the type of disease present. Organizationally, abdominal pain is best separated into regions. Right and left upper quadrant abdominal pain can reflect ipsilateral renal and proximal ureter abnormalities. Right and left lower quadrant abdominal pain can reflect ipsilateral distal ureteral, testicular, and epididymis disease. Bladder disease may result in right, left, or midline lower abdominal pain. Each of the urogenital system structures has the potential to refer pain to the remainder of the trunk, groin, or buttock regions. Table 5-1 shows the possible areas of pain referral from these various structures. Figure 5-5 illustrates the specific referral pattern for the kidneys and ureters. Pain complaints noted in any of these areas should direct the therapist to ask questions regarding the behavior (provocation or palliation) of these symptoms related to urogenital system function in addition to the usual questions relating behavior of symptoms to assumption of specific postures and carrying out specific movements. On the basis of these pain complaints, questions regarding urinary or sexual dysfunction should also be asked.

Besides pain, additional information regarding the function of the urogenital system can easily be collected by the physical therapist. It is necessary to screen patients with the above-described complaints for disorders of voiding. Changes in frequency of urination from a patient's normal pattern can be suggestive of disease. Therefore, questions related to noted increase or decrease of the number of times a day a patient urinates are important.

Increased frequency at night, or nocturia, often reflects a bladder outlet obstruction disorder such as prostatism. Urinary urgency, sometimes to the point of incontinence, is often associated with infection, primarily of the bladder, urethra, and prostate. Complaints of pain and burning while voiding is known as dysuria and often reflects a urinary tract infection or outlet obstruction. Hematuria is always abnormal and a sign associated with serious pathology; any patient who describes his urine as being red should be referred immediately to a physician.[4]

Questions related to sexual function can also provide important information regarding the health of the urogenital system. These questions should address such issues as impotence, pain with ejaculation, premature ejaculation, and inability to maintain an erection.[4] Physical therapists may find it awkward at times to ask patients about sexual dysfunction, but if these questions are not specifically asked, the patient might not volunteer this information because of embarrassment or because he is unaware of the importance and relevance of these data. Figure 5-6 presents a checklist of items related to the urogenital system that should be included in the history if the patient describes pain in the areas previously discussed or has a significant medical history of involvement of this organ system, such as cancer or repeated infection.

Objective Examination

Few physical therapy objective examination techniques provide specific information regarding the status of the urogenital system. Physical therapists evaluate the abdomen by observation, palpation, and possibly percussion. Clinical findings may require the use of soft tissue mobilization techniques, to increase the extensibility of restricted tissue (e.g., scars) and to decrease the resting tone of muscles (e.g., abdominals, iliopsoas, and respiratory diaphragm). Physical therapists must be aware of the nonmusculoskeletal system structures, within this region, that they may also be affecting with the assessment technique and soft tissue mobilization techniques. Of the urogenital system

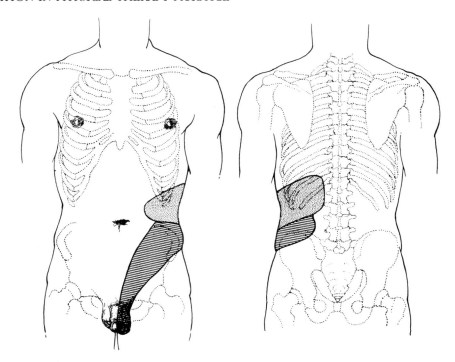

Fig. 5-5. Pain referral patterns for the kidneys (dotted areas) and ureters (horizontal lines). (From Smith,[12] with permission.)

structures described, only the bladder (if distended) and the kidney may be palpable externally. When the therapist detects increased muscle tone or fullness in the suprapubic region associated with tenderness or provocation of symptoms, the therapist must differentiate between the abdominal muscle wall and pubic symphysis as the structures involved versus a deeper visceral structure (including the bladder). One of the special tests a therapist can use is to have the patient perform a partial curl-up (if cervical and upper thoracic spine flexion is not contraindicated) and to palpate the same area. If the area is no longer tender and then is tender again when the superficial muscle wall is more relaxed with the patient fully supine, a structure deep to the abdominal muscle wall should be suspected to be involved.

The therapist must be cognizant of the location of the kidney when assessing and possibly mobilizing the lower thoracic and upper lumbar spine areas, including the 11th and 12th ribs. Pressure on the kidney could also possibly occur with soft tissue mobilization techniques for the quadratus lumborum, lumbar par-

aspinals, and the psoas muscle groups. Palpation of the kidneys is most easily done with the patient supine. The therapist places one hand under the patient just below the lower ribs (see Fig. 5-2 for anatomic location of the kidneys). The therapist places the other hand over the corresponding upper abdominal quadrant, beneath the costal margin. While applying deep pressure with the hand on the abdomen, the patient inhales deeply, causing the kidney to descend, possibly permitting palpation. One of the goals of the physical therapy examination process is the alteration of symptoms by selectively stressing different tissues of the body. Palpation of the kidneys along with clinically stressing the musculoskeletal structures in the region should help the therapist attain this goal. Finally, related to palpation, the testes and penis should be considered. It is considered inappropriate for physical therapists the palpate these structures during an examination process, but the therapist should ask the patient whether he has noted any abnormal masses in the scrotum or change in size of the testicles upon self-examination. If the patient is unclear as to what is normal or abnormal, a description by the therapist of what

Review of systems checklist: Male urogenital system			
Item	Yes	No	Comments
1. Dysuria	___	___	_____
2. Hematuria	___	___	_____
3. Incontinence	___	___	_____
4. Frequency of urination	___	___	_____
5. Urinary urgency	___	___	_____
6. Decreased force of urinary flow	___	___	_____
7. Impotence	___	___	_____
8. Pain with ejaculation	___	___	_____
9. Difficulties with maintaining an erection	___	___	_____
10. Urethral discharge	___	___	_____
11. History of urinary infection	___	___	_____
12. History of venereal disease	___	___	_____

Fig. 5-6. Checklist for review of male urogenital systems. (From Boissonnault and Bass,[11] with permission.)

is normal would be indicated. The description provided should include oval-shaped, smooth, and elastic in texture, but also noting that the right and left testicle might not be the same size.

A correlation of the findings from the history and physical examination may provide the therapist with enough information to suspect involvement of the urogenital system. These specific findings should be communicated to the physician to decide whether the patient should see the doctor at that time for a detailed medical examination.

UROGENITAL SYSTEM DISEASE

Physical therapists should be knowledgeable of certain medical conditions in relationship to the male urogenital system. Infections, tumors, and impotence are the most common disease entities likely to confront physical therapists when treating patients with abdominal, lumbar spine, pelvic, and/or groin pain. This section discusses the etiology and symptoms and signs of these pathologic conditions. A brief overview of the medical testing procedures used to diagnose the conditions and of the common medical treatment approaches for these conditions is presented. Also addressed is chronic renal failure. The emphasis is on the secondary changes commonly associated with the disease, as well as their impact on physical therapy management.

Infections

Urinary tract infections are the second most common infection, after upper respiratory infections. Infections of the solid organs (i.e., kidney, prostate, testicles, and epididymis) will generally be associated with fever, chills, and malaise, with fever being the hallmark symptom.[2] Renal pain is often experienced in the ipsilateral lumbar region caudad to the rib cage. Table 5-1 and Figure 5-5 show additional possible areas of pain perception in the presence of kidney infection. Patients often describe the pain as being a dull constant ache.[4] Pyelonephritis, the most common renal disease, generally follows an untreated bladder infection. This disease should be strongly considered in immunocompromised patients, (e.g., a diabetic or cancer patient on chemotherapy) or in a patient with recent instrumentation (including cystoscopy or catheterization). Other factors predisposing to the onset of pyelonephritis include the presence of metabolic disease (e.g., diabetes mellitus), long-term immobilization, and medications (e.g., analgesics and corticosteroids).[2] A perinephric abscess, an abscess surrounding the kidney, lies in close proximity to the psoas muscle. Therefore, ipsilateral hip flexion may cause local pain secondary to psoas contraction. Pyelonephritis is not common in men but should be considered when a patient complains of unilateral lumbar pain associated with the presence of fever.

Prostatic pain is often experienced as a dull, diffuse, perineal pain. Pain referral patterns besides the perineal pain associated with prostate conditions are presented in Table 5-1. The intensity of the pain may vary with functions, such as bowel movements, urination, and intercourse. Certain perirectal conditions such as rectal fissures and hemorrhoids can mimic this disease, but a medical examination can quickly out rule these entities. Infections of the prostate behave much like bladder infections in that there may be a sense of urgency to void and increased frequency of urination. The increased frequency may be most noticeable to the patient at night as he may be waking two to three times a night to urinate compared with the usual pattern of sleeping through the night. In addition, fever and chills may be present as well as dysuria, urge to defecate, and urethral discharge.[2,4]

Infections of the testicles (orchitis) and epididymis (epididymitis) are associated with rapid local swelling and scrotal tenderness. The patient may also present with fever and malaise. Testicular pain is usually experienced as a local dull ache, but pain can be referred to the lower abdominal or sacral regions. Patients with suspected involvement of the testicles should be seen immediately by a physician to rule out the presence of torsion of the testicle. This condition can compromise the local blood supply requiring immediate medical attention and surgical release. Pain from epididymitis can be difficult to differentiate from testicular pain. Epididymitis causes pain secondary to swelling of the organ and is tender to touch. These infectious processes may be preceded by urethritis or prostatitis.

Infections of the hollow organs of the urogenital system (i.e., the ureters, bladder, and urethra) are associated with pain and other urinary tract symptoms, such as increased urinary frequency and urethral discharge. The hallmark symptom of infection of the solid organs, fever, is often absent.[2] Ureteral pain is often experienced as wavelike (colic) discomfort that can spread from the flank to the ipsilateral lower quadrant of the abdomen and into the ipsilateral testicle[4] (see Fig. 5-5). In the presence of a kidney stone, movement of the pain reflects movement of the stone as it traverses the ureter and bladder. Infection of the ureters can be secondary to multiple organisms, including *Gonorrhoeae*, *Chlamydia*, *Trachamatis*, *Trichomonas*, *Vaginalis*, Herpes simplex, *Candida albicans*, and such bacteria as *Escherichia coli*. Effective treatment includes treatment of the patient's sexual partner, to prevent recurrence.

As with pyelonephritis, bladder infections (cystitis) are not common in men. When present, however, the pain is usually constant and can be located in the suprapubic, sacral, or thoracolumbar regions. The pain may be associated with a sense of urgency to void. Although the pain may be constant, the intensity may vary, being wavelike (colicky), with urination intensifying the symptoms and possibly producing radiation of pain to the penis. Besides dysuria and urgency, other symptoms related to voiding may be increased frequency, including nocturia. Urethral pain associated with infection is often a burning sensation associated with urination. The patient may volunteer that he had urethral discharge.

In summary, although relatively uncommon in men, physical therapists should be familiar with the symptoms associated with urogenital system infections. Medical referral should be accomplished when these symptoms are present. The physician will make the diagnosis on the basis of urinalysis, urine culture, and other tests such as intravenous pyelogram and ultrasound of the kidneys, depending on the situation. The treatment is generally antibiotics depending on the bacterial pathogen. In the case of infections of the solid genitourinary organs, it is often necessary to institute intravenous treatment initially. In immunocompromised patients, immediate consultation should be sought.

Cancer

Tumors of the male urogenital system can be either benign or malignant. Figure 5-7 indicates possible locations of the primary urogenital system tumors. Initially, most malignant tumors are clinically silent, but general symptoms, such as fatigue and malaise, may be present. Only after the mass has reached a certain size will the symptoms and signs of urogenital system involvement become apparent.[2] Of the body neoplasms, there is a high incidence of cancer of the prostate, bladder, and kidney. Neoplasms of the ureter, urethra, penis, epididymis, and seminal vesicles are rare.[4] As with tumors elsewhere in the body, the prognosis for treatment is enhanced by early detection. The physical therapist may be in a position to initiate referral to a physician for diagnosis on the basis of clinical findings.

Kidneys

Cancer of the kidneys can be divided into renal parenchymal and renal pelvis neoplasms. The most common renal tumor is renal cell carcinoma.[5] This disease rarely occurs before the age of 30, with increased incidence noted between the ages of 45 and 75. Peak incidence occurs during the sixth decade affecting men two to three times more frequently than women.[5] The lungs, liver, and bony elements of the musculoskeletal system are the most common sites of metastasis.[4] The tumor may initially be asymptomatic, with sudden onset of painless hematuria precipitating concern on the patient's part. Pain is the most commonly described symptom. Usually a dull ache is noted in the body regions described in Table 5-1 and Figure 5-5. Complaints of malaise, weakness, weight loss, and fever may also be a part of the patient's clinical picture.[4] A correlation between tobacco use and a higher incidence of renal cell carcinoma has been noted.[5] Enlargement of the kidney may make the structure palpable during the objective examination. Medical diagnosis is made by tests, including sonography, angiography, and computed tomography (CT) scanning. Treatment consists of nephrectomy, lymph node dissection, and postoperative radiation.

The renal pelvis (interior of the kidney) may also be a site of cancer development. This disease is also rare before the age of 30 with peak incidence during the sixth decade. Males are affected two times as frequently as women.[5] Carcinomas and papillomas present with a similar clinical picture. Hematuria of unknown cause is the primary finding of clinical concern since enlargement of the kidney does not occur.[4] Pain, colicky in nature, though, may also be present. Other symptoms may include urinary frequency, malaise, weight loss, or fever. A medical diagnosis is made by intravenous or retrograde pyelography, which permits visualization of the ureter and renal pelvis. Treatment would consist of nephroureterectomy, lymph node dissection, and postoperative radiation. Metastasis from this lesion may occur in the ureters and the bladder.

Bladder

Bladder cancer is the fifth most common cause of cancer death in men. Overall, bladder cancer is the second most common cancer of the urogenital system. The incidence is much higher in men than in women (ratio 3-6:1) and affects whites more often than blacks (ratio 4:1).[5] The incidence of bladder cancer is also higher in people in certain occupations (e.g., those exposed to chemicals, dyes, leather products, and rubber) and among cigarette smokers.[4] Cigarette smokers have an incidence of bladder cancer two to five times greater than that of the nonsmoking population.[5] Generally a poor prognosis is associated with bladder carcinoma, as most of the tumors are malignant. Metastasis can occur to the lungs, bony elements of the musculoskeletal system, and the liver. Presenting symptoms may include hematuria, dysuria, nocturia, and urinary urgency.[4] Diagnosis is made by tests including cystogram, cystoscopy, and biopsy. Treatment includes surgical resection of the tumor and postoperative radiation.

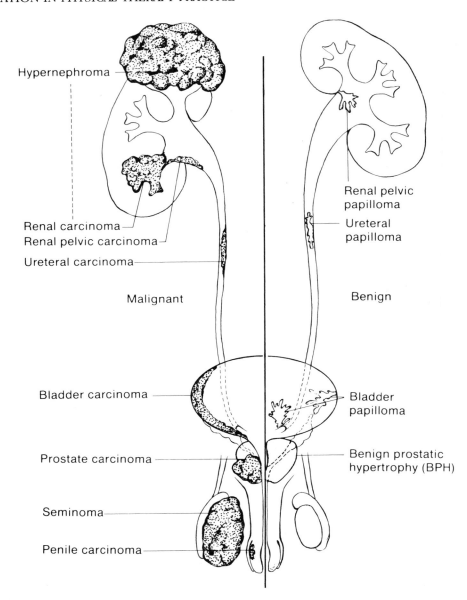

Fig. 5-7. Anatomic locations of malignant and benign lesions of the male urogenital system. (From Skögeland,[2] with permission.)

Prostate

After lung and gastrointestinal tract cancer, carcinoma of the prostate gland is the third leading cause of cancer death in men.[2,6,7] Prostate cancer is the second most common cancer in males.[5] The incidence of prostatic carcinoma and adenoma progressively increases after the age of 50 years.[7] Often no symptoms are noted in the early stages of this disease. The first symptom could be a dull, vague, diffuse ache localized to the central low lumbar spine or upper sacral regions. Early metastasis to the lumbar spine and pelvis (bony elements) is not uncommon. Besides these two sites, the femurs (proximal portion), thoracic spine, ribs, and sternum are sites of metastasis.[6] The most common visceral structures involved with metastasis are the lung, liver, and the adrenal glands. These pathologic lesions resulting in local pain may be the initial symptoms noted by the patient. Only after the tumor is of sufficient size to compromise the urethra will urinary dysfunction be noted by the patient. The early stages of urinary dysfunction may include a sense of urinary urgency and possibly hematuria. In the more advanced stages of this disease, increased frequency of urination, particularly nocturia, slowing of the urine stream, and difficulty in starting the urine stream may also be present. In the early stages of cancer, palpatory abnormalities of the prostate are the primary diagnostic findings. Needle biopsy of the mass would then follow. Treatment may include prostatectomy, radiation treatment, chemotherapy, or hormone therapy.

Testes

Testicular tumors are relatively rare but, when present, are associated with a poor prognosis unless diagnosed early. They tend to be very malignant with peak incidence occurring between the ages of 20 and 40.[2] Testicular tumors are generally marked by painless but slow progressive swelling of a testicle. Other symptoms may include abdominal pain, nausea, vomiting, and weight loss.[4] Owing to the endocrine function of the testicles, a tumor may result in gynecomastia (breast enlargement) and/or impotence.[2] Self-examination may reveal a unilateral, smooth, enlarged testicle or a testicular mass. Further diagnostic testing may include ultrasound, CT scan, and biopsy. Treatment consists of radical orchiectomy. Prompt surgical removal of the tumor may be life saving with early detection paramount for a better prognosis. Therefore, men, especially between the ages of 20 to 40 years, should be encouraged to perform self-examination. Besides a tumor, scrotal enlargement may be caused by a hydrocele (benign fluid collection) or a spermatocele. An evaluation by the physician would help differentiate these entities from a neoplasm.

Chronic Renal Failure

Renal failure is defined as the deterioration of renal function associated with the accumulation of nitrogenous wastes not attributable to extrarenal factors.[8] Chronic renal failure is marked by irreversible loss of kidney function, resulting in a wide range of complications that affects numerous body systems. Patients prediagnosed as having chronic renal failure may be referred for physical therapy for conditions related or unrelated to renal disease. Regardless of why the patient has been referred, the therapist should understand the impact that the disease and associated secondary changes may have on the prognosis and outcome of the therapy sessions.

Chronic renal failure is marked by progressive loss of nephrons. The causes are numerous, with glomerulonephritis, interstitial renal disease, and polycystic kidney disease the most common.[9] Since the kidney functions to regulate the body's extracellular fluid composition, thereby influencing intracellular fluid composition, chronic kidney disease can have a wide-ranging effect on multiple body systems. These secondary manifestations of chronic renal failure can often be mistaken for primary conditions.

A number of symptoms and signs associated with chronic renal failure may interfere with physical therapy or may result in a confusing clinical picture. Common gastrointestinal system complaints associated with chronic renal failure include nausea and vomiting. Insomnia, inability to concentrate, and lack of alertness may also be present.[9] All these symptoms may interfere with the patient's ability to participate in a rehabilitation program, including tolerating exercises in the clinic as well as following through with a home exercise program. Neurologic changes may result in increased deep tendon reflexes,[8] intermittent paresthesias and hypesthesias of the hands and feet, cramping of limb musculature, and absence of sweating.[9] Proximal muscle weakness may also be present making it difficult for patients to rise up from a chair or bed.[9] Differentiating these neurologic changes from those that occur from spinal or peripheral nerve entrapment may be difficult. Generally neurologic changes secondary to a systemic disorder will not follow the pattern of specific dermatomal or myotomal involvement. They will also not follow the pattern of a specific peripheral neuropathy. The therapist must be cautious though, as a common clinical error may be to attribute a patient's complaints of numbness, weakness, or pins-and-needles sensations to the presence of chronic renal failure. Detailed investigation of the behavior of the symptoms may demonstrate changes in intensity or provocation of symptoms related to movements or assumption of specific postures. Similar findings may occur as active and passive range-of-motion (ROM) testing and special tests are implemented in the objective examination. These findings may lead the therapist to suspect that all of or a part of the patient's complaints are not related to the kidney pathology but rather to nerve involvement secondary to mechanical dysfunction. (See Patient Case History 2, Ch. 7, for an example.)

Other changes associated with chronic renal failure may have an impact on physical therapy management as well, including osteodystrophy. Elevated levels of parathyroid hormone secondary to the renal pathology can lead to increased bone resorption. The decreased bone density may lead to microtrauma of the bone resulting in local pain complaints. The most commonly involved bony elements include the vertebral column and femurs.[9] These patients will be more susceptible to fractures as well as other skeletal deformities. The therapist should be cautious when passively assessing spinal mobility, especially the thoracic spine, when using techniques such as central and unilateral pressures as described by Maitland[10] with the patient in a prone position. With the thorax stabilized anteriorly by the table and then stressed in a posterior to anterior direction by the therapist's pressure, the structurally weakened rib cage could be injured. Obtaining information regarding spinal segmental mobility and provocation of symptoms is an important goal of the objective examination. With patients coming to the clinic prediagnosed as having chronic renal failure, alternative patient positions and methods of passive intervertebral testing should be considered to protect the patient.

Finally, cardiovascular complications accompanying the chronic renal failure must be considered. Hypertension is commonly associated with chronic renal failure. Control of high blood pressure is important, to prevent the acceleration of nephrosclerosis and decrease the likelihood that other cardiovascular system disorders will develop.[9] Communication between the physician and physical therapist is important for setting the appropriate aerobic exercise workloads, using pulse rate and blood pressure measures to monitor the patient. Finally, pericarditis can occur in up to one half of undialyzed patients.[9] This condition may de-velop while the patient is being treated by the physical therapist. (See Ch. 2 for a description of symptoms and signs associated with pericarditis.)

Impotence

In our fast-paced world, impotency is becoming a much more common problem. Many men will be reluctant to volunteer the fact that they are impotent, but will be relieved to discuss it if they are suffering from the problem. It is best to be sympathetic and not judgmental and suggest that they discuss it with their physician or urologist. In most cases, the problem is primarily psychological. Organic problems must be ruled out, however. Impotency can be secondary to a neurogenic problem such as polio, multiple sclerosis, tabes dorsalis, spinal trauma, or diabetic neuropathy. It can also be secondary to vascular conditions such as arteriosclerosis or thrombosis. Lastly, it may be secondary to endocrine conditions such as hypogonadism and hypopituitarism. It is also commonly associated with such drugs as sedatives, antidepressants, antihypertensives, as well as estrogens which are often given in the presence of prostate cancer. Alcohol excess can also be associated with the presence of impotency. A careful screening of the patient's past and current medical history could be extremely helpful in directing the patient to the appropriate physician for a diagnostic examination.

SUMMARY

This chapter discusses the male urogenital system as it relates to the practice of physical therapy. The therapist must understand the basic anatomy of the urogenital system as it relates to other organ systems of the body, including the musculoskeletal system. It is important to remember that the signs and symptoms of disease, especially early stage disease of the urogenital system, are often nonspecific and general in nature. Since physical therapists are called on most frequently to help resolve pain or dysfunction, it is also helpful to remember that the original diagnosis may be mistaken and a careful examination on the physical therapist's part may be extremely important in directing the patient to the appropriate physician and subsequent medical treatment. A patient case history follows.

PATIENT CASE HISTORY*

History

The patient was a 58-year-old commuter van driver for a hospital who was referred to the clinic with a diagnosis of mechanical low back pain syndrome and cervical strain secondary to a motor vehicle accident. His van had been struck on the passenger side by a car as he pulled out of a parking lot 3 weeks before the evaluation. His chief complaints were left posterior/lateral cervical spine and left shoulder pain and central low lumbar spine pain. The patient described the left shoulder pain as a constant dull aching that was aggravated by driving for more than 1 hour. Limiting the driving time was his only method of controlling the symptoms. He also experienced intermittent sharp left cervicothoracic junction pain, which interfered with driving. This symptom was solely aggravated by left rotation of the cervical spine. He experienced significant stiffness in the cervical spine and slight aching early in the morning. A hot shower significantly reduced the stiffness, while the aching intensity varied with the amount of driving he did later that day. The cervical spine and left shoulder pain did not interfere with sleeping. The patient had never experienced cervical or shoulder symptoms before the motor vehicle accident.

The low back pain was described as a constant, low-intensity ache occasionally aggravated by repetitive lifting. He was able to obtain slight relief of the aching by assuming a supine or side-lying position for short periods. Driving did not seem to aggravate the lumbar symptoms. The patient stated that the low back pain was most intense early in the morning. He noted he was waking consistently around 3:00 AM with severe low back pain. Getting out of bed and walking for 15 to 20 minutes decreased the ache sufficiently so that sleep was possible again. He has experienced numerous episodes of low back pain over the past 5 to 6 years. None of the episodes was pre-

ceded by a traumatic incident or accident, but this most recent episode, which began 3 to 4 months before the evaluation, was the first marked by severe night pain. When questioned further, the patient revealed that the motor vehicle accident had not changed his low back condition.

The patient's medical history included surgical repair of a right lower abdominal hernia and an appendectomy. He was taking medication for high blood pressure, and ibuprofen had been prescribed since the motor vehicle accident. He denied any visual, auditory, or cognitive changes since the accident. The patient denied bowel dysfunction but had noted increased frequency of urination, including waking two to three times a night to urinate, and difficulty in starting the urine stream. He had not seen a physician specifically for the urogenital problems and had forgotten to tell the physician he saw following the motor vehicle accident. Radiographs were taken of the cervical spine after the accident revealing degenerative disc disease at C5–C6.

Objective Examination

The objective examination revealed significant muscle guarding throughout the left posterior/lateral aspect of the cervical spine. There was also slight muscle guarding noted in the paraspinals, L4–L5. A moderately increased cervicothoracic junction kyphosis and decreased low lumbar lordosis was observed. Sharp left lower cervical spine pain and an increase in the left shoulder ache was noted with one repetition of cervical spine left rotation. Left rotation ROM was decreased by approximately 90 percent. Cervical left side bending and backward bending were moderately reduced with the patient describing a "blocked" sensation in the left lower cervical region at end range. A slight to moderate loss of active backward bending and left and right side bending of the lumbar spine was also observed. The low lumbar symptoms were not provoked with any active movements of the trunk, nor with overpressures. The sharp left cervical pain was provoked with left unilateral pressures on C6.

---

*From Boissonnault and Bass,[11] with permission.

Segmental joint mobility testing also revealed hypomobility at C5, C7, and T1. In the lumbar spine, segmental hypomobility was noted at the L5–S1 segment but, as with the active movements and overpressure in standing, there was no provocation of lumbar symptoms with segmental vertebral provocation or mobility tests.

Assessment and Outcome

The referring physician was contacted after the initial evaluation to discuss the discrepancy between the cervical and lumbar findings. There appeared to be a clear correlation between the motor vehicle accident and the cervical symptoms. The accident had precipitated the cervical and shoulder pain, whereas the lumbar complaints had been present before the accident and had not been changed by the accident. The primary reasons for referring the patient back to the physician, were insidious onset of low back pain, low back pain being the most intense in the early morning (night pain), and dysuria marked by increased frequency, nocturia, and difficulty in starting the urine stream. It should be noted that when the patient was asked originally if he was experiencing any bowel or bladder dysfunction, he answered no. Further questioning regarding specific examples of bladder dysfunction, such as frequency, waking at night to urinate, and difficulty in starting the urine stream, revealed the important medical information. Clinicians should not assume that the patient understands such terms as bowel and bladder dysfunction. Further medical tests revealed that the patient had prostate cancer.

This case history demonstrates the importance of a thorough investigation of the behavior of all symptoms, including symptom variation over a 24-hour period. The report of severe low back night pain was the initial significant warning or suspicious clue picked up during the evaluation. This finding dictated that a very thorough review of organ system questioning be carried out that

ultimately revealed the urinary system complaints. Also demonstrated during this case is the importance of investigating the chronologic history of all symptoms. It was clear that while the traumatic incident was responsible for the upper-quarter complaints, the accident had nothing to do with the lumbar complaints. The last important factor differentiating the two primary symptomatic regions was being able to reproduce the upper quarter symptoms with an active movement and passively stressing a cervical vertebral segment, while not being able to reproduce the lumbar symptoms with any of the objective tests.

REFERENCES

1. Berne RM, Levy MN (eds): Physiology. 2nd Ed. CV Mosby, St. Louis, 1988
2. Skögeland J: Urology. 2nd Ed. Thieme Medical, New York, 1989
3. DeGroot LJ (ed): Endocrinology. Vol. 3. 2nd Ed. WB Saunders, Philadelphia, 1989
4. Tanagho EA, McAninch JW (eds): General Urology. 12th Ed. Appleton & Lange, E. Norwalk, CT, 1988
5. Schrier RW, Gottschalk CW (eds): Diseases of the Kidney. 4th Ed. Vol. 1. Little, Brown, Boston, 1988
6. Catalona WJ: Prostate Cancer. Harcourt Brace Jovanovich, Orlando, 1984
7. Rous SN: The Prostate Book. WW Norton, New York, 1988
8. Walsh PC, Gittes RF, Perlmutter AD, Stamey TA (eds): Campbell's Urology. Vol. 3. 5th Ed. WB Saunders, Philadelphia, 1986
9. Stein JH (ed): Internal Medicine. 2nd Ed. Little, Brown, Boston, 1987
10. Maitland GD: Vertebral Manipulation. 5th Ed. Buttersworth, London, 1986
11. Boissonnault B, Bass C: Pathological origins of trunk and neck pain: part 1—pelvic and abdominal disorders. JOSPT 12(5):192, 1990
12. Smith DR: General Urology. 11th Ed. p. 28. Lange Medical Publications, Los Altos, CA, 1984

SUGGESTED READING

Wilson JD, Braunwald E, Isselbacher KJ: Harrison's Principles of Internal Medicine. 12th Ed. Vols. 1, 2. McGraw-Hill, New York, 1991

6

Screening for Female Urogenital System Disease

FRANK W. LING, M.D.
PATRICIA M. KING, M.A., P.T.
CRAIG A. MYERS, P.T.

The female urogenital system includes anatomic structures of both the female reproductive tract and the urinary system. The former consists of the uterus, fallopian tubes, ovaries, vagina, external genitalia, and perineum, while the latter includes the kidney, ureters, bladder, and urethra. The anatomy of the upper urinary tract and conditions that affect the kidney and ureters are not discussed in this chapter (see Ch. 5, for a full discussion of these areas). Because of their common embryologic origins, as well as their anatomic juxtaposition, lower urinary tract disorders are discussed in conjunction with those of the female genital tract. As a result, the overriding view here is that of a primary care practitioner of obstetrics/gynecology or family medicine.

Abdominal, pelvic and back pain are common symptoms encountered by these medical practitioners. They are potential points of interface between the physical therapist and these physicians. It behooves the physical therapist to be aware of obstetric and gynecologic concepts that might affect his or her encounter with these patients. This chapter focuses on (1) normal anatomy and physiology of the female reproductive tract, including the normal physiology of pregnancy; (2) the relationship of normal physiology to signs and symptoms frequently seen in a physical therapy evaluation; (3) specific diseases of the female reproductive tract that may be seen by the physical therapist, including common clinical signs and symptoms associated with each; (4) signs and symptoms associated with

pregnancy; and (5) a summary of historical keys and physical examination findings that will assist the physical therapist in identifying the patient who may require gynecologic evaluation.

NORMAL ANATOMY AND PHYSIOLOGY

The bony pelvis consists of the sacrum, coccyx, and the two innominate bones. The latter is composed of the ilium, ischium, and pubis, which are fused in the adult patient. Mobile articulations remain throughout adult female life at the pubic symphysis and the sacroiliac joints. The articular surfaces of the female sacrum are irregularly shaped, with considerable variation from individual to individual. The female sacrum is usually wider and has a shorter articular surface with the ilium than does the male sacrum.[1] The irregular design of the sacrum and its articular surfaces creates sacroiliac articulations that present with the mobility necessary to accommodate the changes in pelvic position associated with pregnancy, labor, and delivery. Weight-bearing of the trunk is provided by the ischium when the patient is sitting, while the lower limbs share in the support of the trunk when the patient is standing. Figures 6-1 and 6-2 depict these structures.[2]

The muscles of the pelvic wall are illustrated in Figures 6-3 to 6-5.[2] The primary musculature supporting the

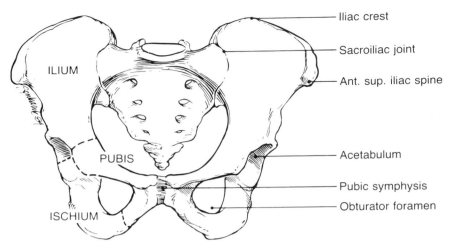

Fig. 6-1. Osseous anatomy of the pelvic girdle. (From Gould,[2] with permission.)

pelvic floor is the levator ani, which has three components: the iliococcygeus, the pubococcygeus, and the puborectalis muscles. These muscles provide the primary support for the pelvic viscera discussed below. The fascial sheath surrounding these muscles is derived from the transversalis fascia. The musculature of the perineum is shown in Figures 6-6 and 6-7. The primary neurologic supply for this area is demonstrated in Figure 6-8. The pudendal nerve, supplied by the 2nd, 3rd, and 4th sacral nerve roots, is the pri-

mary motor and sensory nerve to the perineum. The pelvic viscera is supported anteriorly by the abdominal musculature which derives innervation from spinal nerve root levels T7–L1.

The internal genital organs are pictured in Figures 6-9 and 6-10. The organs of the female reproductive tract are the ovaries, the fallopian tubes, the uterus and cervix, and the vagina. The bladder, distal aspects of the ureter, and the urethra lie in close proximity to these

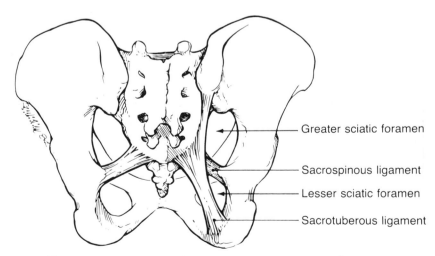

Fig. 6-2. Osseous and ligamentous anatomy of the pelvic girdle. (From Gould,[2] with permission.)

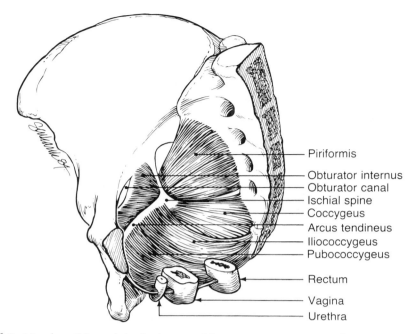

Fig. 6-3. Muscles of the pelvic diaphragm, oblique view. (From Gould,[2] with permission.)

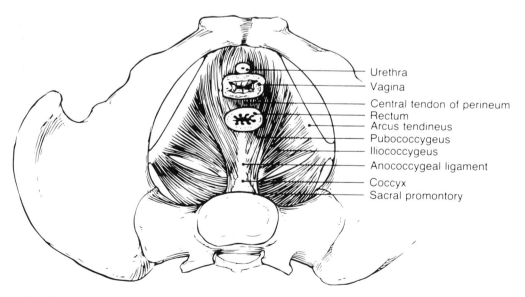

Fig. 6-4. Muscles of the pelvic diaphragm, superior view. (From Gould,[2] with permission.)

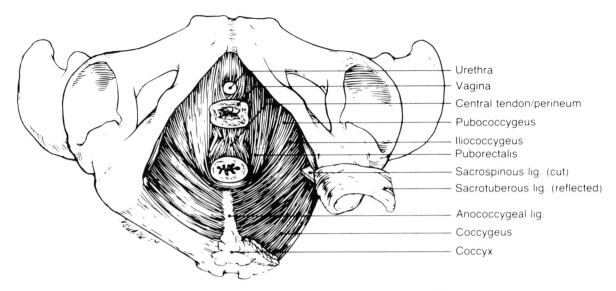

Fig. 6-5. Muscles of the pelvic diaphragm, inferior view. (From Gould,[2] with permission.)

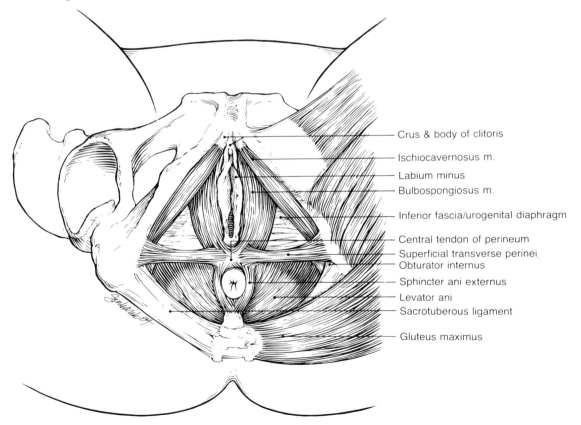

Fig. 6-6. Muscles of the perineum, inferior view. (From Gould,[2] with permission.)

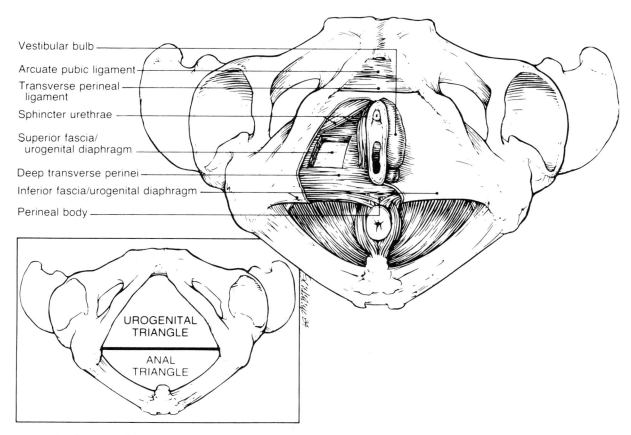

Vestibular bulb

Arcuate pubic ligament

Transverse perineal
   ligament

Sphincter urethrae

Superior fascia/
   urogenital diaphragm

Deep transverse perinei

Inferior fascia/urogenital diaphragm

Perineal body

UROGENITAL
TRIANGLE

ANAL
TRIANGLE

Fig. 6-7. Muscles of the perineum, inferior view; urogenital triangle. (From Gould,[2] with permission.)

internal genital organs. Also in close anatomic proximity are loops of small intestine, the ileocecal junction on the right and the sigmoid colon and rectum on the left. The ovaries are normally 1 cm × 2 cm × 3 cm and lie against the lateral pelvic sidewall. These are the female gonads, the organs of the female reproductive tract that produce hormones, primarily estrogen and progesterone. The fallopian tubes are attached medially to the uterus and open distally at their fimbriated end. The fallopian tube is normally approximately 10 cm in length. Its location in the pelvis varies, as it is fairly free to move about within the pelvis. The uterus is the organ in which a normal pregnancy implants and develops. It is also the origin of menstrual flow. It is situated between the rectum posteriorly and the bladder anteriorly. The uppermost portion is termed the fundus. The junction between the uterus and the vagina is the cervix, the portion of the uterus visible upon vaginal inspection. The vagina (birth canal) is the fibromuscular tube that connects the internal genital organs with the labia. It is in close contact posteriorly with the rectum, as it is with the bladder anteriorly. The internal female genital organs are palpable during a routine bimanual pelvic examination. Unless the anatomy is altered by pregnancy or pathologic enlargement, they should not be palpable by abdominal palpation.

The nerves of the pelvis are illustrated in Figure 6-11. The lateral pelvic wall is the site of the nerve plexuses that supply the pelvic structures. Table 6-1 (see p. 149) illustrates the nerve root values for innervation of the pelvic viscera and related structures as well as potential sites of referred pain from each structure.

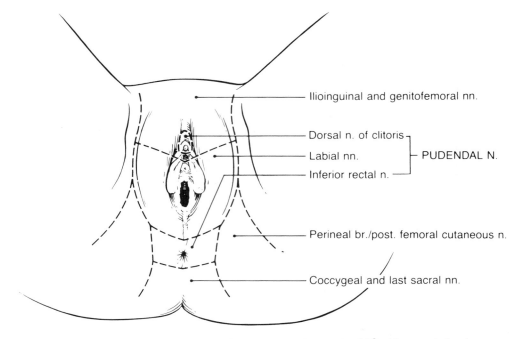

Fig. 6-8. Neurological supply to the perineum. (From Gould,[2] with permission.)

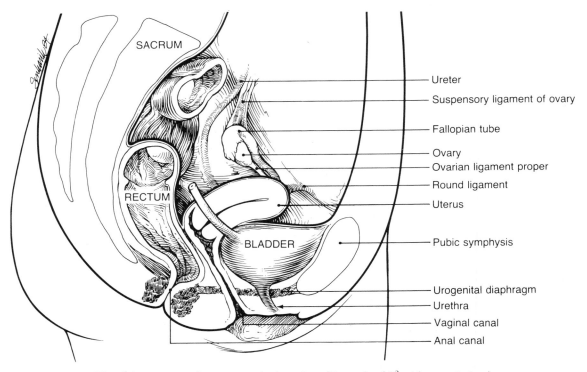

Fig. 6-9. Urogenital organs, sagittal section. (From Gould,[2] with permission.)

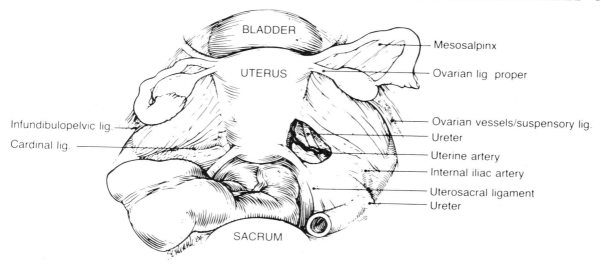

Fig. 6-10. Urogenital organs, posterior view. (From Gould,[2] with permission.)

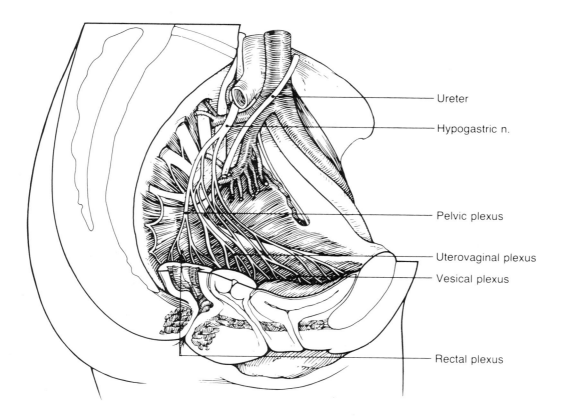

Fig. 6-11. Neurologic supply to the urogenital organs, lateral view. (From Gould,[2] with permission.)

Menstrual Physiology

The normal menstrual cycle and its hormones are depicted in Figure 6-12. The menstrual cycle is functionally divided into three phases: the menstrual phase (when menses occurs), the proliferative phase (during which time the ovarian follicle develops in preparation for ovulation), and the luteal phase (during which time the endometrium of the uterus is prepared for possible implantation of a pregnancy). The entire cycle lasts an average of 28 days. Ovulation occurs at what is termed the mid-cycle, an event that occurs typically 2 weeks before any subsequent menstrual flow. The primary hormone of the follicular (proliferative) phase is estrogen, specifically estradiol, produced by the ovary. Progesterone is the predominant hormone of the luteal phase and is produced by the corpus luteum of the ovary. Relaxin is also produced in the corpus luteum during the luteal phase and is responsible for the ligamentous laxity noted primarily in the pelvic articulations during this phase.[4,5] If no pregnancy occurs, hormonal support of the lining of the uterus (endometrium) is withdrawn and a menstrual flow results. If pregnancy does occur, hormonal support for the endometrium is provided by the placenta.

Physiology of Pregnancy

The physiologic changes during pregnancy that occur in the female patient are necessary to support the growth of the fetus. As a result, anatomy and physi-

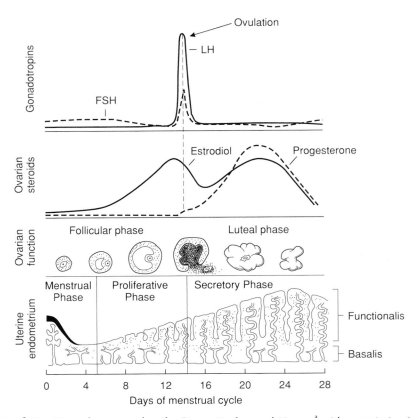

Fig. 6-12. Normal menstrual cycle. (From Hacker and Moore,[3] with permission.)

ology is markedly altered from that of the nonpregnant patient. The mother is forced to adapt both physically as well as physiologically to these changes.

The Spine

The increasing girth of the abdomen that contributes to the progressive development of lumbar lordosis posture is considered a normal feature of pregnancy. Of particular interest to the physical therapist is a noted increase in mobility of the pubic, sacrococcygeal, and sacroiliac joints that manifests during pregnancy apparently in response to increased progesterone and relaxin levels.[5] This increased mobility appears to contribute to the typical maternal posture, which is dominated by the development of an anterior pelvic tilt and an exaggerated lumbar lordotic curve. Discomfort in the lower portion of the back is a common symptom throughout pregnancy associated with these changes.

Late in pregnancy, weakness and paresthesia of the upper extremities are also frequently reported. This may be as a result of a forward head and thoracic kyphotic posture that usually develops along with lumbar and pelvic postural changes. This posture may cause compression of the neurovascular structures of the thoracic outlet and the carpal tunnel regions. Physical therapists are familiar with the sensory and motor changes associated with thoracic outlet and carpal tunnel syndromes, all of which may manifest during pregnancy.

Weight Gain

The average weight gain during pregnancy is 25 to 30 pounds, with individual variations commonly seen. The sheer weight increase is manifest as easy fatigability and pressure sensations of the lower abdomen and lower back. During pregnancy, ovulation obviously ceases, and the corpus luteum of the ovary supports the pregnancy only during the first 6 to 7 weeks of the pregnancy. Hormonal support thereafter is provided by the placenta. During pregnancy, there is increased blood flow and vascularity in the skin of the vagina and the perineum. The skin becomes markedly pigmented in the midline (linea nigra), and angiomas (vascular spiders) develop in many patients. There is also development of diastasis of the abdominal wall musculature.

Blood Pressure

During pregnancy, blood pressure typically drops, with a maximum change seen at 20 to 24 weeks. A gradual rise to prepregnancy levels occurs as the patient approaches term. The mean drop in blood pressure is approximately 8 to 10 mmHg. Heart rate typically increases 12 to 18 bpm, and cardiac output is increased by approximately one-third. Many biochemical and hematologic blood indices are changed during normal pregnancy. These include the urine chemistries, serum chemistries, serum enzymes, and serum hormones.

The enlarging uterus also compresses the iliac veins and inferior vena cava, thereby reducing venous return from the lower extremities. Supine hypotension is of significant concern, as fetal and uterine weight gain increase throughout pregnancy. There is some disagreement as to the point in pregnancy at which the supine position becomes a significant risk. The guidelines for exercise published by the American College of Obstetricians and Gynecologists[6] suggest that exercise should not be performed in the supine position after completion of the fourth month of gestation. Others suggest that exercising in the supine position is not a risk until after the seventh month of pregnancy.[7,8] All pregnant women should be advised, however, to change positions if they become faint, dizzy, or nauseous while in the supine position.

Increases in the pressure in the veins of the pelvis and legs also result from venous compression in the trunk. In response to these changes, an increase in the incidence of hemorrhoids and varicose veins is seen during pregnancy.

Urinary Tract

The urinary tract is dilated during pregnancy, more prominently on the right than on the left, and probably occurs secondary to both hormonal and biomechanical factors. Progesterone relaxes the smooth muscle of these organs and others throughout the body and is therefore responsible for part of the distension. Partial obstruction of the ureter is also induced by the enlarging uterus. Women should be encouraged to empty the bladder completely before and after exercise. The physiologic effects of pregnancy result in an intravascular volume increased 50 percent, with the plasma component increasing approximately twice as much as the red cell mass, resulting in a physiologic fall in hematocrit during pregnancy.

Diabetes

Pregnancy is also a diabetogenic state. Insulin resistance occurs after the first trimester of pregnancy, so that there is prolonged elevation of glucose after meals. A series of hormonal factors have been implicated, with the resultant increased need for the use of insulin in pregnant patients who do not display a predisposing factor for diabetes in the nonpregnant state. Although the thyroid gland normally enlarges during pregnancy, the free, biologically active concentration of both T3 and T4 is unchanged from the nonpregnant state.

Respiration

Respiratory changes occur during pregnancy as a result of the mechanical effects of the enlarging uterus, the increase in oxygen consumption, and the stimulatory effect of progesterone on respiration. The enlarging uterus interferes with the activity of the diaphragm, particularly during the last trimester, causing an increased demand on the accessory muscles of respiration such as the scalenes and pectoralis minor. The increased activity in these muscles may contribute to the development of thoracic outlet syndrome symptoms, along with the postural changes previously mentioned.

PHYSICAL THERAPY EVALUATION

As the physical therapist evaluates a patient, historical and/or physical findings are often elicited in addition to those communicated from the referring practitioner. Knowledge of the fundamental changes that occur in a woman's menstrual cycle and during normal pregnancy will help the physical therapist determine what may be pathologic as opposed to what may be physiologic.

Pain

Pain is the most common history presenting to the physical therapist. With regard to the normal menstrual cycle, the pattern of pain must be determined,

---

Common Physical Findings

Pain
Bleeding
Vaginal discharge or burning
Breast tenderness
Urinary changes
Dyspareunia
Nausea and vomiting

---

that is, whether the pain is chronic or periodic. If periodic, it is useful to determine whether it is cyclic and predictable or whether it is unpredictable and noncyclic. Often a calendar of symptoms helps the patient determine when the pain becomes bothersome. Mild discomfort associated with the menstrual period (dysmenorrhea) is common. Pain that lasts 1 or 2 days at ovulation (*Mittelschmerz*) is normal and is associated with peritoneal irritation caused by ovulation. Pain that cannot be attributed to either of these entities (e.g., excessive dysmenorrhea) should be looked on as pathologic and requires further investigation. If pain is aggravated by particular activities and relieved by rest, a musculoskeletal component may be suspected as either a primary or secondary factor. Aching in the low back, buttocks, and posterior and anterior thighs are common complaints during the luteal phase, apparently associated with the hormone-induced musculoskeletal laxity. Many patients are diagnostically labeled as having chronic pelvic pain by the gynecologist. This usually refers to the presence of lower abdominal pain that is either cyclic or noncyclic for a period of more than 6 months. Endometriosis, pelvic relaxation disorders, pelvic inflammatory disease (PID), musculoskeletal dysfunction and other conditions may be responsible for such symptoms.

Bleeding

Bleeding is considered normal only as part of the normal menstrual cycle. There should, therefore, be a cyclic predictability of the timing, amount, and duration of bleeding. The number of days from the first day of one period to the first day of the next period should be fairly constant. Women occasionally have anovulatory cycles in which a period is delayed or skipped because she failed to ovulate that month. There may, occasionally, be mid-cycle spotting just after ovulation. This is due to the sudden drop in estrogen at the time of ovulation (shown in Fig. 6-12). Bleeding that does not conform to these guidelines, sudden changes in a patient's bleeding pattern, or any bleeding during pregnancy should be looked on as abnormal. It should be remembered that anovulatory cycles are more common and frequent in women during adolescence as well as during the years when ovarian function is waning, a time of life also known as the *perimenopause*. The latter typically occurs after the age of 40, leading to menopause at an average age of 51.

Vaginal Discharge or Burning

Vaginal discharge is also a common complaint. Occasionally, patients complain of a discharge that is actually physiologic. Physiologic leukorrhea is an exaggeration of the normal moisture in the vagina. Physiologic discharge is produced by a combination of mucus secreted from the glands of the cervix mixed with the desquamated cells from the vaginal walls. This appears as a white, curdlike discharge that reaches a maximum at the time of ovulation, when there is a maximum of mucus stimulated by estrogen production. This decreases during the luteal phase of the cycle and becomes more sticky and opaque because of the effects of progesterone.

Vaginal burning and vaginal discharge are commonly associated with one another. Patients often describe a yellow or greenish discharge which may be foul smelling. These symptoms are commonly associated with urinary symptoms as the discharge irritates the urethral meatus. *Vaginal dryness* in menopausal patients is often associated with a lack of estrogen support. The vaginal dryness can also be seen in conjunction with urinary frequency and dysuria in the postmenopausal patient.

Breast Tenderness/Abdominal Bloating

Breast tenderness is occasionally seen in women with fibrocystic breasts. Because of the hormonal changes of the menstrual cycle, there is an exaggeration in tenderness of the breast tissue during the luteal phase of the menstrual cycle. Typically, this pain should resolve shortly after the onset of the menstrual flow. Similarly, some women complain of lower abdominal swelling and bloating on a cyclic basis. Again, these typically occur in the luteal phase and resolve after the onset of menses. Breast symptoms or lower abdominal swelling that do not follow a cyclic pattern should be investigated as possible manifestations of significant pathology.

Breast pain other than the cyclic pain of fibrocystic breasts as described above should be looked on as abnormal. Often, however, patients are unable to differentiate breast pain from chest wall pain. Palpation of the affected area can often differentiate musculoskeletal pain from the pain of the primarily fatty tissue and glands of the breasts in female patients. The thoracic spine, costochondral, and costovertebral articulations may all refer pain into the anterior chest. These should be evaluated by the physical therapist in patients who have been cleared of breast disease or normal breast tenderness but continue to complain of anterior chest wall pain. All women should participate in a monthly breast self-examination routine to screen for breast cancer. Routine gynecologic consultation includes instruction in breast self-examination.

Urinary Changes

Urinary signs and symptoms should always suggest a possible problem, with the exception of those described as a normal part of pregnancy. The following symptoms may suggest a urinary tract infection that should be evaluated using urinalysis and possible culture and sensitivity: pyuria (cloudy urine), dysuria (pain with urination), hematuria (bloody urine), frequency (frequent need to urinate), urgency (immediate sense of the need to void), and incontinence (loss of the normal control of micturition). Incontinence can also be evidence of symptomatic pelvic relaxation (see under Specific Disorders) or of a loss of neurologic control of the bladder. In addition, it is seen in patients with urethral diverticula (outpouching of the urethra). Because of the proximity of the vagina and the urethra, patients with pathologic vaginal discharge can also present with symptoms simulating a urinary tract infection.

Dyspareunia

Dyspareunia (painful intercourse) is associated with both physiologic and psychologic factors. Superficial or "entrance" dyspareunia is most commonly associated with a lack of arousal, as manifested by a lack of vaginal lubrication. This type of dyspareunia may also be associated with vaginitis, urethritis, vaginismus (an involuntary contraction of the pelvic musculature), or other dysfunctions of the pelvic floor. Significant problems of the urethra or bladder can be associated with entrance dyspareunia. Deep thrust dyspareunia is seen with conditions of the pelvis, such as endometriosis, pelvic infection, fibroid tumors, or ovarian cysts.

Nausea and Vomiting

Nausea and vomiting are most commonly associated with early pregnancy. If pregnancy is not a possibility or has been ruled out, it should be remembered that nausea may be associated with any significant pain. Nausea may also present as a symptom of supine hypotension along with faintness and fatigue. Nausea and vomiting should otherwise be looked upon as a manifestation of gastrointestinal disease and appropriate referral for medical evaluation of such symptoms is indicated (see Ch. 4).

SPECIFIC DISEASES

Hormonal Dysfunction

Hormonal dysfunction is a vague term that does not have a specific diagnosis tied to it. It does, however, tend to be a catchall for any female problems that may even remotely be associated with the menstrual cycle. As a result, should the physical therapist encounter problems that appear to be limited to a history of abnormal uterine bleeding, it would not be uncommon for the patient to have had a physician evaluate her hormonal status. Because the normal menstrual cycle is regular and predictable, irregular and unpredictable periods are indicative of anovulation. Most commonly, this is due to stress or a temporary failure of the intricate neuroendocrine feedback loops. Occasionally, other endocrine abnormalities may affect ovulation

(e.g., thyroid or adrenal dysfunction or a pituitary tumor). A patient will typically have sought out medical evaluation long before an impact would be expected on the musculoskeletal system. An example is premature menopause, a condition in which the patient is no longer producing any estrogen as the ovaries have, for whatever reason, ceased to function. Longstanding lack of estrogen could result in a significant decrease in bone density (osteoporosis), increasing the risk of pathologic fractures. It is for this reason that women who have undergone a surgical or natural menopause are often given exogenous estrogen replacement therapy.

Endometriosis

Endometriosis is a condition typically confined to the pelvis in which tissue from the endometrium is present outside the endometrial cavity, typically in the peritoneum, around the fallopian tubes, ovaries, and rectum. It is a source of symptoms, including bilateral lower abdominal pain, dysmenorrhea, painful intercourse (dyspareunia), abnormal bleeding, premenstrual staining, and infertility. This history in a woman in her 20s or 30s should suggest this diagnosis. Clinical suspicion leads to the diagnosis, which can only be confirmed by direct observation of endometriotic lesions. These lesions are classically described as brownish, bluish, or black lesions, the color a result of recurrent hemorrhage in the area. Intense fibrosis is also associated with these lesions. Since the lesions are typically in the pelvis, visualization by means of a surgical operation is usually necessary .Under unusual circumstances, endometriosis can be visualized externally, for example, on the perineum or at the site of a previous abdominal incision. Other than visualization or histologic confirmation on biopsy, or both, no other tests are available to make this diagnosis.

Pelvic Inflammatory Disease

Pelvic inflammatory disease (PID), either acute or chronic, is infection of the reproductive tract. The two most widely reported organisms causing the infection are *Neisseria gonorrhoeae* and *Chlamydia trachomatis*. Either of these organisms can be cultured from the cervix or from the pelvic cavity, if surgery is necessary. The infection is typically a sexually transmitted disease (STD). It is diagnosed as patients present with acute bilateral lower abdominal tenderness, fever, and an elevated white blood cell (WBC) count. The tenderness is commonly rebound tenderness, an indication of peritoneal irritation, found when there is active infection or blood in the abdomen. By pressing and then suddenly releasing the pressure, intense pain can be elicited. All sexually active women from the teenage years through the fifth decade are at risk, but those who have sex with multiple partners and those with a previous history of pelvic infection are at highest risk. The residua of acute infection are primarily adhesions that can cause chronic pelvic pain as well as infertility. Chronic pain caused by adhesions either from PID or endometriosis cannot be diagnosed except by visualization during surgery, specifically laparoscopy. Laparoscopy permits visualization of the pelvic cavity through a fiberoptic instrument, through a small subumbilical incision; this technique avoids the risks, expense, and morbidity of laparotomy.

Fibroids

Leiomyomata uteri, or fibroids, are benign muscle tumors most commonly found in the uterus. They are found more commonly in blacks than in whites, in approximately one-third of all reproductive age women and are commonly associated with symptoms such as heavy menstrual bleeding (menorrhagia), irregular bleeding (metrorrhagia), as well as intermenstrual bleeding. Women in their 30s and 40s are more likely to have fibroid tumors. Fibroids can also cause acute pain at the site of the tumor if they undergo cellular degeneration. They may also be a source of chronic pelvic pain, particularly when they reach larger sizes. A sense of pelvic heaviness, abdominal bloating, or pressure symptoms on the rectum or bladder, or both, are not uncommon with large fibroid tumors. Physical examination of the abdomen can palpate these masses if they are greater than the size of a 4-month pregnancy. Vaginal examination will demonstrate the presence of these fibroid tumors if they are smaller than that. Ultrasound is the most commonly used imaging technique to determine the size and location of these tumors. Fibroid tumors are also an occasional source of back or sacral pain as well as abdominal pain.

Symptomatic Pelvic Relaxation

Symptomatic pelvic relaxation is typically manifested by uterine prolapse or stress urinary incontinence or both. As a result of loss of pelvic support, typically attributable to childbirth or through the aging process, the pelvic organs can begin a descent through the vagina and possibly be visible from the outside. This results in low back pain or the sensation of pressure or falling out. There is also heaviness of the upper thighs. The physical examination reveals findings compatible with a loss of the normal ligaments and muscular support for the bladder, uterus, or rectum, or both. No blood tests or radiographs are necessary to make this diagnosis, and repair is usually surgical, although occasionally supportive mechanisms such as pessaries may be helpful. This diagnosis should be suspected in older patients. Strengthening of the pelvic floor musculature and posture correction may also prove beneficial in the management of these patients.

Neoplasms

Neoplasms of the female reproductive tract present in various fashions, depending on the organ from which they arise. A general rule of thumb suggests that the older the patient, the more likely it is to be a neoplasm. Tumors of the ovary are often asymptomatic and are found only incidentally on pelvic examination. These tumors can present as acute symptoms of pain if they happen to rupture, twist, or bleed. Advanced ovarian malignancies will present with vague symptoms, such as abdominal bloating or early satiety or if the patient's clothes no longer fit. Ultrasound of the pelvis is the typical fashion in which ovarian neoplasms are visualized. Malignancies of the uterine lining usually present as abnormal bleeding, especially in the postmenopausal patient. A biopsy of the endometrial lining in any postmenopausal bleeding patient is necessary to rule out this condition. Cancer of the cervix also presents as bleeding, classically described as postcoital. These lesions are visualized on speculum examination of the cervix, where biopsy reveals the diagnosis without difficulty. Preinvasive cervical lesions are often asymptomatic and are initially picked up by routine Papanicolaou smears and by biopsies often performed under colposcopic visualization. The diagnosis of cancer of the vulva is made by biopsy of the affected area.

Patients often present with subtle symptoms, such as vulvar itching or irritation. On gross inspection, these areas may look normal, appear red and inflamed or pale and thin, or have gross lesions visible. Unfortunately, cancer only infrequently presents with pain as a symptom.

Ectopic Pregnancy

Ectopic pregnancy occurs in reproductive-age women. It is a pregnancy that implants and grows outside the uterine cavity. More than 95 percent of ectopic pregnancies are in the fallopian tube. The typical presentation is menstrual irregularity associated with unilateral or bilateral acute abdominal pain. Occasionally there is also referred shoulder pain. A positive pregnancy test in association with these symptoms warrants immediate gynecologic evaluation.

SIGNS AND SYMPTOMS OF NORMAL PREGNANCY

Nausea and vomiting are common during the first trimester. Small, frequent meals with bland foods are a typical solution to the problem. Bland snacks such as soda crackers are also helpful. These symptoms typically resolve after the first trimester. Urinary frequency is seen throughout pregnancy, especially later in pregnancy, as the enlarging uterus and fetus impinge on the bladder. Supine hypotension is also common as pregnancy progresses. Low back pain, hip pain, as well

---

Signs and Symptoms of Normal Pregnancy

Nausea and vomiting
Frequent urination
Supine hypotension
Posture and mobility changes
Thoracic outlet syndromes
Carpal tunnel syndrome
Edema in hands and feet
Breast Tenderness
Fatigue
Dyspnea

---

as leg pain are caused by the increasing abdominal girth and extra weight that the patient must endure. Posture and mobility changes in these areas were previously discussed in association with the normal physiology of pregnancy. Signs and symptoms associated with thoracic outlet and carpal tunnel syndromes also occur in pregnancy in response to vascular and postural changes. Edema of both the hands and the feet are common complaints. Breast tenderness is an early sign of pregnancy; later in pregnancy, it may be due to engorgement of the breasts. Generalized fatigue is a common finding throughout pregnancy and is best managed with additional rest. Dyspnea is also a common complaint during pregnancy as a result of biomechanic and physiologic changes.

SUMMARY

Normal anatomy and physiology of the female urogenital system have been reviewed along with the clinical signs and symptoms that may be seen as a result of normal physiologic activity in this system. Clearly, the hormonal influences on muscle tone and ligamentous laxity during the normal course of pregnancy and in the luteal phase of the menstrual cycle are of concern to the physical therapist, as they may reduce musculoskeletal stability. Physical therapists have not traditionally questioned patients regarding the onset of last menstrual period or the characteristics of the menstrual cycle. This information should be collected, as it may be beneficial in physical therapy treatment of musculoskeletal dysfunction. Exercise should be modified during times of "normal" increased instability. It is also important to note whether a patient is undergoing hormone therapy and, if so, which specific hormones are involved.

In addition to the signs and symptoms associated with normal physiology, signs and symptoms that indicate pathology in the female urogenital system are presented in this chapter. It is clear that female patients with abdominal pain or anterior pelvic pain (or persisting pain in any of the referred areas noted in Table 6-1) should be questioned about abnormal bleeding, dyspareunia, dysuria, and other signs and symptoms listed in Table 6-2. The signs and symptoms presented in Table 6-2 are most commonly associated with pa-

Table 6-1. Referred Pain: Female Urogenitical System

Structure	Segmental Innervation	Potential Site of Referred Pain
Ovaries	T10–T11	Lower abdomen, low back
Uterus	T10–L1	Lower abdomen, low back
Fallopian tubes	T10–L1	Lower abdomen, low back
Perineum	S2–S4	Sacral apex, suprapublic, rectum
External genitalia	L1–L2, S3–S4	Lower abdomen, medial anterior thigh, sacrum
Kidney	T10–L1	Ipsilateral low back and upper abdominal
Urinary bladder	T11–L2, S2–S4	Thoracolumbar, sacrococcygeal, suprapubic
Ureters	T11–L2, S2–S4	Groin, upper and lower abdomen, suprapubic, anterior-medial thigh, thoracolumbar

Table 6-2. Femal Urogenital System: Review of Systems Checklist

Sign/Symptom	Yes	No	Comments
1. Dyspareunia	⎯	⎯	⎯
2. Dysmenorrhea	⎯	⎯	⎯
3. Amenorrhea	⎯	⎯	⎯
4. Abnormally heavy menstrual bleeding	⎯	⎯	⎯
5. Abnormal bleeding pattern	⎯	⎯	⎯
6. Vaginal discharge	⎯	⎯	⎯
7. Vaginal burning/itching	⎯	⎯	⎯
8. Dysuria	⎯	⎯	⎯
9. Urinary frequency	⎯	⎯	⎯
10. Urinary urgency	⎯	⎯	⎯
11. Urinary incontinence	⎯	⎯	⎯
12. Abdominal pain not associated with menstruation	⎯	⎯	⎯
13. Abdominal bloating	⎯	⎯	⎯
14. Postural hypotension	⎯	⎯	⎯
15. History of infertility	⎯	⎯	⎯
16. History of infection	⎯	⎯	⎯

thology in the urogenital system. Their presence indicates the need for gynecologic evaluation. Therapists working under physician referral should provide the referring practitioner with any new information collected with regard to the urogenital system. Therapists in practice without referral situations should refer patients presenting with such signs and symptoms for gynecologic evaluation.

Many trunk, pelvic, and lower-extremity structures share innervation with the structures of the female urogenital system and are potential sites of referred pain (Table 6-1). Certain pathologic processes, such as pelvic relaxation, cystocele, or retrocele, may mimic the musculoskeletal pain pattern of symptomatic relief with rest and worsening with specific activities. It is important that physical therapists managing patients with pain complaints in these areas have knowledge of normal gynecologic and pregnancy physiology and of common pathologic signs and symptoms, so that pertinent information can be elicited from patients and appropriate referrals made to other practitioners.

Table 6-2 should assist the physical therapist in developing historical questions to be included in their clinical evaluation and re-evaluation of patients who present with signs and symptoms related to the female urogenital system.

PATIENT CASE HISTORY*

History

The patient was a 39-year-old housewife who came to the clinic with a diagnosis of mechanical low back pain syndrome with left gluteal muscle trigger points. Her chief complaint was constant left buttock aching and intermittent sharp pain in the left posterior superior iliac spine (PSIS)

*From Boissonnault WG, Bass C: Pathological origin of trunk and neck pain: part I—pelvic and abdominal visceral disorders. J Orthop Sports Phys Ther 12(15):206, 1990.

area. The left buttock aching intensity varied little but seemed to increase slightly if she was in any single position for more than 30 minutes. She stated that she was forced to change positions constantly. The sharp pain was provoked immediately with weight-bearing on the left lower extremity, both during standing and ambulation. The sharp pain could be relieved within minutes by lying down in any position. The patient woke up in the morning with the left buttock aching and severe left hip stiffness. After soaking in a hot shower, the stiffness, but not the aching, resolved.

The left buttock aching began insidiously 10 weeks before the initial evaluation. She had experienced similar symptoms periodically for the past 2 years. The initial episode also began insidiously. The sharp pain had begun 3 weeks before the initial evaluation. The patient described a fall on her left buttock that preceded the onset of the sharp pain. Until this recent flareup, her symptoms had gradually improved with bed rest and heat.

The patient's general medical and surgical history was negative and the patient was taking naproxen (Naprosyn). The patient stated that she had been constipated and had noted increased frequency of urination during the past 8 weeks. Upon specific questioning, she indicated that there was an increase in the aching of the left buttock when she was severely constipated and a concurrent decrease in the aching after a bowel movement. She stated that the referring physician was aware of the bowel and bladder dysfunction.

Physical Examination

In standing, the patient had difficulty with unilateral weight-bearing on the left lower extremity caused by provocation of the sharp pain. There was a significant increase in muscle tone of the left lumbar paraspinals and gluteals with weight shift on to the left lower extremity. There was a decreased lumbar lordosis in the low lumbar spine, and the bony landmarks of the iliac and greater trochanters were symmetric. There was significant tenderness with palpation from the left inferior lateral angle of the sacrum to the caudal aspect of the left PSIS. Active movement testing of the trunk on standing revealed decreased low lumbar spine motion during backward bending with provocation of sharp discomfort medial to the left PSIS. Also, a significant pulling sensation extending from the left low lumbar spine to the left buttock was noted at the end range of right-side bending. The patient had a positive sitting-forward bending test on the left for sacroiliac joint mobility. Left ilial shear test (passive spring test) provoked sharp left PSIS pain and a spasm end feel. Palpation revealed a significant left on right sacral torsion lesion and increased muscle tone of the left hip flexor and buttock musculature. Moderate to severe tightness was noted in the left hamstring and rectus femoris muscles.

Assessment and Outcome

The physical examination indicated that an apparent left sacroiliac joint dysfunction was responsible for the sharp left buttock symptoms. The aching pain was not altered during any of the components of the physical examination. Also of concern was the recent onset of constipation and urinary frequency and the insidious onset of the aching pain, in addition to the apparent correlation between severe constipation and increased buttock aching. After the left sacral base was mobilized, the sharp pain associated with the left lower-extremity weight-bearing resolved almost immediately, as did the sharp pain noted during active backward bending. The next two sessions consisted primarily of treating the muscle imbalances and residual increased muscle tone of the left hip flexors and buttock muscles. At the end of the 2-week period, the patient noted a 80 percent decrease in the intensity of the buttock aching, no sharp pain with standing and ambulation, and a significant improvement of the constipation and urinary frequency problems. After a weekend, the patient returned to the clinic, stating that all her symptoms had returned, as severe as ever. Specific questioning indicated that only the aching pain had worsened and the constipation and dysuria had returned to the pre-evaluation level. No sharp PSIS pain had returned. The patient could not relate the return of symptoms to any incident or accident. Physical examination revealed virtually no change in signs from her last visit when she was doing so well, and again the symptoms could not be altered.

It was recommended that the patient see her internist, because of the clinical findings. She called 6 weeks later to report that she had undergone abdominal surgery to remove an ovarian cyst. She stated she had been completely asymptomatic for the past 4 weeks.

REFERENCES

1. Williams PL, Warwick R: Gray's Anatomy. 36th Ed. WB Saunders, Philadelphia, 1980, pp 280–282
2. Gould SF: Anatomy. p. 3. In Gabbe SG, Niebyl JR, Simpson JL (eds): Obstetrics: Normal and Problem Pregnancies. 2nd Ed. Churchill Livingstone, New York, 1986
3. Hacker N, Moore GJ: Essentials of Obstetrics and Gynaecology. WB Saunders, Philadelphia, 1986.
4. Pernoll ML, Benson RC (eds): Current Obstetric and Gynelogic Diagnosis and Treatment. 6th Ed. Appleton & Lange, E. Norwalk, CT, 1987, pp 115–120
5. Fenlon A, Lovell D, Oakes E: Getting Ready for Childbirth—A Guide for Expectant Parents. Prentice-Hall, Englewood Cliffs, NJ, 1976, p. 6
6. Pre- and Post-Partum Exercise Guidelines. American College of Obstetricians and Gynecologists, 1985
7. Riczo DB: ACOG's guidelines for exercise during pregnancy and postpartum: Accepted or contested? J Obstet Gynecol Phys Ther 13:6, 1989
8. Perinatal Exercise Guidelines. Obstetrics and Gynecology Section. American Physical Therapy Association, 1986

7
Screening for Endocrine System Disease

JILL S. BOISSONNAULT, M.S., P.T.
DIANE MADLON-KAY, M.D.

The impact of disease within the endocrine system on physical therapy practice may be considerable or relatively uncommon, depending on the physical therapy setting. The therapist practicing within a rehabilitation or geriatric setting may have a large caseload of diabetic patients with a wide variety of complications necessitating physical therapy intervention: cerebrovascular accident (CVA), amputation, diabetic ulcers, and peripheral neuropathies. The signs and symptoms are overt and the conditions prediagnosed. This endocrine system disease presents challenges to the therapist with regard to exercise physiology, wound healing, and sensory integration. Other diseases of the endocrine system are less common but, when present, may also have an impact on physical therapy. Previously undiagnosed signs and symptoms of these diseases may be discovered during subjective and objective portions of the physical therapy evaluation, thus requiring referral back to the physician. Endocrine system diseases include dysfunction of the thyroid gland, parathyroid glands, adrenal glands, and pituitary gland.

Therapists working primarily in an outpatient setting, especially in those states that allow direct access, may encounter a patient who presents with symptoms of weakness, arthralgias, paresthesias, or diffuse pain, the actual etiology of which is metabolic in nature. The therapist may be the patient's sole contact with the medical community. This chapter assists the therapist in differentiating symptoms and signs of metabolic disease from those of musculoskeletal origin, as well as learning the cardinal signs of the more common metabolic diseases.

Two patient case studies are presented, both dealing with the diabetic patient. These case illustrations demonstrate the confusion over the presentation of symptoms and their etiology. Although the discovery of metabolic disease rarely prevents a fatality, it can be tremendously gratifying for both the patient and the therapist. The quality of life is surely diminished when one suffers from diseases such as Graves', Cushing's, or acromegaly. Therapists must avoid mistakenly treating what appear to be dysfunctions of the musculoskeletal system but which are in fact symptoms or signs of metabolic disease. The goal of this chapter is to help avoid that scenario, to aid in differentiation of signs and symptoms of metabolic disease from primary dysfunction of the neuromusculoskeletal system, and to understand the implications of these diseases on physical therapy practice, should they be prediagnosed in a patient.

PHYSIOLOGY OF THE ENDOCRINE SYSTEM

The endocrine system is composed of various glands that secrete substances called hormones into the bloodstream. The hormones are transported to their sites of action elsewhere in the body. The hormones then act on other cells to regulate their functions. Hormones may act on the cells of a specific organ or on cells widely distributed throughout the body. Figure 7-1 shows the location of the major endocrine glands. Table 7-1 summarizes the major endocrine glands,

153

Table 7-1. Summary of Hormonal Function[a]

Site Produced (Endocrine Gland)	Hormone[b]	Major Function
Hypothalamus	Releasing hormones	Secretion of hormones by the anterior pituitary
	Oxytocin	See posterior pituitary
	Vasopressin	See posterior pituitary
Anterior pituitary	Growth hormone (somatotropin, GH)	Growth: secretion of IGF-I; organic metabolism
	Thyroid-stimulating hormone (TSH, thyrotropin)	Thyroid gland
	Adrenocorticotropic hormone (ACTH, corticotropin)	Adrenal cortex
	Prolactin	Breast growth and milk synthesis; permissive for certain reproductive functions in the male
	Gonadotropic hormones: Follicle-stimulating hormone (FSH); luteinizing hormone (LH)	Gonads (gamete production and sex hormone secretion)
	β-Lipotropin	Unknown
	β-Endorphin	Unknown
Posterior pituitary	Oxytocin[c]	Milk "let-down"; uterine motility
	Vasopressin (antidiuretic hormone, ADH)[c]	Water excretion by the kidneys; blood pressure
Adrenal cortex	Cortisol	Organic metabolism; response to stresses; immune system
	Androgens	Sex drive in women
	Aldosterone	Sodiums, potassium, and acid excretion by kidneys
Adrenal medulla	Epinephrine	Organic metabolism; cardiovascular function; response to stress
	Norepinephrine	
Thyroid	Thyroxine (T_4)	Metabolic rate; growth; brain development and function
	Triiodothyronine (T_3)	
	Calcitonin	Plasma calcium
Parathyroids	Parathyroid hormone (parathormone, PTH, PH)	Plasma calcium and phosphate
Gonads		
Female: ovaries	Estrogen	Reproductive system; breast; growth and development
	Progesterone	
	Inhibin	FSH secretin
	Relaxin	Relaxation of cervix and pubic ligaments
Male: testes	Testosterone	Reproductive system; growth and development
	Inhibin	FSH secretion
	Müllerian-inhibiting hormone	Regression of müllerian ducts
Pancreas	Insulin	Organic metabolism; plasma glucose
	Glucagon	
	Somatostatin	
	Pancreatic polypeptide	
Kidney	Renin ($\rightarrow$angiotensin II)[d]	Aldosterone secretion; blood pressure
	Erythropoietin	Erythrocyte production
	1,25-Dihydroxyvitamin D_3	Calcium absorption by the intestine
Gastrointestinal tract	Gastrin	Gastrointestinal tract; liver; pancreas; gallbladder
	Secretin	
	Cholecystokinin	
	Glucose-dependent insulinotropic peptide (GIP)	
	Somatostatin	
Liver (and other cells)	Insulin-like growth factors (IGF-I and -II)	Growth

(*continued*)

Table 7-1. Summary of Hormonal Function[a] (continued)

Site Produced (Endocrine Gland)	Hormone[b]	Major Function
Thymus	Thymosin (thymopoietin)	T-lymphocyte function
Pineal	Melatonin	? Sexual maturity; body rhythms
Placenta	Chorionic gonadotropin (CG)	Secretion by corpus luteum
	Estrogens	See ovaries
	Progesterone	
	Placental lactogen	Breast development; organic metabolism
Heart	Atrial natriuretic factor (ANF, atriopeptin, auriculin)	Sodium excretion by kidneys; blood pressure
Monocytes and macrophages	Interleukin-1 (IL-1)	See Ch. 19 in Vander et al.[26]
	Tumor necrosis factor (TNF)	
	Other monokines	
Multiple cell types	Growth factors (e.g., nerve growth factor)	Growth of specific tissues

[a] Not all functions of the hormones are listed here.
[b] Names and abbreviations in parentheses are synonyms.
[c] The posterior pituitary stores and secretes these hormones; they are made in the hypothalamus.
[d] Renin is an enzyme that initiates reactions in blood that generate angiotensin II.
(From Vander et al.,[26] with permission.)

the hormones they secrete, and the hormonal functions.

The release of a hormone is often triggered by a change in the concentration of some substance in the body fluids. The hormone has a corrective effect, eliminating the stimulus, which then leads to a reduction in hormone secretion. This process is called a negative feedback homeostatic control system. Hormones control and integrate many body functions with this system. In general, hormonal control regulates the metabolic functions of the body, such as moderating chemical reactions in the cells, controlling the transport of substances through cell membranes, and partaking in various aspects of cellular metabolism. The types of effects that occur inside the cell are determined by the character of the cell itself. For example, when the kidneys are stimulated by vasopressin, or antidiuretic hormone (ADH), the vasopressin binds with a receptor causing a biochemical reaction resulting in a conversion of cytoplasmic adenosine triphosphatase (ATP) into cyclic adenosine monophosphate (cAMP). This reaction is believed to be the common process for many hormones and target organs. It is the cAMP that causes the hormonal effects inside the cell, such as increasing the number of enzymes in a cell or changing cell permeability. In the case of vasopressin, the cAMP affects the epithelial cells of the renal tubules by increasing their permeability to water.[1]

Many of the body's metabolic functions are under the influence of the pituitary gland, or hypophysis, which in turn is influenced by the hypothalamus. The pituitary gland is connected to the hypothalamus by the pituitary stalk. Connections to the posterior pituitary or neurohypophysis from the hypothalamus occur through a nerve tract. The hormones released through hypothalamic-neurohypophyseal interaction are vasopressin, which controls the rate of water excretion into the urine, and oxytocin, which, among other functions, helps deliver milk from the glands of the breast. The anterior pituitary gland, or the adenohypophysis, is connected to the hypothalamus by the hypothalamic-hypophyseal portal vessels. Six major hormones are secreted by the anterior pituitary gland: growth hormone, corticotropin (influencing the adrenocortical hormones), thyrotropin (controlling the rate of thyroxine secretions by the thyroid), and the three gonadotropins: follicle-stimulating hormone, luteinizing hormone, and luteotropic hormone.[1]

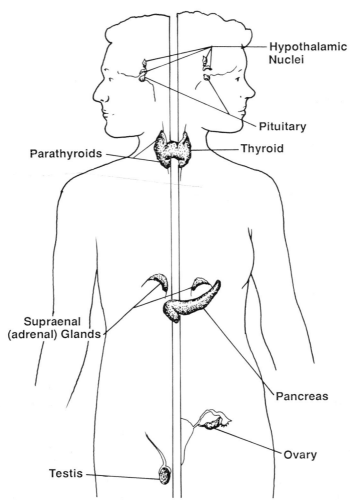

Fig. 7-1. Location of the major endocrine glands, male and female. Not shown are the liver, gastrointestinal tract, pineal gland, thymus, and placenta, all of which secrete hormones.

DISEASES OF THE ENDOCRINE SYSTEM

This chapter covers those diseases of the endocrine system that have an impact on physical therapy, with the exception of metabolic disease of the female genitourinary system (see discussion in Ch. 6; further information about metabolic disease of the female genitourinary system can also be found in the texts listed under Suggested Readings). The information presented on the diseases discussed here is intended as an overview of pathology and treatment as relevant to physical therapy. The diseases covered include diabetes mellitus, hypothyroidism and thyrotoxicosis (hyperthyroidism), hypoparathyroidism and hyperparathyroidism, Cushing's disease, Addison's disease, and acromegaly.

Disease of the pituitary gland itself is limited to discussion of acromegaly. The pituitary gland secretes many trophic hormones, which in turn cause secretion of hormones from target glands. Interference with the pituitary can cause many of the same signs and symptoms as those resulting from actual disease of the target gland. For example, a benign tumor of the pituitary, the most common pathology seen in this gland, could result in diminished secretion of thyrotropin. Since this hormone stimulates production of thyroxine, decreased secretion results in hypothyroidism. Blood tests can distinguish the source of the pathology, so that treatment can be instituted. Occasionally, pituitary enlargement is great enough to cause headaches and may interfere with the optic nerve as it courses by the gland. This would result in visual field disturbances. The headache or visual problems would aid the physician in diagnosing pituitary versus target gland disease.

While reading this section of the chapter, the therapist will note the common subjective patient complaints of lethargy, fatigue, and muscle weakness. Many of our patients complain of such symptoms, and we tend to pay them little heed. It is important to realize that they can be symptoms of real pathology, as evidenced by their presence in many of the following metabolic diseases.

Diabetes Mellitus

Diabetes mellitus is a chronic disease characterized by abnormal glucose utilization with inappropriately elevated blood glucose levels. Most diabetic patients have abnormal insulin secretion, leading to deranged metabolism of carbohydrates, fats, and proteins. Insulin deficiency results in decreased utilization of glucose by the body cells, with a resultant increase in blood glucose concentration. Abnormal metabolism of lipids and proteins results in increased deposition of lipids in the vascular walls and decreased deposition of proteins in the body tissues. The former leads to atherosclerosis and the latter to microangiopathy secondary to thickened basement membranes from excess glycoprotein. Over time, this leads to complications involving the eyes, kidneys, nerves, and blood vessels.

Diabetes is classified into two major categories. Type I or insulin-dependent diabetes mellitus (IDDM) is characterized by an absolute insulin deficiency and a dependence on insulin therapy for the preservation of life. About 10 percent of cases of diabetes are type I.

The onset is generally in childhood or early adulthood. Patients with type II, or non-insulin-dependent diabetes mellitus (NIDDM), do not require insulin therapy for the maintenance of life. However, insulin may be necessary to control symptoms or to correct disordered metabolism. Most type II diabetics are obese.

The prevalence of diabetes is thought to be about 1 percent. The diagnosis can be made in several ways: (1) unequivocal elevation of plasma glucose levels associated with classic symptoms of diabetes mellitus, (2) elevation of fasting plasma glucose on more than one occasion, and (3) elevation of plasma glucose after an oral glucose challenge on more than one occasion.

Treatment may be a combination of diet, oral hypoglycemic medications, and insulin. For the obese NIDDM patient, the immediate and long-term goals are weight reduction. NIDDM patients whose condition cannot be controlled by diet often respond to oral hypoglycemic medications. However, a high percentage of NIDDM patients will require insulin to control their symptoms. Insulin is required for the treatment of all type I patients.

Clinical Features

Diabetes is now most often diagnosed when the patient is asymptomatic as a result of routine blood tests showing an elevated glucose level. Most patients who are symptomatic complain of increased frequency of urination and excessive thirst with increased fluid intake. In severe cases, the patient may have increased appetite and food consumption with weight loss. Symptoms are usually present for weeks or months and have an insidious onset. Occasionally, patients present with no diabetic symptoms but complications have already developed such as neuropathy or vascular disease.

Subjective and/or objective examination by the physical therapist might pick up previously undiagnosed diabetes. For example, a patient may have been referred for physical therapy for a misdiagnosed diabetic peripheral neuropathy. A patient's diabetic symptoms may be subtle enough not to have aroused concern on the part of the patient. A patient may be referred for a separate problem, such as low back pain, with diabetes picked up as an incidental finding. In any case, a careful history and thorough objective examination may yield findings suggestive of diabetes, with necessary referral to a physician.

In the subjective examination, complaints of orthostatic hypotension, blurred vision, sensory deficits, extremity pain, weakness, diarrhea, various bladder problems, impotence, or dysphagia can all be related to diabetes. They can be signs and symptoms of other disease processes or sequelae of primary neuromusculoskeletal dysfunction. Response of these complaints to physical therapy treatment will help determine which of these possibilities is truly the culprit. Should any of these symptoms remain unchanged with physical therapy, referral to a physician would be indicated. Certainly a therapist would want a referring physician to be aware of some of the more viscerally related complaints right away.

Findings on objective examination that might warrant referral back to a physician would be foot ulcerations, muscle atrophy, elevated resting heart rate, or signs of cranial nerve involvement. Other findings, such as absent or diminished ankle jerk, edema, impaired vibratory sense, or decreased muscle strength, if found to be unrelated to the therapist's working diagnosis, should also be cause for referral.

The chronic complications of diabetes are now the major source of morbidity and mortality in both type I and type II diabetics. A broad spectrum of clinical syndromes are potential sequelae. This discussion focuses on the peripheral neuropathy and vascular complications.

Diabetic Neuropathy

Diabetic neuropathies pose considerable challenge to the clinician in terms of differentiation between mechanically and metabolically induced signs and symptoms. It is easy to overlook the possibility of mechanical sources of lower-extremity symptoms, such as numbness and tingling, when the patient presents with a diagnosis of diabetes because peripheral neuropathy is so common in this population. These neuropathies can be responsible for a wide range of symptoms. A case study presented at the end of this chapter illustrates this point.

Diabetic neuropathies are uncommon in young patients, and the incidence rises with the duration of the disease. The liability to neuropathy appears to be similar in both sexes. This discussion classifies diabetic neuropathies by division between symmetric and focal or multifocal lesions, according to the system adapted from Thomas[2] and presented by Dyke et al.[3]

The causation of diabetic peripheral neuropathy is neither well understood nor agreed upon. There is also disagreement in the literature regarding the primary site of pathology, be it peripheral nerve, dorsal root ganglion, or spinal cord.[3] There is a relationship between the degree of control of the disease and occurrence of neuropathy. Some of the signs and symptoms can abate or diminish in intensity once control is restored or attained. The symptoms and signs of diabetic neuropathy that might be found in a physical therapy assessment are summarized in Table 7-2.

Symmetric Polyneuropathies

Peripheral Sensory Neuropathy

The most common form of diabetic neuropathy is a distal symmetric predominantly sensory polyneuropathy. In most cases, symptoms are absent. Routine physical examination demonstrates a loss of vibratory sense, of tactile or proprioceptive sensation, or of ankle reflexes. When symptoms are present, patients complain of paresthesias described as numbness, coldness, or tingling, mainly of the feet. If pain is present, it may be disabling. The pain is typically worse at night.

Neuropathic arthropathies (Charcot's joint) are also possible but uncommon and are present only in association with established sensory polyneuropathy. Possible sites of joint pathology include interphalangeal and metatarsophalangeal joints of the foot, less commonly the ankle joints, knee joints, and rarely, the joints of the spine.[3] Most commonly, the patient presents with a swollen foot that may be painful. The foot is deformed with "rocker-bottom" subluxation of the mid-tarsal region or subluxation of the metatarsophalangeal joints. The foot is usually erythematous and warm. An infected neuropathic ulcer may be present. In the early stages, radiographs show severe arthritis. As the disease progresses, there is complete destruction of the involved joints with resorption of the met-

Table 7-2. Signs and Symptoms of Diabetic Neuropathy

Classification of Diabetic Neuropathy	Subjective Complains Commonly Found in Physical Therapy Evaluation	Objective Signs Commonly Found in Physical Therapy Evaluation
Symmetric polyneuropathies		
Peripheral sensory polyneuropathy	Paresthesias: numbness, coldness, tingling, (mainly in the feet)	Absent ankle jerk Impairment of vibration sense in feet Foot ulcers—often over metatarsal heads

Peripheral motor neuropathy	Pain, often disabling, worse at night
	Complaints of weakness
		Bilateral
		  Interosseous muscle atrophy
		  Claw or hammer toes
		  Decreased grip strength
		  Decreased muscle strength on manual muscle testing

Autonomic neuropathy	Orthostatic hypotension PM diarrhea, after meals Bladder problems Distal anhidrosis—symmetric Impotence Dysphagia	Elevated resting heart rate Peripheral edema
Focal and multifocal neuropathies		
Cranial neuropathy	Pain behind or above the eye Headaches Facial pain	Palpebral ptosis Inward deviation of one eye
Trunk and limb mononeuropathy	Abrupt onset of cramping or lancinating pain, hyperalgesia with hyperesthesia Cutaneous hyperesthesia of the trunk	Peripheral nerve specific motor loss Abdominal wall weakness
Proximal motor neuropathy or diabetic amyotrophy	Pain in proximal lower limbs—worse at night	Asymmetric proximal weakness, atrophy in lower limbs Absent or diminished knee jerk

atarsal heads. Fractures and joint effusions occur as well.[4]

The decreased sensory perception of diabetic neuropathy may lead to unperceived injury to the skin and joints. Insensitivity to heat can result in severe burns. Caution must be used by the therapist when applying physical agents. Unrecognized pressure from poorly fitting shoes can lead to ulcers and infection.

The diabetic patient may benefit from custom-fit foot orthoses. Chronic foot ulcers are generally found over the metatarsal heads. Loss of sensation and pain may be primarily responsible for their development, but ischemia, motor weakness (see peripheral motor neuropathy), the liability of diabetic tissues to infection, and anatomic deformity may also contribute to their development.[3]

Peripheral Motor Neuropathy

Motor abnormalities are much less common than sensory abnormalities. The small muscles of the feet and hands are most commonly involved. Interosseous

muscle atrophy allows the foot to assume abnormal positions with "claw" or "hammer" toes. New pressure points develop, leading to callus formation and ulceration. Hand involvement leads to weakness of grip. Diffuse weakness of the legs and upper extremities may also occur.

Autonomic Neuropathy

Diabetic autonomic neuropathy, like symmetric sensory polyneuropathy, is also probably length related; the longer fibers are initially affected. Thus, the earliest changes affect the lower extremities rather than innervation to the heart or great vessels.[3] Segmental demyelination is the predominant pathologic change. Disturbances of autonomic function often occur late in the disease process and pose an increased risk of mortality. The more common clinical manifestations of diabetic autonomic neuropathy include abnormal pupillary findings, such as a reduction in pupillary size and reduction in pupillary response to light, and the cardiovascular disturbances of orthostatic hypotension, elevated resting heart rate, and peripheral edema. Other common findings of diabetic autonomic neuropathy include poor thermoregulatory function, such as anhidrosis and abnormal vasomotor responses (the patient loses the normal reflex vasoconstriction and vasodilation of skin vessels to elevation or reduction of central body temperature), and atony of the esophagus, stomach, gallbladder, colon, and bladder. Gastrointestinal disturbance may include diabetic diarrhea,[3] which usually occurs at night or after meals. Bladder disturbances usually begin with lengthening intervals between voiding and progress to problems of micturition with straining, weakness, and intermittency of stream, as well as postmicturition dribbling. The final stage involves overflow incontinence.

Focal and Multifocal Neuropathies

Cranial Nerve Lesions

It is possible to see isolated or multiple palsies of the nerves to the external ocular muscles in older diabetics. The most common disturbance is of an isolated third nerve lesion resulting in palpebral ptosis that may be partial or total. The sixth nerve is less commonly affected and presents with an inward deviation of the eye on the affected side. The onset is generally abrupt and may be painless, though pain has been reported to occur in about half the cases and may precede paralysis by several days. The pain may be quite intense and can be felt behind or above the eye. Headaches may also occur. Other cranial nerves may be affected, but less frequently than those to the external ocular muscles. In almost all cases the paralyzed extraocular muscle recovers function in 4 to 8 weeks with improved diabetic control and symptomatic treatment.

Facial nerve paralysis is also possible secondary to diabetic cranial neuropathy, although less common than paralysis to ocular musculature. Clinical progress is similar to lesions of nerves III and VI.

Trunk and Limb Mononeuropathies

Mononeuropathies can affect any part of the body. This complication is characterized by involvement of a single nerve or its branches. The lower extremities are more commonly involved, specifically the femoral, lateral cutaneous or peroneal nerve. In the upper extremity, the ulnar, median, and radial nerves are most commonly affected. The onset is usually sudden with intense cramping or lancinating pain. Symptoms can involve sensory, motor, or mixed manifestations. The pain is typically worse at night and may be relieved by pacing when the lower extremities are involved. Sensory loss produces a clinical picture of hyperalgesia with hyperesthesia.

A diabetic truncal mononeuropathy has also been seen. Presentation is of abdominal wall weakness or cutaneous hyperesthesia with electromyographic evidence of paraspinal denervation. The prognosis for recovery is reported to be good for both the trunk and peripheral mononeuropathies.[3,5]

Proximal Motor Neuropathy or Diabetic Amyotrophy

Amyotrophy is a form of neuropathy that resembles a primary muscle disease. Severe proximal asymmetric muscle weakness and pain usually affect the pelvic girdle and thigh muscles through a disturbance of the lumbosacral plexus. The knee jerk is depressed or abolished but sensory loss is not prominent. The condition primarily affects the iliopsoas, quadriceps, and adductor musculature. The anterolateral muscle group in the lower leg may simultaneously be involved producing what has been termed the anterior compartment syndrome.[3] The typical patient is an elderly NIDDM male patient with mild disease. The onset may be rapid and accompanied by low-grade fever. Patients may have profound weight loss and severe depression. Function is often recovered spontaneously with the aid of good diabetic control.[6,7]

Diabetic Vascular Disease

Macrovascular or Macroangiopathy

The pathology of atherosclerosis in the diabetic patient is quite similar to that in the general population; however, it's rate is severely accelerated. Complications due to macrovascular disease in the diabetic include myocardial infarction (MI) which is more likely to be painless in a diabetic due to associated autonomic neuropathy affecting the pain fibers to the heart, CVA, and peripheral vascular disease. (Further reading on signs and symptoms of these processes can be found in Ch. 2.)

Microvascular or Microangiopathy

Microangiopathy is considered to be a lesion of the capillaries unique to diabetics. The basement membranes of the capillaries thicken. This is seen primarily in the retina, glomeruli, skin, and muscle. Increased permeability occurs and eventually ischemic and hemorrhagic complications occur. These lesions are particularly threatening to the type I diabetic. (See Ch. 5 for a discussion of the signs of kidney disease and Ch. 8 for a further assessment of vision in relationship to cranial nerve function.)

Diseases of the Thyroid Gland

The thyroid gland is composed of two lobes lying on either side of the trachea and connected in the midline by a thin isthmus. The isthmus lies just below the cricoid cartilage of the larynx. The examination of the thyroid begins with inspection. The patient is asked to extend his neck. The normal thyroid is barely visible. If sufficiently enlarged, a mass may be observable within the jugular notch, rendering the borders of the notch indistinct. The patient is asked to swallow. Normally, the thyroid rises during swallowing. Any mass or enlargement that moves upward is likely to be within the thyroid. Any enlargement of the thyroid gland is termed a goiter, except in pregnancy or menstruation, when enlargement is normal. The parathyroid glands are usually related to the posterior borders of the lobes of the thyroid gland.

Palpation is best done from behind the patient. The posterior approach involves placing the examiner's two hands around the neck of the patient whose neck is slightly extended. The index fingers are placed just below the cricoid (Fig. 7-2). As the patient swallows, the thyroid isthmus should rise under the fingers. The fingers are then rotated slightly downward and laterally, so that one can feel as much of the lateral lobes as possible. The normal thyroid is often not palpable.

The size, shape, and consistency of the gland, as well as any nodules or tenderness, should be noted. The normal thyroid gland has the consistency of muscle tissue. Unusual hardness may be due to cancer or scarring. A toxic goiter may be soft or spongy. Tenderness of the gland may be due to infection or hemorrhage

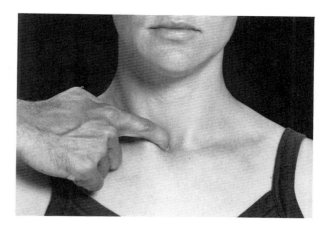

Fig. 7-2. Palpation of the thyroid gland. The examiner's finger is placed below the cricoid cartilage in the space just above the sternal notch and medial to the sternocleidomastoid muscle.

into the gland. If the thyroid is enlarged, it should also be auscultated. The bell of the stethoscope is placed over the lobes. A systolic bruit suggests a toxic goiter.

Physical examination of the thyroid reveals little about the function of the gland. Symptoms and signs elsewhere in the body provide clues to the functional status of the thyroid.

Thyrotoxicosis

Thyrotoxicosis (hyperthyroidism) is a syndrome that results from an excess of thyroid hormone. Thyrotoxicosis has several causes, the most common of which is Graves' disease, an autoimmune disease. Thyrotoxicosis is also commonly caused by a hyperfunctioning nodular goiter. Less frequently, the cause is a solitary hyperfunctioning adenoma, thyroiditis, or related to iodine.

The incidence of thyrotoxicosis in the United States is 2 per 10,000 cases, with a strong female predominance. The diagnosis is made by thyroid function blood tests. Treatment varies with the etiology and may include antithyroid medications (propylthiouracil or methimazole), adjunctive medications (iodine, adrenergic antagonists), radioactive iodine, or surgery.

Clinical Features

The clinical presentation of thyrotoxicosis is variable and dependent on the degree of hormone excess, rapidity of onset, duration, and age of the patient (Table 7-3). The typical patient presents with at least one of the following complaints: nervousness, weight loss, palpitations, enlarging neck mass, change in the appearance of the eyes or symptoms of heart failure or fatigue. Muscle weakness and bony and trophic changes also occur and, along with fatigue, are the signs and symptoms most likely to be picked up in physical therapy evaluation. Since these findings are also representative of many other diseases and dysfunctions, the therapist would probably need to rely on the patient's response to therapy for guidance regarding further medical evaluation; that is, if muscle strength were to return to normal levels after a conditioning program, no further referral would be necessary, but unchanged or worsening complaints would warrant referral to a physician.

Weakness and fatigability are frequent symptoms. Usually there is no evidence of local muscle disease other than a general wasting associated with weight loss. The weakness is most prominent in the proximal muscles of the extremities. Occasionally proximal muscle wast-

Table 7-3. Incidence of Symptoms and Signs Observed in 247 Patients with Thyrotoxicosis

Symptom	%	Symptom	%
Nervousness	99	Increased appetite	65
Increased sweating	91	Eye complaints	54
Hypersensitivity to heat	89	Swelling of legs	35
Palpitation	89	Hyperdefecation	33
Fatigue	88	(without diarrhea)	
Weight loss	85	Diarrhea	23
Tachycardia	82	Anorexia	9
Dyspnea	75	Constipation	4
Weakness	70	Weight gain	2

Sign	%	Sign	%
Tachycardia[a]	100	Eye signs	71
Goiter[b]	100	Atrial fibrilation	10
Skin changes	97	Splenomegaly	10
Tremor	97	Gynecomastia	10
Bruit over thyroid	77	Liver palms	8

[a] In other studies, thyrotoxic patients patients with normal pulse rate have been observed.

[b] Enlargement of thyroid is reported lacking in approximately 3 percent of patients with thyrotoxicosis in other studies.

(From Wilson and Foster,[27] with permission.)

ing may be seen. The myopathy affects men more than women and may be the most prominent symptom. The contraction and relaxation phases of deep tendon reflexes are shortened due to weak contractions of skeletal muscles.[8,9]

Hypokalemic periodic paralysis (resulting from abnormally small concentrations of potassium ions in the circulation) may occur, particularly in Oriental patients. The attack of paralysis may be generalized or localized and may be precipitated by exercise or high carbohydrate or high sodium meals. The attack may last for minutes to days and is associated with a lowering of the serum potassium level.[8,9]

Thyrotoxicosis may be associated with demineralization of bone and pathologic fractures, particularly in elderly women. Though not a contraindication to passively stretching a patient, this condition would warrant caution on the therapist's part when using passive accessory or physiologic techniques. Osteopathy with subperiosteal bone formation and swelling is rare but, when present, may be particularly evident in the metacarpal bones.

Thyroid dermopathy consists of a thickening of the skin, particularly over the lower tibia. Occasionally it also involves the entire lower leg and may extend into the feet. It is caused by an accumulation of glycosaminoglycans and is found in only 2 to 3 percent of patients with Graves' disease. Onycholysis, separation of the nail from its bed, is a much more common finding.[10]

Hypothyroidism

Hypothyroidism results from decreased thyroid hormone production. In about 95 percent of cases, the hormone deficiency is caused by a disease within the thyroid gland itself. Only 5 percent of cases are caused by pituitary or hypothalamic disease. The most common single cause is treatment of hyperthyroidism with radioiodine or surgery. Another common cause is autoimmune destruction of the thyroid, such as in Hashimoto's thyroiditis.

Hypothyroidism is very common. Community surveys find that about 8 percent of women and 1 percent of men have subclinical hypothyroidism. Overt hypothyroidism is reported in about 1 percent of patients seeking medical care. The diagnosis is made by thyroid function blood tests. Treatment is with synthetic thyroid hormone. The symptoms of hypothyroidism in adults are largely reversible with this medication.

Clinical Features

The clinical manifestations of hypothyroidism are variable, depending on its cause, duration, and severity (Table 7-4). Thyroid hormone is required for the normal functioning of most organ systems. Therefore thyroid hormone deficiency results in slowing of physical and mental activity, cardiovascular, gastrointestinal, and neuromuscular function. Deposition of glycoaminoglycans in the intracellular spaces, particularly in skin and muscle, along with the generalized slowing down of the organism, results in the clinical picture of myxedema.

Many of the symptoms and signs of hypothyroidism, such as fatigue, lethargy, constipation, and dry skin, are nonspecific. The most helpful symptoms and signs that aid in the diagnosis are slow movements, coarse skin, decreased sweating, hoarseness, paresthesias,

cold intolerance, periorbital edema, and slow reflex relaxation. The thyroid gland may be diffusely enlarged or may not be palpable, depending on the etiology. Since the incidence of hypothyroidism is so great, especially in women, it is not unlikely that therapists would come upon this either previously diagnosed or undiagnosed. The trophic changes of dry skin or periorbital puffiness may be observed during the objective examination, and reflex testing might elicit the slowed relaxation response. Muscle testing might reveal a pattern of weakness (see below). The subjective examination would probably elicit the complaints of fatigue and possibly complaints of arthralgias or specific weakness.

Patients often complain of extremity paresthesias but usually have no objective neurologic abnormalities other than slow deep tendon reflexes. These characteristic "hung-up" reflexes result from a decrease in the rate of muscle contraction and relaxation. Carpal tunnel syndrome may occur because of mucinous edema of the wrist. Some patients have a polyneuropathy because of myxedema of peripheral nerves. Movements are slow and clumsy. Signs of cerebellar dysfunction may occur, such as ataxia and intention tremor.[9,11]

Muscle cramps, myalgias, and stiffness are frequent symptoms. Subjective weakness and fatigability are common. Some objective muscle weakness may be noted in the shoulder and pelvic regions. Muscle mass may be slightly increased, and the muscles tend to be firmer than normal. Rarely, a large increase in muscle mass accompanied by slowness of muscular activity may be the predominant finding. Elevated serum creatine phosphokinase (CPK) levels are commonly found even in patients without muscle symptoms.[9,12,13] Patients may have arthralgias with synovial thickening and effusions, usually of the knees or small joints of the hands and feet.[14]

Diseases of the Parathyroid Gland

Hyperparathyroidism

Hyperparathyroidism is caused by an increased secretion of parathyroid hormone by the parathyroid gland. Parathyroid adenomas or, less commonly, carcinomas

Table 7-4. Frequency of Signs and Symptoms of Hypothyroidism[†]

	Frequency (%)	Diagnostic Weight Present	Diagnostic Weight Absent
Symptoms			
Dry skin	60–100	+3	−6
Cold intolerance	60–95	+4	−5
Hoarseness	50–75	+5	−6
Weight gain	50–75	+5	−1
Constipation	35–65	+2	−1
Decreased sweating	10–65	+3	−6
Paresthesias	50	+5	−4
Decreased hearing	5–30	+2	0
Weakness	90		
Signs			
Slow movements	70–90	+11	−3
Coarse skin and hair	70–100	+7	−7
Cold skin	70–90	+3	−2
Periorbital puffiness	40–90	+4	−6
Bradycardia	10–15	+4	−4
Slow reflex relaxation	50	+15	−6

[†] In patients with no other illness and receiving no medication, a total score of +19 or greater indicates hypothyroidism and a score of −24 or less excludes it.

(From DeGroot et al.,[28] with permission.)

are the cause. The incidence is about 1 per 1,000 persons. The excess hormone usually leads to elevated calcium and decreased phosphate levels in the blood. With the widespread use of multiphasic screening blood tests, most patients have no symptoms, but are diagnosed on the basis of elevated calcium. Other patients present with recurrent kidney stones, peptic ulcers, mental changes, or extensive bone resorption.

The diagnosis of hyperparathyroidism is confirmed by an elevated blood parathyroid hormone level. Treatment varies with the severity of the hypercalcemia. Medical management followed by surgery is required for patients with severe symptomatic hypercalcemia. Many patients can be followed with periodic testing of bone and kidney function and no specific therapy.

Clinical Features

Osteitis fibrosa cystica is the classic skeletal disorder of hyperparathyroidism. Patients may have subperiosteal resorption, bone cysts, brown tumors, fractures, deformities, and marked replacement of bone marrow by fibrous tissue. In mild cases, the subperiosteal resorption may be limited to the radial side of the middle phalanges. The skull is the next most frequently involved area. Increased bone resorption in the skull leads to a salt-and-pepper appearance on skull radiographs. Later resorption may be seen close to the acromioclavicular joint, symphysis pubis and sacroiliac joints. Patients may also have diffuse osteopenia which is indistinguishable from postmenopausal osteoporosis.[15,16]

Several joint disorders are frequently associated with hyperparathyroidism: chondrocalcinosis, gout, juxta-articular erosions, subchondral fractures, traumatic synovitis and calcific periarthritis.[15] Symptoms also include proximal muscle weakness and easy fatigability, particularly in the lower extremities. Gross motor atrophy may be present on biopsy. Electromyograms are abnormal.

Occasionally patients complain of dysesthesias. The patient may have abnormal tongue movements and atrophy. The neurologic exam may show decreased vibratory sense in the feet and glove-and-stocking sensory loss.[17,18] As seen in patients with thyroid disease, hyperparathyroid disease presents with muscle weakness and fatigue. Bony loss may be present, similar to the demineralization of hyperthyroidism. Physical therapy evaluation should reveal the reflex changes, muscle weakness, and sensory changes. Most patients are asymptomatic, and the disease is found during a routine physical examination through blood work.

Hypoparathyroidism

Hypoparathyroidism is caused by a decreased or absent secretion of parathyroid hormone by the parathyroid gland. Hypoparathyroidism may be hereditary or acquired. The hereditary form may first become manifest in adult life. It may be an isolated abnormality or associated with other endocrine and skin disorders. Acquired hypoparathyroidism is usually the result of inadvertent surgical removal of all of the parathyroid glands. This may occur during surgery for hyperthyroidism or hyperparathyroidism.

The reported incidence of permanent hypoparathyroidism after thyroidectomy ranges from 0.2 to 33 percent. The incidence is 1 percent after surgery for hypoparathyroidism. The diagnosis is made by finding a low serum calcium level with a low serum parathyroid hormone level. Patients are treated with calcium and vitamin D.

Clinical Features

Mild symptoms are nonspecific and include psychological symptoms, such as irritability and depression, paresthesias, and muscle cramps. More severe symptoms are delirium, psychosis, tetany, and seizures. Left untreated, the severe form can lead to death.

The most common manifestations of hypoparathyroidism are neurologic. A typical attack of overt tetany begins with tingling in the fingertips and around the mouth. This gradually increases in severity and spreads proximally along the limbs and over the face. The muscles of the extremities and face feel tense and then go into spasm. Pain may be very severe, depending on the degree of tension developed in the muscle.

Provocative tests may demonstrate the presence of latent tetany. A positive Chvostek's sign is obtained by a sharp tap given over the facial nerve just anterior to

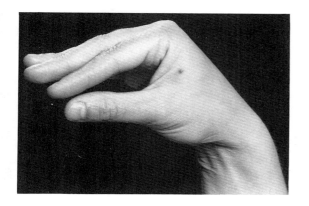

Fig. 7-3. Hand of a patient with a positive Trousseau's sign.

the ear, which produces a contraction of the facial muscle around the lip. The sign may be noticed by the patient during shaving. This test is also positive in up to 25 percent of normal people.[18]

Another diagnostic maneuver, Trousseau's sign, is compression of the upper arm by a blood pressure cuff with the pressure elevated above the systolic pressure. The test is positive when spasm of the hand occurs within 3 minutes (Fig. 7-3). This test is more reliable but may occur in about 4 percent of normal people. When the cuff is released, the muscles take about 5 to 10 seconds to relax.[18]

Many variations in clinical expression of tetany are possible. The patient may describe the muscle spasm as a cramp or stiffness or clumsiness. The patient may have continuous mild paresthesias or cramps rather than clearly defined attacks of tetany. Some patients develop carpal spasm only during prolonged use of the hand. If the spasm is more severe in the legs, the patient may have a limp or difficulty walking or fall frequently. Only one side of the body may be affected in some patients.[18]

Calcification of the basal ganglia may occur. There may be no neurologic disability associated or a variety of extrapyramidal symptoms such as chorea, tremors, dystonia, spasms, oculogyric crises, and parkinsonism. Age-related bone loss proceeds more slowly. Paravertebral ligamentous ossification can cause spinal nerve root compression and back stiffness.[19]

Fatigue and weakness are common symptoms. Rare patients may have a true myopathy.[18,20]

Patients with hypoparathyroidism would normally proceed to a physician with their complaints rather than seeking assistance from a physical therapist. Should a patient present first to a therapist, the objective and subjective signs and symptoms mentioned above would be unusual enough to immediately suggest a disease process and warrant referral to a physician.

Diseases of the Adrenal Gland

Cushing's Syndrome

In Cushing's syndrome (adrenocortical hyperactivity), an excess amount of glucocorticoid is secreted by the adrenal gland, along with a varying amount of adrenal androgens. Most cases are due to oversecretion of adrenocorticotropic hormone (ACTH) from a pituitary tumor, which then leads to adrenal hyperplasia. This etiology is termed Cushing's disease. Other less common causes of adrenal hyperactivity are adrenal adenomas or carcinomas or a malignant tumor elsewhere in the body that produces ACTH. The incidence is 10 cases per million people per year.

Patients with suspected Cushing's syndrome can be screened by an overnight dexamethasone suppression test or measurement of the 24-hour urinary excretion of cortisol. Treatment varies with the cause of the syndrome. Adrenal adenomas are surgically removed. Pituitary tumors can also be surgically removed. An alternative treatment is pituitary irradiation in combination with an adrenal suppressing medication.

Clinical Features

The typical patient with Cushing's syndrome is a middle-aged woman with truncal obesity, hirsutism (the presence of excessive body or facial hair, especially in women), a ruddy round face, and hypertension. Almost every organ system can be affected.

The effect on the muscles is variable. Patients may have marked muscle wasting. Weakness may also be due to low serum potassium. Patients with longstanding Cushing's syndrome will have demineralization of bone. Osteoporosis produces back pain, kyphosis, and loss of height. As many as 40 percent of patients have pathologic fractures of the ribs or vertebrae. Occasionally patients develop avascular necrosis of the femoral and humeral heads.

Dilation and thinning of blood vessel walls occur, increasing their fragility, leading to a significant increase in bruisability. Poor wound healing is a particular problem for postsurgical patients.

The significance of this disease to a manual therapist is the necessity of avoidance of techniques which might cause pathologic fractures secondary to osteoporosis. Here the emphasis should be placed on understanding and respecting the disease process in a previously diagnosed patient who presents to the clinic for pain management or for any other physical therapy intervention.

Addison's Disease

Addison's disease (adrenocortical insufficiency) is the primary inability of the adrenal gland to make sufficient quantities of adrenal steroid hormones. It is most commonly due to an autoimmune process, with antibodies present in adrenal tissue. Addison's disease is uncommon, with a prevalence of 4 per 100,000 persons.

It is difficult to diagnose early Addison's disease because nonspecific weakness and fatigue are the most frequent symptoms. Screening for Addison's disease may be done by ACTH stimulation testing, which measures the reserve capacity of the adrenal for steroid production. Treatment is specific hormone replacement with cortisol and often fludrocortisone.

Clinical Features

All patients with Addison's disease complain of weakness and fatigue. Gastrointestinal symptoms such as anorexia, vomiting, and diarrhea are common, and most patients will have a history of weight loss. Most patients will have signs of hyperpigmentation, most noticeably on the extensor surfaces, the creases of the palm, and the buccal mucosa.

Serum calcium is frequently elevated, leading to calcification of cartilage. The ears may be hardened to a stonelike consistency. The costal cartilage may also be calcified. Serum potassium elevation may produce an ascending neuromyopathy that ultimately causes flaccid paraplegia or quadriplegia. Addison's disease may also be associated with spastic paraplegia and polyneuropathy, called adrenomyeloneuropathy.

Once again, weakness and fatigue are the symptoms most relevant to diagnosis and most likely to be found on physical therapy assessment. Response to treatment, as mentioned with regard to disorders of other endocrine glands, is a key to deciding on referral of the patient for further physician follow-up.

Diseases of the Pituitary Gland

Acromegaly

Acromegaly is a disease caused by an excess production of growth hormone after adolescence. Pituitary tumors are the most common cause. This chronic, slowly progressive, debilitating disease is characterized by overgrowth of the skeleton and enlargement of soft tissues. Acromegaly occurs most often in middle age. The annual incidence is estimated to be 3 cases per million persons.

Patients with acromegaly often have symptoms for many years before the diagnosis is made. The diagnosis is confirmed by an elevated serum growth hormone level that does not suppress with an oral glucose load. Treatment options include surgery, radiation, and medical therapy with bromocriptine.

Clinical Features

The most common clinical feature suggesting the diagnosis is a coarsening of facial features over many years. Multiple organ systems can be adversely affected by acromegaly. The physical therapist rarely has the opportunity to see a patient over a course of years and therefore would not notice this coarsening of features. The symptoms and signs of skeletal changes with associated weakness and pain should clue the therapist into the possibility of acromegaly if these skeletal changes are overtly observable.

Patients with acromegaly tend to be tall. The mandible enlarges, resulting in prognathism (an underbite). The frontal, malar, and nasal bones are overgrown. As the metacarpals, metatarsals, and phalanges increase in thickness, the patient may notice an increased glove and shoe size. The ribs elongate and result in a barrel-shaped chest. The vertebral bodies of the spine elongate and widen and develop hypertrophic spurs. Thoracic kyphosis is common. Joint symptoms are prominent and vary from backaches and arthralgias to severe degenerative osseous overgrowth. As the disease progresses, degenerative arthritis of the hips, knees, shoulders, and elbows may develop.[21] Muscle weakness is primarily due to neuropathies. There may also be a proximal muscle myopathy.[22,23]

Patients may have compression of the nerve roots at the vertebral foramina with resultant spinal stenosis from overgrowth of the bony canal. Acroparesthesias are due to entrapment of nerves by bone or connective tissue overgrowth. Paresthesias of the hand are particularly common resulting from compression of the median nerve at the wrist.[23–25]

SUMMARY

This chapter covers those diseases of the endocrine system that might have an impact on physical therapy care or outcome. Diabetes mellitus, thyrotoxicosis (hyperthyroidism) and hypothyroidism, hyperparathyroidism and hypoparathyroidism, Cushing's syndrome, Addison's disease, and acromegaly have been discussed. The most common subjective and objective changes found in patients suffering from these diseases are summarized in Table 7-5. Many of these diseases present with common subjective complaints of weakness, fatigue, and lethargy. It is therefore important to pay heed to these complaints, especially if they are accompanied by unexplained objective findings or when seemingly explainable objective findings do not respond to physical therapy.

The goals of this chapter have been to provide the physical therapist with the information necessary to determine when referral to a physician might be warranted in the case of metabolic disease. Additionally,

the discussion of these diseases and their signs and symptoms should aid the clinician in appropriate treatment planning and goal setting.

PATIENT CASE HISTORY 1
History

A 52-year-old male tool and dye worker was referred by physician to physical therapy with a diagnosis of cervical and lumbar spondylosis. His chief complaints were of right neck, posterior shoulder, and low back pain. He was seen a year after involvement in a motor vehicle accident. He had been in another vehicle accident 1 year before this second one and suffered a work-related low back injury 9 years before therapy. Previous physical therapy did help but did not relieve his symptoms. In addition to the neck, shoulder, and arm symptoms, he complained of some dizziness and discomfort in the medial aspect of both great toes.

The patient's neck pain was aggravated by pulling, picking things up, or turning his head too fast. The low back discomfort was brought on by quick forward bending or by sitting in a car for more than 1 hour. The patient was unaware of what increased or brought on his dizziness. Medications and assuming a non-weight-bearing position diminished his neck and back symptoms. The patient denied any general medical problems and had a surgical history of tonsillectomy and vasectomy.

Objective Examination

Observation demonstrated the patient's head to be slightly rotated to the right and that he had scoliosis of the lumbar spine convex to the right. Increased muscle tone was noted throughout the paraspinal musculature: motion testing revealed restriction in C1–C2 joint mobility and decreased anterior glide at the cervicothoracic

Table 7-5. Subjective and Objective Changes Associated with Common Endocrine Disease

Disorder	Subjective	Objective
Diabetes mellitus	Orthostatic hypotension Blurred vision Sensory deficits Extremity or truncal pain Weakness Diarrhea Bladder complaints Impotence Dysphagia	Edema Foot ulcerations Muscle atrophy Elevated resting heart rate Deviation of the eye inward Diminished ankle jerk Impaired virbratory sense Decreased muscle strength
Thyrotoxicosis (hyperthyroidism)	Nervousness Weight loss Palpitations Muscle weakness Fatigue	Enlarging neck mass Decreased muscle strength Trophic changes—thickening of the skin Pathologic fractures
Hypothyroidism	Fatigue, lethargy Constipation Paresthesias Cold intolerance Arthralgias, myalgias Stiffness, muscle cramps	Dry, coarse skin Slowed movements Decreased sweating Hoarseness Periorbital edema Slowed reflex relaxation Decreased muscle strength
Hyperparathyroidism	Weakness Fatigue Nausea, vomiting Joint complaints, bone aches Memory loss, confusion	Decreased muscle strength Glove and stocking sensory loss Ostopenia, subperiosteal resorption, bone cysts
Hypoparathyroidism	Irritability Depression Paresthesias Back stiffness Muscle cramps	Tetany (initially tingling in fingertips and mouth) Seizures Stiffness upon passive spinal mobilization
Cushing's syndrome (adrenocortical hyperactivity)	Back pain Increased bruising	Truncal obesity Hirsutism Hypertension Muscle atrophy Decreased muscle strength Osteoporosis with increased thoracic kyphosis and pathologic fractures of ribs or vertebrae Poor wound healing
Addison's disease (adrenocortical insufficiency)	Weakness Fatigue Weight loss GI synmptoms	Hyperpigmentation Decreased muscle strength
Acromegaly	Backache Arthralgias Muscle weakness Paresthesias of the hand	Coarsening of facial features over many years Overgrowth of manible, frontal, and nasal bones Thickening of metacarpals, metatarsals, and phalanges Barrel-shaped chest Increased thoracic kyphosis Decreased muscle strength Sensory changes

junction. Various muscle length restrictions were found, including bilateral tightness of gastroc-soleus, hip flexors, rectus femoris, hamstrings, and hip adductors. Disruption of normal mechanics was found at the L5–S1 motion segment. Neurologic examination was negative.

Assessment and Outcome

The patient was seen for 10 physical therapy visits. He was treated with soft tissue mobilization, joint mobilization, muscle energy techniques, muscle stretching, and strengthening. He was provided with a home program for stretching and strengthening and given guidance regarding a previously established general conditioning program. The patient's low back and neck pain abated after the 10 visits to physical therapy. His dizziness remained. During the course of treatment the patient complained of blurred vision which came on while doing push-ups, bicycling, and home exercise program. The therapist suggested the patient contact his physician, which he did. He was then diagnosed with diabetes and when discharged was working to get it under control through insulin injections and diet. He was still having dizziness and blurred vision when discharged.

The patient's diabetic complications did interfere with his physical therapy treatment in that his exercise program had to be postponed due to his inability to regulate his insulin during these periods, at least initially. The important point of this case is that the therapist initially paid little attention to the dizziness because the patient had a cervical problem that could have been responsible for this symptom. Fortunately, the therapist recognized the complaint of blurred vision with exercise as being unexpected and referred him back to a physician. The dizziness did not change with manual therapy even though the cervical pain and dysfunction abated. Had the blurred vision not signaled the diabetes, at the end of treatment the therapist might have realized that the dizziness did not fit a musculo-skeletal diagnosis and referred him back to the physician in any case.

PATIENT CASE HISTORY 2

History

A 54-year-old man was seen in October 1989 by physician referral with a diagnosis of degenerative disc disease at L5–S1 and a small herniated nucleus pulposis on the left. When initially evaluated in physical therapy he was not working his light duty airport commission job secondary to uncontrolled diabetes. The patient complained of constant deep aching in the central low lumbar spine, sometimes spreading into the buttocks, left greater than right. In addition, he complained of a constant numblike sensation in the lateral aspect of the left thigh and calf extending to the left heel. The patient noted an increase in the lower-extremity symptoms with an increase in the low back ache. The low back and buttock symptoms were aggravated by sitting greater than 60 to 90 minutes or with walking greater than two blocks. Forward bending or reaching activities also increased his low back pain. Diminishment of the low back ache could be attained through self-traction achieved by putting his weight on his arms in the sitting or standing positions, through a constant change of position, or by assuming any recumbent position. His symptoms began in 1985 when he was pulling on a heavy wrench trying to loosen a lock and felt a sharp stabbing pain in the low back. The next morning he could not get out of bed. He stated that he had progressively gotten worse as the pain had spread into his buttock and left leg, and he felt stiffness up through the trunk to the cervical region.

The patient was a diabetic under the care of a physician for the condition. When initially seen, his diabetes was out of control and he was attempting to remedy this. The patient also suffered from high blood pressure. He had been told by another physician that his low back and buttock pain were the result of his herniated disc and that his left lower extremity complaints were the results of his diabetes. The patient denied any previous surgeries of any kind.

Objective Examination

Observation in the standing position revealed a loss of lumbar lordosis, moderate lateral shift to the right, and an increase in cervicothoracic junction kyphosis. A compensatory lateral curvature was present in the thoracic spine, convexity to the right. The patient was unable to forward bend without pain and backward bending provoked sharp pain in the low back and numbness in the left lower extremity. Straight leg raising was positive on the left at 45 degrees for increased buttock and low back pain. There was a slight hyposensitivity to pin prick in the left lateral calf and the S1 ankle jerk reflex was slightly decreased as well. Myotome testing for the lower quarter was negative. Central pressures at L5 and prone press-ups both provoked his symptoms at the lumbosacral area and into the left buttock. There was extensive muscle guarding in the left lumbar paraspinals from S1 to L3 and on the right from S1 to L4.

Treatment

On the first visit the patient was treated by attempting to correct his lateral shift in standing against the wall. This alleviated all of the patient's symptoms including the "numbness" of the left leg. He was fit with a lumbar support with a hard insert and given a home program for the shift correction. Follow-up visits included a progression through extension exercises; he was given soft tissue mobilization to the right lateral trunk, buttock, and hip flexors.

Assessment and Outcome

At discharge the patient was back at work, wearing the lumbar support, and complaining only of some intermittent left lateral thigh numbness and occasional low back ache. His lower leg numbness had subsided. This case demonstrates the need to pursue conservative care, including physical therapy, for complaints of distal pain or altered sensation, even when systemic disease might seem to conveniently explain away those symptoms. Diabetic peripheral neuropathy can explain many lower extremity and, less commonly, upper extremity complaints, but not all. Provocation of this patient's lower extremity symptoms through movement of the lumbar spine and by direct pressures at the L5–S1 motion segment established a direct correlation between the patient's low back and leg complaints. In this case, the patient was already under the therapist's care and was going to receive therapy, regardless of this correlation. However, when we as therapists have the opportunity to screen patients for physical therapy without prior physician referral, we should always maintain the possibility that symptoms common to the patient's known disease process may not be a result of that disease, but may instead result from a neuromusculoskeletal dysfunction amenable to our care.

REFERENCES

1. Guyton A: Human Physiology and Mechanisms of Disease. WB Saunders, Philadelphia, 1982
2. Thomas P: Metabolic neuropathy. JR Coll Physicians Lond 7:154, 1973
3. Dyck P, Thomas P, Lambert E, et al (eds): Peripheral Neuropathy. Vol. II. 2nd Ed. WB Saunders, Philadelphia, 1984
4. Sinha S, Munichoodappa CS, Kozak GP: Neuro-arthropathy (Charcot joints) in diabetes mellitus. (Clinical study of 101 cases.) Medicine (Baltimore) 51:191, 1972
5. Podolsky S: Clinical Diabetes: Modern Management. Appleton & Lange, E. Norwalk, CT; 1980
6. Chokroverty S, Reyes MG, Rubino FA, Tonaki H: The syndrome of diabetic amyotrophy. Ann Neurol 2:181, 1977
7. Asbury AK: Proximal diabetic neuropathy. Ann Neurol 2:179, 1977
8. Engel AG: Neuromuscular manifestations of Graves' disease. Mayo Clinic Proc 47:919, 1972
9. Swanson JW, Kelly JJ, McConahey WM: Neurologic aspects of thyroid dysfunction. May Clin Proc 56:504, 1981

10. Greenspan F, Forsham P: Basic and Clinical Endocrinology. 2nd Ed. Lange Medical Publications, Los Altos, CA, 1986

11. Sanders V: Neurologic manifestations of myxedema. N Engl J Med 266:547, 1962

12. Khaleeli AA, Griffith DG, Edwards RHT: The clinical presentation of hypothyroid myopathy and its relationship to abnormalities in structure and function of skeletal muscle. Clin Endocrinol (Oxf) 19:365, 1983

13. Klein I, Parker M, Shebert R, et al: Hypothyroidism presenting as muscle stiffness and pseudohypertrophy: Hoffmann's syndrome. Am J Med 70:891, 1981

14. Dorwart BB, Schumacher HR: Joint effusions, chondrocalcinosis and other rheumatic manifestations in hypothyroidism: A clinicopathologic study. Am J Med 59:780, 1975

15. Steinbach HL, Gordan GS, Eisenberg E, et al: Primary hyperparathyroidism: A correlation of roentgen, clinical, and pathologic features. AJR 86:329, 1961

16. Dauphine RT, Riggs BL, Scholz DA: Back pain and vertebral crush fractures: An unemphasized mode of presentation for primary hyperparathyroidism. Ann Intern Med 83:365, 1975

17. Patten BM, Bilezikian JP, Mallette LE, et al: Neuromuscular disease in primary hyperparathyroidism. Ann Intern Med 80:182, 1974

18. Frame B: Neuromuscular manifestations of parathyroid disease. In Vinken PJ, Bruyn GW (eds): Handbook of Clinical Neurology. Vol. 27. North-Holland, Amsterdam, 1976

19. Okazaki T, Takuwa Y, Yamamoto M, et al: Ossification of the paravertebral ligaments: A frequent complication of hypoparathyroidism. Metabolism 33:710, 1984

20. Kruse K, Scheunemann W, Baier W, Schaub J: Hypocalcemic myopathy in idiopathic hypoparathyroidism. Eur J Pediatr 138:280, 1982

21. Detenbeck LC, Tressler HU, O'Duffy JD, Randall RV: Peripheral joint manifestations of acromegaly. Clin Orthop 91:119, 1972

22. Mastaglia FL, Barwick DD, Hall R: Myopathy in acromegaly. Lancet 2:907, 1970

23. Pickett JBE, Layzer RB, Levin SR, et al: Neuromuscular complications of acromegaly. Neurology (NY) 25:638, 1975

24. Epstein N, Whelan M, Benjamin V: Acromegaly and spinal stenosis. J Neurosurg 56:145, 1982

25. O'Duffy JD, Randall RV, MacCarty CS: Median neuropathy (carpal-tunnel syndrome) in acromegaly. Ann Intern Med 78:379, 1973

26. Vander AJ, Sherman JH, Luciano DS: Human Physiology—The Mechanism of Body Function. 5th Ed. McGraw-Hill, New York, 1990

27. Wilson JD, Foster DW (eds): Williams Textbook of Endocrinology. 7th Ed. WB Saunders, Philadelphia, 1985

28. DeGroot LJ, Besser GM, Cahill GF, et al (eds): Endocrinology. 2nd Ed. WB Saunders, Philadelphia, 1989

SUGGESTED READINGS

Barker LR, Burton JR, Zieve PD (eds): Principals of Ambulatory Medicine. 2nd Ed. Williams & Wilkins, Baltimore, 1986

Bates B: A Guide to Physical Examination and History Taking. 4th Ed. JB Lippincott, Philadelphia, 1987

Berkow R (ed): The Merck Manual. 4th Ed. Merck & Co, Rahway, NJ, 1982

Braunwald E, Isselbacher KH, Petersdorf RG, et al (eds): Harrison's Principles of Internal Medicine. 11th Ed. McGraw-Hill, New York, 1987

Kohler PO, Jordan RM (eds): Clinical Endocrinology. John Wiley & Sons, New York, 1986

8

Screening for Pathologic Origins of Head and Facial Pain

EDWARD R. ISAACS, M.D., F.A.A.N.
MARK R. BOOKHOUT, M.S., P.T.

Physical therapists are increasingly confronted by patients with headache or facial pain as a consequence of musculoskeletal system dysfunction. During this era of direct access, patients may not be screened by a physician before treatment is initiated by a physical therapist. Patients who have been referred by a physician may develop new medical conditions during a course of physical therapy treatment that require a physician's attention. It has therefore become mandatory to broaden the knowledge of the therapist to consider other diseases involving the cranial structures and nervous system which may manifest as head or facial pain, such as tumors, vascular diseases, infections, neuralgias, endocrine and ophthalmologic disorders. The goal of this chapter is to provide the physical therapist with a means of identifying those potentially serious conditions which are beyond the scope of physical therapy practice. Once a disease of this sort is suspected, an appropriate referral to a physician can be made in a fashion that would enhance meaningful communication.

Although headache is a very common affliction, only recently has the role of the physical therapist been recognized in its treatment. In 1944 Campbell and Parsons[1] demonstrated that irritation of both joint and ligamentous structures of the upper cervical spine resulted in referral of symptoms to the cranium and therefore can be a potential source of head and facial pain (Fig. 8-1). Edeling[2] and Jull[3] have described the use of manual therapy directed to the upper cervical spine in the treatment of chronic headaches. Myofascial spray and stretch techniques directed toward the skeletal muscles that refer pain into the head or the facial area have been extensively documented by Travell and Simons.[4] Any multidisciplinary approach to the evaluation and treatment of pain caused by temporomandibular joint dysfunction now includes the participation of a physical therapist.

The following characteristics have been associated with headaches related to cervical spine dysfunction[5,6]:

1. Headaches precipitated by movements of the neck or pressure on trigger points in the neck
2. Pain, stiffness, and decreased range of motion (ROM) of the cervical spine
3. Asymmetric or unilateral symptoms
4. Occasional associated ipsilateral shoulder or arm pain

When the signs and symptoms are atypical for head pain from cervical spine dysfunction, or if the patient's response to treatment is not as expected, other reasons for the pain should be considered. An organized systematic approach to this kind of problem will by necessity emphasize an assessment of the nervous system.

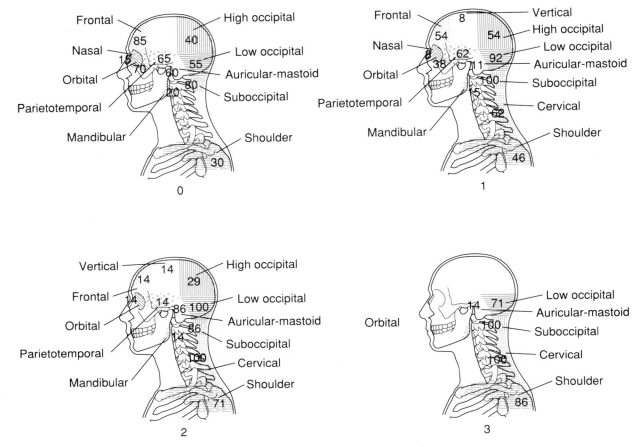

Fig. 8-1. Charts of head, neck, and shoulder regions, illustrating schematically the distribution and frequency of pains referred from the following sites: 0, basal occipital region; 1, occipitoatlanto region; 2, interspinous space C2; 3, interspinous space C3. (From Campbell and Parsons,[1] with permission.)

PHYSICAL THERAPY EVALUATION FOR DISEASES OF THE CRANIUM THAT PRESENT AS HEAD OR FACIAL PAIN

Subjective Examination

History of Present Illness

The patient's history with regard to head pain is especially important, since many diseases of the cranium and cranial nerves can only be diagnosed on the basis of history, as there may be no physical or laboratory manifestations to rely on. While taking the history, the examiner also has an opportunity to assess cognitive and language ability, speech patterns and articulation, and mannerisms. Descriptions of head pain should be directed to include location, quality, frequency, duration, progression, peak intensity, and consistency of symptoms, when pain is recurrent. Associated symptoms that are important include loss of concentration and memory ability, numbness, weakness, incoordination, and any cranial nerve dysfunction affecting sense of vision, smell, hearing and taste, swallowing and speech (Table 8-1). Any determination of an al-

Table 8-1. Questions to Ask During the Subjective Examination Pertaining to Cranial Nerve Function

Question	Cranial Nerve(s) Involved
Any loss of smell?	I
Any loss of taste?	VII, IX
Any loss of vision or visual acuity?	II
Double vision?	II, IV, VI
Numbness of face or frontal scalp?	V
Hypersensitivity to sound?	VII
Any loss of hearing or ringing in the ears?	VIII
Difficulty swallowing?	IX, X
Chronic cough, loss or impairment of voice?	X

teration of mentation or cognitive ability, especially when associated with nausea, vomiting, and/or loss of consciousness, indicates the need for referral to a physician.

Symptoms that emerge with postural or positional change may sound mechanical in nature but may also be caused by changes in intracranial pressure, which, when abnormally elevated, can be further increased during a strenuous activity or when the patient is lying down. Pathologic processes within the cranium produce symptoms by disturbing blood vessels, dura, periosteum, sinus membranes, and cranial nerves. Screening of the nervous system should be a priority during the initial evaluation, especially if the patient describes any of the following symptoms:

1. Headaches that worsen with activity or excretion
2. Headaches that begin suddenly and that are immediately severe and generalized in location
3. Headaches which begin after lying down, especially if they awaken the patient from sleep
4. Headaches associated with projectile vomiting, but no nausea
5. Headaches that begin with, or remain as, unilateral pulsating pain in synchrony with the heartbeat
6. Focal tenderness over the temporal artery in any patient past the age of 60 (Fig. 8-2)
7. Sudden, intense, lancinating, brief pain that is either spontaneous or triggered by a mild stimulus
8. Intense pain localized over a sinus or around the teeth
9. Headaches associated with other symptoms
   a. Altered ability to think or personality change
   b. Visual disturbance (i.e. blindness, double vision,

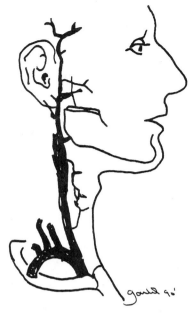

Fig. 8-2. Temporal artery distribution. Palpable anterior to the ear and in the temporal region. (From Boissonnault and Bass,[11] with permission.)

   distortions, spots, or jagged scotoma; loss of vision to one side)
   c. Numbness or altered sensibility defined by a cortical (hemisensory), brain stem (bilateral), or spinal (disassociated) pattern
   d. Loss of strength or coordination ability
   e. Loss or alteration of sense of smell or taste
   f. Loss or alteration of hearing ability
   g. Fever or associated systemic illness

A complete history regarding the events preceding the development of head pain is just as important as the descriptive analysis of the events during and after the onset of symptoms. Any history of head or neck injury close to the time of onset should raise suspicion of subdural hematoma or undiagnosed fracture of the odontoid process and/or loss of integrity of the alar ligaments. Recent dental treatment may be a cause of focal sinus infection or temporomandibular joint dysfunction. Any previous malignancy, especially carcinomas of the breast, lung, kidney, bowel, prostate, and malignant melanoma, must be considered as they metastasize to the skull or brain.

Past Medical History

Past medical history reviews previous as well as ongoing illnesses that might affect treatment plans or provide additional information that may not have seemed relevant to the history concerning the primary complaint. A history of heart disease becomes important when one considers that the pain of angina often is referred outside of the chest and can localize to the jaw and occasionally the forehead.[7] Patients with diabetes are more susceptible to infection, vascular disease, and cranial neuropathies. Taking a past history also gives the practitioner an additional opportunity to screen for history of malignancy and trauma that may have been missed.

Family History

The family history is of limited value in the diagnosis of head pain outside of migraine, in which 66 percent of patients with this complaint report a history of migraine in another close family member.[7] Recurrent Bell's palsy and adult-onset diabetes also have some familial tendencies.

Social History

The social history describes habits, hobbies, work, and home environment and can provide additional useful information. Questions are directed toward detecting potential sources of support and stress. Pressures and stresses from work, marriage, and family strife, as well as other social relationships may be disclosed. Habits concerning the use and abuse of alcohol, tobacco, or drugs not only directly affect health but also suggest deficiencies in coping mechanisms. Descriptions of work requirements and work environment provide information about potential injury, physical demands, and possible toxic exposure.

Review of Systems

As part of a complete history, the patient is asked about organ or body system functions in an organized manner designed to elicit other pertinent information. Questions about head, eyes, ears, nose, and throat should have been covered but can be asked again in regard to other problems, such as allergies. Chest function is discussed in terms of chest pain, cough, and/or shortness of breath and might uncover potential infection or malignancy. Symptoms of heart disease include chest pain, angina, shortness of breath, and edema in the extremities, and may also be associated with other vascular complaints. Problems affecting the gastrointestinal system cause altered appetite, weight loss, nausea, vomiting, diarrhea, and abdominal pains. Painless bleeding from the bowel may produce red or black stools, depending on the site of bleeding. Constipation may be a cause of headache, since increased intra-abdominal pressure can be directly transmitted centrally through the paraspinal venus plexus, which is unique in its absence of intraluminal valves. Genitourinary system disorders affect bladder dysfunction either in regard to control or pain on voiding. Recurrent urinary tract infections in the male suggest neurogenic bladder dysfunction or chronic infection associated with systemic disease. An obstetric/gynecologic history can be an easy way of learning about an early pregnancy as well as endocrine function. The neurological system review was done as part of the history of present illness. A suggested checklist of items to be covered during history taking to screen for diseases of the cranium is outlined in Table 8-2.

Physical Examination

Observation is an integral part of any physical examination and can be accomplished indirectly as the patient walks into the examination/treatment area and during the taking of the history, and then directly during the formal examination. Particular attention should be paid to head and neck posture, which provides the first suggestion of dysfunctional cervical spine mechanics. A head tilt might also be the result of diplopia (double vision) or extraocular eye muscle weakness (cranial nerve IV). Drooping of an eyelid and lateral eye deviation are indicative of oculomotor dysfunction (cranial nerve III). Viewing the open mouth is a part of the assessment of the temporomandibular joint, as it provides an opportunity to visualize the tongue for atrophy and the health of the gums and teeth. Missing teeth and malocclusion should be noted, as well as unhealthy gum tissue that does not appear to be a firm or a pink fleshy color. Drooping of one shoulder may be the consequence of abnormal thoracic or scapular mechanics or may be due to atrophy of the trapezius secondary to a peripheral lesion of cranial nerve XI.

Table 8-2. History Taking to Screen for Diseases of the Cranium

1. Date of onset
2. Mode of onset
3. Location of pain
4. Character and intensity of pain
5. Duration of pain
6. Aggravating or relieving factors
   Postural/positional
   Activity/rest
   Medication
   Previous therapy or treatment
   Diet
   Associated complaints (i.e., numbness, pins-and-needles sensation, tingling)
7. Special senses
   Vision
   Hearing
   Smell
   Taste
8. Past medical history
   Cancer
   Head injury
   Heart disease
   Stroke
   Allergy
   Ease in frequency of infection
   Dental history
   Surgical history
9. Family history
10. Social history
    Work
    Toxic exposure
    Habits (tobacco, alcohol, drugs)
    Marital status or living arrangement
11. Review of systems
    Chest pain
    Shortness of breath
    Chronic cough
    Edema in extremities
    Weight loss
    Abdominal pain/vomiting
    Bloody stool
    Pain on voiding
    Ob/gyn problems

Active and passive range of motion (ROM) of the cervical and thoracic spines should be assessed with an attempt made to provoke the patient's symptoms either partially or wholly, while searching for a musculoskeletal cause for this complaint. Particular attention should be paid to the upper cervical spine segments, since these are most commonly the origin of referred pain to the cranium.[2,3] Functional mobility of the temporomandibular joint should also be examined.

A neurologic screening examination may be necessary to confirm suspicions of serious illness or simply to satisfy the therapist that there are no obvious contraindications to proceeding with therapy directed toward the patient's complaint. The purpose of the examination is to alert the therapist to the presence of neurologic dysfunction, necessitating the attention of a physician skilled in diagnosing and treating diseases of the nervous system. The basic screening neurologic examination can be done in any sequence, but establishing one pattern of examination to be used over and over again can ensure a consistently complete examination that should take no more than 15 minutes. The examination outlined here is designed to minimize frequent changes in the patient's position and the need to use the same diagnostic tools again at different points of the examination.

Neurologic Examination: Standing*

1. *Gait and Station:* Observe for posture, balance, limping, circumduction, heel-strike, toe-off, and so forth. A spastic gait pattern occurs when there is corticospinal tract dysfunction, which can be cortical, brainstem, or spinal in origin. A wide-based and unsteady gait that is easily improved with one-finger assistance denotes cerebellar disease. Stooped posture, shuffling steps, and tremor in hands held in arms that do not swing are typical of extrapyramidal disease, while small, quick unsteady steps indicate frontal lobe dysfunction. A footdrop may be due to peripheral nerve, radicular, and/or corticospinal tract dysfunction.
2. *Walk on toes:* Observe for balance and gastrocnemius/soleus strength. Tests the S1 peripheral nerve root.
3. *Walk on heels:* Observe for balance and foot extensor strength. Tests the L5 peripheral nerve root.
4. *Walk in tandem, heel to toe:* Observe for balance and coordination ability. Assesses for spasticity, ataxia, and extrapyramidal dysfunction.
5. *Hop or skip on either foot or tap alternate feet rapidly on the floor:* Tests coordination, strength, bal-

*While it is most likely to have ambulatory patients in an outpatient clinic, occasional patients are chair bound, and the examiner simply begins the examination with the patient in the seated position.

ance, and fine motor skills. Assesses for cortical, brainstem, extrapyramidal, cerebellar, spinal, and peripheral nerve function.

6. *Romberg test:* Patient stands with feet together while eyes are closed with the examiner prepared to catch the patient if balance is lost. If the patient is unable to stand with feet together while eyes are opened, do not test with eyes closed. Assesses the posterior spinal tracts and peripheral nerves for lower extremity positional sense.

Neurologic Examination: Sitting

1. Coordination, fine motor ability, and strength testing of the upper extremities; assesses corticospinal, cerebellar, and extrapyramidal function.

   a. *Finger-nose-finger testing:* Patient uses the tip of own finger to touch own nose, then examiner's fingertip and back to own nose again, repeated several times while the examiner moves the finger to present a moving target for the patient. Observe for accuracy (cortical or cerebellar), speed (extrapyramidal), static and end-point tremor (cerebellar and extrapyramidal), while observing inactive contralateral extremity and legs for resting tremor (extra-pyramidal).

   b. *Alternate motion rate:* Patient rapidly pats flat palmar surface of hand on thigh for several seconds with each hand, then rapidly pats thigh by alternating dorsal and palmar surfaces of the hand. Observe for speed, consistency, and rhythmicity of motion (cerebellar, extrapyramidal, and cortical).

   c. *Thumb tap:* Ask the patient to tap the extended thumb with index finger of same hand rapidly and repeatedly, without moving thumb, to assess fine motor skills.

   d. *Muscle tone:* Assess by passive movement at the shoulder, elbow, and wrist, observing for spasticity (corticospinal), "leadpipe" or "cogwheel" rigidity (extrapyramidal), or reduced tone (peripheral system).

   e. *Muscle strength:* Best tested bilaterally and simultaneously or alternately for the same muscles using sustained maximal contractions comparing strength bilaterally as well as the examiner's ability to overcome the muscle being tested. Test in a pattern that screens all my-

otomes, e.g., deltoids (C5,C6), supraspinatus and infraspinatus (C5,C6), biceps (C5,C6), triceps (C7,C8), wrist extensors (C6,C7,C8), grip (C6,C7,C8,T1), finger adductors and abductors (C8,T1), and thumb opposition and flexion (C8,T1).

2. Coordination testing, strength, and fine motor testing for the lower extremities

   a. *Heel-shin:* Have the patient tap below the ipsilateral knee with contralateral heel, then slide heel gently and slowly down the edge of the shin to the ankle. Repeat by switching legs, and observe for ability to maintain heel contact with the leg.

   b. *Toe-finger:* Patient tries to touch the examiner's finger with the tip of the great toe in a similar fashion as the finger-nose-finger test.

   c. *Foot tapping:* This is done against the examiner's hand for alternate motion rate unless already tested while standing.

   d. *Muscle tone:* Assess by passive motion at the hips, knees, and ankles, or by shaking the lower leg and observing for freedom of motion.

   e. *Muscle strength:* May have already been tested during the gait analysis; no muscles in the lower extremities should be overcome by the examiner's upper extremity unless they are of comparable size. Test again in myotomal patterns, e.g. iliopsoas (L2,L3), quadriceps (L2,L3,L4), hamstrings (L5,S1,S2), foot extensors (L4,L5), and toe extensors (L5,S1).

3. Deep tendon reflexes assess the peripheral system as well as the corticospinal tracts since uninhibited reflex pathways are hyperactive. Any deep tendon reflex which is so hyperactive as to initiate clonus is abnormal. The deep tendon reflexes are also compared on the basis of presence or absence and symmetry. Proper testing of the deep tendon reflexes is best done with a rubber hammer that enables the examiner to easily strike and stretch the tendon, and may be achieved most consistently with a rounded rubber head on top of a long and flexible handle. Proper and bilaterally consistent limb positioning allows for maximal relaxation prior to tendon strike and elimination of extraneous factors which may introduce asymmetry of the response. The following tendon reflexes should be tested:

a. *Upper extremity:* Biceps (C5,C6), triceps (C6,C7), brachioradialis (C6).

b. *Lower extremity:* Quadriceps (L2,L3,L4), gastrocnemius/soleus (S1,S2).

4. While still holding the reflex hammer, three other reflexes may be checked:

a. *Snout reflex:* Done by gently tapping over the patient's lips and observing for reflex puckering which can be normal or represent diffuse cortical or bilateral corticospinal tract dysfunction originating above the cervical spine.

b. *Plantar responses,* e.g., Babinski sign (Fig. 8-3): Done by stroking the plantar surface of the foot with the sharp end of the reflex hammer moving from heel to heads of the metatarsals along the lateral border, then across the metatarsal heads medially to the great toe; observe for a positive response, which is fanning of the lateral four toes and extension of the great toe. Normally all toes will plantar-flex or curl, but occasionally uncontrollable withdrawal of the foot will mimic an abnormal response and other variations may be needed (e.g., lightly stroke from the base of the fifth toe back toward the heel). If peripheral disease is causing loss of strength in the toe extensors, an abnormal or positive response is not possible, even if there is sufficient dysfunction within the corticospinal pathways to allow this primitive reflex response to resurface. This reflex should disappear once an infant begins to walk.

c. *Abdominal reflexes:* Done by gently stroking

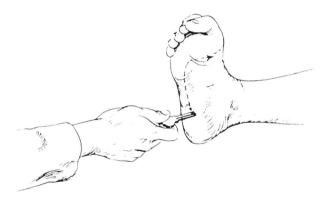

A negative Babinski

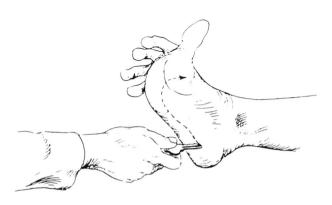

A positive Babinski

Fig. 8-3. Babinski test. (From Hoppenfeld,[12] with permission.)

each abdominal quadrant with the end of the reflex hammer and noting the umbilicus deviating towards the stimulus. Upper abdominal quadrants: T7–T10, lower abdominal quadrants: T10–L1.

5. Sensory examination:
   a. *Position sense testing:* Done while already in position for testing plantar responses; grasp the lateral margins of the great toe to avoid providing clues by finger pressure and slowly move the toe up (cephalad) or down (caudad), asking the patient to keep the eyes closed and indicate the direction that the toe is being passively moved. Fingers can be tested in a similar fashion, especially if there is indication of dysfunction in the peripheral system, posterior spinal columns or contralateral cortex.
   b. *Vibratory sense:* Test distally with 128-Hz tuning fork on all fingers and toes; if abnormal test proximally as well (useful in checking the same pathways as for positional sense).
   c. *Temperature sense:* Test over various dermatomes of the face, head, trunk, and extremities by simply placing a tuning fork in the freezer for a short while and testing for cold sensibility which may be a sensitive indicator of segmental, central spinal cord, or brainstem dysfunction.
   d. *Pinprick:* Sharp versus dull best tested with disposable safety pin discarded after one patient examination. Test the extremities for relative and absolute sensory changes considering dermatomes (Fig. 8-4), peripheral nerve innervation zones (Fig. 8-5), cortical and spinal patterns, and hemianesthesia versus defined loss to a segmental level. Test the head for cranial nerve patterns as well.

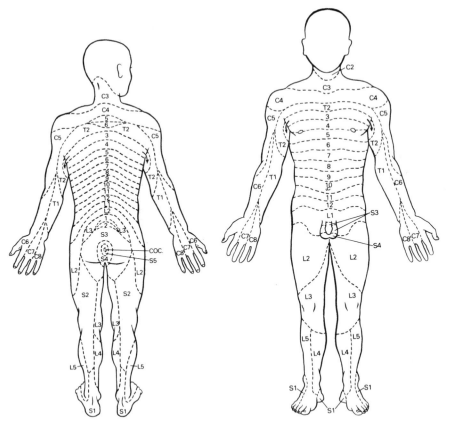

Fig. 8-4. Dermatome charts. (From Devinsky and Feldmann,[13] as modified from Haymaker and Woodhall,[14] with permission.)

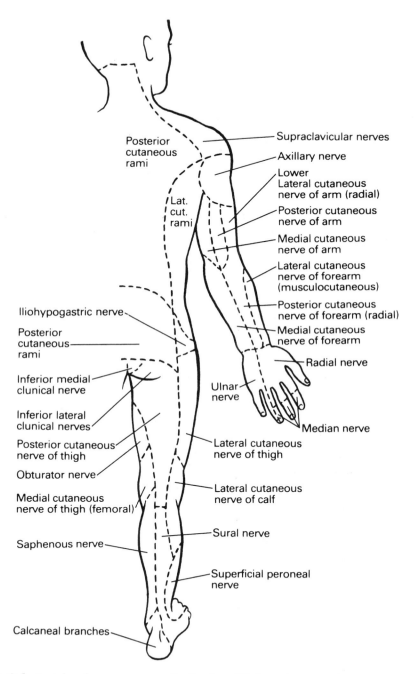

Fig. 8-5. Peripheral nerve sensory distribution. **(A)** Posterior view. (*Figure continues.*)

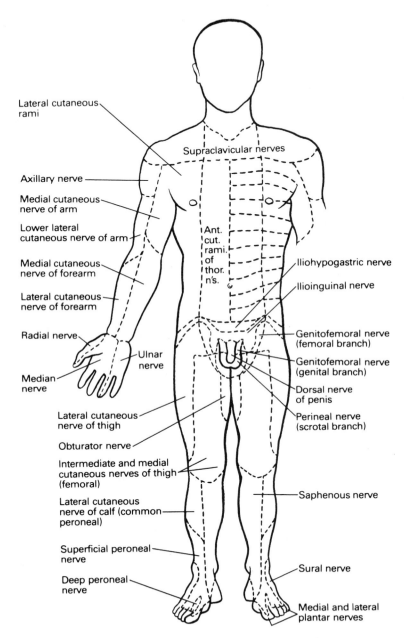

Fig. 8-5. (*Continued.*) **(B)** Anterior view. (From Devinsky and Feldmann,[13] as modified from Haymaker and Woodhall,[14] with permission.)

e. *Light touch:* Use a wisp of cotton or pulled tip of the cotton swab and test the same patterns as with pin prick, asking the patient to respond affirmatively when sensing light touch. Eyes of the patient should remain closed during sensory testing (observe for dermatome versus cord/segmental pattern versus hemisensory/cortical).

f. If a wooden cotton applicator was used for light touch testing, it can be turned around and used to trace a single digit on the patient's palm. The patient, with the eyes still closed, is then asked to identify the number that was traced in the palm of the hand. Any similar instrument can be used (screens for parietal lobe function provided all other sensibilities are intact).

6. Cranial nerve testing:

a. *Oculomotor, trochlear, abducens:* Cranial nerves III, IV, and VI are usually assessed together, since they control ocular motion. A wooden cotton-tip applicator can still be used. This time, the white cotton tip becomes a visual target that is followed by the patient's eyes, as it is moved laterally left to right and right to left. Then it is moved vertically and obliquely to assess the full range of eye motion, while observing for symmetry of range, speed of motion, and the presence or absence of nystagmus (rhythmical oscillating, rapid, low-amplitude motion, which may not be abnormal at the extremes of lateral gaze unless it is pronounced). Figures 8-6 to 8-8 demonstrate evaluation of the right visual fields. The same tests should be done to the left side as well to test the corresponding cranial nerves. Dysfunction usually creates diplopia (double vision) with both eyes open and improvement by closing or covering one eye. A head tilt is common when a lesion of cranial nerve IV causes vertical diplopia. Lesions of cranial nerve VI are common with increased intracranial pressure for any reason and present with double vision when looking at a distance rather than close up and a loss of the ability to move the eye laterally. Lesions of cranial nerve III cause double vision for near rather than far objects and may be associated with drooping of the eyelid and dilation of the pupil as well as loss of vertical and medial gaze. Often this is associated with laterally placed intracranial masses,

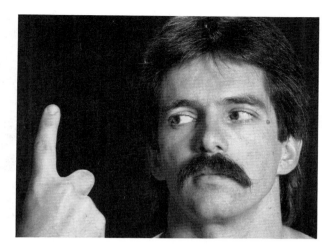

Fig. 8-6. Eyes following the target laterally to the right. Assessment of intact cranial nerve VI (right) and cranial nerve III (left).

intracranial aneurysms and systemic disease associated with cranial neuropathies. *Any dysfunction that affects ocular motion requires ongoing assessment and management by a competent physician.*

b. *Optic nerve (cranial nerve II):* Testing for optic nerve function requires an evaluation of visual acuity, color vision, visual fields, and a fundoscopic examination. Since this type of examination is well beyond the scope of physical therapy, testing in the clinic would necessarily be brief and not inclusive. Again using the cotton-tip applicator as a target, have the patient cover one eye while fixating vision with the uncovered eye on the examiner's nose. The tip of the applicator is moved from the periphery (lateral, medial, above, below) toward the center of vision asking the patient to indicate when the tip is first seen. Compare the patient's response with the examiner's own visual field tested at the same time by placing the target equidistant between the examiner and the patient. Color vision can be grossly tested and is absent in certain males (inherited for red and green) or in patients with loss of central vision, in which case acuity will be very poor or absent. The pupils should constrict simultaneously and consensually when a bright light shines into either eye.

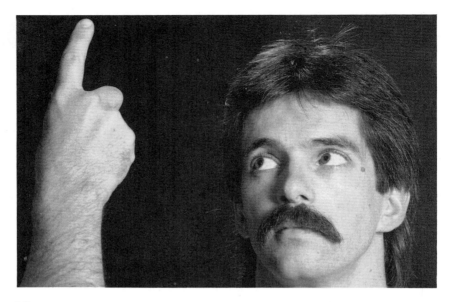

Fig. 8-7. Eyes following the target laterally and superiorly. Assessment of intact cranial nerve III (right) and cranial nerve III (left).

It is helpful to know that the patient has had a recent thorough professional eye exam.

c. *Olfactory nerve (cranial nerve I)*: Olfactory nerve function is best tested by presenting a familiar odor to each nostril individually and ask-

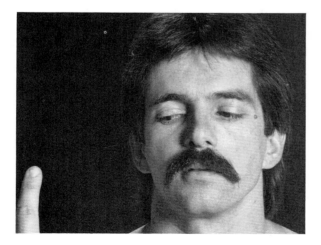

Fig. 8-8. Eyes following the target laterally and inferiorly. Assessment of intact cranial nerve III (right) and cranial nerve IV (left).

ing the patient to identify; if unable to do so then provide multiple choices. (Test odors can be obtained by buying a small bottle of flavoring from any grocery store.) Olfactory nerve dysfunction can be described as either a loss of sense of smell, altered sense of smell, or, more often, alteration or loss of sense of taste of salty, sweet, bitter, and sour. Elderly patients may suffer loss of taste because of loss of function of the taste end organs innervated by cranial nerve VII or loss of cranial nerve I function because of altered sinus and nasal membranes or chronic nasal obstruction. Unilateral loss of sense of smell is more significant because it is a more localized finding of olfactory dysfunction as a consequence of direct compression from a subfrontal brain tumor such as olfactory groove meningiomas, which might also cause personality changes and seizures as well as severe frontal headaches. Bilateral loss of sense of smell can also be a permanent consequence of head injury, either coup (deceleration/acceleration or direct injury to the side of blow) or countercoup (acceleration/deceleration or injury to the side opposite from where the head strikes) and should alert the examiner to additional injuries to the cranium, brain, cervical spine, and spinal cord.

d. *Trigeminal nerve* (*cranial nerve V*): All sensation for the face and the anterior half of the scalp except for the angle of the mandible and the ear is mediated by the trigeminal nerve (Fig. 8-9). Motor fibers of the trigeminal nerve innervate the muscles of mastication and can be tested by palpation of the masseter and temporalis muscles comparing tone when the jaws are clenched tightly together. Cranial nerve V is more commonly assessed by testing sensibility over the face, forehead, and under the chin as well as the inside of the cheek, tongue, teeth, and gums. The production of intense, brief pain in testing would suggest a neuralgia of this nerve. While loss of sensation to the face is unusual for the nontraumatized nerve, transmission of appropriate painful sensations, especially from the mouth, eyes, sinuses, cranial bones, meningeal membranes, and vessels, is part of its normal function. Chronic persistent pain requires neurodiagnostic investigation to rule out destructive or invasive lesions and may necessitate the use of radiographs and computed tomography (CT) and magnetic resonance imaging (MRI) scans, before a definitive diagnosis can be made. The trigeminal nerve is most often irritated by an aberrant, tortuous, arterial branch from the basilar artery. It can also be infected by herpes zoster virus, which results in more constant, intense, burning neuritic pain. Trigeminal neuralgia occurs spontaneously in adults over the age of 40 years and may be part of the clinical picture in younger patients with multiple sclerosis.

e. *Facial nerve* (*cranial nerve VII*): The facial nerve innervates all the muscles responsible for facial expression, as well as the platysma and the muscle to the tympanic membrane. Aside from the obvious facial weakness (noted when the patient speaks, smiles, furrows the brow), paralysis of the tensor tympani muscle permits the eardrum to continue to vibrate with each sound, causing an echo or hypersensitivity to sound. Within the auditory canal, the facial nerve joins with the sensory nerve (chordi and tympani) that transmits the basic sense of taste from the anterior two-thirds of the tongue. The sense of taste can be tested by asking the patient to identify the nature of a test solution placed on the antero-lateral aspect of the tongue and comparing the response when the other side is tested (dilute salt or sugar solutions work well and can be easily and appropriately placed on the tongue by

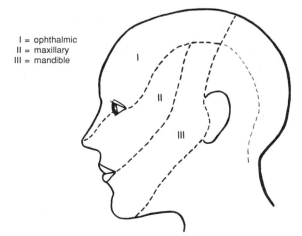

I = ophthalmic
II = maxillary
III = mandible

Fig. 8-9. Sensory distribution of the three divisions of the trigeminal nerve. (From Devinsky and Feldmann,[13] with permission.)

using a medicine dropper). The most common affliction of this nerve is caused by swelling and inflammation within the facial canal, possibly the result of a viral infection causing weakness of all ipsilateral facial muscles and loss of sense of taste from the ipsilateral half of the tongue. This syndrome, also known as Bell's palsy, is often preceded or accompanied by pain in the region of the ipsilateral ear. Occasionally the appearance of a typical Herpetic rash around the external auditory canal identifies the causative agent. Mononeuropathy due to vascular compromise to the nerve can also occur in diabetes and sarcoidosis. The nerve can also be affected by disease originating in the parotid gland, such as infection or tumor, in which case taste would not be affected. Tumors that grow in the cerebellopontine angle, especially acoustic neuromas, can produce unilateral facial weakness. Recent rapid development of bilateral facial weakness is an uncommon but extremely ominous presentation of acute polyradiculoneuropathy (Guillian-Barré syndrome). The facial muscles can be involved in generalized myasthenia gravis, as well as myotonic and facioscapulohumeral muscular dystrophy. Lower facial weakness that disappears when the patient smiles spontaneously suggests a cerebral and not a peripheral cause.

f. *Acoustic nerve (cranial nerve VIII)*: The acoustic nerve consists of two separate parts known as the cochlear and vestibular nerves. The hearing and vestibular functions of this cranial nerve are tested separately and are best done in audiovestibular laboratories. Hearing can be screened grossly by judging the patient's response to the examiner's voice or by comparing the ability to hear the sound made when the examiner rubs adjacent fingers together next to each ear. The first sign of dysfunction of the cochlear portion may be a gradual loss of hearing which begins with the higher frequencies and is accompanied by annoying tinnitus (ringing). Unexplained unilateral hearing loss must be investigated to exclude early development of a small acoustic neuroma.

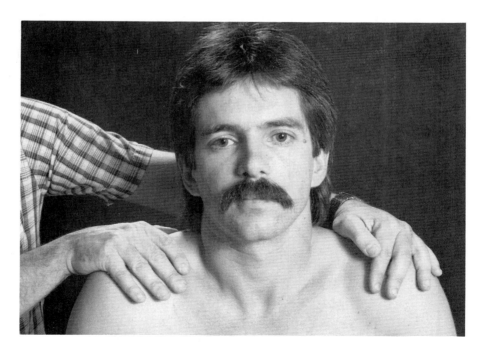

Fig. 8-10. Bilateral assessment of cranial nerve XI. The patient shrugs the shoulders and holds against resistance as the tester attempts to depress the shoulders.

g. *Glossopharyngeal and vagus (cranial nerves IX and X)*: The glossopharyngeal nerve has both motor and sensory functions. The pharyngeal (gag) reflex depends on an intact sensory component of cranial nerve IX, as does transmission of taste from the posterior one-third of the tongue. The vagus nerve (cranial nerve X) is the major source of parasympathetic innervation to the viscera. Cranial nerves IX and X can be tested together by asking the patient to swallow small quantities of water or by inducing a gag reflex (cotton applicator). There is a branch of the vagus nerve which innervates the epithelial lining of the external auditory canal which, when irritated, can be the source of unexplained chronic coughing. Shortly after exiting the cranium, the recurrent laryngeal nerve branches from the vagus to innervate the ipsilateral vocal cord. Interruption of this branch by injury or tumor results in chronic hoarseness. Other motor branches are necessary for proper swallowing in the transition from skeletal to smooth muscle contraction.

h. *Accessory nerve (cranial nerve XI)*: The accessory nerve is a motor nerve to the sternocleidomastoid and upper trapezius muscles that can be assessed by asking the patient to shrug the ipsilateral shoulder and/or rotate the head to the opposite side (Fig. 8-10). Pathology of the accessory nerve is uncommon, when it does occur, it is usually due to injury during a surgical biopsy of a superior clavicle lymph node, usually distal to the branch to the sternocleidomastoid. Since cranial nerves IX, X, and XI all exit the cranium through the jugular foramen, any dysfunction of all three at the same time will indicate a process localized to this region.

i. *Hypoglossal nerve (cranial nerve XII)*: The hypoglossal nerve innervates the tongue and exits the cranium through its own foramen in the occipital bone. Tongue strength can be measured by having the patient push against a tongue blade (Fig. 8-11) or simply the inside of the cheek with counterresistance applied from outside of the mouth. Inspection of the tongue will provide direct observation for possible atrophy and fasciculation. Tongue weakness is first suspected by the typical speech pattern caused by talking with-

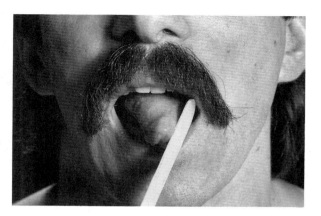

Fig. 8-11. Assessment of cranial nerve XII. Pressure is applied against the lateral aspect of the tongue and the patient asked to hold. Both sides of the tongue should be tested.

out moving the tongue. Dysfunctions that primarily cause tongue weakness occur because of direct nerve compression, most commonly from regional or metastatic tumors. The tongue can be selectively or jointly affected along with other skeletal muscles in such diseases as myasthenia gravis, and especially amyotrophic lateral sclerosis. Unilateral weakness of the tongue without atrophy is most probably due to an upper motor neuron dysfunction such as cerebral infarction.

The examination concludes with palpation of the cranium, seeking painful areas especially over blood vessels, or for enlarged and possibly tender lymph nodes which may reflect local infection or systemic disease. (See Ch. 1 for a description of the characteristics associated with lymph node abnormalities.) Areas to be palpated for lymph nodes include the submental, submandibular, periauricular, and posterior cervical regions (Fig. 8-12). Table 8-3 outlines the neurologic screening examination.

DISEASES OR DISORDERS THAT CAN CAUSE HEAD OR FACIAL PAIN

After taking the history and completing an examination of a patient with head pain, therapy is initiated unless there is concern about a disease or disorder that is

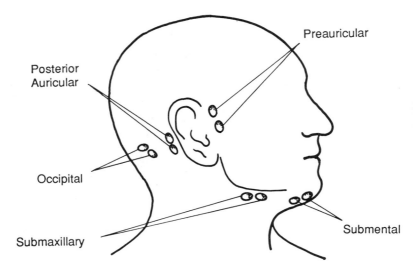

Fig. 8-12. Lymph nodes of the head and neck.

not amenable to physical therapy. The following section is not meant to provide information from which the physical therapist might make a diagnosis. Greater difficulties might arise if the patient is referred to the physician with a particular diagnosis rather than a report outlining concerns about particular history and/or findings on examination.

Headache: General Considerations

The most common headache types are migraines, tension headaches, and headaches arising from either mechanical cervical or cranial dysfunction, or both. Despite overlap of these categories, it is possible to define these types of headaches within a diagnostic framework that would encourage the most appropriate therapy. Any text or paper that reviews headache emphasizes the need to consider what structures are pain sensitive (i.e., have nociceptor innervation). Generally those structures with the capability of generating painful sensation include blood vessels, dura, ligaments, fascia, periosteum, muscles, joints, skin, subcutaneous tissues, glandular tissue, sinus and nasal mucosa, dental pulp, gums in the lining of the oropharynx, endoneurium, epineurium, and perineurium of the cranial and cervical nerves.[7] Pain can also be referred into the cranium from structures located elsewhere, but pain-sensitive structures are still primarily involved.

The term *migraine* refers to headaches believed to be of vascular origin. The name itself derives from the term hemicrania, suggesting an asymmetric, unilateral location of the pain. This derivation can be appreciated if the "he" is dropped from the hemicrania, leaving "micrania" from which emerges *migraine*. Migraines may be associated with a severe tension headache especially if there is photophobia, nausea, and vomiting. More recent research and theories would suggest that migraine is really a brainstem dysfunction involving serotinergic pain pathways with the vascular changes reflecting only epiphenomena.[8] True migraine is further classified into subcategories of typical, classic, and complicated forms, depending on the presence of an aura and associated symptoms. Migraine is a familial disorder, with fairly stereotypical headaches recurring at various frequencies, often before or during menstrual periods or after periods of stress or precipitated by certain foods containing tyramine (aged cheese, red wine) or other vasoactive substances, (e.g., chocolate). The typical migraine begins with unilateral discomfort, which is pulsatile and associated early on with nausea, often followed by vomiting. The pain usually increases, and the sense of illness pervades and incapacitates. Some patients with typical migraine note inexplicable alterations of mood beginning about 1 day before onset. Interestingly, in support of the central brainstem dysfunction theory, many migraineurs find relief of

Table 8-3. Outline for Neurologic Screening of a Patient with Head and/or Facial Pain

A. In standing
  1. Gait and station
  2. Toe walk
  3. Heel walk
  4. Tandem walk
  5. Hop or skip
  6. Romberg
B. In sitting
  1. Coordination, fine motor, and strength of upper extremities
    a. Finger-nose-finger
    b. Alternate motion rate
    c. Thumb tap
    d. Muscle tone
    e. Muscle strength
  2. Coordination, fine motor, and strength of lower extremities
    a. Heel-shin
    b. Toe-finger
    c. Foot tapping
    d. Muscle tone
    e. Muscle strength
  3. Deep tendon reflexes
    a. Upper extremities
    b. Lower extremities
  4. Other reflexes
    a. Snout
    b. Babinski
    c. Abdominal
  5. Sensory examination
    a. Position sense
    b. Vibratory sense
    c. Temperature sense
    d. Pinprick
    e. Light touch
  6. Cranial nerve testing
    a. Cranial nerves III, IV, VI: Test ocular motility (follow your finger)
    b. Cranial nerve II: Check peripheral vision and pupil constriction to light
    c. Cranial nerve I: Check sense of smell
    d. Cranial nerve V: Check sensation of face; palpate temporalis and masseter tone with teeth clenched
    e. Cranial nerve VII: Check facial expressions, check for hypersensitivity to sound (hyperacousis), check taste anterior two-thirds of tongue
    f. Cranial nerve VIII: Check hearing by rubbing fingers together
    g. Cranial nerve IX, X: Check for difficulty with swallowing water
    h. Cranial nerve XI: Check contralateral head rotation and shoulder shrug
    i. Cranial nerve XII: Check protrusion of tongue for deviation to the weaker side

symptoms after sleeping. This usually requires assistance from some medication. There may be some underlying cervical mechanical dysfunction that can be treated, but treatment will not significantly reduce the discomfort. Classic migraine differs from typical migraine by the occurrence of a preceding or associated aura that usually affects vision with perception of a central or peripheral bright scotoma that may have a geometric configuration. Occasionally the aura is olfactory, with a migraineur sensing a peculiar, usually unpleasant, aromatic hallucination. Complicated migraine is noteworthy in that the aura consists of more significant neurologic dysfunction, including ophthalmoplegia, hemisensory loss, and even hemiplegia. Often the epiphenomena persist well into the headache and occasionally occur without associated headache, nausea, or vomiting and are then called "migraine equivalents."

In 1962 the ad hoc committee on the classification of headache adopted the term *muscle contraction headache* for conditions previously referred to as tension or nervous headaches.[9] Pain generation is then defined as being derived from sustained contraction of skeletal muscles of the head and neck as the primary source of pain. Trott[10] believes that the diagnosis of a tension headache or muscle contraction headache presents a problem to clinicians, as it is often clouded by either a vascular element or a triggering mechanism, or both. She defines underlying trigger factors as anxiety, depression, poor posture, occlusal problems, and disorders of the upper cervical spine. It is not clear whether frequent tension in the suboccipital muscles leads to stiffness in the underlying joints or whether the muscle tension is secondary (reflexive) to dysfunction of the cervical joints. Typically the pain is described as a dull ache that may be located frontally or in the occipital and posterior upper neck regions; it then builds in intensity while spreading in distribution around the scalp and neck. The pain builds slowly and steadily, usually over hours and sometimes days. At its peak there is usually some throbbing or pulsatile quality noted especially with motion and, if severe enough, nausea, vomiting, and fainting can occur. With intense pain, the ciliospinal reflex adds blurred vision and photophobia by causing pupillary dilatation. Tension headaches can last hours to days, being most responsive to nonprescription drugs if taken early or close to the onset.

Stress is often cited as one of the major causes of the pain, but it would seem more appropriate to consider the alerting response as the mechanism that first tightens the posterior neck, frontal, and periaurical muscles as noted in other mammals.[7] Once these muscles cause discomfort, the alerting response continues and a self-aggravating situation ensues. Adding to the building headache is a tendency to be more concerned and distracted by the headache as well as becoming increasingly more irritable and less tolerant of environmental stress, which again feeds into the alerting response. Some of this behavior is a consequence of "psychic investment" in the head, which is a measure of importance placed on the structure that is most closely identified with personality and self-image. A similar pain located in the leg, for instance, would not be as distracting or disabling. As with migraine, underlying mechanical restrictions subjected to the stress of increased muscle tone and shortening might well further decompensate and predispose to a more asymmetric presentation which will require some direct manual therapy treatment.

Edeling[2] argues that tension or muscular contraction headaches and headaches of cervical origin are one and the same. Physical therapy directed at treating the muscle is ineffective, since the reflex muscle contraction is in response to abnormal and dysfunctional upper cervical spinal mechanics. Patients with headaches of cervical origin often have a history of preceding cervical strain. In a retrospective study of 96 patients with headache complaints, Jull[3] found that the onset of headache was directly related to a neck injury in 40 percent of the patients studied, 16 of the patients having been involved in motor vehicle accidents. Headaches of cervical origin are usually sensitive to positions of sustained neck flexion or changes in posture. Pain is most commonly referred into the frontal, retro-orbital, occipital, or suboccipital areas with neck pain as a frequent accompaniment of the headache.[3] Edeling[2] and Jull,[3] among others, have found that manual therapy treatment directed at restoring the accessory movements of the upper cervical spine, specifically C0–C1, C1–C2, and C2–C3, have been very effective in successfully managing headaches of cervical origin. Temporomandibular joint pain must be also considered as a special form of head pain of musculoskeletal origin and treated appropriately.

Tumors and Headaches

Perhaps the greatest fear among patients and those not trained in the neurosciences is that a persistent, recurrent, or severe headache is associated with a brain tumor. Actually brain tumors rarely cause headaches either early on or even after they are well established and diagnosed. Brain tumors produce symptoms of neurologic dysfunction far more often and consistently than they produce headache. The absence of pain should be of no surprise, since brain tissue is not a pain-sensitive structure, there being no nociceptors within the central nervous system (CNS). When it occurs, pain is due to a distortion of the supportive pain-sensitive structures, such as dural membranes, blood vessels, and periosteum. Intracranial brain tumors cause symptoms of brain or CNS dysfunction either by directly compressing or destroying tissue or by interfering with blood supply to brain tissue. Irritation of the brain tissue is not uncommon and may lead to the onset of seizures.

As the tumor increases in size and the surrounding cerebral edema produces increased intracranial pressure, alterations in mentation and progressive neurologic dysfunction develop, but usually without head pain. Head pain as a result of increased intracranial pressure occurs as a consequence of pressure elevations at a rate that is faster than accommodating mechanisms. Any further increase in pressure caused by physical exertion, postural changes, or lying down (which eliminates the negative intracranial pressure affects of gravity) will not be tolerated, and the headache will increase in severity. The increase in intracranial pressure causes reduced mentation, vomiting without nausea, nonlocalized dull headache, blurred vision, and a loss of lateral gaze with the eyes deviated medially (cranial nerve VI).

Tumors that are considered to be benign include meningiomas and neurofibromas. They grow relatively slowly and do not invade brain tissue but grow by displacing and pushing normal tissue aside. This characteristic enables potential total removal without disrupting brain tissue. Meningiomas are troublesome because they are usually highly vascular and may calcify because they are slow growing. These tumors may also grow around vital arteries or venous sinuses, making removal difficult. Meningiomas arise from arachnoid villi and can grow from any surface area or from the sagittal sinus. Those that grow under the brain tend to invade bone and may be impossible to remove. One such tumor tends to grow in the olfactory groove, causing an ipsilateral loss of sense of smell long before frontal headache develops. Meningiomas are most commonly found incidentally during the examination of a brain scan or as part of an evaluation for adult-onset seizures with little in the way of neurologic deficit.

Neurofibromas are most commonly diagnosed as acoustic neuromas and first cause unilateral hearing loss (bilateral if they are present at multiple sites). Growth begins in the internal auditory canal expanding into the cerebellopontine angle. Large tumors compress cranial nerve VII and then V but eventually compress the brainstem and cause increased intracranial pressure as a result of noncommunicating hydrocephalus. Head pain is not common before this late stage. Interestingly, there is a decreased incidence of multiple intracranial tumor formation when the patient has a preponderance of external skin lesions and tumors.

Tumors that grow within the pituitary gland can affect the endocrine system either by producing hormones or by destroying the functioning part of the gland. As these tumors grow, sudden swelling can occur with rapid onset of dysfunction. Because the tumors grow into the bone and up into the dura, pain is not uncommon, referring to the occiput or frontal regions. As these tumors grow upward, pressure is applied to the underside of the middle of the optic chiasm. The result is compression that directly affects the crossing nerve fibers that provide lateral peripheral vision for each eye. The visual field deficit affecting bilateral lateral vision is therefore very specific for a lesion affecting the optic chiasm. Plain lateral skull radiographs may demonstrate an enlarging sella turcica.

Primary malignant brain tumors are graded on the basis of local invasiveness and rapidity of growth and usually originate from the supporting glial tissues rather than the neurons. These tumors grow within the substance of the brain, destroying neurons and interrupting connecting pathways. Headache is an extremely rare complaint attributed to these tumors. The diagnosis is usually made as part of an evaluation for seizures with the development of neurologic dysfunction. Metastatic brain tumors from outside the nervous system behave in much the same way and also generally do not cause headaches. The onset of neurologic dysfunction in a patient with a history of carcinoma of the breast, lung, kidney, bowel, or oropharynx necessitates diagnostic scanning of the brain.

Tumors that originate within sinuses or oropharynx may cause local or referred pain before their presence is obvious. Early diagnosis is best made by skilled examination and by radiographic scanning techniques.

Although not a neoplasm, subdural hematomas develop as extracortical masses after head trauma and act like rapidly growing tumors. By the time symptoms develop, cognitive dysfunction may interfere with the ability to present an accurate history. Usually there is a headache, fluctuating focal neurologic signs including dysfunction of cranial nerves III or VII, excessive drowsiness, worsening of symptoms on lying down, and occasionally scalp tenderness to percussion over the region of the hematoma. Because of the unstable nature of the condition and the erratic growth pattern, the sooner diagnosis is made and proper management instituted, the better the outcome. When it is difficult to obtain a reasonable history from the patient, it is best to try to obtain some history from anyone who knows the patient and who can at least describe the usual level of mentation and ability.

Increased intracranial pressure associated with severe headache and transient visual loss, especially with postural changes and without any focal neurologic deficit except for weakness of the lateral rectus muscle (cranial nerve VI), can occur without the ability to demonstrate any intracranial tumor or mass. This condition is known as pseudotumor cerebri. The pain characteristics conform to the consequence of rapidly increasing intracranial pressure. Blindness is a possible outcome in the untreated patient as a result of increasing pressure on the optic nerve. The condition can be suspected during periods of rapid weight gain, especially pregnancy.

Vascular Disease Causing Headache

Aside from brain tumor, stroke is also often feared as a cause of recurrent or chronic severe headache. Most feared is the possibility of an aneurysm and intracranial headache. The headache associated with aneurysmal rupture is sudden, immediately severe, and often associated with a transient loss of consciousness, followed by reduced mentation, drowsiness, and usually nausea and vomiting. Nuchal rigidity is usually too severe to permit neck flexion, but this may not be true when there is depressed mental function or coma. There may or may not be any other neurologic signs, except for a positive Babinski or loss of either cranial nerve III or VI, because of the close proximity to the aneurysm or because of hematoma formation and/or increased intracranial pressure. There are no signs, clues, or reliable noninvasive ways to diagnose this type of aneurysm before rupture; even if diagnosed before hemorrhage, there is no way to predict if and when the rupture will occur. It is not uncommon to find other aneurysms that have not ruptured during diagnostic arteriography of the intracranial vessels. The aneurysm remains fairly asymptomatic until rupture.

Arteriovenous malformations are capable of causing severe recurrent headaches, especially if there is recurrent leakage of blood into the subarachnoid space. These malformations tend to cause some form of neurologic dysfunction and seizures, affecting brain function and tissue by altered local blood supply as well as by small hemorrhages. As with any cause of meningeal irritation, neck stiffness to flexion far exceeds resistance to neck rotation, thereby differentiating meningeal irritation from mechanical dysfunction of the cervical spine.

Migraine headaches were well described earlier. Other forms of vascular headaches include cluster headaches and lower-half headaches. Cluster headaches usually occur in males who smoke cigarettes. The headache lasts less than 2 hours and localizes behind one eye with associated redness and tearing and occasionally a Horner's syndrome (small pupil, mild ptosis, and shrinkage of the globe). Cluster headaches are excruciating and usually begin in the early morning, awakening the patient from sleep. They may occur more than once a day and recur daily for weeks to months. Between these clusters of headaches, the patient is headache free, except for the common tension type. Lower-half headaches usually occur in women with many of the features of migraine except that the pain is localized to the lower half of the face extending into the anterior neck and associated with tenderness over the carotid artery.

Extremely rare before the age of 60, temporal arteritis is always of concern when headaches begin later in life. This syndrome is usually associated with diffuse muscle and joint pains typified as polyarthralgia rheumatica. It is similar to migraine in that unilateral throbbing head pain recurs. Tenderness may be palpated over the temporal artery. The danger of delayed diagnosis or misdiagnosis by failure to obtain an erythrocyte sedimentation rate and/or biopsy of the artery with subsequent appropriate steroid therapy is progression to retinal ischemia and blindness or cerebral ischemia and stroke, or both.

Neck pain and headaches have been reported during carotid artery occlusion or after emboli, but the neurologic deficit will be obvious and will overshadow this complaint. Atherosclerotic disease or stenosis of either carotid or vertebral arteries does not cause headache, nor can headache be generated by a mechanical distortion of these structures alone.

Throbbing, severe, focal, or generalized headaches occasionally will follow a convulsive or nonconvulsive seizure and may last for hours. The headaches probably result from postictal alterations of pain pathways perhaps in a way similar to migraine. These headaches occur in the absence of any obvious head trauma and do not respond to physical treatment.

Infection

Probably the most self-diagnosed cause of headache is sinus headache, which the patient typically attempts to self-treat by the use of over-the-counter remedies.

True sinus infection is uncommon and is accompanied by fever, severe localized pain, and systemic generalized aches, pains, and malaise. Such conditions are usually diagnosed by plain radiographs and are not the cause of recurrent or chronic headache. Other sinus headaches may be better described as allergic headaches.

Cranial infection caused by a virus or bacteria is an acute or subacute illness with severe pain, nausea, vomiting, and signs of meningeal irritation. On examination, varying degrees of resistance to neck flexion will be palpated, yet no such resistance will accompany neck rotation. Associated fever and systemic signs usually require evaluation at a local emergency room. Chronic meningitis caused by fungal infection leads to chronic headache but little early on in the way of focal findings or neck stiffness. Such infections occasionally present in diabetics and in immunocompromised patients, now much more frequently seen in those patients suffering from acquired immune deficient syndrome (AIDS). Any form of meningitis may also result in increased intracranial pressure and present with additional signs and symptoms appropriate to this condition. Encephalitis is not usually associated with neck stiffness, but instead presents with headache and varying degrees of neurologic deficit, usually nonfocal and cognitive in nature.

SUMMARY

During the evaluation and treatment of patients presenting with head and facial pain, the physical therapist must be aware of the signs and symptoms of conditions that are not of musculoskeletal origin.

The following conditions require referral to a physician:

1. Head or facial pain associated with trauma not responding to therapy and associated with focal neurologic signs or symptoms or an alteration of personality and mental status
2. Head pain preceded by or associated with a loss of consciousness

3. Head pain associated with tenderness of a scalp artery in any patient past the age of 60 years.
4. Head or facial pain in any patient with focal cranial nerve dysfunction
5. Head or facial pain in any patient with neurologic dysfunction involving corticospinal, extrapyramidal, cerebellar, and spinal or radicular dysfunction

PATIENT CASE HISTORY 1
History

The patient was a 46-year-old bookkeeper who came to the clinic with a diagnosis of spastic torticolis. She had been treated previously at the physical therapy clinic, with the last visit occurring 4 months before her return. At the end of her previous physical therapy program, her chief complaint of left posterolateral cervical pain and stiffness and left occipital and temporal headaches had improved considerably. She had returned to the clinic stating that her headaches had returned and were much more severe than before. She had not seen her physician since this recent flare-up, having called his office only. The patient had spoken to someone on the physician's staff stating, "My headache came back. Can I see my physical therapist, since the treatment helped last time?" Permission was granted.

The patient's current chief complaint was daily, constant headaches. This was in contrast to her previously described chief complaint of left cervical pain and stiffness. When asked about the location of symptoms, she stated that it was primarily facial pain that hurt, specifically in the frontal and orbital regions bilaterally. She described the headaches as being a deep pressure sensation, severe at times. Again, this was in contrast to her previous description of headaches located in the left occipital and temporal region and described as tension or tightness.

The current headaches were constant, but the intensity quickly increased with the assumption of a forward-flexed head and neck posture when sitting or standing. The facial pressure subsided within a few minutes of returning the head and neck to an upright position. She noted a slight decrease in the pressure and intensity when she would lie down supine or side lying. The previously described left temporal and occipital headaches were aggravated by sitting more than 90 to 120 minutes, including driving. Forward-flexed postures had not influenced these headaches.

The facial pain had begun insidiously 3 weeks before re-evaluation. The patient could not recall any incident or accident that may have precipitated the onset of these symptoms. She noted there had not been a concurrent increase in left cervical symptoms. She recalled having similar pressure-like symptoms in the frontal and orbital regions two to three times in the past, although this pain was much more intense. The previous facial headaches seemed to have disappeared when the patient was given medication for sinus infections.

The patient's medical history had not changed over the 4 months between physical therapy sessions. She had not seen a physician for a medical condition, nor had her medications changed. She acknowledged a past history of recurrent sinus infection, in fact, she felt as though she had had a cold for the past month.

OBJECTIVE EXAMINATION

The objective examination findings were very similar to the presentation 4 months earlier regarding postural assessment, active and passive range of motion (ROM) findings, and special tests. Differences were noted, however, including swelling in the orbital regions, the eyes being red and teary, and the patient sounding very congested. Forward-bending ROM had not changed, but a sustained forward-flexed posture caused a significant increase in facial pressure within 10 to 15 seconds. The patient's previous left-sided headaches did not change in the past with cervical active ROM or sustained head and neck postures. Specific palpation or other active or passive cervical or cranial maneuvers did not alter the patient's current chief complaint. Cranial nerve assessment was negative.

ASSESSMENT AND OUTCOME

The pattern of evaluation findings suggested that the patient's current chief complaint was probably unrelated to what she had been treated for previously. In fact, the symptoms noted in the past had remained significantly improved over the previous 4 months. The referring physician was called regarding the patient's current status and the concern about the origin of these new complaints. It was communicated to the physician that the headaches were of new location and description as compared to what she had been treated for previously, and the previous symptoms remained improved from when she was last treated; also reported were insidious onset of the new headaches, inability to alter the facial pain except with sustained forward-flexed postures during the objective examination, the swelling noted around the eyes and redness of the eyes, the feeling that the patient had a cold for 4 weeks, and the fact that she has had similar symptoms previously that had resolved with taking medications for sinus infections. The physician saw the patient immediately, made the diagnosis of sinus infection, and placed the patient on antibiotics. The patient was called in 2 weeks later, and she reported complete relief of the facial pain and had resumed all normal activities. She did not feel the need to return for physical therapy.

The main point of this patient case presentation is that it represents a common mechanism of how certain medical conditions can arrive at the doorstep of the physical therapy clinic. This patient had developed new symptoms and failed to relate this information to the physician's office when she called. She did not realize that they were unrelated to her previous condition, treated by the physical therapist and physician. She also did not make the realization that these new symptoms were similar to the type of pain she had experienced previously and subsequently treated with antibiotics. Therefore, the patient called the physician stating that her headaches were back and could she go see her physical therapist again. In her case, the condition was not life threatening and was easily diagnosed and treated by the physician.

True sinus infections are relatively rare, but they should be considered if orbital or maxillary pain is noted; if the pain is described as aching, throbbing, or pressure; if the pain is accompanied by fever; if local edema in the area of the sinus is noted; and if a sense of nasal congestion or copious amounts of nasal discharge are noted by the patient. Allergic rhinitis (e.g., hay fever) may result in similar symptoms, such as nasal congestion, watery eyes, and nasal discharge. The congestion may lead to complaints of pressure or tension in the facial or frontal regions. The frontal, orbital, and maxillary regions are not uncommon referral areas for cervical structures. A patient may present with a chief complaint of headaches with discomfort located in the occipital, temporal, and frontal regions. The therapist must consider all local structures, as well as structures from adjacent regions (cervical area), as a source of symptoms. In this case, the left temporal and occipital headaches were related to cervical mechanical dysfunction, while the facial pain was related to involvement of local structures—the sinuses.

PATIENT CASE HISTORY 2
HISTORY

The patient was a 47-year-old receptionist who came to the physical therapy clinic on the recommendation of a friend. Her chief complaint was intermittent but severe right-sided head-

aches. The aching and throbbing pain was most intense in the right parietal, temporal, and frontal regions of the cranium. The headache seemed to start in the right cervicothoracic and upper scapular regions, and spread to the cranial areas described above. In the past 6 months, the headache would be present and severe for 3 to 4 days; the patient would then be pain free for up to 7 to 10 days. The patient could not relate the onset of the headaches to any particular incident or accident, nor could she explain why the headaches disappeared.

When present, the headaches were most intense when the patient would lie down. She woke up two to three times per night due to the severity of the headaches. The intensity of the throbbing and aching would decrease when she got up to walk around. Neck movements and activities such as tennis would increase the stiffness in the right cervical spine and cause a slight increase in the headache intensity.

The patient stated that the headaches began years ago following an automobile accident. During the past 18 months, the headaches had increased in frequency and severity, and seemed more intense in the temporal and frontal regions. Soon after the automobile accident, the headaches were more localized to the cervical and occipital regions. The patient could not relate the increase in headache frequency or severity to a particular incident or accident that might have happened 18 months ago. During the 12 months prior to the physical therapy evaluation, the patient went to a chiropractor and received adjustments of the cervical spine and shoulder girdle exercises. She had also gone to a dentist and was fitted with a mouth appliance for a temporomandibular joint condition. Neither the chiropractic care nor the appliance helped the patient's condition.

Besides the chief complaint, the patient also described left-sided headaches similar to the right-sided symptoms, but they were very infrequent and not intense. They were only present when the right-sided symptoms were at their worst. She stated that both arms felt weak even though she had been exercising them for months using free weights. Although she denied problems with vision, taste, smell, or swallowing, she had noticed a decrease in her hearing ability, especially the right side, over the past 12 months. She had not seen a physician for her current condition.

The patient stated that her current medical history was negative. The only medication she was taking was estrogen replacement which she had taken since her hysterectomy. Surgical history also included a craniotomy to remove a benign cyst from the right frontal lobe region. When asked about symptoms leading up to the craniotomy, the patient described headaches and cervical pain very similar to her current symptoms. After the surgery, the headaches were significantly reduced.

PHYSICAL EXAMINATION

Postural assessment revealed that the occiput was side bent left and right rotated on the cervical spine. The right shoulder girdle was elevated compared to the left. There was moderate muscle guarding noted in the right posterior suboccipital, upper trapezius, and levator scapulae regions. Cervical spine active ROM testing revealed right upper cervical spine discomfort (posterior aspect) with forward and backward bending and right rotation. Left rotation and backward bending were the most restricted. Vertical cervical compression and distraction were negative. Mandibular depression was of functional ROM and caused slight discomfort in the right temporomandibular joint region.

Passive accessory vertebral motion testing (PAVM) revealed significant hypomobility of C1, right and left side, and of C7, T1, and T2 centrally. Symptoms were not altered with the PAVM testing of the temporomandibular joint and the cervical and upper thoracic spine. Sensory and motor testing of the upper extremities revealed no abnormalities, but cranial nerve assessment

revealed a significant deficit in hearing of the right ear. There was also slight weakness noted when assessing cranial nerve XII.

ASSESSMENT AND OUTCOME

Despite the dysfunction noted during the evaluation (i.e., segmental vertebral hypomobility, postural faults, muscle guarding, etc.), the patient was advised to see a neurologist before any further physical therapy was administered. Numerous findings (described earlier in this chapter) caused concern and the therapist had more questions than answers regarding the patient's condition after the evaluation. The history revealed a condition marked by intermittent but severe headaches, aching and throbbing in nature, which insidiously worsened 18 months ago. The onset and cessation of the headaches could not be explained mechanically. When present, the headaches were most intense when the patient was lying down, and they woke her at night. She had a previous history of craniotomy for a benign cyst, and with specific questioning, the patient admitted her current symptoms were similar to symptoms she experienced prior to the craniotomy. After the surgery, she had noted a dramatic decrease in the intensity and frequency of her symptoms.

Raising concern in the physical examination was the significant hearing loss on the right side and possible weakness of the tongue. Also of importance was the inability of the therapist to alter the headache during the physical examination. Being unable to alter the patient's headache by stressing musculoskeletal structures locally or in the cervical/thoracic region raised questions regarding the relevance of the findings of mechanical dysfunction as they related to the patient's complaints.

The patient scheduled an appointment with a neurologist and was instructed to contact the therapist after her visit. The therapist contacted the neurologist and the above information was communicated. After not hearing from the patient 3 weeks after her scheduled physician visit, the therapist called the patient. She stated that she had to cancel her physician appointment because of her busy schedule. The therapist encouraged the patient to reschedule the appointment as soon as possible, and the reasons for the referral to the neurologist were reviewed with her. Three months later, the therapist met the friend who initially referred the patient to the physical therapy clinic. The friend stated that since the physical therapist evaluation the patient had been hospitalized for depression and further testing had been done by a neurologist. The test revealed the presence of numerous brain tumors.

REFERENCES

1. Campbell DG, Parsons CM: Referred head pain and its concomitants. J Nerv Ment Dis 99:544, 1944
2. Edeling J: Manual Therapy for Chronic Headache. Butterworths, London, 1988
3. Jull GA: Headaches associated with the cervical spine—A clinical review. p. 322. In Grieve GP (ed): Modern Manual Therapy of the Vertebral Column. Churchill Livingstone, Edinburgh, 1986
4. Travell JG, Simons DG: Myofascial Pain and Dysfunction. The Trigger Point Manual. Williams & Wilkins, Baltimore, 1983
5. Fredriksen TA, Sjaastad O: Cervicogenic headache: A clinical entity. Cephalgia 7(suppl 6):171, 1987
6. Jaeger B: Cervicogenic headache: Relationship to cervical spine dysfunction and myofascial trigger points. Cephalgia 7(Suppl 6):398, 1987
7. Dalessio DJ (ed): Wolff's Headache and Other Head Pain. 5th Ed. Oxford University Press, New York, 1987
8. Raskin N, Appenzeller O: Major Problems in Internal Medicine. Vol. XIX: Headache. WB Saunders, Philadelphia, 1980
9. Blumenthal LS: Tension headache. p. 157. In Vinken PJ, Bruyn GW (eds): Headaches and Cranial Neuralgias: Handbook of Clinical Neurology. Vol. 5. John Wiley & Sons, New York, 1968
10. Trott PH: Tension headache. p. 336. In Grieve GP (ed): Modern Manual Therapy of the Vertebral Column. Churchill Livingstone, Edinburgh, 1986
11. Boissonnault W, Bass C: Pathological origins of trunk and neck pain. Part 2. JOSPT 12(5):208, 1990
12. Hoppenfeld S: Physical Examination of the Spine and Extremities. Appleton & Lange, E. Norwalk, CT, 1976
13. Devinsky O, Feldmann E: Examination of the Cranial and Peripheral Nerves. Churchill Livingstone, New York, 1988
14. Haymaker W, Woodhall B: Peripheral Nerve Injuries. WB Saunders, Philadelphia, 1953

SUGGESTED READINGS

DeJong RN: The Neurologic Examination. 3rd Ed. Harper & Row, New York, 1967

Dalessio DJ: Wolff's Headache and Other Head Pain. 5th Ed. Oxford University Press, New York, 1987

9

Screening for Musculoskeletal System Disease

TERRY RANDALL, P.T. A.T.C. *
KEVIN McMAHON, M.D.

"The Scientist is not content to stop at the obvious."
Charles H. Mayo

Physical therapists devote most of their time to treating impairments of the musculoskeletal system. The evaluation of specific deficits, such as muscle strength or proprioception, is becoming increasingly sophisticated. At times it seems very difficult to keep pace with the latest innovations in rehabilitation. However, this is not the only area of practice that is changing rapidly. The development of direct access will alter the methods of the physical therapist's evaluation and scope of practice.

With expanding roles and increasing responsibilities, physical therapists must expand their knowledge base beyond that of traditional practice. Functioning in a direct access mode "assumes that we desire to achieve an even greater degree of excellence and accountability...."[1] Physical therapists will find themselves functioning in the role of primary care provider more often in the future. Clinicians who practice in more traditional, referral-based settings must also recognize their increasing responsibility. The quality of evaluation is not dependent on the mode of practice.

To achieve this level of excellence and practice, we must be more aware of the role of the physical therapist in view of the entire medical system. "Physical therapy is part of the health-care system, not the whole thing. If all we do is provide excellent physical therapy, the independent practitioner will not be a door into the health-care system but a dead end."[2] The expansion of physical therapist's responsibilities must be associated with broadening the physical therapist's view of the patient. No longer can patients be viewed as just having an ankle sprain, or back pain. The goal of physical therapy evaluation should be to formulate an unambiguous diagnosis that demonstrates specific impairments and disabilities.[3]

The precise terminology of this diagnosis is controversial.[4-6] However, the value of making a clinical assessment concerning the patients complaint and basing a treatment plan on that assessment should be universally acceptable. It stands to reason that a definitive assessment will lead to a more precise treatment. Clinical evaluation models can assist in formulating a thought process to assist in formulating a specific diagnosis.[7,8]

This chapter, provides an overview of musculoskeletal system diseases that, while not always amenable to physical therapy treatment, can be seen in our patients. Descriptions of the more common primary skeletal neoplasms, skeletal metastasis, infections, and metabolic disorders are included. While these musculoskeletal disorders may be relatively uncommon, they are serious conditions for which early detection is cru-

---

* The opinions or assertions contained herein are the private views of the author and are not to be construed as official or as reflecting the views of the Department of the Army or the Department of Defense.

199

cial to effective treatment. Information is provided concerning the pathogenesis of each disorder so that clinicians will have a common background as to their origins.

The epidemiology and clinical features of the disease are of primary importance to the physical therapist. Special attention has been given to situations in which these diseases may present as more typical or common disorders routinely treated by physical therapists. A brief description of appropriate treatment techniques is included. This book is not intended to be a treatment manual, but physical therapists do need to be familiar with the extent and forms of treatment available so they may educate their patients.

The conditions presented in this chapter require consultation or referral for further diagnostic tests. Physical therapists must develop the skills needed to function within the framework of medical specialties. For these reasons, the appropriate referral process is discussed as well.

PRIMARY SKELETAL NEOPLASMS

The diverse nature of musculoskeletal pathology makes the differential diagnosis elusive. Zohn[9] describes five pathologic conditions that can affect seven anatomic structures (Table 9-1). Cross-matching these lists produces an extensive list of musculoskeletal problems that must be considered during an evaluation. Neoplasms are but one small, albeit important, part of the spectrum.

Table 9-1. Summary of Cross-matching Anatomic Structures and Pathologic Conditions

Anatomic Structures That May Be the Seat of Pain-Producing Pathology	Pathologic Changes or Conditions That May Affect These Structures
Bone and periosteum	Trauma (extrinsic and intrinsic)
Hyaline cartilage	Inflammation
Synovial capsule	Metabolic disease
Ligaments	Neoplasms
Muscles, tendons, and tendon sheaths	Congenital anomalies
Intra-articular menisci	
Bursae	

(From Zohn,[9] with permission.)

Primary tumors of the musculoskeletal system are a very rare finding. Thus, it is easy to become complacent in our daily practice, comforted in the knowledge that the odds are against us ever seeing a primary neoplasm. From time to time, it is important to reiterate the significance of these lesions and the catastrophic ramifications that can ensue if treatment is delayed unnecessarily. For these reasons, physical therapists must be familiar with the clinical features of the more common of these lesions. In an area where clinicians claim a wide disparity of experience, it may be best to begin with commonly used terms.

The following definitions are taken from Salter.[10] *Tumor* is a commonly used word that may be used in rather imprecise ways to describe any localized swelling or mass. *Neoplasm* has more meaning in describing a new and abnormal formation of cells. *Metastasis* refers to the ability of a neoplasm to initiate independent growth at a distant site, therefore being malignant.

Many of the symptoms that physical therapists are accustomed to dealing with on a daily basis can also be manifestations of the presence of neoplasms. Pain, swelling, and loss of function may represent the body's reaction to mild trauma. However, these same symptoms can also be the primary warning signs of far more serious pathology. For this reason, neoplasms are often missed at the initial presentation. This fact also emphasizes the importance of physical therapist continually re-evaluating their patient's response and progress to treatment. An unexpected or unexplained response to treatment should generate suspicion that may lead to further evaluation or referral. Likewise, symptoms that do not lead to a specific diagnosis must be suspect. This important concept should be an integral part of the clinician's evaluation and documentation process.[11]

Many different classifications for tumors have been used. Even the broad distinction between malignant and benign is not always straightforward. Consideration of the tissue of origin of a neoplasm can provide a useful classification. Most primary neoplasms can therefore be divided into osteogenic, chondrogenic, collagenic, and myelogenic.[12] Neoplasms can also have a neurogenic, vascular, or adipose origin.[13]

Fortunately, the malignant neoplasms are less common than benign bone lesions. Both types are serious, however, and even benign lesions can jeopardize the affected limb. It is important to know the incidence of neoplasms if one expects to avoid missing subtle physical signs. Some lesions are correlated with, but not limited to, a specific age group; for example, osteosarcoma is most commonly seen in childhood.

Clinical Features

The clinical features are of particular interest to anyone involved in evaluation of musculoskeletal conditions. While trauma is a common complaint of patients with neoplasms, this only serves to focus the evaluation to a specific area and is not associated with the type, location, or progression of the lesion.

Pain, while not universal, is by far the most common symptom in all neoplasms and, unlike trauma, may be directly linked to a neoplasm. Pain is more likely to occur with rapidly growing neoplasms, such as osteosarcoma. The characteristics of the pain, as always, can vary but may evolve from mild and intermittent to more intense and constant. In aggressive malignant lesions, the pain can be caused by the rapidly expanding mass. Pain does not occur in the same stage of development for all lesions. In some cases, pain may present very early in the course, and hence be helpful in early detection. In other instances, the neoplasm may progress significantly before the development of pain. This varied response is due to the nature, location, and rate of growth of the neoplasm. It is vital, therefore, for physical therapists to be aware of the subtle differences in the description of pain and how our patients react to it. It is also important to remember the patterns of referred pain. A careful examination, both distal and proximal to the painful area, must be done. Constant vigilance is required to detect cases of pain that are uncharacteristic of common musculoskeletal conditions. The expected response to treatment must also be known and monitored.

The use of percussion can also aid in the assessment of pain. Both direct and indirect methods can be used.[14] By generating a firm, sudden force from one hand, a specific bone or portion of bone can be assessed through the fingers of the other hand. Joint dysfunction may cause a sharp pain of short duration, while disease may produce a deep throbbing pain that persist for several minutes.[15] These general descriptions do not apply in all situations.

Swelling can be present with many different neoplasms, but it is not always detectable clinically. The swelling can be localized or diffuse, tender or painless, warm or neutral. The nature of the swelling is a function of the vascularity, the proximity of the lesion to the surface, and the rate of growth. Palpation can also help discern whether a mass is present, as well as the consistency, mobility, location, dimensions, and growth rate of the neoplasm.[16] These ordinary clinical signs may be the only clue to the severe nature of the underlying pathology. Therefore, some of the more common neoplasms and their specific characteristics are presented.

Most neoplasms have an age group where the incidence is highest (Table 9-2). This does not mean that a specific lesion cannot occur outside this range. In general, primary neoplasms of bone occur in children and young adults. It has been suggested that this is due in part to the higher rate of growth in the bones in this age group.

Neoplasms that are destructive to bone in weight-bearing areas may cause weakening, leading to pain. If the destruction continues, a pathologic fracture may occur. Pathologic fracture occurs when destructive characteristics of the neoplasm weaken the cortex. A history of insignificant trauma along with pain in the area before the fracture should raise suspicion.[17] In this case, the physical therapist may require further consultation to rule out a pathologic fracture.

Referral

Proper referral for the patient with a suspected neoplasm should contain some basic information that can be gathered from a thorough physical examination. The physician will be interested in the general health of the patient. A detailed history and review of all systems is appropriate[18] (see Ch. 1).

If a mass is present, its characteristics should be noted.

Table 9-2. Characteristics of Bone Tumors

Type of Tumor	Age of Patient (yr)	Site of Tumor	Radiographic Features	Histopathologic Features	Comments
Benign					
Osteochondroma	5–35	Metaphyseal	Cancellous and cortical	Normal bone and cartilage	Malignant transformation in <1%
Osteoid osteoma	15–30	Femur, tibia posterior elements of spine	Sclerotic area surrounding lytic nidus	Disorganized, thin osteoid trabeculae with or without mineralization	Painful, relieved by aspirin
Osteoblastoma	10–30	Vertebrae, long bones	Destructive with or without sclerosis >2 cm	Thicker osteoid trabeculae with mineralization	Differential diagnosis includes aneurysmal bone cyst and osteosarcoma
Chondroblastoma	15–30	Epiphysis of long bones	Central bone destruction surrounded by a thin sclerotic rim	Chondroblasts in chondroid matrix	Giant cells may be present
Giant cell	20–40	Epiphysis of long bones	Eccentric expanding zone of radiolucency	Benign giant cells with oval or spindle-shaped stromal cells	7.5% may behave as a malignant lesion
Malignant					
Osteosarcoma	15–30	Metaphysis of long bone	Destructive lesion with or without an ossified matrix	Malignant connective tissue cells producing osteoid	Most common primary malignant bone tumor
Ewing's sarcoma	10–20	Diaphysis of long bones	Permeative destructive lesion with or without periosteal "onion skin"	Monotonous pattern of cork staining small cells	May mimic infection
Myeloma	40–80	Spine, ribs, pelvis	"Punched-out" areas of destruction with or without cortical expansion	Sheets of closely packed plasma cells	Most common neoplasm of bone

(From Wilkins and Sim,[19] with permission.)

Descriptions of size, location, mobility, tenderness, and texture are important in the differential diagnosis. While the size of the mass may not be an indicator of the severity of the condition, the change in size over time is very important. The location of the lesion must be determined as accurately as possible. The type of bone involved and even the specific location within the bone can provide information concerning a possible diagnosis.

If the mass is located within the muscle belly, it may become fixed when the muscle is contracted and mobile when the muscle is relaxed. Neoplasms that are deep and connected to fascia or bone are not usually mobile. In this way, palpation alone can distinguish a soft tissue neoplasm from a bone lesion.[19]

Most physical therapists cannot order radiographs, but films may be available for review. Despite many of the newer, highly sophisticated imaging equipment available today, the plain radiograph remains the standard for the initial workup in suspected neoplasms. Wilkins and Sim[19] alert the examiner to four features to be noted when a lesion is detected radiographically.

OSTEOGENIC NEOPLASMS

Osteoid Osteoma

Jaffe[21] is credited with describing a benign, bone-forming tumor that is characteristically found in the long bones of the lower extremity. This neoplasm, like

Features to Note in a Radiographically Detected Lesion

1. *Location:* The specific bone, and location within the bone (epiphysis, metaphysis, or diaphysis) can be determined.
2. *Effect on normal bone:* The effect the lesion has had on the normal bone should be checked. Both osteolytic and osteoblastic changes can be present with neoplasms.
3. *Local response:* The local response to the presence of the lesion should be assessed. Sclerotic borders and periosteal reactions give indications of the growth characteristics.
4. *Presence of a matrix:* The presence of a matrix is determined. An ossified matrix can be seen on either bone or soft tissue lesions. A more detailed description of the radiologic findings in bone lesions can be found in Madewell et al.[20]

many others, is most common in boys and young adults, but the precise etiology is unknown. The lesion, like many tumors, can affect joint function, which may lead to a misdiagnosis of musculoskeletal origin on the basis of subjective complaints of pain and some loss of function in the associated joint. Because joint pain and injury are common, especially in an active population, more mundane types of problems are usually implicated as the source of pain.

Clinical Features

Pain is associated with this lesion. It can be described as a dull ache that may increase in severity over several months. An important quality of the pain is that it is often worse at night and is alleviated with salicylates. No systemic symptoms such as weight loss or fever are present. Males between the ages of 5 and 30 years are most susceptible.

This lesion is seen on radiographs, but it may not appear for several months after the onset of symptoms. Therefore, it is important to obtain repeated films when symptoms are persistent. The appearance of an

osteoid osteoma is that of a small (<1-cm) translucency called a nidus[22] (Fig. 9-1). This is surrounded by sclerotic bone.[23] Treatment is usually successful but requires excision of the entire nidus. Patients can expect to return to normal function after complete excision.

Physical Therapy Evaluation

Physical therapists should be aware of the osteoid osteoma because a patient with this lesion may have had multiple evaluations that indicate few objective findings, yet the symptoms continue. The presence of associated trauma or possible overuse only confuses the presentation further. Years can pass with continued symptoms before a correct diagnosis is made.[24] The presence of gradually increasing night pain relieved with aspirin should clue the clinician to this possible alternative diagnosis. There are no reported malignant tendencies associated with this neoplasm, but it must be treated by an orthopaedic surgeon.

Osteoblastoma

A neoplasm that has many similarities to the osteoid osteoma is the osteoblastoma. The World Health Organization (WHO) recognizes the common characteristics and places both lesions under a common heading.[25]

Clinical Features

Most patients with osteoblastoma are under 30 years of age. Osteoblastoma differs from osteoid osteoma in that the most common location is in the spine. The posterior elements are frequently involved. Pain is common to both types of neoplasms, but the osteoblastoma is considered less painful and more difficult to localize. This may result in longer elapsed time before the lesion is detected. Typically, several months and up to 2 years may pass before the lesion is detected. Thirty-four percent of osteoblastomas are located in the spine, and of those, 50 percent will cause neurologic symptoms.[26]

Radiologically, the lesion does not produce the reac-

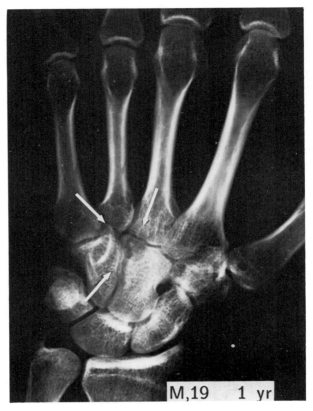

Fig. 9-1. Anteroposterior radiograph of the wrist and hand of a 19-year-old man with wrist pain and median nerve paresthesias of 1-year duration. The capitate bone shows a small area of increased density surrounded by a radiolucent area (arrows). The osteoid osteoma was excised. (From Cohen et al,[22] with permission.)

tion in surrounding bone seen in osteoid osteoma. Therefore, the dense sclerotic margin surrounding osteoid osteoma is not seen in the osteoblastoma. When present in the posterior elements of the spine, the affected area may appear enlarged.[27]

Treatment

Treatment principles are the same as those for osteoid osteoma in that the best prognosis occurs when the lesion can be excised. Because of the predilection for the spine, excision may be a challenging procedure.

Osteosarcoma

Osteogenic sarcoma is one of the more common primary malignant bone neoplasms, representing 25 percent of primary malignant tumors.[28] The lesion itself has an extremely rapid growth rate. It is often found in areas such as the metaphysis of long bones, which also have a rapid growth rate. The most common sites include the lower femur or upper tibia and the proximal humerus. In one series of 243 patients, 80 percent had lesions in these locations.[29]

Children and adults in their 20s and 30s are most susceptible; another rise in incidence is seen in adults over the age of 50. This may be due to an association with Paget's disease. Males are twice as likely to have osteosarcoma than are females.

Clinical Features

The most consistent clinical finding is that of pain. The pain is usually described in a classic pattern of progression from mild and intermittent to severe and continuous. Some alteration in function can be expected because this neoplasm is found in the metaphysis, hence close to the joint. A mass may be one of the initial findings. If present, it may vary from soft and fluctuant to very firm. The skin overlying the tumor may be warm to the touch because of the increased vascularity associated with the rapid growth.[10]

Radiography shows cortical destruction early during the course of the lesion,[16] predisposing the bone to pathologic fracture. Another radiologic sign associated with osteosarcoma is Codman's angle.[30] This refers to the area of periosteal bone that lifts from the cortex as a malignant tumor breaks into the surrounding soft tissue (Fig. 9-2). Further studies such as tomograms, bone scans, computed tomography (CT), and magnetic

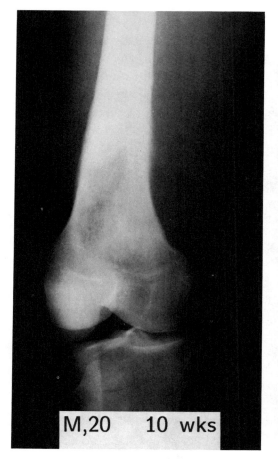
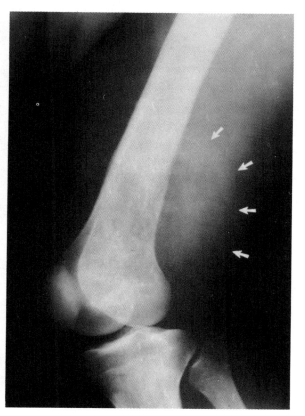

Fig. 9-2. Anteroposterior **(A)** and lateral **(B)** radiographs of the right femur showing a lytic osteosarcoma with posterior extension into soft tissue (arrows). (From Cohen et al,[22] with permission.)

resonance imaging (MRI) are used for diagnosis and staging.

Treatment

Treatment for osteosarcoma, like that of many tumors, has evolved rapidly over the past 10 years. A survival rate of less than 10 percent was the prognosis only a decade ago. Left untreated, death occurs in less than 2 years.[31,32] The poor prognosis was in part due to the fact that osteosarcoma metastasizes to the lungs through the bloodstream early in its course. With state-of-the-art treatment using surgery and chemotherapy, the survival rate is improving,[33] thanks to advances in chemotherapy, better staging of the lesion, and improved surgical techniques and equipment.

The most widely accepted method of staging was developed by Enneking.[34] The purpose of a staging system is to enable clinicians to predict the course of disease. The most efficacious treatment can then be chosen, depending on the classification. Characteristics used to stage a neoplasm include a histologic grade, location, and presence or absence of metastasis. Histologic grade is subdivided into two categories according to the aggressiveness of the lesion. The location also has two levels: intracompartmental and extracompartmental. The presence or absence of metas-

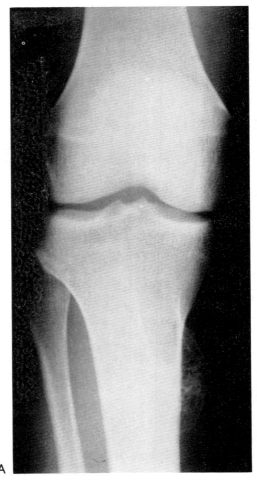

A

Fig. 9-3. Osteocartilaginous exostosis. A 20-year-old man presented with complaints of pain and of a mass about the proximal aspect of his right tibia. Anteroposterior **(A)** and lateral. (*Figure continues.*)

tasis is also an important variable in predicting outcome.

CHONDROGENIC NEOPLASMS

Osteochondroma

The most common benign primary neoplasm of the bone is osteochondroma. It is formed by an osseous outgrowth that is continuous with the host bone. The outgrowth is composed of spongy bone with a cartilaginous cap. It occurs in adolescence and rarely con-

tinues to develop once skeletal maturity is reached. The metaphysis of the long bones is affected. The knee and elbow are commonly affected.

Clinical Features

Initial symptoms may be associated with a bursitis or localized inflammatory response caused by friction from the overlying tissues. A firm, stable, nontender mass may be palpated. Because the cartilaginous cap is not visible on radiography, the mass will feel much larger than it appears on the x-ray film[35] (Fig. 9-3). The outgrowth always points away from the nearest epi-

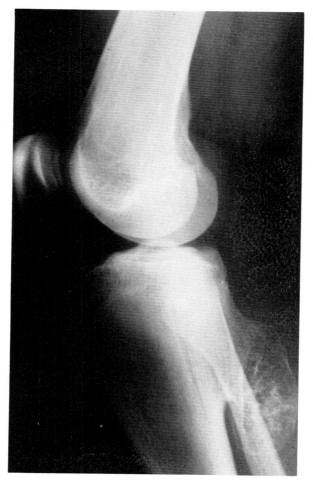

B

Fig. 9-3. (B) radiographs showing an osteochondroma arising from the posterior medial aspect of the proximal tibial metaphysis with continuity of the host cortex sweeping into the cortex of the osteochondroma. (From McGuire et al,[35] with permission.)

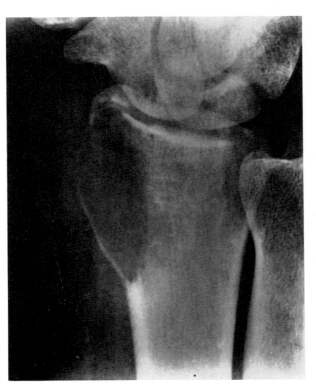

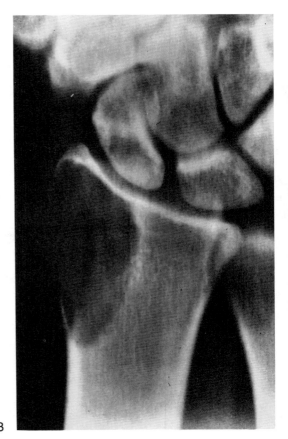

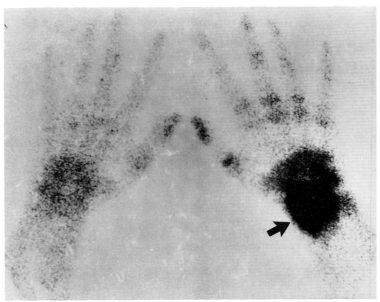

physis.[10] Trabeculated bone will be seen within the outgrowth.

Treatment

Treatment of osteochondroma is largely symptomatic. Surgical excision is considered if the lesion interferes with the normal function of the muscle-tendon units in the area. If no symptoms are present, no definitive treatment may be needed. The lesion does need to be followed because of the risk of malignant change, although this risk is very small.

Chondroblastoma

A chondroblastoma is a rare primary neoplasm of cartilaginous origin. It is most often found in the epiphyseal region of long bones, primarily the femur and humerus. Often the lesion can cross the epiphysis into the metaphysis. Most chondroblastomas are detected in males under the age of 30. Clinical symptoms include pain and tenderness and, because the lesion is close to a joint, limitations in movement or function may be seen. A joint effusion may also be detected.[19] There have been reports of neurologic involvement; this finding is related to the location of the lesion.[36]

Clinical Features

A chondroblastoma will appear as an oval translucent area in the epiphyseal region and will have a thin sclerotic margin. This sets it apart from more malignant lesions, such as osteosarcoma, which is usually isolated in the metaphysis and has a wide sclerotic rim.[37] The lesion is contained by the cortex, but some thinning may occur.

Treatment

Treatment of chondroblastoma usually includes curettage and bone grafting. A chondroblastoma is a be-nign lesion that generally does not require radiation or chemotherapy. Results of treatment are generally good, and patients may eventually resume a normal activity level. In a recently reported case, a college football player returned to competitive athletics 1 year after excision and bone grafting of a chondroblastoma from the proximal humerus.[36]

Osteoclastoma/Giant Cell

Four to 5 percent of all primary neoplasms of the bone in the United States are giant cell tumors.[38] The epiphysis of the long bones, such as the distal femur, radius, and the proximal tibia, are likely areas in which it occurs. Osteoclastoma develops after the epiphysis is closed and therefore is generally seen in people over the age of 20. The incidence decreases after 40 years of age. Pain is the most prevalent symptom initially. A soft tissue mass may be palpable, and pathologic fractures do occur.[19] This type of involvement in the proximity of the joint may impair function.

There is a tendency for the neoplasm to cross the epiphyseal line to involve the subchondral bone. Radiography will show a large, osteolytic, lesion that may expand the cortex outward but not penetrate it[39] (Fig. 9-4). Treatment has progressed from amputation to more functional limb- and joint-sparing procedures. Radiation is also an adjunct treatment, especially in those cases in which complete excision is not possible.

Enchondroma

A very common benign neoplasm is the enchondroma. This lesion is found in both men and women, ages 10 to 50 years. It usually occurs in the hands or feet, forming in the medullary cavity and expanding slowly. Over

Fig. 9-4. Giant cell tumor in the distal radius of a 29-year-old man. **(A)** Plain film showing an unmarginated geographic lesion with a sharp zone of transition extending from the metaphysis into the epiphysis. **(B)** Conventional tomogram showing the lesion extending distally to the subchondral bone. **(C)** Radionuclide bone scan showing increased activity in the lesion (arrow). (From Chew,[39] with permission.)

many years, the cancellous bone is replaced with cartilage, and the cortex thins; this will be indicated by the lucency on the radiograph.[40] Most enchondromas are asymptomatic. The difficulty in management is establishing the diagnosis. The presence of a malignant lesion must be ruled out. Eventually the patient may notice a firm swelling, which is due to the expanding bone. Pathologic fractures may also occur (Fig. 9-5). Treatment consists of curettage and packing the defect with bone. The prognosis in solitary lesions is excellent.

MYELOGENIC NEOPLASMS

Plasma Cell Myeloma

The most common primary neoplasm of bone is the plasma cell myeloma. Myeloma is a neoplastic proliferation of plasma cells in the bone marrow. It can be multifocal (multiple myeloma) or solitary. It is likely that the solitary lesions will become multicentric over time. This is one neoplasm that is apt to be found in people over 40 years of age. The peak incidence appears to occur during the sixth decade.[41] In this age

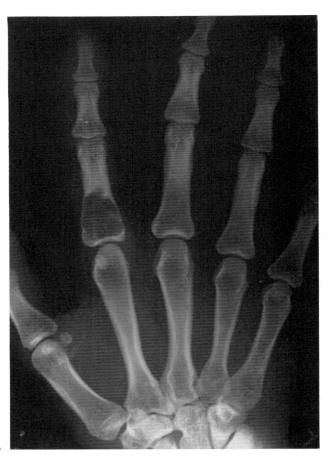

A

Fig. 9-5. Solitary enchondromas. **(A,B)** Radiographic appearance of solitary enchondromas of the short tubular bones of the hands. The lesion of the proximal phalanx of the index finger has thinned the cortex and is radiolucent in nature. The lesion of the fifth metacarpal has markedly expanded the cortex and has small calcific densities within the lesion itself. This picture would be considered diagnostic of enchondroma. (From McGuire et al,[35] with permission.)

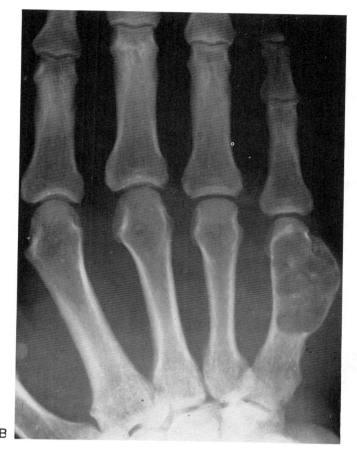

B

Fig. 9-5. (*Continued.*)

group, the largest concentration of bone marrow is in the spine, pelvis, and skull—the most common sites of involvement.[10] Clinical findings include pain, bone tenderness, weight loss, and anemia with a normal white blood cell (WBC) count. Pathologic fractures are common.[42]

Clinical Features

The pain associated with plasma cell myeloma is described as deep and may increase with activity. Back pain is a common complaint because the location of the lesion is frequently in the spine. Compression of the cauda equina by the lesion can cause radicular symptoms. Turek[27] describes a situation in which a patient may present with symptoms very similar to those of a disc herniation. Although initially episodic, the pain eventually becomes constant.

The initial radiographic finding may be osteopenia of the spine. In the flat bones, cystic or punched-out areas may appear (Fig. 9-6). Eventually, the osteolytic effects extend to the cortex and beyond.

Treatment

Treatment for plasma cell myeloma has not proved successful. Most patients succumb to the disease within 11 to 32 months of detection.[43]

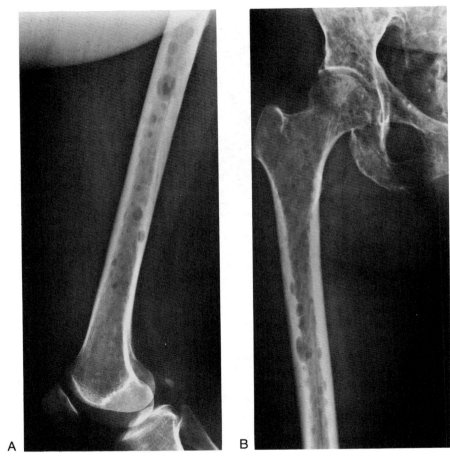

Fig. 9-6. Multiple myeloma in a 44-year-old woman. **(A,B)** Radiographs of the femur showing multiple lytic lesions of varying size throughout. Bone destruction has proceeded from the endosteal side of the cortex. The pelvis is diffusely involved. (From Chew,[39] with permission.)

Ewing's Sarcoma

Like multiple myeloma, Ewing's sarcoma arises in the bone marrow. Myeloma develops directly in the marrow cells; Ewing's sarcoma develops in the marrow support structure or reticuloendothelial tissue.[27]

Clinical Features

Ewing's sarcoma is a highly malignant primary bone neoplasm that occurs in children and young adults. Ninety percent of these neoplasms occur between the ages of 5 and 30 years. In 25 percent of cases, metastatic disease will develop.[44] It does appear to be rare in the black population. The diaphysis of the femur is the most likely site, but the pelvis, tibia, and humerus can also be involved.[19] Pain and swelling cause these patients to seek medical care. The pain may be intermittent early in the course but usually becomes constant. A mass may be palpable and can be tender. Systemic symptoms such as fever and malaise are common.

The term "onion peel" is often applied to the radiographic appearance of Ewing's sarcoma, attributable to the formation of new periosteal bone in multiple layers parallel to the bone shaft. The destructive nature of this lesion can lead to cortical thinning, leaving the patient susceptible to pathologic fractures (Fig. 9-7). The use of braces or crutches may be indicated during treatment if the weight-bearing bones are involved.

Treatment

Surgical treatment for Ewing's sarcoma has not played as important a role as have radiation and chemotherapy. However, as more is learned about the significant limitations of chemotherapy, surgical intervention is increasing. Late effects of radiation and chemotherapy include stiffness, asymmetry, and limb shortening. These can all pose problems for the physical therapist who is trying to improve function.

MISCELLANEOUS LESIONS

Lipoma

The most common tumor of the musculoskeletal system is the lipoma. This mass of mature fat appears in adults after the second decade. The mass is usually asymptomatic, soft, and highly mobile. Physical therapists will undoubtedly palpate many lipomas during their evaluations. The mass may be noted to harden significantly after the application of ice.[19] The physical therapist should palpate the entire area of the body to be treated with any modality in order to detect post-treatment changes.

Although lipomas rarely cause problems, the patient should be questioned as to the progression of the mass. Patients who are unaware of its presence should be taught to palpate and recognize any changes that might develop. Pain is associated with lipomas only when nerve compression is involved. In these cases, excision may be required.

Dermatologic Lesions

Other lesions that physical therapist should be aware of are those affecting the skin. Physical therapists often see a large number of patients and have the opportunity to screen for skin lesions during the evaluation of the patient's musculoskeletal problem. While the presentation of skin lesions is varied, a few points must be emphasized.

Dermatologic Screening

1. *Know the types of lesions:* There are many different types of skin lesions. Many do not represent conditions that warrant further evaluation or treatment. But as with the neoplasms previously discussed, the value of an appropriate referral of a potential malignancy is immeasurable.

2. *Ask about the nature of skin lesions that are present:* Any change in the size, color, texture, or shape should be noted. If the lesion has changed, the rate of change may be important. Tendencies for the lesion to ulcerate or bleed may be an indication for referral. Some skin lesions, such as basal cell carcinoma, rarely metastasize, while metastasis from a melanoma is common.[45]

3. *Know skin cancer risk factors:* Certain patients are more at risk of the development of skin cancer. A fair complexion and exposure to excessive sunlight will increase the risk. Biopsies are routinely performed for definitive diagnosis. Excision may be indicated, and radiation is sometimes used in treatment.

PHYSICAL THERAPY TREATMENT

The physical therapist must proceed with caution in treating the patient with a known or suspected neoplasm. Many of the modalities frequently used in physical therapy are contraindicated in the presence of neoplasms. The more common modalities to be concerned with include ultrasound, electrical stimulation of various types, and diathermies. Various types of manual therapy and spinal traction are also contraindicated in patients in whom tumor or infections may be aggravated by the treatment.[46] The need for physical therapists to be aware of the signs related to primary neoplasms should be obvious.

It must be emphasized once again that primary tumor of the bone is a rare condition. It is estimated that only

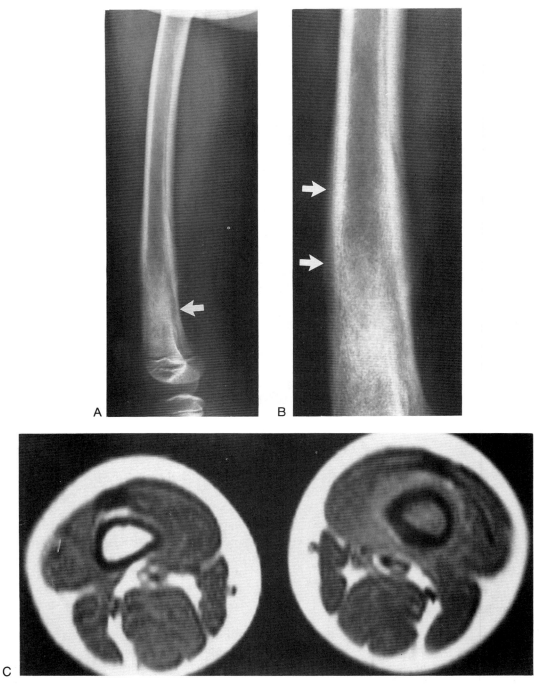

Fig. 9-7. Ewing's sarcoma in the femoral shaft. **(A)** Lateral radiograph showing a region of sclerosis in the distal femoral shaft (arrow). **(B)** Photographic enlargement showing cortex thickened by periosteal new bone (arrows). **(C)** MRI scan with T_1 weighting showing abnormal marrow signal in the left femur. Soft tissues surrounding the bone also have abnormal signal. (*Figure continues.*)

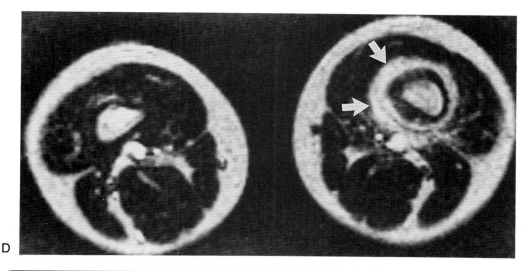

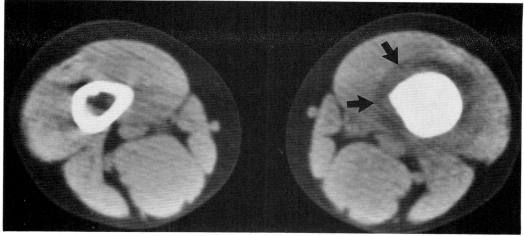

Fig. 9-7. (*Continued.*) **(D)** MRI scan with T_2 weighting showing a rim of abnormal signal surrounding the femur (arrows) and areas of high signal in the thickened cortex. These findings correspond to cortical penetration of tumor from the marrow space into the surrounding soft tissues. **(E)** CT scan showing increased attenuation in the marrow cavity and decreased attenuation in the surrounding soft tissues (arrow), indicating marrows pace involvement and cortical penetration, respectively. (From Chew,[39] with permission.)

10,000 new cases of primary bone neoplasms occur in the United States each year.[45] Therefore, most physical therapists will not have the unenviable experience of finding these lesions in their patients. This fact does not excuse us from knowing the signs and symptoms of these conditions.

SKELETAL METASTASES

Secondary neoplasms refer to the development in bone of cancerous lesions that have their origin in other organs of the body. Relative to primary tumors, skeletal metastases are much more common. All malignant tumors have the capability to metastasize to bone. Patients usually succumb to their primary cancer but, because of advances in treatment, they are now often able to live longer, more productive lives. This has led to increased interest in the disability caused by skeletal metastases and appropriate treatment. The incidence of skeletal metastases is increasing because of increased life expectancy and improved methods of detection.

The incidence of metastases for any given type of cancer has been difficult to assess, as suggested by the wide spectrum of reported values.[47] For example, carcinoma of the breast has been reported to metastasize within a range of 47 to 85 percent of cases. The site of metastasis is somewhat predictable. Overall, the spine, particularly the lumbar vertebral body, is the most common area.

Metastases to the skeleton are of interest to the physical therapist because patients may present with complaints of musculoskeletal pain that could be the first sign of an undiscovered carcinoma elsewhere in the body. If a patient is known to have cancer, it behooves the physical therapist to be aware of the incidence of metastases and the most likely site. Knowledge of the possibility of skeletal metastases in a patient could therefore dramatically affect the assessment and treatment of many musculoskeletal complaints.

Skeletal metastases are most often seen as secondary lesions from the breast, prostate, lung, kidney, and thyroid. All the factors involved in the development of metastasis in certain locations are not known. The location of a metastasis is dependent on the vascular supply to the area, proximity to the primary growth, environment of the host, and probably many other factors of both chemical and mechanical nature that are not well understood at this point.

Neoplasms can spread and develop in secondary locations by transport of the tumor emboli through the bloodstream or lymphatic system or by direct extension. It appears that the vascular system is of primary importance when considering skeletal metastases. The bloodstream is responsible for the spread of most can-

cerous growths. Most likely sites include those bones that have the greatest amounts of bone marrow, such as the vertebrae, pelvis, and proximal portion of the femur and humerus. Along with the many necessary functions, such as the production of antibodies and transportation of lymphatic fluid, the lymph system serves as one of the avenues for the spread of malignancy. The circulatory and lymphatic systems are intimately linked, and the method of transporting the cancerous cells is probably similar. The direct extension of neoplastic growths to the skeletal system can be seen in several locations. Breast cancer often spreads to the rib cage or the thoracic vertebrae. The pelvis and skull are also susceptible to this type of metastases.

Clinical Findings

Although not universal, the hallmark of skeletal metastases is severe, incessant, pain. The specific characteristics of the pain depend on the bone involved. Pain can also have a variety of sources other than bone. Nerve compression, soft tissue involvement, and the viscera must be considered as possible sources of pain.[48,49] As with primary neoplasms, pathologic fractures occur when the metastasis is responsible for cortex thinning in a weight-bearing bone. This type of fracture is most often seen as a result of metastasis from mammary carcinoma. The proximal femur is the most likely location.[50]

Swelling and tenderness are less common clinical findings in patients with skeletal metastases. Radiography may show either osteolytic or osteoblastic reactions in the host bone. In reviewing spinal films, scrutiny of the pedicles may indicate destruction as an initial finding. As in primary neoplasms of bone, sophisticated studies are becoming more useful in diagnosing, staging, and planning the treatment of skeletal metastases. These studies include scintigraphy, computed tomography (CT), and magnetic resonance imaging (MRI) (see Ch. 13).

Physical therapist can have a significant effect on the outcome of many malignancies when consulted early in the treatment course.[51] For example, establishing a baseline for pulmonary status, teaching proper breathing techniques, and assessing the fitness level can provide valuable data that will aid in the rehabilitative effort. Specific evaluations depending on the source of the cancer may be appropriate. Shoulder range-of-motion (ROM) and circumferential measurements are necessary for patients undergoing treatment for breast cancer. Along with other standard contraindications for the use of modalities, caution should be exercised in the application of heat to areas that have had recent irradiation.[51]

Breast

Carcinoma of the breast is the third most common type of cancer, with 130,000 new cases seen every year.[52] Only cancer involving the lung and skin is seen more frequently. Breast cancer is the most common primary lesion that will metastasize to bone. Occasionally, the metastasis will be the first indication of carcinoma.[53] When the cancer does metastasize, it will likely be seen in the pelvis, ribs, vertebrae, or proximal femur.

The etiology of breast cancer is unknown, but many risk factors have been identified. Both genetic and environmental influences are being studied. A positive family history of breast cancer and the presence of benign breast disease are two important factors that certainly increase the risk. International differences in the incidence of breast cancer implicate environmental and dietary factors.[54] Breast malignancy is seen most often in women between the ages of 40 and 60.[55] In this age group, breast cancer is the leading cause of death.[56] Many times a painless lump is detected by the patient as the initial sign. This underscores the importance of teaching patients self-examination and encouraging them to perform it on a monthly basis. A benign breast cyst is differentiated from a malignancy through palpation and aspiration. The aspirate can be examined if there is suspicion of malignancy.[57]

The use of screening mammograms is becoming more popular in an attempt to detect this carcinoma in an earlier stage, when treatment is more successful. The American Cancer Society currently recommends that women obtain their first screening mammography between the ages of 35 and 40.[58] For women with higher risk, mammography should be performed much earlier.

Cancer of the breast has a high rate of recurrence, therefore, patients who have had treatment should be followed on a regular basis. The opposite breast is a very likely location for the development of cancer. Physical therapists should be aware of the possibility of recurrence when examining patients with a history of breast cancer.

Treatment

Various combinations of radiation, chemotherapy, and surgery are used in the treatment of breast cancer. The extent of both surgery and radiation is dependent on many factors, including the stage of the cancer. The size, location, and number of metastases will also direct the treatment plan. Biopsy is performed to determine the characteristic of an abnormality in the breast. Not only masses, but nipple discharge and local skin changes, can be a sign of cancer.

The success of treatment seems to be highly correlated with the stage of the disease when detected. When found in the initial stages, treatment can be promising. In general, the earlier the diagnosis, the less extensive the surgical procedures needed to control the disease.

Prostate

In the United States, 20 percent of all new cancers in men will be found in the prostate. The distinctive characteristic of prostate cancer is its relationship to advancing age. Ninety-nine percent of prostate cancer detected is found in men over the age of 50.[59] Other risk factors have been studied, but no definitive conclusions can be made. Carcinoma of the prostate will metastasize to bone in about 50 percent of cases.[60] The lumbar vertebrae, proximal femur, and pelvis are commonly involved. If the pain from metastases is treated as a musculoskeletal complaint, progression may occur undetected. Screening is considered important for the early detection of this disease (see Ch. 5). Rectal examination should be included in all routine physical examinations for men over the age of 50.[61]

Treatment

If the cancer is detected early, radical prostatectomy can remove all of the lesion, which may cure the disease. While prostatectomy may be successful in removing the cancer, it is not without significant morbidity. Urinary incontinence and impotence are common sequelae. The use of transrectal ultrasound may offer advances in the ability to diagnose and stage prostate cancer. In more advanced cases in which the cancer has progressed, radiation or chemotherapy will be added to the treatment. When metastasis is found in bone outside the pelvis, the prognosis is poor. Bone scans will usually detect metastasis before routine radiography. Hormonal therapy is often begun in an effort to decrease the level of serum androgens.

Kidney

Renal cell carcinoma is found primarily in the 50- to 60-year-old group. The clinical presentation of renal carcinoma includes pain, hematuria, fever, and weight loss. Unfortunately, these symptoms may not occur until the disease has progressed significantly. The pain, when present, may be found directly over the kidney. The kidney can be examined with palpation and percussion.[62] Kidney tenderness can be elicited by striking the hand placed over the costovertebral angle. This should produce a solid blow to the patient, but not pain. Direct palpation can also be performed with an anterior approach. The right kidney is more often palpable than the left (see Ch. 5).

Primary neoplasms in the kidney will spread to the vertebrae, pelvis, and proximal femur in about 40 percent of cases. It can also be seen in the lung, and liver. The intravenous pyelogram (IVP) and ultrasound are used to examine the kidney initially. Biopsy and CT are also used in diagnosis and staging. Renal carcinoma is unique in its unpredictability. Both the rate and pattern of growth can be erratic.[63]

Treatment

Treatment often consists of surgical excision of the tumor in conjunction with chemotherapy. Survival rates are probably related to the localization of the tumor. If the disease has spread beyond the local area or has metastasized to distant sites, the prognosis is not favorable.

Lung

Nearly 150,000 new cases of lung cancer are detected every year in the United States. It has been estimated that the incidence would be only 15 to 20 percent of the current rate if smoking were eradicated.[65] Cigarette smoking has been strongly linked to most cases of lung cancer. The strength of this correlation is seen in the dramatic rise in the incidence of lung cancer in women that corresponded with the increase in women smokers. It now ranks ahead of breast cancer as the leading cause of death in women.

Screening has not been found effective in early detection of lung cancer. Symptoms such as a change in cough, sputum production, shortness of breath, or pneumonia may not surface until the disease is advanced. It is not uncommon for the initial symptoms to be related to the presence of metastasis in the skeleton. Because metastasis occurs relatively early in the disease, treatment is often unsuccessful.

Thyroid

Cancer of the thyroid is not a common occurrence but can be associated with metastasis to bone. Two or three new cases in 100,000 are reported every year.[65] Women are affected three times more often than men. Pain is rarely associated with thyroid cancer, but hoarseness and a palpable mass may be present (see Ch. 7). Carcinoma of the thyroid typically follows a slow progression over many years. Metastases are commonly found in the skull, ribs, sternum, and spine; these metastasis are osteolytic. It is important to remember that the development of metastasis can be delayed and can even occur after removal of a cancerous thyroid.

Summary

The goals for treatment for skeletal metastasis are quite different from those directed toward primary neoplasms of bone. For metastasis, the goal shifts from affecting life expectancy to improving function and relieving pain as the primary benefits. The same methods

Screening for Cancer

1. *History:* A thorough history will elicit considerable information relevant to the patient's relative risk factors for many forms of cancer. Information such as the age and sex of the patient is important. The incidence of most cancers increases with advancing age, especially with those malignancies associated with a high mortality rate. Patients must be queried specifically concerning previous detected cancer in themselves and their families. Insight regarding their life-style may reveal excessive exposure to sun, tobacco, or alcohol. Nutritional status may have implications both for medical screening and for physical therapy evaluation. Specific questions should address the presence of other treated illnesses or symptoms. Any changes in the patient's bowel or bladder habits (e.g., frequency, urgency, bleeding, or pain) must be noted. Recent weight loss, presence of fever, and persistent fatigue, may be warning signs.

2. *Characteristics of pain:* The characteristics of pain, as always, are vitally important. The clinician must obtain an exhaustive description of the location, severity, frequency, and variability of the patient's pain. Pain that increases at night or that is not associated with activity should be suspect. Migrating pain or pain of insidious onset that covers large unrelated areas can have a systemic or visceral origin.

3. *Palpation:* If possible, all structures, both superficial and deep, should be identified and palpated. However, palpation must not be restricted to the patient's area of complaint. Information from the history may warrant examination of unrelated symptoms at various locations.

4. *Additional screening:* A more thorough medical screening may include inspection of the mouth and throat, breast and pelvic examination, rectal and testicular evaluation, and appropriate laboratory studies. As in many other situations, however, it may be helpful for the physical therapist to explain procedures and their purpose. It is crucial that the physical therapist be aware of normal procedures in a physical examination. Allaying patient fears may encourage them to seek an appropriate medical evaluation.

are used: surgery, irradiation, and chemotherapy. Treatment of a pathologic fracture requires consideration of more factors than in traumatic fractures of the same type. The source of the primary tumor, stage of the cancer, and life expectancy of the patient must be weighed.

As with primary neoplasms of bone, the fundamental concept in screening patients for cancer and skeletal metastasis is that of awareness. Being cognizant of the possibility for carcinomas to mimic musculoskeletal complaints will improve evaluation and influence clinical decisions.

Physical therapists who are aware of the characteristics associated with malignant disease may easily increase their screening effectiveness using skills normally possessed by clinicians. Observation and palpation are skills that physical therapists must develop and use to the fullest. Physical therapists sometimes have the opportunity to observe their patients repeatedly over time. This allows for the identification of changes in the general condition of the patient as well as specific points such as skin lesions.

Complaints or symptoms that do not appear to be related specifically to the physical therapy problem should not be dismissed; rather, they should be investigated to ascertain their significance. Many cancers are detected during the course of a regular physical examination. Again, it must be emphasized that the physical therapist's role in medical screening is not to replace physicians, but to augment their efforts. Physical therapists can increase patient awareness relative to the benefits of screening, regular medical examinations, and self-examination. Physical therapists have a unique opportunity to intervene with their patients on a level that can lead to many health benefits.

METABOLIC BONE DISEASE

The processes of bone formation and resorption can be altered in many different disease processes. Rickets is caused by a lack of calcification of the bone matrix, which is regulated by the amount of serum calcium and phosphorus. Scurvy is a disease that decreases the osteoblastic formation of the bone matrix. The resorption rate is normal in both cases, but the change in balance causes osteopenia. Both rickets and osteomalacia can be caused by either vitamin D deficiency or malabsorption, or both. Although dietary changes have reduced the incidence of these disorders, it can still be present in mild forms in patients who do not eat a balanced diet and who have little exposure to the sun. The diffuse demineralization seen with osteomalacia can cause bone pain and tenderness. The possibility of pathologic fractures also exists. Treatment with increased vitamin D is usually effective.

Many diseases that cause hormone imbalances have their primary effect in bone. Hyperpituitarism produces various skeletal abnormalities from gigantism to acromegaly. Diseases of the adrenal cortex and thyroid can also cause generalized bone disturbances. While physical therapists may treat patients with these diseases for secondary problems, their clinical presentation is usually not mistaken for a musculoskeletal disorder.

Osteoporosis

Osteoporosis is the most common metabolic bone disease. The quality of bone present is normal, but the quantity is decreased. It is a growing concern because of the effects of the disease and the increasing number of elderly Americans who may be affected. More than 20 million Americans are affected every year. The associated fractures can lead to extreme disability or death. The costs of treatment and follow-up care are increasing annually.

Physiology of Bone

To treat osteoporosis and its effects, the underlying physiology must be understood. Cortical bone is solid and dense and is found in the outer walls of bones. It is most abundant in the shafts of the long bones. The haversian system, made up of concentric rings of lamellae arranged around a central canal, is found in the cortical bone. The trabecular, or cancellous, bone is found in the ends of long bones and is more common in the axial skeleton. It is described as porous or as resembling a honeycomb. The size and number of trabeculae are related to the magnitude and direction of force placed on the bone. The trabecular bone has a higher metabolic rate than that of cortical bone, which means that metabolic disturbances will be seen initially in the trabecular bone.

Bone consists of highly differentiated types of cells. Osteoblasts are responsible for bone formation, which is accomplished by synthesizing various collagens, alkaline phosphatase, and other chemicals. The counterpart to the osteoblast is the osteoclast. Resorption of calcified bone is accomplished by the acid produced by the osteoclasts. All bone undergoes an ongoing process of resorption and bone formation. In response to an abnormal stimulus, either the rate bone resorption or bone deposition can be altered. Localized cell death (avascular necrosis) can also occur.[66]

Osteoporosis is characterized by a decreased bone formation as well as increased resorption. The clinical symptoms of osteoporosis may include chronic back pain. This can be caused by the anterior wedge compression fractures commonly seen in the thoracic spine. In the lumbar spine, the vertebral bodies may develop a concavity on both superior and inferior surfaces. This biconcavity is called a codfish vertebrae and is present when the central portion of the lumbar vertebral body is 80 percent or less than the height of the posterior aspect of the body. As the disease progresses, there is a characteristic increase of the dorsal kyphosis (Fig. 9-8). Radiographs will show the decreased bone density as well as changes in the lumbar spine. The vertebral bodies may develop a concavity on both the superior and inferior surfaces.

Etiology

There are numerous causes of osteoporosis; among these are disuse and hormonal imbalance. Two important factors determine the extent and development of the disease. One factor is the amount of peak bone mass attained early in adult life. This level is affected by dietary habits, life-style, and hormonal status. For this reason, adequate nutrition is important long before the earliest signs of the disease are manifested. Of particular interest is the calcium intake from early childhood. The recommended daily allowance for calcium in the young adult is 1,200 mg/day.[68]

Exercise is also a factor in the development of peak

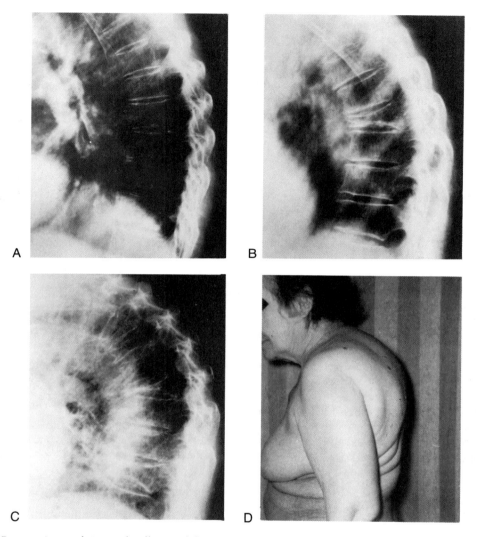

Fig. 9-8. Progressive wedging and collapse of thoracic vertebrae **(A–C)** in a postmenopausal woman from the age of 68 over a period of 4 years. This led to marked loss of height, as well as hyphosis and **(D)** the development of abdominal creases caused by impaction of the lower ribs onto the pelvic brain. Risk factors were menopause at age 36 and smoking. (From Woolf and Dixon,[67] with permission.)

bone mass.[69] Weight-bearing activity is thought to be especially helpful in bone development. Weight lifters have been found to have increased bone density, whereas swimmers may not show this increase.[70]

A major factor in the development of osteoporosis is the rate of bone loss. When the rate of bone deposition is less than bone resorption, there will be an overall loss of bone density. If the process continues, this will be visible as a decrease in radiographic density, or rarefraction.

These rates will vary depending on the age, sex, and health of the patient, as well as many other variables. Bone mass usually reaches its peak at about age 30. Bone density tends to decrease after the age of 40 in both sexes. In women, bone density decreases dramatically during the decade after menopause. The changes in bone density are important because density is correlated with fracture rate. Fractures are most often seen in areas that have a high percentage of trabecular bone, such as the distal radius, vertebral bodies, and femoral neck. It is the treatment and resultant disability stemming from these fractures that makes osteoporosis so costly, not only in terms of dollars but in life-style changes as well.

There is not total agreement in the literature concerning the level of correlation of peak bone mass and resorption rates with the prevention and development of the disease or with treatment. This is due to many variables that are difficult to control in research studies. Even the method of measurement of bone density is sometimes questioned. Conventional radiography is the most frequently used method of assessing osteoporosis in clinical practice. Osteopenia is the term used to describe the appearance of decreased bone density on radiography. The spine is often examined radiographically; in osteoporosis, the vertebral bodies will eventually show the decreased density. There is a tendency to lose the horizontal trabeculae first; and height of the body will also decrease (Fig. 9-9). This will be evident on the lateral view, where only the faint vertical trabeculae may be seen. Unfortunately, significant bone loss has occurred before the radiograph shows osteopenia.

Other methods of assessment using radiography include comparison of vertebral body height in the lumbar spine, noting trabecular patterns in the proximal femur and measurement of cortical thickness of the metacarpals. These methods are easy to use clinically but have limitations.

Single- and dual-photon absorptiometry, dual-energy x-ray absorptiometry, and quantitative CT are just a few of the other common methods of assessment.[71] The proper use of these tests in screening or treatment has not been standardized. Other discrepancies in the research can be attributed to the fact that changes in bone metabolism are multifaceted. Diet, hormones, exercise, and genetics as well as research design can affect the findings.

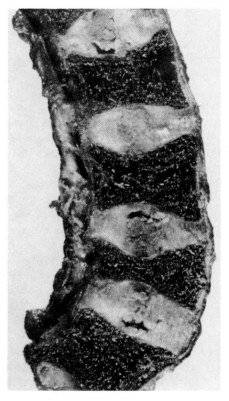

Fig. 9-9. Cross section of an osteoporotic spine showing loss of trabeculae, especially horizontally, and loss of height of vertebrae. (From Woolf and Dixon,[67] with permission.)

Physical Activity

While evidence is accumulating that physical activity and muscle strength are correlated with bone density, specific recommendations concerning intensity, duration, and frequency cannot be made with certainty.[72–74] This is an area that should be of special interest to physical therapists because exercise may play a vital role in prevention and treatment of osteoporosis. It is likely that proven principles used in cardiovascular conditioning and strengthening will be used in modified forms, depending on the individual needs of the patient.

The important factors to be considered before making recommendations are the relative risk of the development of osteoporosis (Table 9-3), the extent and rate of progression, and the risk of fracture. With these

Table 9-3. Risk Factors for Osteoporosis

Female	Long-term calcium
Aging	deficiency
Early menopause	Ectomorphic body type
Caucasian or Asian race	Cigarette smoking
Genetic predisposition	Long-term use of steroids

factors in mind, the specific exercise program may include a program that emphasizes balance and strength to reduce the risk of falls for patients who have significant progression of the disease.[75] The tendency to develop compression fractures of the spine dictates that flexion exercises for the spine may not be desirable. Modifications may also be necessary in the daily routine. Avoidance of sudden forceful contractions, especially in a flexed posture and emphasis on proper lifting techniques are indicated. For those at risk of the development of osteoporosis later in life, a consistent exercise program should be initiated along with proper dietary counseling.

Identifying those at risk is extremely important because prevention will become more important in the management of this disease as further studies are analyzed. The single most important variable is the onset of menopause in women. A rapid loss of bone is seen in women near the onset of menopause. The decrease in bone density can continue at a rapid rate for a decade after menopause. Other factors that can influence the development of osteoporosis are race, nutritional status, and exercise habits.

Treatment

Trends in treatment include various recommendations concerning the use of dietary supplements, hormonal therapy, and exercise. The importance of dietary calcium appears to be greatest in the development of peak bone mass in early adulthood. The effect of dietary calcium in postmenopausal women is controversial. Combining calcium supplements with estrogen replacement therapy appears to give better results in slowing the rate of bone loss in older women.[76]

Of the many types of osteoporosis, that resulting from disuse and immobilization will be encountered most often by the physical therapist. Disuse can be a result of pain, joint pathology, paralysis, or immobilization.

The bone loss will be more rapid in weight-bearing and trabecular bone. While mobility will restore bone density, the process is much slower.[77] The implications for the physical therapist should be obvious. Activity levels must be monitored and patients educated concerning appropriate limitations.

Treatment of osteoporosis is a good example of physical therapist working concurrently with the physician to implement a total treatment regimen that will have a positive effect on the patient. Patients who have been diagnosed as having osteoporosis as well as those who have not been evaluated but who are at great risk should be encouraged to have regular follow-up visits with their physician. For these patients, it is important to have a medical evaluation before the implementation of an exercise program addressing osteoporosis. Physical therapists can take an active role in educating patients of the risks and preventive measures they might use to lessen their chance of the development of osteoporosis and to minimize the effects of the disease process. Patients who present with significant clinical risk factors should be encouraged to have further testing to ensure proper treatment and follow-up management.

Paget's Disease

Although Paget's disease (osteitis deformans) is quite common, the actual cause is unknown. A viral origin may be implicated, but more study is needed. Males are affected more often than females. It is usually seen in patients over the age of 50.

Osteitis deformans is best considered a disease that progresses through several phases. Initially, osteoclast activity results in areas of osteolysis. These weakened areas then go on to fill with fibrous tissue. Haphazard attempts at repair leave the bone susceptible to fracture. Later the bones become enlarged and more dense. The femur, tibia, vertebral bodies, and skull are commonly affected. Conversely, the hands and feet are rarely affected.

Often the symptoms are so mild as to go unrecognized. The disease may be discovered as an incidental finding when the patient is examined for other problems. The diagnosis is made with the aid of radiographic and biochemical findings. While plain radiography may establish the initial diagnosis, a radionuclide bone scan can localize all sites of involvement. The initial symptom may be pain at the involved site, which can be a dull ache. The pain is not necessarily constant and can in fact subside spontaneously. When the skull is involved, headache is a common complaint. As the disease progresses, the enlargement of the bones may be noticed. The long bones of the lower extremities tend to bow anteriorly (Fig. 9-10). The spine will become more kyphotic. Although the disease is disabling to varying degrees, patients can expect a normal life span, unless malignant degeneration occurs. The affected bones become thicker, which is obvious in the jaw, skull, and extremities. The enlargement can also lead to nerve impingement. Hearing impairment can develop as a result of either the nerve compression or bone enlargement.[78]

The secondary development of osteosarcoma is the most serious complication of Paget's disease. It may be found in the early stages of the disease and is a very malignant type of neoplasm. The most common complication of Paget's disease is fracture of the weight-bearing bones. Successful healing depends on the stage of the disease. Fractures that occur late, when the bone is dense and vascularization is poor, may result in delayed union.

Treatment

There is no specific treatment to reverse or prevent Paget's disease. Treatment to alleviate disability as a result of fracture or pain is common. Calcitonin in-

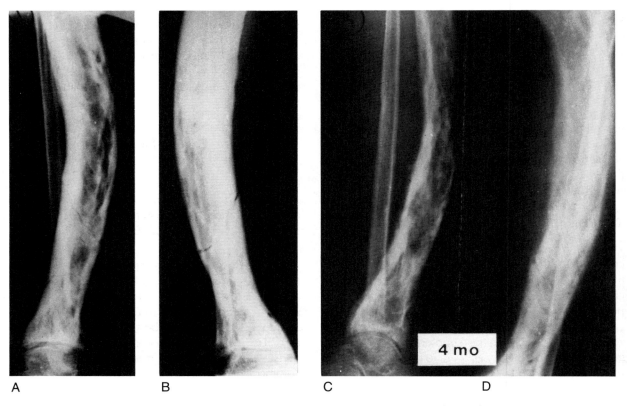

A   B   C   D

Fig. 9-10. Anterior **(A)** and lateral **(B)** radiographs showing Paget's disease of the tibia, with anterior bowing and fracture of the junction of the middle and distal thirds. **(C,D)** At 4 months, the fracture is healed. (From Cohen et al,[22] with permission.)

hibits bone resorption and is used along with other medications that affect the osteolytic process.

INFECTIONS

Physical therapists are accustomed to treating a wide variety of inflammatory disorders and should be aware of the normal responses the body has to these reactions. There are general features common to different types of inflammation. Response to inflammation at the tissue level sets off a predictable course of events and typical symptoms. Rubor (redness) and calor (heat) are a result of the increase vascularity, which is an immediate response of the body to irritation. Vascular changes are primarily due to hemodynamic adjustments, such as arteriolar dilation, increased blood flow, and increased permeability of the small vessels. Neurogenic and chemical mediators, such as histamine and kinins, also contribute to the vascular changes by dilating arterioles and increasing permeability.

Tumor (swelling) indicates the presence of an exudate. The characteristics of the exudate, such as duration, type, and composition, are important in classifying the inflammation. Dolor (pain) has many characteristics and it is very important to assess both the quantity and quality of the sensation. The pain can be a result of direct pressure on nerve endings or can be caused by chemical irritation. Most infections have this inflammatory response in common. Other characteristics may differentiate the infections into very diverse types. Infections such as osteomyelitis and septic arthritis can produce pus, thereby being pyogenic. Pyogenic infections are serious conditions. Not all bacteria cause infection, but many produce toxins that can stimulate an inflammatory response. The bacteria can spread through the lymph system and eventually reach the bloodstream. If the bacteria enters the bloodstream (bacteremia), continued buildup of toxins may result in septicemia. This progression can actually occur quite rapidly, requiring immediate intervention. With acute pyogenic infections, surgery is often necessary to remove the pus and hasten the effect of antibiotics.

Acute Osteomyelitis

Acute osteomyelitis is a rapid, progressive infection of the medullary cavity of bone. The infection can also involve the cortex and periosteum. It is seen primarily in children and more often in boys. The metaphyses of the long bones are affected, especially the femur, tibia, and humerus.

Staphylococcus aureus is responsible for the infection in more than 90 percent of cases. This bacteria can enter the body through infected scratches on the skin or through the mucous membranes in the presence of an upper respiratory infection. If not recognized or left treated, the infection can spread rapidly, from a small localized area of bone to the bloodstream, resulting in septicemia. Often the initial focus is in the metaphysis, which may permit direct access for the bacteria to enter the joint, producing a septic arthritis. During this process of expansion through the cortex and periosteum, pain will be the significant finding.

Diagnosis

The clinical findings are most important in this diagnosis because the radiographic and laboratory values will be normal in the early stages. Radiographic evidence of the infection may not be visible for 1 week. Symptoms may include pain, fever, local tenderness, and swelling.[79] The presentation of acute osteomyelitis usually includes a highly febrile child with intense, deep, or throbbing pain in the affected limb. Blunt trauma may be included in the history. Occasionally a patient presents with pain and decreased function or limp, but no fever. Again, the infection spreads quickly, and this will cause an associated increase in the patient's systemic symptoms of fever and fatigue.

Acute osteomyelitis can also be seen after a focal infection, which is common after surgical procedures, prosthesis implantation, puncture wounds, or comminuted fractures. After the insertion of prosthetic material, clinicians should be more alert to signs of infection. Daily inspection will indicate signs of acute osteomyelitis, such as recurrence of inflammation along the scar, discharge at a wound edge, pain with physical therapy exercise or movement, and low-grade fever. Any of these signs warrants further inspection.[80]

Treatment

Acute osteomyelitis is best evaluated and treated by collaboration between an orthopaedic surgeon and an internist. Immediate treatment with appropriate antibiotics is indicated. Some cases require early surgery if septic complications occur. Prognosis is related to the speed with which the infection is diagnosed and appropriate treatment initiated. Both early and late complications can materialize. Septic arthritis or abscess formation can occur. Chronic osteomyelitis and local growth disturbances may complicate the treatment course over the long term.

Chronic Osteomyelitis

The demarcation line between acute and chronic osteomyelitis is not well defined. Chronic osteomyelitis can be a result of a delay in the diagnosis of acute osteomyelitis or of inadequate treatment in the early phases. The classification is sometimes based on prior diagnoses, the type of organisms found, or the presence of later-stage sequelae, such as radiographic changes.

Often the patient will have none of the symptoms commonly seen in acute cases. The findings are much more vague and are often mistaken for other musculoskeletal pathology. Wound drainage should always alert the clinician. Loss of function and local signs of pain and swelling may still be present but are usually less dramatic than in the acute phase. The diagnosis is made with various imaging studies, blood cultures, and biopsies.

For treatment the use of appropriate antibiotics is important. Once again, surgery may be indicated to remove all necrotic bone and infected granulation tissue.

Vertebral Osteomyelitis

Vertebral osteomyelitis is very difficult to diagnose because the primary complaint is back pain with no history of infection. There may be no associated fever or radiographic signs, and rest may actually improve the symptoms of pain, as in the more common musculoskeletal conditions. With pyogenic osteomyelitis, the pain is not always severe but may be continuous. The picture of fever, chills, and severe back pain is probably the exception rather than the rule. The patient may have a positive straight leg-raising test. The onset of back pain in conjunction with a history of a recent infection elsewhere, such as urinary or respiratory tract infection and folliculitis, should raise the level of suspicion. Obviously, recent surgery, intravenous catheterization, or drug abuse may also be implicated. Any procedure that might have punctured the disc space, such as acupuncture, discography, or laminectomy, should be noted. Exquisite spinal tenderness or a fluctuant mass suggests spinal epidural abscess.

Osteomyelitis of the vertebrae usually occurs through the hematogenous route, probably related to the pattern of blood supply in the vertebrae. Tiny branches of the vertebral intercostal or lumbar arteries supply the anterior body. These vessels also give branches to the anterior longitudinal ligament. The vascularity of the disc changes with age, decreasing markedly when the vessels that pass through the cartilaginous plate in children disappears. In addition, the vertebral body is mostly cancellous bone, which may be a conducive environment.

Radiographs may show symmetric destruction of two adjacent vertebral bodies with a narrowed disc space. Unfortunately, significant bone destruction may take place before radiographic documentation because visible changes may not be detected for 4 to 12 weeks after onset of symptoms. The earliest radiographic changes may be erosion or rarefaction of the cortical margin of the vertebral body.[81]

Infections of Bursae and Tendons

Acute infections located in the bursae and tendons are not commonplace, but the serious sequelae that can result demand attention. Infections are usually seen in the more superficial structures. Bursae and tendons lying close to the skin are susceptible to direct contact with microorganisms when even a minor insult to the skin occurs. Less commonly, the infection can begin as a result of transmission from the bloodstream.

Infections of certain bursae and tendons can be suspected quite easily from knowledge of the local anatomy. But many times the clinical picture is not clear. Aspiration and inspection of fluid must be done to rule out septic infection. The fluid is cultured and a cell count performed to determine the characteristics of the fluid. Once this is completed, appropriate treatment can be initiated.

The bursae are filled with synovial fluid and are located throughout the body. They are susceptible to inflammation and infection from many sources. In many cases, the inflammation is due to repetitive motion. The friction causes inflammation of the bursae. This type of bursitis is often seen and treated quite successfully by physical therapists. The most common site of infection of the bursae is the elbow.

The olecranon bursa is superficial and subject to trauma in many situations. Certain activities, such as wrestling, may predispose this bursa to injury. The onset of symptoms is usually sudden and may be extremely painful. The elbow will be held in a flexed position, and movement will be guarded. Swelling is localized to the bursal area rather than the elbow joint. Examination of the aspirate is necessary to determine whether the swelling is caused by a septic infection. Culture will also indicate the proper antibiotic therapy.[82] Immediate treatment is indicated. Left untreated, a bacterial olecranon bursitis may not resolve. Fortunately, the infection does not readily develop into osteomyelitis.[83]

The subdeltoid bursa plays a crucial role in the normal function of the shoulder. It is one example of a bursa that lies deep to muscle and is therefore protected from direct contact. It is still possible to have an infected subdeltoid bursa, but it may be secondary to an infection in the glenohumeral joint that reaches the bursa through a tear in the rotator cuff.

Tendon sheaths in the distal extremities can also become infected. This is a common occurrence because of the many injuries seen involving the hand. Lacerations and abrasions permit direct access for the microorganisms to pass through the skin. *Staphylococcus aureus* is a common bacterium responsible for serious infections in the hand. The reaction of the tendon sheath to infection is quite predictable. Because of the pyogenic nature of the infection, the tendon sheath

---

Kanavel's Four Cardinal Signs of Suppurative Tenosynovitis[84]

1. Slight flexion of finger
2. Fusiform swelling of finger
3. Pain on extension (passive or active)
4. Tenderness along tendon sheath into palm

---

becomes distended and the finger assumes a flexed posture. Localized swelling and severe pain that occur with passive motion are the most important clinical features. Treatment for pyogenic tenosynovitis must not be delayed and entails operative management for drainage and the use of antibacterial drugs.

The physical therapist must remember the four cardinal signs and consider consultation or referral when they are present in patients for whom a diagnosis has not been confirmed.

Pain with passive extension of the finger is thought to be the most reliable sign of acute tenosynovitis of the flexor tendons. Patients will usually complain of swelling and pain associated with activity. Pain will soon increase, and patients often seek medical treatment within 2 to 3 days after onset. Operative intervention is commonly required. Thorough irrigation of the tendon sheath is critical. Normal motion can be expected within 1 week of drainage.[85]

Besides the tendon sheath, the paronychia and felon can be involved. The felon is primarily fat, and the

---

Differential Diagnosis of Suppurative Tenosynovitis

1. Reaction to local calcific deposits
2. Gout
3. Reiter's syndrome
4. Collagen vascular diseases

infection gains access through puncture or extension of a paronychia. Treatment consists of proper antibiotics along with incision and drainage.

CONSULTATION AND REFERRAL

Physical therapists are accustomed to receiving referrals from all types of physicians and specialties. In some instances, referrals follow rigid guidelines concerning appropriateness and format. In other cases, a more informal system is employed between practitioners who use each other's services regularly. Referrals range from requests for specific treatments to open consultation and treatment as indicated.

In general terms, consultation entails asking for another opinion or point of view on a particular patient or finding. It may include collaboration and discussion. This can occur within the specialty or from another source. Generally, physical therapists work closely with their colleagues, and consultations are routine within the confines of their clinic. Consultation with other health professionals is sometimes not as convenient, and many physical therapists do not have the opportunity to engage in this beneficial process. Both parties benefit from consultation because in many instances it is a sharing of knowledge. In no way should a physical therapist feel inadequate because the expertise of a colleague is needed. On the contrary, responding to the needs of the patient in this way is exemplary.

The better the physical therapist's understanding concerning the expertise and perspective of the potential consultation source, the more meaningful the information will be. Many differences exist between specialties concerning evaluation and management of patients. For example, Figure 9-11 presents an algorithm that a primary care physician may consider when evaluating a patient with low back pain. It is worthwhile for the physical therapist to consider the different perspective that this algorithm reveals and to contemplate how a physical therapy evaluation could complement it.[87] Physical therapists must broaden their perspective if medical disease is to be recognized early and treatment provided by the appropriate physician.

> **Four Functions of a Consultant.[86]**
>
> 1. *Evaluation:* Diagnostic skills are applied to analyzing and assessing the problem. The need for additional data is identified.
> 2. *Advice:* A course of action is recommended and additional studies of value in resolving the problem are specified. Alternative approaches to the solution and the potential outcomes of each are identified.
> 3. *Teaching:* The role of continuing education in the consultative process is recognized. The consultant contributes on-the-spot teaching or other appropriate approaches.
> 4. *Liaison:* Ongoing availability and liaison are offered with the consultant's own professional group and with other consultants in that group or elsewhere.

A referral may take on a slightly different meaning. When a patient is referred to physical therapist, generally a working diagnosis has been made and the need for treatment or specialized evaluation has been recognized. Traditionally, this referral does not mean that the referral source, whether it be a physician or physical therapist, is no longer interested in the well-being of the patient. The accepting health professional may take responsibility for the specific treatment or evaluation requested, but the referring source should be kept informed. The relationship between two practitioners may dictate the exact referral process, but general guidelines are helpful. A pertinent history leading to the reason for the referral is necessary.

Results of previous examinations and tests that may aid in the evaluation must be included. At the same time, extraneous information must be eliminated to provide a succinct clinical picture. The patient must also be aware of the specific reasons this referral is being considered. Vague excuses (e.g., "I just want another opinion") may not be appropriate and will not justify the patient's trust.

Physical therapists will also find the need to refer pa-

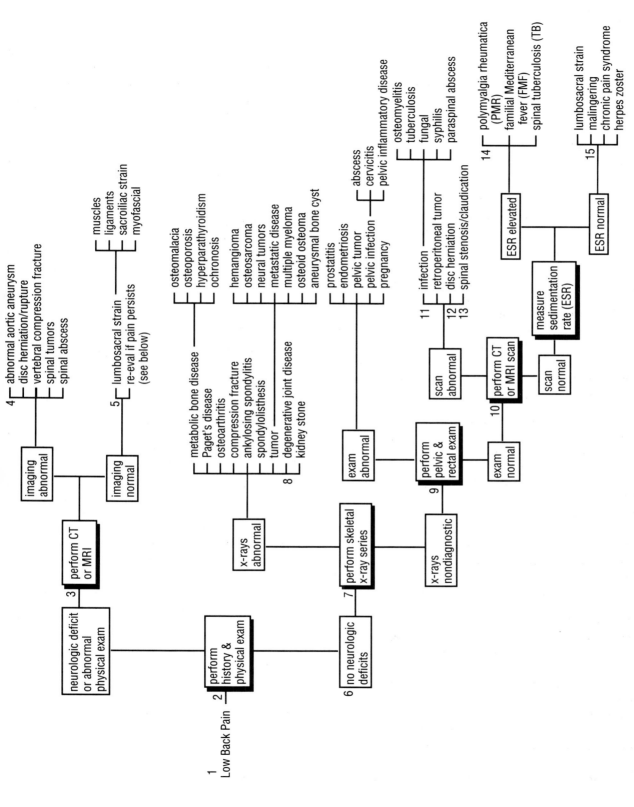

Fig. 9-11. Algorithm for low back pain. (From Healey and Jacobson,[87] with permission.)

tients to outside sources more frequently as their roles expand. Soon it may be commonplace for physical therapists to have a vast network of referral sites that will provide a wide variety of services. From a simple technical request for bracing to the complex examination for suspected musculoskeletal disease, referrals and consultations must take place efficiently and accurately if patients are to receive the highest quality care.

SUMMARY

Although the foundations of physical therapy were laid thousands of years ago, in many ways physical therapists have only just begun to realize the important role that they have in patient care. The training and expertise of physical therapists must advance along with the expectations and responsibilities if the profession is to continue to prosper and gain the esteem it deserves. Continued progress will only come with the cooperation and partnership of the entire medical community.

Medical technology has pushed life to the limits and brought to the surface ethical dilemmas that were science fiction a decade ago, yet patients with low back pain suffer daily without the proper treatment that comes from a sound understanding of the pathology. Physical therapists must foster closer working relationships with physicians not only for the treatment of their patients but also for collaboration in research. Independent practice must not develop into isolated practice. Without close ties to the medical community, the open communication necessary for the optimal treatment of patients will not be present.

Disease of the musculoskeletal system should be a familiar topic to the physical therapist. The existence of these disorders underscores the importance of a thorough evaluation. Both subjective and objective portions are extremely valuable. Expertise in conducting a thorough examination can only be developed with experience. It is recommended that the physical therapist become familiar with one examination sequence and develop the specific techniques to a high level.[88]

Supervision is also important. Direct feedback concerning technique and methods can be of great value in developing a proficient examination. The use of intake forms and examination work sheets can also be important adjuncts to the examination process. Upper- and lower-quarter screening examinations should be required with all extremity evaluations.

Attempts should be made to gather objective and subjective data that are measurable. The more reliable the measurements, the more meaningful the data will be. It will also help the therapist assess progress or changes in patient status. Continuous re-evaluation is crucial to detection of subtle changes in a patient's symptoms or response to treatment. The following case history demonstrates the importance of these principles.

PATIENT CASE HISTORY
History

The patient was a 75-year-old tool-and-die maker who was referred to the clinic with a diagnosis of mechanical low back pain syndrome. His chief complaint was intermittent sharp, stabbing pain in the right low lumbar spine and a constant throbbing pain across the lumbosacral junction. The sharp, stabbing pain was aggravated with coughing and sneezing, bending, and transitional movements such as sit-to-stand movements and bed mobility. Because the patient was unable to assume any recumbent position because of the sharp pain provoked, he had been sleeping in a lounge chair. The throbbing pain did not appear to vary in intensity, regardless of posture.

The sharp pain began approximately 4 weeks before the initial evaluation. While the patient was pulling up fence posts, he felt a tug in the low lumbar area. The sharp right lumbar pain began shortly after the incident and was primarily noted with sit-to-stand movements and bed mobility.

---

* From JOSPT 12:219, 1990

The intensity of the sharp pain had increased steadily over the next 4 weeks. The deep throbbing pain began 1 to 2 days after the original incident and has steadily increased in intensity as well. Initially the patient went to a chiropractor for four sessions receiving hot packs, electrical stimulation, and adjustments to the lumbar spine. After obtaining no relief from chiropractic care, the patient went to a physician and was placed on pain medication and referred for physical therapy. This patient had a 30-year history of low back pain episodes. The precipitating incident was usually repetitive lifting and bending, but the symptoms usually would be gone within a few days. The pain associated with the fence post-pulling incident was much sharper than usual and had lasted much longer. Also, the patient noted that during the previous episodes, lying down generally helped improve symptoms, but he could not lie down in any position during this most recent episode because of the excruciating pain.

The patient's medical history included current treatment for high blood pressure (medication) and a slight diabetic condition (diet controlled). He stated that he had had a stomach tumor removed surgically 1 year earlier. He was not scheduled to be checked by an oncologist for another 6 months. He had not undergone any radiologic testing following his most recent episode of low back pain. He also denied any bowel or bladder dysfunction.

Objective Examination

Observation indicated a significant reduced lumbar lordosis with significant muscle guarding noted with palpation from L2 to S2, left and right sides. Active backward bending caused immediate sharp right low lumbar pain, as the patient was barely able to move beyond the neutral position. He was able to reach his knees with his fingertips during forward bending, but he had great difficulty returning to an upright position because of sharp right low lumbar pain. Active side bending and rotation of the trunk caused

soreness in the low lumbar region and were moderately restricted. Right unilateral pressures on L5 done in a sitting position provoked the sharp right low lumbar pain with a spasm end feel. Vertical trunk compression (downward pressure applied to the shoulders with the patient sitting) produced a slight increase in the patient's throbbing pain. Passive vertebral segmental testing done in sitting demonstrated general hypomobility throughout the lumbar spine.

Assessment and Outcome

The referring physician was aware of the patient's previous history of cancer but wanted to avoid medical testing such as radiologic testing if possible. Owing to the patient's 30-year history of low back pain episodes and the fact that this episode was precipitated by a specific event (a lift), the physician considered a trial of physical therapy to be warranted. The physician requested physical therapy for 2 weeks with weekly correspondence scheduled between the therapist and physician.

Because cancer had not been ruled out, joint mobilization for the hypomobile segments was not used. Soft tissue mobilization for the areas of muscle guarding and gentle manual traction for the lumbar spine in sitting were carried out. Hot packs were also used for the lumbar spine. A soft lumbar corset was tried but provided no relief of symptoms. After the third visit, he reported that the sharp pain was virtually gone but that the throbbing and aching pain across the lumbosacral junction still prevented him from lying down. During the fourth visit, significant edema was noted in the lower legs and feet; the patient stated that he had noted the development of swelling over the past 24 hours. He also reported having a very difficult time with a bowel movement. The physician was contacted regarding these new developments, and medical tests were ordered. The test showed numerous metastatic lesions and pathologic fractures in the rib cage, thoracic spine, and lumbar spine, including L5.

This case demonstrates some of the inherent dif-

232 EXAMINATION IN PHYSICAL THERAPY PRACTICE

ficulties of differentiating between disease of the musculoskeletal system and mechanical musculoskeletal system dysfunction as the source of symptoms. Generally the onset of symptoms from mechanical musculoskeletal dysfunction is associated with an incident, accident, or repetitive overuse-type of insult to a body region, while symptoms from a disease process are thought to begin insidiously. This patient's history included a very specific precipitating incident, the lift and pull of a fence post. In addition, the behavior of symptoms from mechanical musculoskeletal system dysfunction is generally thought to include a change of body/limb position or movements altering the symptoms, while symptoms from a disease process are thought to vary little with movement or changes in posture. This patient reported very specific positions (recumbent) and movements (sit to stand and bed mobility) that would cause sharp right low back pain. In addition, backward bending caused the same right low back pain, as did right unilateral pressures on L5, but he did state that the deep throbbing pain varied little initially, regardless of posture. Diseases of the musculoskeletal system, such as cancer, that cause a change in the local anatomy and therefore a change in ability to function, clinically present differently than diseases of the urogenital or pulmonary systems. As with conditions of mechanical musculoskeletal dysfunction, certain body positions or movements will stress the diseased area (in this case, sites of pathologic fracture), while other postures or movements will not. Therefore, the symptoms of the two clinical entities may have similar behavior. Often other subjective information or objective examination results do not fit the usual pattern of findings associated with mechanical musculoskeletal dysfunction. Such was the case with this patient, who presented with an unusual pattern of symptoms not normally associated with mechanical musculoskeletal dysfunction condition resulting from a lifting injury. This patient could not lie down in any position because of severe pain. Patients with back pain from mechanical dysfunction may have pain moving from a sitting to recumbent position, but once lying down can get comfortable to some degree.

A good general rule to follow is that if a patient presents with a history of cancer, the symptoms should be assumed to have a pathologic etiology until proved otherwise. In this case, the referring physician was aware of the patient's past medical history and the potential of disease being responsible for the symptoms, hence the physician's request for frequent communication between himself and the therapist, in addition to careful monitoring of the patient's status. If this patient had not been seen by a physician before physical therapy, he would have been referred to one after the initial evaluation.

REFERENCES

1. Mathews JS: Preparation for the Twenty-First Century: The educational challenge. Phys Ther 69:981, 1989
2. Watts NT: The privilege of choice. Phys Ther 63:1802, 1983
3. WHO: International Classification of Impairments, Disabilities, and Handicaps. World Health Organization, Geneva 1980
4. Sahrmann SA: Diagnosis by the physical therapist: A prerequisite for treatment. Phys Ther 68:1703, 1988
5. Jette AM: Diagnosis and classification by physical therapists. Phys Ther 69:967, 1989
6. Rose SJ: Diagnosis: Defining the term. Phys Ther 69:162, 1989
7. Harris BA, Dyrek DA: A model of orthopaedic dysfunction for clinical decision making in physical therapy practice. Phys Ther 69:548, 1989
8. Shenkman M, Butler RB: A model for multisystem evaluation, interpretation, and treatment of individuals with neurologic dysfunction. Phys Ther 69:538, 1989
9. Zohn DA: Crossmatching anatomy with pathology as a means to differential diagnosis. p. 35. In Diagnosis and Physical Treatment. Little, Brown, Boston, 1988
10. Salter RB: Neoplasms of the musculoskeletal tissues. p. 304. In Textbook of Disorders and Injuries of the Musculoskeletal System. Williams & Wilkins, Baltimore, 1970
11. Echternach JL, Rothstein JM: Hypothesis-oriented algorithms. Phys Ther 69:559, 1989
12. Sweet DE, Madewell JE, Ragsdale BD: Radiologic and pathologic analysis of solitary bone lesions III. Radiol Clin North Am 19:785, 1981
13. Spjut HJ: Histologic classification of primary tumors of bone. p. 57. In Management of Primary Bone and Soft Tissue Tumors. Year Book Medical Publishers, Chicago, 1977

14. Siedal HM, Ball JW, Dains JE, Benedict GW: Examination Techniques and Equipment. p. 21. In Mosby's Guide to Physical Examination. CV Mosby, St. Louis, 1987
15. Zohn DA: Clinical observations aiding diagnosis. p. 71. In Diagnosis and Physical Treatment. Little, Brown, Boston, 1988
16. Barbera C, Lewis MM: Office evaluation of bone tumors. Orthop Clin North Am 19:821, 1988
17. Cohen J, Bongiflio M, Campbell CJ: Special fractures and injuries. p. 121. In: Orthopedic Pathophysiology in Diagnosis and Treatment. Churchill Livingstone, New York, 1990
18. Siedal HM, Ball JW, Dains JE, Benedict GW: The history and interviewing process. p. 1. In Mosby's Guide to Physical Examination. CV Mosby, St. Louis, 1987
19. Wilkins RM, Sim FH: Evaluation of bone and soft tissue tumors p. 189. In D'Ambrosia R (ed): Musculoskeletal Disorders: Regional Examination and Differential Diagnosis. 2nd Ed. JB Lippincott, Philadelphia, 1986
20. Madewell JE, Ragsdale BD, Sweet DE: Radiologic and pathologic analyisis of solitary bone lesions I. Radiol Clin North Am 19:715, 1981
21. Jaffe HL: Osteoid osteoma: A benign osteoblastic tumor composed of osteoid and atypical bone. Arch Surg 31:709, 1935
22. Cohen J, Bonfiglio M, Campbell CJ: Musculoskeletal tumors. p. 397. In: Orthopedic Pathophysiology in Diagnosis and Treatment. Churchill Livingstone, New York, 1990
23. Freiberger RH, Loitman BS, Helpern M, Thompson JC: Osteoid osteoma: A report of 80 cases. AJR 82:194, 1959
24. Wuisman P, Harle A, Frohberger U: Parosteal osteosarcoma as a cause of chronic knee pain in an athlete. Sportverletz Sportschaden 3(1):37, 1989
25. Schajowicz FL, Ackerman LW, Sisson HA: Histologic Typing of Bone Tumors. International Histologic Classification of Tumours No. 6. World Health Organization, Geneva, 1972
26. Healy JH, Ghelman B: Osteoid osteoma and osteoblastoma. Ten most common bone and joint tumors. Clin Orthop 204:76, 1986
27. Turek SL: Tumors of bone. p. 537. In Orthopaedics Principles and Their Application. 3rd Ed. JB Lippincott, Philadelphia, 1977
28. Klein MJ, Kenan S, Lewis MM: Osteosarcoma, clinical and pathological consideration. Bone tumors: Evaluation and treatment. Orthop Clin North Am 20:327, 1989
29. Romsdahl MM, Ayala AG: Surgical Management of Osteosarcoma. p. 137. In Management of Primary Bone and Soft Tissue Tumors. Year Book Medical Publishers, Chicago 1977
30. Ragsdale BD, Madewell JE, Sweet DE: Radiologic and pathologic analysis of solitary bone lesions. II. Radiol Clin North Am 19:772, 1981
31. Dahlin DC, Coventry MA: Osteosarcoma: A study of 600 cases. J Bone Joint Surg 49A:101, 1967
32. Sweetnam R: Osteosarcoma. Ann R Coll Surg 44:38, 1969
33. Mankin HJ: Forward. In Lewis MM (ed): Bone Tumor Surgery. JB Lippincott, Philadelphia, 1988
34. Enneking WF: A system of staging musculoskeletal neoplasms. Ten most common bone and joint tumors. Clin Orthop 204:9, 1986
35. McGuire MH, Mankin HJ, Schiller AL: Benign cartilage tumors of bone. p. 4717. In Evarts C (ed): Surgery of the Musculoskeletal System. 2nd Ed. Churchill Livingstone, New York, 1990
36. Barton B, Clifton EJ: Chrondroblastoma in a college athlete. Athletic Training 24:342, 1989
37. Nolan DJ, Middlemiss H: Chondroblastoma of bone. Clin Radiol 26:343, 1975
38. Eckardt JJ, Grogan TJ: Giant cell tumor of bone. Ten most common bone and joint tumors. Clin Orthop 204:45, 1986
39. Chew FS: Skeletal Radiology—The Bare Bones. Aspen Publishers, Rockville, MD, 1989
40. Spjut HJ, Dorfman HD, Fechner RE, Ackerman LV: Tumors of Bone and Cartilage. Armed Forces Institute of Pathology, Washington, DC, 1971
41. Goodman MA: Plasma cell tumors. Ten most common bone and joint tumors. Clin Orthop 204:86, 1986
42. Kapadin S: Multiple myeloma: A clinical pathological study of 62 consecutive autopsied cases. Medicine (Baltimore) 58:380, 1980
43. Durie B, Salmon S: The current status and future prospects of treatment of multiple myeloma. Clin Heamatol 11:181, 1982
44. Neff JR: Nonmetastatic ewing's sarcoma of bone; the role of surgical therapy. Ten most common bone and joint tumors. Clin Orthop 204:111, 1986
45. Roaten S, Lea WA: Dermatology. p. 1111. In Rakel RE (ed): Textbook of Family Practice, 4th Ed. WB Saunders, Philadelphia, 1990
46. Yates D: Indications and contraindications for spinal traction. Physiotherapy 58:55, 1972
47. Galasko CSB: Incidence and distribution of skeletal metastasis. p. 14. In Skeletal Metastases. Butterworth, Boston, 1986
48. Twycross RG, Fairfield S: Pain in far-advanced cancer. Pain 14:303, 1982
49. Foley KM: The treatment of cancer pain. N Engl J Med 313:84, 1985
50. Glasko CSB: Local complication of skeletal metastastis. p. 125 In Skeletal Metastases. Butterworth, Boston, 1986

51. Gunn AE, Dickison EM, McBride CM: Physical rehabilitation. p. 23. In Gunn AE (ed): Cancer Rehabilitation, Raven Press, New York, 1984

52. Spratt JS, Donegan WL, Greenberg RA: Epidemiology and etiology. p. 46. In Donegan WL, Spratt JS (eds): Cancer of the Breast. WB Saunders, Philadephia, 1988

53. Giuliano AE, Sparks FE, Morton DI: Breast cancer presenting as renal colic. Am J Surg 135:842, 1978

54. Mettlin C: Breast cancer risk factors. p. 35. In Ariel IM, Cleary JB (eds): Breast Cancer: Diagnosis and Treatment. McGraw-Hill Book Co., New York, 1987

55. Siedal HM, Ball JW, Dains JE, Benedict GW: Breasts and axillae. p. 339. In Mosby's Guide to Physical Examination. CV Mosby, St. Louis, 1987

56. Haskell CM, Giuliano AE, Thompson RW, Zarem HA: Breast cancer. p. 123. In Haskell CM (ed): Cancer Treatment. WB Saunders, Philadelphia, 1985

57. Ariel IM, Teng Pk, Predente R: Fibrocystic breast disease, diagnosis treatment and association with cancer. p. 60. In Breast Cancer; Diagnosis and Treatment. McGraw-Hill Book Co., New York, 1987

58. Mammography 1982: A statement of the American Cancer Society. Ca 32:226, 1982

59. Badalament RA, Drago JR: Prostate cancer. Postgrad Med J 87(5):65, 1990

60. Turek SL: Secondary tumors of bones. p. 587. In Orthopaedics Principles and their Application. 3rd Ed. JB Lippincott, Philadelphia, 1977

61. Mueller EJ: Cancer of the prostate. Postgrad Med J 86(7):115, 1989

62. Siedal HM, Ball JW, Dains JE, Benedict GW: Abdomen p. 363. In Mosby's Guide to Physical Examination. CV Mosby, St. Louis, 1987

63. Neuwirth H, Figlin RA, deKernion JB: Kidney. p. 769. In Haskell CM (ed): Cancer Treatment. WB Saunders, Philadelphia, 1985

64. Kessel KF, Leslie WT, Rossof AH: Neoplastic diseases. p. 583. In Taylor RB (ed): Family Medicine Principles and Practice. Springer-Verlag, New York, 1988

65. Donald PJ: Thyroid p. 196. In Head and Neck Cancer. Management of the Difficult Case. WB Saunders, Philadelphia, 1984

66. Salter RB: Reactions of the musculoskeletal tissues to disorders and injuries. p. 17. In Textbook of Disorders and Injuries of the Musculoskeletal System. Williams & Wilkins, Baltimore, 1970

67. Woolf AD, Dixon AS: The prevention of osteoporosis. p. 146. In Osteoporosis: A Clinical Guide. JB Lippincott, Phialdelphia, 1988

68. National Research Council (US): Recommended Dietary Allowances. 10th Ed. National Academy Press, Washington, DC, 1989

69. Halioua L, Anderson JJB: Lifetime calcium intake and physical activity habits: Independent and combined effects on the radial bone of healthy premenopausal Caucasian women. Am J Clin Nutr 49:534, 1989

70. Nilsson BE, Westlin NE: Bone density in athletes. Clin Orthop 77:179, 1971

71. Genant HK, Block JE, Steiger P, et al: Appropriate use of bone densitometry. Radiology 170:817, 1989

72. Halle JS, Smidt GL, O'Dwyer KD, Lin S: Relationship between trunk muscle. Torque and bone mineral content of the lumbar spine and hip in healthy postmenopausal women. Phys Ther 70:690, 1990

73. Smith E, Reddan W, Smith P: Physical activity and calcium modalities for bone mineral increase in aged women. Med Sci Sports Exerc 13:60, 1981

74. Sinaki M, Offord K: Physical activity in postmenopausal women: Effect on back muscle strength and bone mineral density of the spine. Arch Phys Med Rehabil 69:277, 1988

75. Dalsky GP: The role of exercise in the prevention of osteoporosis. Comp Ther 15:30, 1989

76. Ettinger B, Genant HK, Cann CE: Postmenopausal bone loss is prevented by treatment with low-dosage estrogen with calcium. Ann Intern Med 106:40, 1987

77. Woolf AD, Dixon AS: Clinical types and associations. p. 73. In Osteoporosis: A Clinical Guide. JB Lippincott, Philadelphia, 1988

78. Woolf AD, Dixon AS: Differential diagnosis of bone pain and fracture. p. 110. In Osteoporosis: A Clinical Guide. JB Lippincott, Philadelphia, 1988

79. Waldvogel FA, Medoff G, Swartz MN: Osteomyelitis: A review of clinical features, therapeutic considerations and unusual aspects. N Engl J Med 282:198, 1970

80. Waldvogel FA: Acute osteomyelitis. p. 1. In Schlossberg D (ed): Orthopaedic Infection. Springer-Verlag, New York, 1988

81. Bonakdor-pour A, Gaines VD: The radiology of osteomyelitis. Orthop Clin North Am 14:21, 1983

82. Ho G Jr, Tice AD, Kaplo SR: Septic bursitis in the prepatella and olecranon bursae: An anslysis of 25 cases. Ann Intern Med 89:21, 1978

83. La Cour EG, Schmid FR: Infections of bursae and tendons. p. 92. In Schlossberg D (ed): Orthopaedic Infection. Springer-Verlag, New York, 1988

84. Kanavel AB: Infections of the Hand. A Guide to the Surgical Treatment of Acute and Chronic Suppurative Processes in the Fingers, Hand, and Forearm. 7th Ed. Lea & Febiger, Philadelphia, 1939

85. Neviaser RJ: Closed tendon sheath irrigation for pyogenic flexor tenosynovitis. J Hand Surg 3:464, 1978

86. Rakel RE, Williamson PS: Use of consultants. p. 190. In Textbook of Family Practice. 3rd Ed. WB Saunders, Philadelphia, 1984

87. Healey PM, Jacobson EJ: Musculoskeletal disorders. p. 186. In Common Medical Diagnoses: An Algorithm Approach. WB Saunders, Philadelphia, 1990
88. Saunders HD: Evaluation and treatment of musculoskeletal disorders. p. 59. Educ Opportun 1982

SUGGESTED READINGS

American Academy of Orthopaedic Surgeons: Orthopaedic Knowledge Update 3. 1st Ed. Vol. 3, 1990

Avioli LV, Krane SH: Metabolic Bone Disease and Clinically Related Disorders. 2nd Ed. WB Saunders, Philadelphia, 1990

Cohen J, Bonfiglio M, Campbell CJ: Orthopedic Pathophysiology in Diagnosis and Treatment. Churchill Livingstone, New York, 1990

Galasko CSB: Skeletal Metastases. Butterworth, Boston, 1986

Schajowicz F: Tumors and Tumor-like Lesions of Bone and Joints, Springer-Verlag, New York, 1981

Schlossberg D: Orthopaedic Infection. Springer-Verlag, New York, 1988

Woods CG: Diagnostic Orthopaedics—Pathology. Blackwell Scientific, London, 1972

10

Screening for Rheumatic Disease

PAUL H. CALDRON, D.O.

The essence of rheumatic disease is inflammation, specifically inflammation that promotes damage to organs in the absence of continuous inciting trauma or an invading pathogenic organism or substance. Such inflammation results from immunologic or metabolic functions intrinsic to the host that have gone awry. The term *inflammation* refers to a set of processes involving cadres of blood and tissue cells and their products that make up a dedicated infantry. This army responds to a great variety of command sources in a rather limited number of ways.

The teleologic missions of these cells are to clean up the aftermath of tissue damage accruing through trauma or an invading organism or substance, to confine the perimeters of the assault, to promote reconstruction and healing, and to formulate recall potential for rapid recognition of recurrent invaders. When the signals for attack continue, or the signals for "cease-fire" by the inflammatory process are not heard, despite the lack of an identifiable invader, then further tissue damage is inflicted by chronic inflammatory cells and their products.

Thus, rheumatic disease therapy pivots on controlling unnecessary inflammation. Rheumatologic practice hinges on identifying clinical syndromes of immune dysregulation and metabolic causes of unhelpful inflammation. The challenge of such practice begins with differentiating which patients have primary mechanical or degenerative dysfunction from those patients with infection, or primary disease in other organ systems, who report similar discomforts as those with untoward inflammation.

This chapter is intended to aid the physical therapist in recognizing rheumatic disease. Several rheumatologic entities selected because of their likelihood of presenting to independent physical therapy practices are described briefly. Subjective and objective clinical clues to help differentiate primary inflammatory disease from mechanical dysfunction and other medical disease are emphasized. Where appropriate, screening or diagnostic laboratory tests are discussed.

GENERAL SYMPTOMS AND SIGNS OF RHEUMATIC DISEASE

The most fundamental aid to recognizing rheumatic disease in people presenting with musculoskeletal discomfort is evaluating for systemic symptoms. Such symptoms may be constitutional, including new-onset fatigue, fever, weight change, or loss of appetite, or may include signs of disease in organ systems other than musculoskeletal. Typical manifestations may include mucocutaneous signs, such as rash, mouth sores, hair loss, skin thickening or tightening, or nodules. Joint pain occurring with diarrhea or dysuria, headaches or scalp tenderness, or pleuritic chest pain should also suggest the possibility of systemic rheumatic disorders. Sensitivity to sun exposure, with resultant rash, fever, abdominal or joint pain, should be noted. Such systemic symptoms are nonspecific and are rarely diagnostic, and often suggest infection. However, the clustering of certain features into groups, in the absence of demonstrable infectious causes, should lead to the suspicion of a rheumatic disorder.

A case in point is that of systemic lupus erythematosus (SLE). This disorder is often considered the prototyp-

237

Table 10-1. Criteria: Systemic Lupus Erythematosus[a]

Criteria	Further Description
1. Malar rash	Fixed erythema, flat or raised, over the malar eminences, tending to spare the nasolabial folds
2. Discoid rash	Erythematous raised patches with scaling and atrophic scarring
3. Photosensitivity	Skin rash
4. Oral ulcers	Usually painless, shallow mucosal ulcers
5. Arthritis	Usually nondeforming
6. Serositis	Pleuritis or pericarditis
7. Renal disorder	Proteinuria or cellular casts
8. Neurologic disorder	Seizures or psychosis
9. Hematologic disorder	Hemolytic anemia, leukopenia, lymphopenia, or thrombocytopenia
10. Immunologic disorder	Positive LE cell preparation, anti-DNA, anti-Sm, or false-positive serologic test for syphilis
11. Antinuclear antibody	Screening test for autoantibodies

[a] Four or more of the 11 criteria support a diagnosis of SLE.

ical systemic rheumatic disease. As in most inflammatory rheumatic disorders, the incidence is higher in women. Patients with SLE often present with nonspecific arthralgias and myalgias, or polyarthritis. The diagnosis is dependent on the demonstration of disease manifestations in several other organs concomitant with certain autoantibodies (Table 10-1). When suspicion of SLE is raised by the clustering of some of these criterion symptoms, testing for antinuclear antibodies (ANA) is essential. This group of autoantibodies is generally felt to play a substantial role in the pathogenic mechanisms in the various diseased organs. Although no particular antibody test is absolutely diagnostic, these and other autoantibody species can provide strong clues to a variety of autoimmune rheumatic disorders.

Another rudimentary task in sorting out rheumatic disease is identifying inflammation in tissues clinically. First, the focus of the complaint must be isolated: Does the discomfort arise from muscle, tendon, bursa, or joint?

In general, pain of *joint* origin is characterized by discomfort throughout the range of motion (ROM). Joint pain is usually accompanied by limitation of range either because of mechanical barrier or because of muscle guarding attributable to pain. Pain is felt throughout the articulation. By contrast, *periarticular tendon or bursal* pain is usually better isolated with a single pointing finger, and more likely to hurt during a definable segment in the ROM. For example, supraspinatus tendon pain is typically located at the subacromial space and occurs most notably between 30 and 60 degrees abduction. By comparison, *muscular* pain may be indicated by local tenderness or by discomfort with a particular isolated motion out of all the available motions of the joint. Muscular pain may be present throughout passive lengthening of an individual muscle or muscle group but is usually worse with active contraction, including isometric contraction. These points on differentiating joint versus tendon or bursa versus muscular origin of pain generally hold true for both inflammatory and mechanical or strain conditions. It is useful to note, however, that the end feel with passive movement testing of inflamed joints is generally more spongy in character than degenerative joint changes because of inflammatory edema.

If the source is indeed articular, the presence of inflammation versus degenerative or mechanical pathology can usually be suggested by historical clues. Typically, patients with noninflammatory conditions will describe "postrest gel," indicating stiffness in a spine region or peripheral joint after a period of immobility. Post-rest gel loosens momentarily, within a few steps or passages of motion. In contrast, inflamed joints may take 30 minutes to several hours of regular motion, particularly in the morning, to feel freely mobile. In the worse scenario, the patient may feel stiff throughout the day.

Next, the observer must seek the presence of the cardinal signs of inflammation at the joints. These signs include soft tissue (especially synovial) swelling, redness, heat, and tenderness, as well as pain on motion at the site. Bony thickening resulting from noninflammatory induced cartilage degeneration typifies osteoarthritis, and the cardinal signs of inflammation are generally absent.

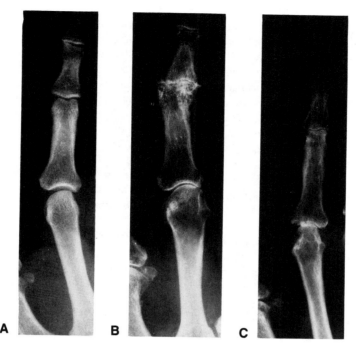

Fig. 10-1. **(a)** Radiograph of normal index finger. **(b)** Osteoarthritis. Note narrowing of joint cartilage space and periarticular bony thickening of the interphalangeal joints, and sparing of the metacarpophalangeal joint. **(c)** Rheumatoid arthritis. Note joint space narrowing with periarticular decrease in bone density and marginal bony erosions. The metacarpophalangeal and proximal interphalangeal joints are involved, while the distal interphalangeal joint is spared. (Courtesy of Arthritis and Orthopedic Center of Excellence, Humana Hospital, Phoenix, Az.)

In the laboratory, acute-phase reactants such as the erythrocyte sedimentation rate (ESR) and C-reactive protein (CRP) are usually increased when substantial inflammation is present. In the absence of known trauma, plain radiographs are generally helpful only when joint pathology has been present for at least several months. By that time, degenerative changes versus inflammatory effects may be differentiated (Fig. 10-1).

Differentiation of Arthritis

It is imperative for the clinician to distinguish an inflammatory from a noninflammatory (degenerative) chronic arthropathy as early and precisely as possible. Without adequate pharmacologic suppression of inflammation in inflammatory disorders, there is little hope of effective symptom control or joint preservation despite the most meticulous attention to physical therapy. Likewise, early recognition of degenerative osteoarthritis can allow for alteration in the mechanical stresses that hasten cartilage and disc breakdown and may demonstrably retard the rate of further deterioration. In community practice, the distinction of degenerative from inflammatory arthritis is rarely difficult if the observer focuses on the aforementioned historical and examination clues, and notes the typical distribution of the involved joints. Distinguishing various subtypes of inflammatory arthritis, again, is aided by the distribution of involved joints, and the concomitant extra-articular manifestations.

Osteoarthritis

If osteoarthritis is "wear and tear" induced, intuitively, the primary weight-bearing joints (i.e., knees, hips, and lumbar and cervical spine) should be the most affected. Such is the case. Similarly, small joints, such as the first carpometacarpal articulation, first metatarsal phalangeal joint, and distal and proximal interphalangeal joints are also commonly involved. In these non-weight-bearing joints, genetic influence and use-intensive accumulated microtrauma lead to narrowing of joint cartilage and bony thickening. Metacarpophalangeal joints, wrists, ankles, elbows, shoulders, and temporomandibular joints are less affected, unless there are occupational or athletic influences promoting trauma specifically to these joints (Fig. 10-2). Predictably, the incidence of symptomatic osteoarthritis increases with age equally in the sexes, affecting one-half the population by age 65.

Management of pain and postrest gel is approached with measures to maintain ROM and muscle tone with the goal of optimizing joint function. Supportive devices, including mobile supports, canes, and proper footwear, may be of significant benefit. Simple analgesic medications can be used. Since some degree of inflammatory cell action may be present as deterioration progresses, presumably in an attempt to remove debris, some patients with osteoarthritis have better symptom control with the judicious use of nonsteroidal anti-inflammatory drugs (NSAIDs) than with simple analgesics. Potent systemic anti-inflammatory drugs or immunomodulatory drug therapy has no role. While radiographs help define and grade degenerative joint disease, there are no other laboratory tests of utility in this process. In the near future, however, blood levels of certain cartilage matrix glycoproteins may give an index of the rate of cartilage deterioration.

Rheumatoid Arthritis

The most common form of inflammatory arthritis resulting from chronic immune dysregulation is rheumatoid arthritis (RA). Occurring at any age, the peak

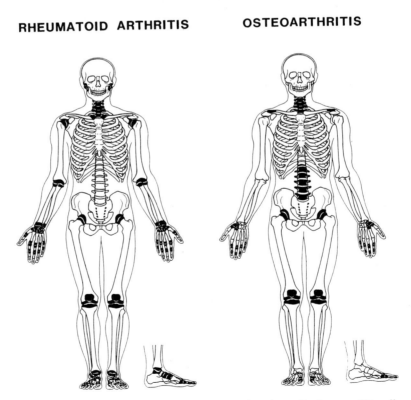

RHEUMATOID ARTHRITIS   **OSTEOARTHRITIS**

Fig. 10-2. Commonly involved joints. (Courtesy of Arthritis and Orthopedic Center of Excellence, Humana Hospital, Phoenix, Az.)

incidence is in the 30- to 50-year-old population, with a 3:1 female predominance. All the cardinal signs of inflammatory synovitis become evident in the untreated patient; when present for more than 6 weeks, most infectious or other extrinsic causes of such inflammation can be excluded. Morning stiffness can be very prolonged. The distribution of RA is peculiarly symmetric in most cases or becomes so with the passage of time. The distribution is not influenced by mechanical stresses but by unknown forces that allow the disease to variably involve virtually any joint, typically metacarpal phalangeal (MCP) joints, wrists, elbows, temporomandibular joints, and cervical spine, while inexplicably sparing the distal interphalangeal (DIP) joints and the rest of the spine and sacroiliac joints (Fig. 10-2).

Several extraarticular manifestations can occur, and virtually all organ systems may be affected in particular ways (Fig. 10-3). Constitutional symptoms of low-grade fever and fatigue are common, as is the presence of rheumatoid nodules. ESR and CRP usually accord a physiologic numerical value to help follow management of inflammation, and low-grade anemia typically develops. There are no diagnostic laboratory tests. So-called rheumatoid factor is an autoantibody that occurs in about 80 percent of RA patients by 1 year of disease but does not occur exclusively in RA, nor does its absence negate the diagnosis. Physical measures combined with aggressive anti-inflammatory and immunomodulatory drug therapy round out disease management.

Spondyloarthropathies

The term *spondyloarthropathies* is given to a group of inflammatory arthritides that are classed together because of certain shared characteristics. These include asymmetric oligoarthritis, sacroiliitis, dactylitis (inflammation occurring in the distal interphalangeal joints), enthesitis (inflammation occurring at the site of tendinous and ligamentous insertion into periarticular bone), absence of rheumatoid factor, and an increased prevalence in persons whose genome codes for the cell surface marker HLA-B27. These entities are separated nosologicaly by the presence of significant inflammatory disease in other organ systems. Psoriatic arthritis, the arthritis of inflammatory bowel disease

(enteropathic arthritis), reactive arthritis (Reiter's syndrome, postdysentric and posturethritic arthritis), and ankylosing spondylitis are the clinical subtypes. Table 10-2 displays the disease associations and extra-articular manifestations that typically occur with each syndrome. There are often overlapping features, raising the likelihood that each syndrome may represent a set of particular disease expressions for closely linked genes associated with immune dysregulation. The symptoms of ankylosing spondylitis, the prototype of the spondyloarthropathies with inflammatory back pain, are further characterized in the section on rheumatoid back and neck pain.

The spondyloarthropathies may occur in females as commonly as males, though the spinal manifestations are usually much less extensively expressed in women. The outcome in ankylosing spondylitis may be rigid fusion of most or all of the spine with a composite flexion posture. Early radiographic changes are typically seen at the sacroiliac joints, and with further fusion of vertebral segments, the characteristic "bamboo spine" may become evident (Fig. 10-4). Limitation of spinal motion is measurable, although nonspecific.

While radiographic changes of sacroiliitis and spondylitis are distinctive in well-established disease, no other laboratory tests are diagnostic. ESR may be moderately elevated with the spondyloarthropathies, and rheumatoid factor is characteristically absent. While HLA-B27 and newer genetic markers may define a population at increased risk of these disease expressions, none as yet is diagnostic. HLA-B27 occurs in about 8 percent of the American Caucasian population, and only about one in five individuals whose genome codes for this cell surface marker has any correlative signs of disease.

Management of inflammatory back disease and associated extraspinal findings, again, revolves around selected pharmacologic interruption of the inflammatory sequence of events. In the psoriatic and enteropathic variants, the back symptoms may improve with suppression of the associated disease. In addition to the usual physical therapy applications for peripheral joint disease, the therapist is called upon to educate the spondylitic patient in an extension maintenance

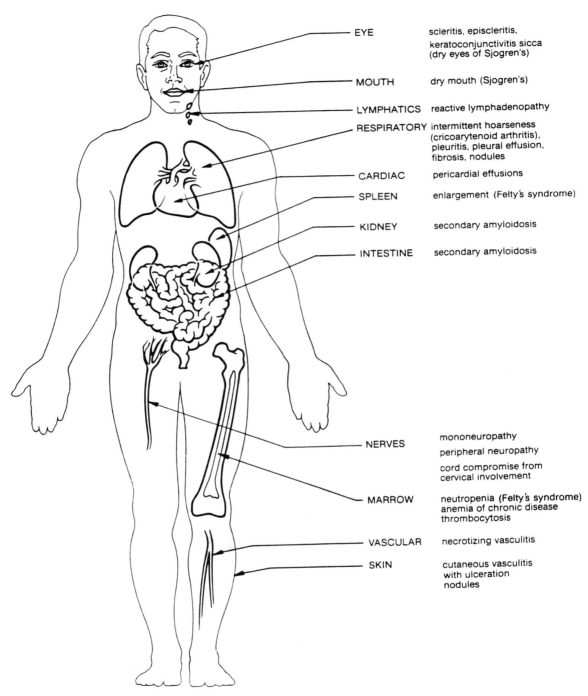

Fig. 10-3. Systemic features that may accompany rheumatoid arthritis. (Courtesy of Arthritis and Orthopedic Center of Excellence, Humana Hospital, Phoenix, Az.)

Table 10-2. Differentiation of the Spondyloarthropathies

Spondyloarthropathy	Principal Disease Manifestations	Distribution of Arthritis	Extra-articular Manifestations
Psoriatic arthritis	Psoriasis	Any small or large joint, including DIP joints (dactylitis), sacroiliitis common	Psoriatic pitting of nails common; eye inflammation
Arthritis of inflammatory bowel disease (enteropathic arthritis)	Crohn's disease; ulcerative colitis	Peripheral oligoarthritis, usually knees, ankles. Unilateral sacroiliitis to extensive spondylitis	Eye inflammation, mouth ulcers, skin ulcers (pyoderma gangrenosum)
Reactive arthritis (including Reiter's syndrome)	After urethritis or dysentery	Sacroiliitis, peripheral oligoarthritis predominantly of large joints of lower extremities, Achilles tendonitis	Eye inflammation urethritis, mouth ulcers, rash, (keratodermia blenorrhagica), penile rash (circinate balanitis)
Ankylosing spondylitis	Primary spinal arthritis	Spinal and pelvis articulations and entheses, including hips; occasional varying peripheral arthritis	Eye inflammation, aortitis with aortic murmur, lung fibrosis

program, so that any eventual axial fusion will occur in the optimally functional position.

Rheumatic Back and Neck Pain

The origins of back pain are myriad and complicated, and the major impact of chronic back pain on health care expenditures and disability has been well recognized. An exhaustive review of back pain etiologies would exceed the scope of this chapter; however, several key aspects in differentiating some sources of back pain merit particular attention when screening for rheumatic disease. Similarly, clinicians seeing patients with rheumatic disorders must be aware of certain concepts regarding the cervical spine.

Inflammatory Back Pain

Fundamental to discriminating back pain of inflammatory versus degenerative origin or musculoligamentous strain is an understanding of the nature of ankylosing spondylitis (AS). This inflammatory condition, which may affect all of the axial skeleton, tends to have a gradual onset invariably below the age of 40, and is usually dated to the second or third decade. In AS, and in the related spondyloarthropathies, when the sacroiliac or spinal segments are involved, pain and stiffness usually last several minutes to hours after rising and tend to improve with exercise. Since onset is insidious, patients generally are seen after several

months of symptoms for which an inciting event cannot be recalled.

Contrast these features with mechanical back pain, which is also quite common in this younger age group who are likely to be engaged in heavy labor or athletic endeavors and at risk for lumbosacral musculoligamentous strain, herniated discs, or stress fractures. These patients would tend to present for evaluations very soon, if not immediately, after an easily recalled task or event that precipitated the back pain. Such conditions would be expected to improve with rest, analgesics, and physical therapy procedures within days to a few weeks. Characteristically, the discomfort associated with such injuries tends to be less after rest and to increase after activity, during the recovery phase. Therefore, the distinguishing clinical features for recognizing inflammatory back pain include (1) pain or stiffness that is worst in the morning and that improves with activity; (2) insidious onset; and (3) pain present for 3 months or more, with an onset of symptoms usually well below the age of 40.

Danger Signs in Back Pain Patients

In relationship to the previous discourse on inflammatory and noninflammatory back pain, a few "red flags" should pique the therapist's attention when interviewing the patient with back pain. Patients should be asked about any known history of cancer. Several

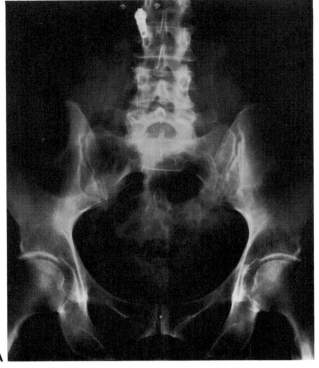

A

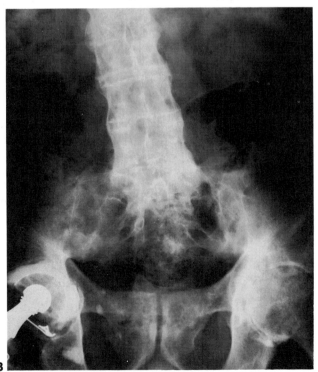

B

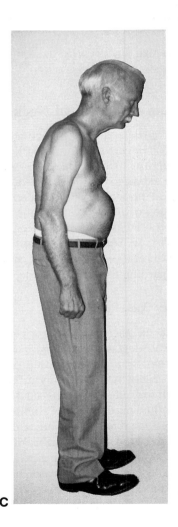

C

Fig. 10-4. **(A)** Normal pelvis and sacroiliac joints. **(B)** Advanced ankylosing spondylitis with fusion of sacroiliac joints and calcification of spinal ligamentous structures. Hips are affected, the right having undergone total hip arthroplasty. **(C)** Patient with fixed spinous posturing typical of ankylosing spondylitis. Note the increased dursal kyphosis and cervical flexion. The protuberant abdomen is often found associated with these spinal changes. (Courtesy of Arthritis and Orthopedic Center of Excellence, Humana Hospital, Phoenix, Az.)

solid tumors, such as breast, lung, prostate carcinoma, and sarcomas, often metastasize to bone. Leukemias, lymphomas, and multiple myeloma may present with periarticular bone pain or back pain and, by the nature of their cellular origin, may produce various systemic autoimmune symptoms, such as fever, vasculitic rash, weight loss, and fatigue. A known history of malignancy should always raise concern for an association with any new skeletal pain. Undiagnosed malignancy should be suspected in the presence of new atraumatic back or bony pain that is constant and that varies little with position or motion. This red flag must not be clouded over by the presence of other established causes of rheumatic complaints.

Elderly postmenopausal women, and those treated with high doses of corticosteroids for prolonged periods may be at risk of osteoporosis (i.e., diminished bone density). The probability of hip, wrist, and other appendicular fractures increases with falls or trauma, but such persons may sustain compression fractures of thoracic or lumbar vertebrae with physiologic events, such as coughing, sneezing, squatting, or lifting very little weight. Acute onset of intense spinal pain

and paraspinus spasm that worsens with the slightest movement, should raise suspicion of compression fracture in these populations. Metastatic pathologic fractures of the spine may be clinically and radiographically identical. In patients not at risk of osteoporosis, further investigation, including computed tomography (CT) scanning or bone biopsy for carcinoma or infection, must be pursued.

Narrowing of the caliber of the spinal canal may result from tumor or abscess, inflammatory diseases including rheumatoid arthritis and ankylosing spondylitis, as well as degenerative changes. Bony facet thickening, disc bulging, posterior longitudinal or ligamentum flavum thickening, and segmental listhesis may compromise the cord or nerve roots (Fig. 10-5). Complaints from the patient of burning, tingling, searing or aching pain in a radicular distribution will easily prompt an evaluation and diagnosis of neural impingement. However, the symptoms of cord compromise in some patients may be other than neuritic. Several historical clues to neural impingement may be available to the clinician, even when neuritic symptoms are absent, and objective changes on sensory, motor, or reflex

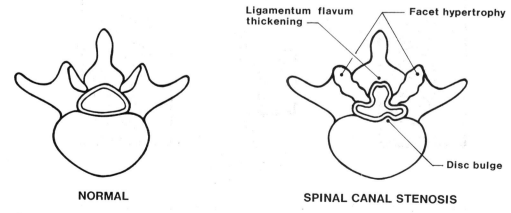

NORMAL   SPINAL CANAL STENOSIS

Fig. 10-5. Compromise of the spinal canal in degenerative disease. (Courtesy of Arthritis and Orthopedic Center of Excellence, Humana Hospital, Phoenix, Az.)

examination or electrophysiologic testing are not evident.

Symptomatic lumbar canal stenosis secondary to degenerative spondylosis, as opposed to intraspinus abscess or tumor, has a gradual onset. Typical symptoms might include worsening of lumbar pain when standing in one place, such as at the kitchen sink or counter, for which the patient relates having to bend forward at the waist and lean on the arms to get relief. In this circumstance, a sense of weakness or "rubberiness" in the legs or burning ache in the buttocks may accompany the increased low back pain. Sitting or lying further relieves these symptoms. In addition, neurogenic claudication may occur (i.e., buttock pain or leg weakness when walking) with or without increased lumbar pain or neuritic symptoms. Neurogenic claudication must always be distinguished from vascular (ischemic) claudication resulting from peripheral vascular insufficiency. An historical clue is that the pain of vascular claudication tends to arise in the buttocks, thighs, or calves more quickly after a reproduceable distance, at the usual walking rate, and likewise tends to subside more abruptly with rest, and often merely by standing still. Neurogenic symptoms, by contrast, tend to wax and wane more gradually with walking and rest. In either disorder, strength and deep tendon reflexes are usually normal, although in lumbar canal stenosis, weakness and transient decrease in reflexes may be detectable if checked immediately after walking. Diminished or absent pedal pulses are a clear indicator of compromised arterial flow. The two conditions not uncommonly coexist in older patients.

Inflammatory Neck Pain

Nontraumatic cervical stenosis occurs usually as a result of advanced degenerative spondylosis but may result from inflammatory disease, particularly rheumatoid arthritis and ankylosing spondylitis. Symptoms of cord and root compromise may run the gamut from radicular symptoms to weakness, areflexia or spasticity, to drop attacks and loss of bowel or bladder control, and potentially to quadriplegia or respiratory arrest. A progressive presentation of cervical cord compromise may mimic the presentation of multiple sclerosis as a group of focal neurologic deficits, initially intermittent, separated by time of onset and neural pathways.

The rheumatoid cervical spine deserves special comment. Facet and ligamentous disruption with shifting of segments and distortion of the canal and neuroforamina may occur, principally in the midcervical seg-

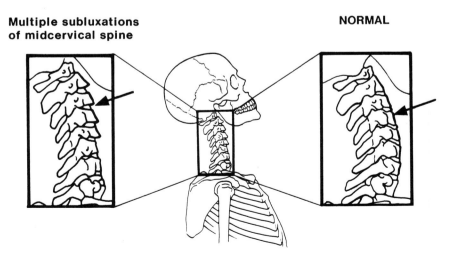

Fig. 10-6. Rheumatoid cervical spine. Multiple segmental subluxations may cause narrowing of the spinal canal and pressure on spinal cord and nerve roots. (Courtesy of Arthritis and Orthopedic Center of Excellence, Humana Hospital, Phoenix, Az.)

ments (Fig. 10-6). This avenue of change usually occurs indolently. Patients typically complain of weakness, often initially attributed to their peripheral arthritis. By contrast, instability of the atlantoaxial articulation often precipitates more acute complaints. The odontoid process of C2 may become loosened from its ligamentous moorings within the anterior portion of the ring of C1 as a result of inflammation (Fig. 10-7). Similarly, erosive synovitis at this rotatory articulation may lead variably to blunting or disintegration of the odontoid or to whittling of this structure to a fine point. This process may allow the odontoid to move posteriorly into the canal, impinging neural tissue, or migrate upward to impale the brainstem. With unchecked motion, especially with forceful or sustained cervical flexion, the results may be devastating, and sudden paralytic respiratory death is a recognized complication. Harbingers of such life-threatening inflammation include severe neck pain and spasm with intense occipital pain, lightning pains into extremities, drop attacks, incontinence, intermittent paresis of any or all extremities, or complaints from the patient of a sense that his or her head may fall off.

Lateral flexion and extension plain radiographs may give a clue to the amount of motion at the odontoid in the anteroposterior plane. Magnetic resonance imaging (MRI) best defines the integrity of the relationships of the bony structures and neural components in this area. Management may require neurosurgical intervention and fusion of C1 and C2, but this must be weighed against the potentially grave surgical risks. Often the most appropriate management is a rigid cervical collar, strict avoidance of cervical manipulation or inertial injuries, and meticulous care to avoid hypermobilization when intubating or moving the anesthetized rheumatoid patient at surgery.

The cervical spine in ankylosing spondylitis may fuse in its entirety, generally with loss of the normal lordotic curve, to form a single osseus beam. Occasionally, fractures through this fusion mass sustained in a fall will give the patient a sense of regained motion in the neck. Such a history should prompt the clinician to evaluate for potential cervical instability.

Muscular Rheumatism

The approach to differentiating the etiology of muscular disorders in screening for rheumatic disease begins with an attempt to clarify the most prominent aspect of the muscular complaint (i.e., weakness or pain). Overlap of these two principal symptoms is extremely common; however, a careful history and examination will most often discriminate the hallmark feature.

Polymyositis

Inflammation in muscle leads primarily to weakness. Polymyositis is a term applied to conditions of inflammatory cell infiltration in muscle tissue, resulting histopathologically in edema of the interstitial zones, with muscle fiber necrosis and regeneration. The release of elevated levels of creatine phosphokinase and aldolase in the blood is typical, although nonspecific. Characteristic features of inflammation are usually detectable by electromyography (EMG), including inser-

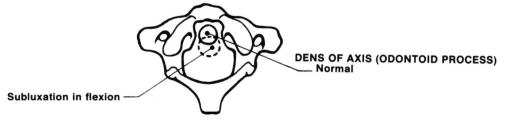

SUPERIOR VIEW -THE ATLAS

DENS OF AXIS (ODONTOID PROCESS)
Normal

Subluxation in flexion

Fig. 10-7. Rheumatoid cervical spine. Remodeling of the dens and loosening of its attachments as a result of inflammation may cause impingement of the spinal cord. (Courtesy of Arthritis and Orthopedic Center of Excellence, Humana Hospital, Phoenix, Az.)

tional irritability, fibrillation potentials, and positive sharp waves.

Polymyositis may occur as a primary disease of unknown etiology. When accompanied by certain skin manifestations, it is called dermatomyositis. A heliotrope rash, appearing as faint erythema and puffiness around the eyes, and Gottron's papules occurring over the dorsum of the metacarpophalangeal (MCP) and proximal interphalangeal (PIP) joints as thick erythematous lesions that commonly ulcerate, are tip-offs to underlying intense chronic muscular inflammation. Polymyositis may also occur as a mild or prominent component of other rheumatic diseases, such as SLE, RA, scleroderma, or vasculitis, or represent a paraneoplastic phenomenon in the presence of recognized or occult malignancy.

Muscular inflammation is typified by several common complaints, signaling predominantly proximal limb girdle weakness. Patients develop difficulty arising from chairs without help, climbing stairs, brushing hair or teeth, or similar activities requiring substantial proximal motor power. Muscle pain and tenderness usually pale by comparison to the aspect of weakness in inflamed muscle. Normal sensory findings and reflexes that persist until muscle weakness is advanced distinguish polymyositis from neuropathic weakness.

Even on muscle biopsy, differentiating inflammatory muscle disease from primary degenerative muscle disease (muscular dystrophy) may be difficult. Tissue that demonstrates an intense chronic inflammatory cell infiltrate supports the former. Other clinical features with respect to age and the involved muscle distribution may help distinguish the various forms of dystrophic muscle disease from typical polymyositis. Special stains and electron microscopy can usually sort out inclusion and storage myopathies and parasitic infection of muscle. Inflammatory muscle disease usually requires potent anti-inflammatory and immunomodulatory therapy for extended periods of time.

Myasthenia Gravis

Myasthenia gravis appears to be an autoimmune disorder wherein antibodies may destroy the myoneural junction. By both EMG and muscle strength testing, these patients display rapidly ensuing weakness after initial strength following a period of rest and may be present in virtually any muscle. Response to cholinesterase inhibitors may be helpful in diagnosis (Tensilon test), as well as in the primary management. The detection of antibodies to acetylcholine receptors is also supportive. Tumors of the thymus, a primary organ of immune lymphocyte development, may accompany myasthenia gravis, and should be sought and potentially resected. Immune modulatory therapy with corticosteroids, immunosuppressive drugs, and plasmapheresis are required in many cases.

Polymyalgia Rheumatica

Pain, rather than weakness, typifies this nosologic entity. Although a diagnosis of exclusion, the usual clinical features of polymyalgia rheumatica (PMR) cry out for recognition that only comes when the clinician is keenly aware of this clinical syndrome. The pathogenesis is not clear but may relate to subclinical synovitis involving the joints of the shoulder and pelvic girdles. Diffuse but predominantly proximal muscular and joint pain on motion, occurring acutely or subacutely in older people, should suggest polymyalgia rheumatica. Tenderness of muscles may be present or absent, typically without joint swelling. Rarely occurring below the age of 60, most patients with this syndrome can recall the day, if not the hour, in which the pain began. These older persons can clearly distinguish subjectively their new pain from previous stiffness of degenerative joint disease. There are no diagnostic tests or findings on muscle biopsy, but as a rule of thumb, the ESR is elevated numerically to approximate or exceed the patient's age. Low-grade fever and anemia with mild elevation in liver function enzymes are common systemic findings, but muscle enzymes are normal, and no autoantibodies are found. Other pulmonary or gastrointestinal influenza-like symptoms are typically absent. A dramatic, often overnight, response to low doses of corticosteroids is very supportive of the diagnosis of PMR. Bacterial infection should be ruled out with blood cultures. Rarely, a PMR-like syndrome may foretell the presence of an occult solid malignancy, and a thorough physical examination is essential.

An important caveat when considering the diagnosis

of PMR is the frequent coexistence in such patients of a specific type of vasculitis referred to as temporal arteritis or giant cell arteritis. New-onset severe headaches, especially temporal, with eye pain, and visual symptoms such as blurring or double vision suggest temporal arteritis. Other key symptoms may include aching in the masseter, temporalis, or tongue muscles with persistent speaking or chewing, neck pain with swallowing during a meal, scalp tenderness with hair brushing, or bulging and tender temporal arteries. Extremely high ESR is common, and a biopsy of temporal artery is needed for confirmation. Without rapid treatment with high doses of corticosteroids, this idiopathic arterial inflammation may result in blindness, stroke, or other vasculopathic outcomes. Other forms of vasculitis may present with muscle pain and tenderness but are usually accompanied by cutaneous signs, such as palpable purpura, skin ulcerations, or ischemic digital infarcts.

Fibromyalgia

Fibromyalgia syndrome, also known as fibrositis, must be distinguished from inflammatory muscle disease and synovitis. Patients with this noninflammatory condition complain of tightness and aching in muscles, and joint stiffness, as well as a subjective sense of swelling in the hands and feet, and at times, variable and fleeting radicular symptoms. Objective signs of joint inflammation are absent, however, and neurologic examination, including motor strength, is normal. Physical examination demonstrates a pattern of tender points (Fig. 10-8) that appears to be reproducible from patient to patient. Several investigators suggest that the symptoms and hypersensitivity of muscles and fibrous tissue are associated with a disturbance of sleep, and a history of nonrestful sleep is usually elicited from such patients. The symptoms may be chronic and ongoing or intermittent in association with stressful times. Laboratory testing, including ESR, should be normal, unless the sleep disturbance is fostered by other medical illness. Recognition and explanation to the patient are of great value toward implementing steps to restore more physiologic sleep. Regular low-impact exercise also appears to be beneficial when other medical conditions allow. Hypothyroidism is a common clinical entity that mimics fibromyalgia and should be screened (see Ch. 7).

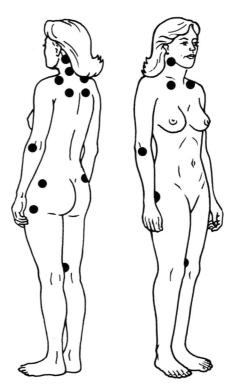

Fig. 10-8. Fibromyalgia, tender points. **Definition:** Pain on digital palpation. **Occiput:** Bilateral, at the suboccipital muscle insertions. **Low cervical:** Bilateral, at the anterior aspects of the intertransverse spaces at C5–C7. **Trapezius:** Bilateral, at the midpoint of the upper border. **Supraspintaus:** Bilateral, at origins, above the scapular spine near the medial border. **Second rib:** Bilateral, at the second costochondral junctions, just lateral to the junctions on upper surfaces. **Lateral epicondyle:** Bilateral, 2 cm distal to the epicondyles. **Gluteal:** Bilateral, in upper outer quadrants of buttocks in anterior fold of muscle. **Greater trochanter:** Bilateral, posterior to the trochanteric prominence. **Knee:** Bilateral, at the medial fat pad proximal to the joint line. (Courtesy of Arthritis and Orthopedic Center of Excellence, Humana Hospital, Phoenix, Az.)

Other Noninflammatory Pain Syndromes

Several clinical entities deserve brief note because of their propensity to present to the physical therapist for management, often under a presumed misdiagnosis. A high index of suspicion is required for each of these nosologies.

Benign Hypermobility Syndrome

Patients with lax joints, such as in Ehlers-Danlos type III collagenosis, or other subtle developmental differences in collagen structure, are at risk of premature degenerative joint disease. Commonly, such patients complain in adolescent years of prolonged aching in the joints and tendons after engaging in activities, but no signs of inflammation or degenerative joint disease are evident. A history or demonstration of excessive joint motion is suggestive and may include the ability to extend the fingers passively for close approximation of the wrist, flexing the thumb to the wrist, hyperextension of the elbows or knees to 190 degrees or more, or placing the palms to the floor from a standing position with knees locked in extension. Patients may be able to sit with legs tightly interlocked (so-called "lotus position"); to lift a foot forward to place it behind the head; or to relate "double-jointedness" with easily subluxed shoulders, hips, or patellae. Maturing collagen begins to lessen such hypermobility. Meantime, efforts to avoid premature degenerative joint disease by counseling toward low-impact conditioning exercises and the avoidance of sports that embody extension stress (gymnastics, ballet) may be helpful.

Reflex Sympathetic Dystrophy Syndrome

Also known as shoulder-hand syndrome, although it occasionally occurs in the foot, reflex sympathetic dystrophy syndrome (RSDS) represents a poorly understood autonomic response in an extremity to a variety of clinical insults. Progressive causalgic (burning) pain and tenderness, especially in the hand or foot, is accompanied early on by diffuse swelling, coolness, and in mottling, and later by atrophy, loss of skin appendages, and contracture. This sequence of events may take weeks or months and must be interrupted by intensive physical therapy. At times corticosteroids and sympathetic blockade are needed to avoid permanent limb dysfunction. Inciting events most commonly include shoulder injury (shoulder-hand syndrome), intrathoracic or intracranial malignancy, stroke, or trauma in the lower extremity.

Aseptic Osteonecrosis

Sudden loss of nutrient arterial flow to subcortical bone may result in flattening of humeral head, femoral head, or femoral condylar bone with acute pain and destruction of these major joints. The typical presentation is that of an adult in the third to sixth decade with atraumatic subacute large joint pain at rest, worsening with motion and weight bearing. Although similar pathology in the wrist or tarsus may follow trauma, the more common settings that should trigger an investigation for osteonecrosis are alcoholism, high-dose corticosteroid use, SLE, and sickle cell disease. Radionuclide bone scanning may suggest osteonecrosis, even before the findings of subcortical lucency or cortical flattening are evident on plain radiographs.

Hypertrophic Osteoarthropathy

Pulmonary, cardiac, or liver disorders may induce this peculiar osseus disease characterized by clubbing of digits, synovitis in distal joints, and aching and tenderness in the shafts of long bones in the extremities. Such tenderness correlates with periosteal thickening seen on radiographs, and even earlier on radionuclide bone scanning. Elevation of the extremities often gives temporary dramatic relief of pain, and this complex of findings may resolve with successful treatment of the underlying visceral pathology.

Referred Pain

Pain referred from intra-abdominal, pelvic, or intrathoracic organs is an important consideration in evaluating atypical musculoskeletal complaints. (This issue is reviewed in Ch. 1.)

Acutely Swollen Joint

Most rheumatologic care is applied to chronic disease entities. While early diagnosis almost universally carries advantages, there is usually time for careful observation of unfolding clinical patterns. By contrast, acute monarthritis with effusion is a clinical presentation that demands urgent clarification and management because of intense pain and the potential for rapid articular destruction.

Acute Septic Arthritis

Bacterial infection in the joint requires prompt and adequate drainage and intensive antibiotic therapy to prevent rapid cartilage destruction and invasion of adjacent bone. The septic joint displays all the signs of inflammation with effusion and is generally accompanied by fever and chills. In addition to immediate aspiration for microbiological studies and joint space decompression, an investigation for the portal of infection is necessary. Even when chronic inflammatory arthritis such as rheumatoid arthritis is present, joint sepsis must be ruled out when an isolated intensely inflamed joint and fever develop. Indeed, joints with preexisting damage from other disorders are more susceptible to hematogenous seeding of bacterial, fungal, or tubercular organisms.

The term crystalline arthropathy principally encompasses gout and pseudogout. Gout is a disorder of purine metabolism resulting in an accumulation of the by-product uric acid. Crystals of uric acid may develop in various tissues, including synovial lining, and may intermittently shower into the synovial fluid, precipitating an intensely painful inflammatory reaction. Any joint may be involved, but the most commonly susceptible seem to be the first metatarsal phalangeal joint, knee, tarsus, and wrist. Men may be affected as early as the second decade, but women rarely before menopause. The blood uric acid level is usually elevated in gout but is not diagnostic, and gout may clearly be present with normal uric acid levels. Definitive diagnosis depends on microscopic demonstration of uric acid crystals in synovial fluid. Acute attacks are managed with anti-inflammatory drugs, and the disease is usually well controlled over the long term with medications to reduce total body load of uric acid.

Pseudogout manifests in a very similar clinical fashion as gout, but is not related to uric acid handling. Rather, the episodes of acute joint inflammation are induced by calcium pyrophosphate crystals. Calcification of joint cartilage may be appreciated on radiographs, and polarized microscopic evaluation of aspirated joint fluid can distinguish the crystal types. Anti-inflammatory drug therapy and analgesics as well as rest are helpful. Some cases of pseudogout are associated with other disorders of metabolism such as thyroid and parathyroid dysregulation or degenerative joint disease.

Hemarthrosis

Hemarthrosis, or bloody joint effusion, must be ruled out in post-traumatic acute effusions of large joints. Spontaneous hemarthrosis can occur in a variety of inherited coagulation disorders. Such effusions are usually warm, tense, tender, and painful with motion. Except in the hip, a bluish hue may be appreciated about the joint.

In the absence of evidence of infection, crystals, or blood, joint aspiration of the acutely inflamed joint will still help differentiate a noninflammatory effusion of injury or degenerative joint disease from the onset of new inflammatory arthritis.

RHEUMATIC SYNDROMES ASSOCIATED WITH INFECTION

Any acutely inflamed joint in the presence of recognized infection in other organ systems is suspect for hematogenous spread of the organism to the joint space. By contrast, as discussed under the spondyloarthropathies, an immunologically mediated reactive arthritis may follow infection with such enteric pathogens as some species of *Salmonella, Shigella, Yersinia, Campylobacter*, and others, or with urinary pathogens such as *Chlamydia* species, without the actual presence of organisms in the joints. Symptoms of intestinal or urogenital infections, therefore, should always be sought in the evaluation of new arthritis (see Chs. 4, 5, and 6).

Similarly, rheumatic fever is an immunoreactive process in susceptible individuals following group A β-hemolytic streptococcal pharyngitis. Along with various cutaneous, cardiac, and neurologic features, acute inflammatory arthritis of one or more joints may occur. Demonstration of high titers of antistreptococcal antibodies (streptozyme test and others) at the peak of joint symptoms is supportive.

Bacterial endocarditis is associated with diffuse myalgias and synovitis of one or more joints. The presence of fever, a new or changing heart murmur and cutaneous signs of septic emboli are highly suggestive of endovascular infection. Blood cultures will usually readily identify the pathogen (see Ch. 2). In endocarditis, a reactive synovitis or true septic arthritis may occur.

Review of systems checklist: Rheumatic disease Item	Yes	No	Comments
1. Constitutional symptoms (fever, weight loss, loss of appetite, fatigue, and malaise) in absence of obvious infection	———	———	——————————— ——————————— ——————————— ———————————
2. Mucocutaneous signs (i.e., mouth ulcers, rash), especially with sun exposure, or on mid-facial area not explained by infection or allergy	———	———	——————————— ——————————— ——————————— ———————————
3. Joint pain not explained by strain or injury, especially with swelling, redness, heat, and stiffness	———	———	——————————— ——————————— ——————————— ———————————
4. Chest pains with deep breathing (pleurisy) or substernal chest pain with lying (pericarditis) in absence of injury or infection	———	———	——————————— ——————————— ———————————
5. Persistent unexplained back or neck pain or stiffness	———	———	——————————— ——————————— ——————————— ———————————
6. Persistent discomfort with urination, hematuria or cloudy urine, not explained by infection	———	———	——————————— ——————————— ———————————
7. Persistent or recurrent diarrhea not explained by infection	———	———	——————————— ——————————— ——————————— ———————————
8. Unexplained progressive weakness	———	———	——————————— ——————————— ——————————— ———————————

Fig. 10-9. Checklist for review of systems in screening for rheumatic disease.

Lyme disease is mediated by the spirochete *Borrelia burgdorferii* and is transmitted by the bite of the *Ixodes dammini* tick. Early manifestations include constitutional symptoms and a violaceous spreading rash, called erythema chronicum migrans. Later manifestations involve a variety of neuropathic and cardiac findings and, weeks to months later, arthritis of one or more joints. Interestingly, some patients are not fully evaluated until seen for arthritis. Because of the increasing incidence and widening endemic areas for this infection, patients with new inflammatory arthritis should be questioned about time spent in wooded areas, tick bites, and the typical rash or antecedent (or concomitant) neurologic or cardiac symptoms. Supportive serology for Lyme antibodies and urine testing for antigens from the spirochete are available. Appropriate antibiotic therapy usually results in cure and appears to be more successful earlier in the disease.

SUMMARY

Rheumatology is the medical subspecialty dedicated to the investigation and clinical management of rheumatic diseases. The key to screening for rheumatic disease is an appreciation of the observable effects of untoward inflammation in synovium, muscle, skin, and other organ systems (Fig. 10-9; see also Fig. 10-3 and Tables 10-1 and 10-2). Combined with a familiarity with the common syndromes outlined here, such an appreciation of inflammation will allow the physical therapist to guide patients toward appropriate medical management. Excellent comprehensive reviews of rheumatic disease are available in the texts listed under Suggested Readings.

SUGGESTED READINGS

Kelly WM, Harris ED, Ruddy S, Sledge CB (eds): Textbook of Rheumatology. 3rd Ed. WB Saunders, Philadelphia, 1989

McCarty DJ (ed): Arthritis and Alllied Conditions. 11th Ed. Lea & Febiger, Philadelphia, 1989

Sheon RP, Moskowitz RW, Goldberg VM (ed): Soft Tissue Rheumatic Pain: Recognition, Management, Prevention. 2nd Ed. Lea & Febiger, Philadelphia, 1987

11

Screening for Psychological Disorders

WARREN J. BILKEY, M.D.

Though poorly understood, the complex interaction between mind and body, psyche and soma, is universally appreciated in health care. Overlapping fields of psychiatry and psychology attempt to describe the process within a diagnostic and treatment framework. The physical therapist is often the first person to confront these issues when dealing with a new patient presenting with complaints of pain and disability.

This poses a seemingly difficult conceptual problem. Physical therapy and psychology are discrete, focused specialties with very different clinical viewpoints and relatively little understanding of each other's methodologies. Many patients are most efficiently addressed by the coordinated input of both disciplines. Early recognition of this need may determine a quick treatment success from a chronic, discomfortingly dependent, seemingly plateaued case that drains the clinician of patience and energy. Such is the subject of this chapter.

This chapter is clinically focused. Rather than present a broad academic view of psychology, the discussion is organized around a particularly difficult clinical problem in physical therapy: the pain patient. Orthopaedic, or manual, physical therapy is emphasized.

The psychological aspects of pain are reviewed, beginning with basic definitions and a general review of the effect of pain on the patient and the family. The relationship between pain and human personality is addressed, as is the diagnosis of specific psychiatric disorders and psychoses and their association with pain. Related concerns of stress, abuse, and chemical dependency are reviewed. Assessment tools for psychopathology, specifically those appropriate to the practicing therapist, are presented and commented on. Finally, chronic pain syndrome and types of chronic pain rehabilitation are reviewed.

ACUTE AND CHRONIC PAIN

Pain is an unpleasant sensory and emotional experience associated with tissue damage or described in terms of tissue damage.[1] Pain may be acute or chronic, each producing different effects.[2] Acute pain, of recent onset, is typically associated with autonomic activity proportionate to the perceived intensity of the stimulus. Measurable increases occur with cardiac rate, stroke volume, blood pressure, palmar sweating, striated muscle tension, oxygen intake, glycogen release into the circulation, and adrenal release of epinephrine and norepinephrine. There are decreases in gut motility and cutaneous circulation.

The pattern demonstrates the fight-or-flight response. Anxiety reactions are associated with the same pattern of events. Indeed, patients with acute pain normally experience anxiety about the intensity of perceived significance of the pain. Therapeutic reduction of anxiety through medication or counseling usually reduces pain.

Chronic pain is of longer but differentially defined duration. In terms of appropriateness for manual intervention, chronic pain lasts beyond normal soft tis-

255

Problems Facing the Chronic Pain Patient

Personal issues
    Loss of mobility
    Physical change
    Psychological distress
    Loss of control of life-style
    Change in body image
    Diminished coping skills
    Fear
Interpersonal issues
    Increased dependency on spouse and family
    Sexual dysfunction
    Diminished role in family functioning
    Marital discord, separation, divorce
    Isolation from family and social interaction
    Impaired interpersonal skills
    Self-defense of psyche in lieu of organic cause of pain
Socioeconomic issues
    Lost income after job loss
    Confusion about eventual financial settlement
    Stressful interactions with distrusting employer and agencies
    Return-to-work issues
    Monetary and social secondary gain

---

sue healing time, ranging from 2 to 12 weeks. In terms of human psychology, chronic pain is of at least 6 months' duration, well beyond the patient's perceived expected time for resolution. A different pattern of normal consequences occurs, including sleep disturbance, change in appetite, decreased libido, irritability, social withdrawal, weakening of relationships, and increased somatic preoccupation. Habituation to the autonomic responses of acute pain may occur if the pain is not intermittent. This pattern of vegetative and other signs is typically seen in depressive reactions.

Psychological testing usually demonstrates depression in chronic pain patients. Depression may be masked by the patient's overwhelming preoccupation with somatic symptoms. Indeed, therapeutic reduction of depression usually results in reduction of pain. Alternatively, treatment of pain will reverse the neurotic depression caused by that pain.

Beyond the normally present depressive response to chronic pain, the afflicted patient is faced by an array of diverse problems.

Persistent pain has a progressive impact on the patient's psychological and social well-being.[3] There is confusion about the organic cause of the problem. Frequent humiliating medical examinations, inconvenient or painful tests, and unsuccessful treatment attempts add to the problem, by causing psychological distress. The result is depression, anxiety, social isolation, lowered self-esteem, and fear. Fear may be spectacular. In spite of their suffering, these patients may be told, directly or indirectly, that the pain is psychogenic, that it is "all in the head." This approach further harms the therapeutic relationship and forces patients to take on the added burden of defending their psyche.

Secondary gain becomes important as a reinforcement for pain complaints. The more chronic the pain, the more extensive the secondary gain issues, and the more resistant the patient is to treatment. The needed disability compensation provides a financial incentive to hurt. Perhaps more powerful are the social responses to the "sick role," which provide for unmet dependency needs, enhancement of self-esteem, stabilization of weakened or immature personality, and conflict resolution of sexual and aggressive drives.

It is generally regarded that persistence of reinforced chronic pain beyond 2 years' duration is not fully curable. Patients rarely return to work if their pain was sufficient to cause them to be unemployed for more than 1 year.

Pain must be distinguished from nociception, suffering, and disability.[4] Nociception is the stimulus that activates A delta and C fibers, which signal the central nervous system (CNS) that tissue damage is occurring. Pain is the unpleasant sensation arising from perceived nociception. Pain may occur in the absence of nociception, such as with couvade syndrome (abdominal pains in men during their wives labors or pregnancies). Nociception may occur without pain, as illustrated in Beecher's observations of nonpainful yet severe combat injuries.[5]

Suffering is the emotional response with attendant psychological distress triggered by perceived nociception.[6] Suffering is intimate and personal and is communicated to society by pain behavior. Disability is the social judgment (partially based on medical judgment and law) placed on the patient as a response to collected pain behaviors.

Pain behavior is influenced by culture, personality, and social context. Culture, or ethnic membership, partially determines the expressive style of suffering.[2] For example, Scandinavian Americans and Irish Americans are notably stoic. They tend to inhibit their pain expression. By contrast, Italian Americans and Jewish Americans demonstrate a lower pain tolerance and encourage its expression. Note that pain threshold, and not pain tolerance, remains stable cross-culturally.

Introversion-extroversion is the psychological continuum correlated with expression of suffering. The neurotic introvert will suffer in silence; the extrovert will tend to overcommunicate concerns. All communication and, more importantly, listener bias occurs within the framework of social context. Personality and psychological disorders have additional influence on somatic tolerance, pain threshold, the likelihood to develop chronic pain, resistance to purely mechanical treatment of pain syndromes, and effectiveness of communication with the clinician.

FAMILY DYNAMICS AND PAIN

Family dynamics have a major impact on the development and maintenance of chronic pain.[7] Marital maladjustment may challenge self-esteem and cause depression, with attendant chronic pain. Alternatively, family dysfunction may create dependency needs or leave existing needs unmet. The patient uses pain complaints to help satisfy these needs. Conflict may arise with unsatisfied aggressive drives, with the outlet being chronic pain. Pain may permit denial of unresolved family conflict. Pain is a powerful tool for manipulation of family members to seek attention and to

avoid normal family role responsibilities while maintaining a sense of self-esteem. Chronic pain syndrome patients often come from families of chronic pain sufferers.

After a patient develops pain, the family, with benign intent, responds with pain-reinforcing behavior. Providing attention by being constantly present, by assisting with essential activities of daily living (e.g., dressing or bathing the patient, feeding or cutting the food, assisting with transfers or gait), and by being verbally sympathetic to disability and irresponsibility ("since the accident happened, you hurt too much to work") reinforces and perpetuates pain, suffering, and pain behavior. In reducing fear, these inputs further reinforce pain. Perhaps also with benign intent, the family may, in effect, "solve" marital dysfunction by making the sick role of the pain patient the scapegoat. This approach has the effect of stabilizing an unstable dysfunctional family relationship.

In the dysfunctional family, the spouse may become overprotective or may reject the patient. The former tends to fixate on pain behavior rather than on the person. The latter fails to offer sufficient support and participation in pain management.

Family dysfunction can be responsible for the chronic pain syndrome or can perpetuate it. These signs do not preclude mechanical treatment of mechanical dysfunction. Rather, they indicate a need for additional input of competent marital counseling, family therapy, or individual psychological consultation.

PERSONALITY ISSUES AND PAIN

As with any stress, patients faced with disabling chronic pain employ adaptive defense mechanisms and available social supports to cope. The adaptive mechanisms depend on personality structure. Along the continuum of increasing pathologic behavioral significance, certain personalities, specific and perhaps odd personality traits, personality disorders, neuroses, and psychoses will modify patient suffering, pain behavior,

Signs of Family Dysfunction That May Have Significant Impact on Chronic Pain

Current or past history of physical abuse or sexual abuse

History of alcohol or other drug abuse

History of criminal activity on the part of children or spouse

History of extramarital affair of patient or spouse

Patient says "family problems" exist or describes many family arguments

Major economic difficulties

History of suicide attempt by spouse/children

Family assists with essential activities of daily living of patient (dressing, bathing, feeding)

Chronic pain for longer than 2 years

Family speaks for patient and attends all physical therapy sessions

Family deserts patient at home

Spouse appears overprotective or over-rejecting of patient

Unemployed spouse

Spouse or children living at home have chronic pain

and prognosis for outcome of an entirely manual approach to the presenting pain syndrome.

There is no accepted "unitary theory" of psychiatry that effectively combines normal behavior, thought and emotion, and psychopathology. It is attractive and useful to conceptualize continua of function (e.g., normal, borderline, severe dysfunction/incompetence) or continua of behavior (e.g., normal social interaction, "different," bizarre/threatening). Such is not the case for diagnosis. Psychosis is not simply a more severe neurosis. Indeed, recent trends in taxonomy view psychopathology as a collection of diseases, disorders, syndromes, traits, states, symptoms, and signs based on level of diagnostic certainty.

Realizing that the psychologically disturbed patient can have either mechanical or "psychogenic" pain, or both, puts the clinician in the difficult role of deciding if and when expert psychology consultation is nec-

essary. This concept is never a clinical problem in the absence of diagnosed mechanical dysfunction. Difficulty arises when the mechanical dysfunctions appear not to fully explain the presented symptoms or when appropriate manual treatment fails to resolve symptoms. Should mechanical treatment proceed? Is concurrent referral to the psychology consultant indicated?

PSYCHIATRIC DISORDERS

What follows is a brief review of psychiatric disorders. Three primary references are drawn from two comprehensive textbooks of Psychiatry[8,9] and the DSM III-R.[10] The American Psychiatric Association Diagnostic and Statistical Manual of Mental Disorders, 3rd edition, revised (DSM III-R) presents the current universally accepted taxonomy of psychiatric disorders. It lists all disorders and defines their diagnostic criteria. Each disorder is briefly discussed as it pertains to chronic pain. The major psychiatric disorders to be concerned with are the somatoform disorders, personality disorders, and affective disorders.

Somatoform Disorders

Somatoform disorders involve the expression of psychological distress through physical symptoms. Affected patients present physical symptoms that suggest a physical disorder for which there are no demonstrable organic findings or physiologic mechanism and for which there is evidence linking symptoms to psychological issues. These include conversion disorder, somatoform pain disorder, somatization disorder, and hypochondriasis. Factitious disorder and malingering are considered different because, in these cases, the patient presumably has voluntary, conscious control of symptoms. Psychophysiologic conditions are also considered a separate entity because a psychologically induced physiologic mechanism is indeed present to explain the etiology of symptoms (e.g., muscle tension headache).

The clinician must be aware of several major conceptual problems. Absence of a demonstrable etiologic physiologic mechanism for the symptom is the essential feature of somatoform disorders. Because classic medical teaching emphasizes the diagnosis of visceral, bone, joint, and nerve pathology and de-emphasizes the diagnosis and treatment of ligament, muscle, and joint motion dysfunctions, there is a very strong likelihood of misdiagnosis. Indeed, follow-up studies of diagnosed conversion disorder cases demonstrate 13 to 64 percent incidence of subsequent diagnosis of neurologic illness.

The manual clinician presents a significant new technology to medical diagnosis. All patients who present to the manual clinician with a diagnosis of somatoform disorder or malingering should be considered "virgin" and should receive a normal comprehensive, biomechanical assessment of their pain symptoms. Likewise, all medical literature to date on the topic of somatoform disorders must be studied with a pervading concern for blatant inaccuracy.

Psychophysiologic conditions present an equally difficult but more subtle problem because they pretend to provide an answer and may erroneously justify nonindicated treatment methodologies. For example, eager acceptance of muscle tension as an etiology of headache risks ignoring other potentially treatable causes, such as upper cervical spine mechanical dysfunction, regional weakness, cranial dysfunction and temporomandibular joint dysfunction. Again, all cases require competent biomechanical examination.

Conversion Disorder

According to the DSM III-R, conversion disorder involves a pain-free loss or alteration of physical function that suggests a physical disorder. These are symptoms that the patient is not consciously producing and that cannot be explained by a known physical disorder. Psychological stressors or conflict must be demonstrably related to the onset or exacerbation of symptoms. Pain symptoms are classified under somatoform pain disorder. Autonomically mediated symptoms (e.g., fainting, palpitations, dizziness, tachycardia, dyspnea) are also excluded from the conversion disorder category.

Somatoform Pain Disorder

Somatoform pain disorder is characterized by the presence of severe pain for longer than 6 months either with no explainable pathophysiologic mechanism or in which the severity of complaints or resulting disability is in gross excess of that expected from the demonstrated organic pathology. This wide-ranging disorder tends to be subdivided by pain location (e.g., abdominal, low back, pelvic). Most chronic pain syndrome cases are considered to be somatoform pain disorders. Depression is frequently manifested in these patients.

Many theories have been offered to explain the psychophysiology of somatoform disorder. Unconscious guilt may be expressed as self-punishment with chronic pain, particularly in patients with life histories of abuse and defeat.[11] Another theory proposes effective noninhibition of autonomic activity and afferent stimulation centrally.[12] Behavioral theory implicates positive reinforcement from family members.[13]

Psychological distress, regardless of cause, may be reflected as pain complaint and suffering because somatic symptoms are culturally more acceptable to society, to the patient, and to co-workers. Somatic symptoms usually engender immediate social and professional attention, which unfortunately may reinforce dysfunctional pain behavior. Perhaps most important, pain complaints permit avoidance of the discomfort of direct confrontation with the psychosocial issues causing the psychological distress. Attention to the pain thus delays appropriate care of the psychological disorder.

Somatization Disorder

Somatization disorder is characterized by a history of multiple somatic complaints beginning before the age of 30 and persisting for several years. The clinical presentation tends to be dramatic and flamboyant with obsessively detailed symptoms and past histories of multiple hospitalizations and excessive surgery. Again, no organic pathology is found. Concerns must be significant enough for the patient to see physicians, take prescribed medication, or alter life-style. Beyond pain, symptoms complained of will range across all organ systems. Somatization disorder has a high frequency of concurrent psychiatric disorder (e.g., depression, chemical dependency, phobia, mania).

Hypochondriasis

Hypochondriasis is characterized by an unrealistic chronic (more than 6 months') preoccupation with fear of having (or belief that one has) a serious disease, based on the patient's interpretation of sensations or physical signs. This fear or belief persist in spite of a negative medical evaluation and reassurance from the physician. The patient with exaggerated somatic awareness, capable of feeling or sensing every minor mechanical dysfunction, may be a borderline or overt hypochondriac. Depression is frequent.

Personality Disorders

Personality disorders are longstanding, inflexible behavior patterns, evident by late adolescence, that cause distress or that impair social and or occupational functioning. These maladaptive, irrational ways of thinking, feeling, and acting significantly impair human interaction far beyond what is normally regarded as an odd character trait.

Personality disorders are divided into four groups: (1) eccentric (includes the schizotypal, schizoid, and paranoid disorders); (2) dramatic, or erratic (includes the histrionic, narcissistic, antisocial, and borderline personality disorders); (3) anxious or fearful (includes the avoidant, dependent, obsessive-compulsive, and passive-aggressive disorders); and (4) self-defeating personality disorder.

Eccentric Personality Disorders

Schizotypal personality disorder typically presents with an eccentric manner of speaking, behavior, and appearance. Patients are nonemotional, paranoid, and socially isolated and have odd beliefs (e.g., superstitiousness: "others can feel my feelings"). By contrast, schizoid personality disorder presents a pervasive indifference to social relationships, and preference for social isolation. These patients are unresponsive to praise or criticism and are aloof and detached. Paranoid personality disorder presents an intense, driven suspiciousness, mistrust, and hypervigilance. A sec-

ondary hostility, irritability, and anxiety may occur when stressed.

The eccentric personality disorders are not frequently associated with chronic pain. The symptoms they present should be considered understated. Mechanical dysfunctions causing pain in this group should be approached in a direct, nonemotional, rational, and scientific manner. There is no benefit in attempting to provide emotional support or friendship. After mechanical problems are corrected, there should be prompt resolution of symptoms. If not, one should assume persistent organic pathology and proceed with further diagnostic study.

Dramatic Personality Disorders

Histrionic personality disorder is a pervasive pattern of excessive emotionality and attention seeking. These patients tend to be dramatic, overly gregarious, seductive, manipulative, exhibitionistic, labile, frivolous, aggressive, and demanding. Narcissistic personality disorder is characterized by a grandiose sense of self-importance, conceit, arrogance, low empathy, and hypersensitivity to criticism and compliment (even if not expressed). These patients seek constant attention and admiration and expect favorable treatment. Antisocial personality disorder is a pattern of chronic, socially irresponsible, exploitative, and shameless behavior. Physical fights, illegal acts, unemployment, substance abuse, and inadequate parent and spouse functions are seen. Borderline personality disorder is characterized by instability of mood; chaotic, unstable interpersonal relationships; and self-damaging impulsiveness. Inappropriate emotional outbursts, suicidal threats or gestures, uncertainty of sexual orientation and long-term goals, and frantic efforts to avoid perceived abandonment may be seen.

The dramatic, or erratic, personality disorders have a direct impact on the management of musculoskeletal pain. Symptoms complained of must be assumed to be exaggerated in description of quality, intensity, and resulting disability. The inadequate ego of these patients responds to verbal sympathy and support. There may be real value in specifically treating symptoms before treating cause. This improves patient tolerance for physical procedures that are typically pain provoking. Aggressive pretreatment with short-term analgesic medication or physical therapy modalities may be indicated. Clinicians must be careful to avoid emotional entrapment by the histrionic and narcissistic behavior of their patients. Pain may be an important defense mechanism that stabilizes a weak ego structure in these patients. On rare occasions, successful, or the threat of successful, treatment of the chronic case will result in florid psychopathology—even a psychotic reaction. Such a response should be assumed to be unavoidable by the clinician; competent psychiatric consultation is needed.

Dramatic personality disorder patients may be particularly distressed by pain because it limits their exhibitionism and attractiveness. By contrast, they may be symptomatically unresponsive to appropriate manual intervention, yet persistently seek caring attention. Discharge from treatment may be interpreted as rejection, criticism, or accusation of psychopathology, with a response of angry, threatening emotional outburst. This situation is best approached by being clear with the patient that (1) symptomatic treatment is only transiently effective, since cause is ignored; (2) treatment must terminate when mechanical dysfunction resolves, or disabling dependence on procedures or medication results; and (3) biomechanical dysfunction does not explain all pain, and persistent symptoms require input of other specialists, perhaps even a chronic pain rehabilitation program. The issue is not whether or not the patient truly hurts, or is being understood; rather, it is whether the clinician can provide any further help. Improved mobility and relief of tissue tension may be the only gains—not pain relief.

Anxious or Fearful Personality Disorders

Avoidant personality disorder is characterized by timidity, social discomfort, fear of criticism or disapproval, fear of social embarrassment, low self-esteem, apprehension, mistrust, and exaggerated fear of potential danger in ordinary activities. Dependent personality disorder presents a pervasive pattern of submissive reliance on others for companionship, emotional support, and everyday decision-making. These patients tolerate mistreatment, are hurt by disapproval, and fear abandonment. Obsessive-compulsive personality disorder is the tendency toward disabling perfectionism; preoccupation with rules, organization, and schedule; indecisiveness, inflexibility, and over-intellectualizing. These stubborn, controlling people are disposed toward power struggles. Passive-aggressive personality disorder involves passive, indirect resistance to authority and responsibility. It is vindictive negativism. These patients procrastinate, forget, become sulky and argumentative when asked to perform, and are critical and disgruntled. A "yes, but" response may follow every suggestion.

Somatic and depressive disorders may accompany these anxious or fearful personality disorders. Persistent pain may offer the avoidant personality a convenient "way out," the dependent personality a ready source of needed social support. The inflexible obsessive-compulsive and the resistive passive-aggressive will tend not to carry out recommended therapeutic activities. They will have plenty of excuses. The clinician must remain aloof to power struggles and be simple, direct, and thorough in explanations and directions (e.g., of exercise programs) discussed with the patient. No room should be left for conceptual misinterpretation and argument. The dependent may do exactly as told but still hurt somewhere. The passive-aggressive will not do as told and still hurt. Persistent symptoms must be assumed to follow appropriate manual intervention. As with the dramatic personality disorders, there must be a clear statement to the patient of separation of symptom and cause, and scientific rationale for termination of treatment.

Self-defeating Personality Disorder

Self-defeating personality disorder is characterized by a pattern of chronic pessimism; resignation to failure, suffering defeat, or exploitation; and tendency to place oneself repetitively in situations that are harmful or painful. These patients reject help or opportunity for pleasure and fail to accomplish crucial tasks they are capable of. Pain patients with self-defeating personality disorder may receive multiple surgeries, setting themselves up for procedures that fail to cure the pain (e.g., by positive symptomatic response to body cast as an indication for surgical fusion). Conversely, they may reject or discontinue effective treatment.

Affective Disorders

In contrast to somatoform and personality disorders, the affective, or mood, disorders consist of depression and bipolar (or manic-depressive) disorder. Of these, depression is significant to chronic pain. Although depression increases pain threshold, it also increases pain complaints. Depression is remarkably prevalent, both causing chronic pain and resulting from chronic pain.[14] Studies with defined criteria for diagnosis of significant depression describe a prevalence of 80 to 100 percent in chronic pain patients. Major depression (psychosis) occurs in 21 to 43 percent of chronic pain patients.

DSM III-R criteria for the diagnosis of minor depression (dysthymia or neurotic depression) in adults include (1) depressed mood for most of the day, for more days than not, for more than 2 years; (2) presence of either poor appetite or overeating, insomnia or hypersomnia, low energy or fatigue, low self-esteem, poor concentration or difficulty making decisions, feelings of helplessness (at least two of these features must be present); and (3) absence of concurrent psychosis, mania, or medication that causes depression.

Depression has been described as a normal patient response in the natural history of all persistent pain.[15] During the acute and subacute stages of pain, the patient is hopeful of a cure. Approximately 6 months to several years after onset, the patient realizes the permanence of pain and becomes hopeless, helpless, and depressed. Eventually, the subchronic phase of pain occurs; the patient accepts the reality of pain and makes positive physical and psychosocial changes to cope. If a chronic, undiagnosed, and untreated mechanical dysfunction is eventually treated successfully, the depression usually resolves. Separate treatment of the depression may or may not be necessary. In depressed chronic pain patients, pain may resolve with treatment of only the depression, particularly if mechanical dysfunctions are relatively mild.

Depression can present initially as hypochondriasis, chemical dependency, behavior disorder, dementia, or psychosomatic disorder or as a specific pain syndrome. The depressed patient will continue to complain of every new discomfort either elicited by physical handling or as depression is unmasked by effective treatment of the primary mechanical problem.

Generalized anxiety disorder involves persistent (more than 6 months) unnecessary worrying about life circumstances. Four types of symptoms are seen: (1) motor tension (shakiness; muscle tension, ache, or soreness; easy fatiguability and restlessness); (2) autonomic hyperactivity (increased perspiration, dry mouth, lightheadedness, nausea, shortness of breath, palpitations, urinary frequency, diarrhea, hot flashes or chills); (3) apprehensive expectation; and (4) vigilance and scanning (irritability, sleep disorder, difficulty concentrating). Complaints of pain are frequent as part of the motor tension symptoms of anxiety. The anxious patient may or may not relax enough to be examined or therapeutically handled. These patients tend to be overly fearful, presenting a verbal nuisance, but also inadvertently prevent their own appropriate treatment.

Malingering

Malingering is fraudulent intentional production of physical or psychological symptoms, motivated by a specific goal. Goals include money, avoiding work, avoiding criminal prosecution, and obtaining medication. Malingering is not a psychological disorder. Opportunistic malingering has been described as taking advantage of an accident or injury by exaggerating symptoms or disability, for financial gain.[16]

Several physical examination findings may be indicative of malingering or psychological disturbance. With muscle strength testing, there is poor pain-free effort, a jerky on-off agonist contraction, or co-contraction of antagonist muscle. "Touch-me-not" syndrome exists when diffuse tenderness prevents accomplishment of even a rudimentary biomechanical examination. Provision of analgesia through medication, accupuncture, or physical therapy modalities does not enhance the ability to carry out the examination. Obviously contradictory findings are demonstrated. An example is a painful spring test of a lumbar spinous process and a

Clinical Markers of Malingering

Symptoms not explainable by examination findings

Symptoms persist after successful treatment of diagnosed problem

Symptoms severe but vague; pain behaviors overdramatized .

Poor cooperation with diagnostic evaluation

History of recurrent accident or injury

Injury presents opportunity for financial gain, work avoidance, or evasion of legal proceedings

Patient requests addictive medication

Antisocial traits demonstrated

---

nonpainful spring test of simultaneous bilateral transverse processes at the same level. Another example is painful bilateral knee-to-chest posture at less than 90-degree hip flexion, in contrast to comfort sitting. Many relatively controversial findings are used by experienced clinicians. For example, it is rare to see a case of purely organic or mechanical low back pain in which radiation of pain into the leg causes the patient to have falls. I have never seen a patient with organic or mechanical low back pain tolerate less than 15-degree straight leg raise.

To minimize conflict from misdiagnosis of malingering, no attempt should be made by the manual clinician to diagnose the patient on a psychosocial basis. The clinical question is not whether malingering or psychogenic pain is present. Rather, can symptoms be explained by organic pathology or mechanical dysfunction? If so, diagnosed problems should be treated. If not, the clinician cannot help, and the patient is discharged or referred to alternative specialist consultation. If signs indicative of a significant psychosocial problem are found, the patient should receive concurrent psychological evaluation and treatment along with whatever mechanical treatment is needed. Some patients will require separate treatment of pain and of their mechanical dysfunction.

OTHER PSYCHIATRIC DISORDERS

Pain is usually not associated with the remaining major psychiatric disorders: schizophrenic disorders, organic mental disorders (dementia), delusional (paranoid) disorders, and dissociative disorders. Schizophrenia is notable for relative insensitivity to pain, which may obscure the presentation of serious organic disease. Rarely, delusional pain will be present in schizophrenia. In these cases, the complaints are highly bizarre and ill defined. For the sake of completeness, the diagnostic features of these disorders are reviewed.

Schizophrenic Disorders

Schizophrenic disorders are a group of disorders characterized by major psychiatric disturbance and severely disordered behavior. Bizarre delusions, prominent hallucinations, incoherence or marked loosening of associations, grossly inappropriate affect, and/or catatonic behavior are present. Types of schizophrenia include disorganized, catatonic, paranoid, undifferentiated, and residual (burned-out psychosis but still functionally disabled).

Delusional (Paranoid) Disorders

Delusional disorders are characterized by nonbizarre delusions, such as involving real-life situations. Delusions are unrealistic, fixed ideas that persist in spite of logic or objective contradictory evidence. Patients with other psychotic disorders and dementia will commonly have delusions. The specific delusional disorder will not have prominent hallucinations or otherwise bizarre behavior and will not meet the criteria for schizophrenia. Types of delusional disorders include erotomanic (believes to be loved by another), grandiose (inflated worth, power, identity), jealous (infidelity), persecutory (belief of malevolent treatment), somatic (believes has defect or disease), and other type not fitting above categories.

Dissociative Disorders

Dissociative disorders are a group of syndromes characterized by a sudden, temporary disruption in identity, consciousness, or motor behavior. These include psychogenic amnesia, multiple personality disorder, psychogenic fugue (sudden travel, new identity, inability to recall one's past), depersonalization disorder (sense of dreamlike automation and detachment from self), and possession/trance disorder (psychogenic altered state of consciousness or possession).

PSYCHOPHYSIOLOGY OF PAIN

An alluring question is whether a psychiatric disorder can cause a segmental or regional mechanical dysfunction that requires psychiatric treatment for the mechanical dysfunction to resolve. Psychophysiologic pain syndromes refer to pain resulting from involuntary psychogenic musculoskeletal dysfunction. The classic example of muscle tension headache presumes stress-induced chronic muscle contraction causing local pain. Undoubtedly, cases do occur even in the absence of cranial dysfunction. Bruxism and chronic tension of masseters and temporalis muscles are considered part of the cause of temporomandibular joint syndrome.

Some patients demonstrate a tendency to contract their cervical paraspinal extensors and trapezii when stressed, or inappropriately so when performing light work with the distal upper limbs. Theoretically, these cases would respond to relaxation training or biofeedback therapy. However, electromyographic (EMG) biofeedback muscle relaxation has been shown, in a large number of cases, to aggravate pain.

Alternative psychophysiologic pain states may be induced by regional fascial restriction, perhaps autonomically mediated. Distant segmental mechanical dysfunction may result and confuse the diagnosis. Finally, a general tension state may exacerbate existing mechanically induced painful muscle spasm or may augment the autonomic effects of mechanical dysfunction. The case history at the end of this chapter suggests a pathophysiologic etiology, through fascial restriction.

Whether there is significant psychopathology or not, if mechanical dysfunctions are diagnosed, they should be treated mechanically. Anyone can develop mechanical pain syndromes, even the psychologically disturbed. The medical literature fails to describe the behavior of patients with psychiatric disorders in whom an organic pain problem develops. There are several suggestions.

Psychopathology is characterized by weak ego structure, poor social support network, insecurity, and immaturity. Thus, pain is perceived as a greater personal threat (there is a limited reserve). Pain more easily disables the psychologically disturbed from an already barely functional level of interpersonal and social relationships.

With organic pain, psychologically disturbed patients have a greater likelihood of being depressed, anxious, or highly fearful. These patients are less likely to decline the relief of addicting analgesic medication or to understand and carry out self-help methodologies (e.g., exercise programs). They may have unrealistically optimistic expectations of success of outcome of therapeutic procedures and may be overly pessimistic about a neutral or negative response. They will tend to challenge the patient-clinician relationship through socially aversive behavior, including bizarre descriptions of pain (heightened or disturbed perceptions), excessive dependency behavior (insecurity, immaturity, and fear), naive attempts to manipulate people and situations (insecurity, immaturity, and fear), "touch-me-not" intolerance to necessary physical handling of the patient in the therapeutic situation (decreased pain threshold of anxiety), and generally increased emotionality of speech and behavior (fear and immaturity).

The medical literature presents confusing data. Waring et al.[17] showed that the mere presence of significant psychopathology fails to predict surgical therapeutic success. However, several retrospective studies demonstrate an association between hypochondriasis, hysteria, anxiety, and depression with poor surgical outcome.[18–20] None of these attempted to rule out mechanical dysfunctions as part of the cause of the symptom complex. As is feasible, the clinician must wade through these issues in attempting to correct mechanical dysfunction.

STRESS AND PAIN

The initial understanding of stress is attributed to the work of Hans Selye. He noted that all human maladies, illnesses, and injuries produced certain common changes within the body or the "syndrome of just being sick." These observed changes were primarily endocrine and visceral, including enlargement of the adrenal cortex, shrinkage of the spleen, and gastrointestinal ulcers, termed the *general adaptation syndrome*.[21]

Allowance is made for specific variations in response to specific stressors. Allowance is also made for individual differences in conditioning factors that selectively enhance or inhibit a particular stress effect. Thus, normally tolerable stress will induce a "disease of adaptation" in a patient predisposed to such. Stressors that produce the stress response include infection, toxin, social environment, physical environment, emotional stimuli, and nervous stimuli.

Stress is divided into eustress and distress. Eustress is the positive successful adaptation to a stressor or challenge, which is helpful and enjoyable. Distress is the negative adaptation to a threat, as well as loss of control, aggression, or failure to cope within the environment. Subsequent to Selye's work, investigators have tended to confuse stress with distress, which is more in line with the generally accepted socially contexted view of the stress response as a purely negative experience.

Sequelae to stress have been described as including medical and psychiatric illness, mood disorders, autonomic dysfunctions, self-defeating behaviors, and pain syndromes.[22] Stress participates in causing illness, possibly delays healing, and complicates coping with the resulting disability. Thus, there is much value to recognizing significant stress and then providing appropriate clinical management to care for the pain patient.

Several associated factors help define stress. Cognition is a powerful mediator of stress, including recognition of the stressor and appraisal of its relative associated harm (threat) or gain (challenge). Response is shaped by personality attributes: motives, beliefs, and emotional life of the person, and relative confidence in one's wealth of coping resources (or self-esteem).[23] The psychological significance of the threat may be more important than the injury itself in effecting a stress response. Indeed, coping is largely anticipatory of the injury.

There are several specific stress-response syndromes[9]: (1) fearful or anxious states of mind, associated with perception of the threat and sense of vulnerability; (2) conditioned emotional response generalized from past danger experience and repeatedly evoked by a memory of that experience (responses may be exaggerated in relationship to the current or potential danger); and (3) signal anxiety or other affect (e.g., guilt, shame, disgust, pride, joy) arising consciously or unconsciously to signal arrival of a stress event.

Stress emotions are complex and troublesome. The person subject to stress may typically fear repetition of the stress, have shame over being helpless against the stressor, be angry toward a symbol of the stress source, and then have shame or fear over aggressive ideations.

Coping with stress may include the typical mechanisms of defense: denial, repression (unconscious unawareness of the stress), suppression (conscious expulsion of distasteful thoughts), displacement (or transfer of concern to another person, situation, or object), projection (of emotion/impulse to others), regression (turning back maturational clock), turning against self, intellectual detachment, rationalization, and acting out. Other defenses include sublimation (replacing an unacceptable thought with one that is socially appropriate), undoing (opposite behaviors), and reaction formation. Reaction formation is the unconscious replacement of a "bad" feeling/thought with a conscious emphasized opposite thought or activity.

Coping represents an effort to postpone or prevent the harm, overcome the injury, or palliate the consequent affective distress. Coping mechanisms may be beneficial, inadequate, or overtly harmful. Examples of the latter would be worsening a problem by ignoring it or adding a new problem to the original stressor, such as chemical dependency added to chronic pain. Success with coping determines the ability to control the effect of a stressor on a person's life. Coping controls whether the stressor is essentially a positive (eustress) or negative (distress) experience in life. The essence of stress is control. Stress is thus best defined as the unpleasant consequence, with attendant emotions, of loss of control over significant aspects of one's life.

Factors that enhance control over stress include strong self-esteem, a positive typical reactive emotion to stress, strong social support network, benevolence of chosen defense mechanism, and perhaps physical fitness and strength. An appropriate assessment of the impact of stress on pain must include these stress-mitigating factors.

In the neurologic rehabilitation setting, the stress-coping process is often referred to as the process of *adjusting to disability*. This frequent complicating factor limits the efficiency and outcome of rehabilitation efforts. In the presence of biomechanical dysfunction, stress should not be considered the sole cause of pain. Stress may delay or limit therapeutic efficacy or may be part of a broader chronic pain disability.

If there is evidence of inadequate control over stress, referral to a psychology consultant is indicated. This would yield a better assessment of control issues, stress emotion, and coping skills. Treatment would enhance coping skills and limit secondary anxiety and depression. This should not be done in lieu of appropriate physical management of mechanical dysfunction associated with the pain complaint. Both treatments should proceed concurrently as feasible.

There are two stress-relevant psychiatric diagnoses: adjustment disorder and post-traumatic stress disorder. Adjustment disorder is a common reactive psychiatric disorder to an identifiable significant stress. This disorder is sufficient to impair occupational or social functioning. Symptoms are in excess of the normal or expected reaction to the stress event. While exclusive of other psychiatric diagnoses, symptom patterns commonly include depressed or anxious mood, disturbed emotion and conduct, work inhibition, physical complaints, and withdrawal.

By contrast, post-traumatic stress disorder is comparatively severe. It occurs from a stress event outside the normal range of human experience that would be considered markedly distressing to almost anyone. The traumatic event is persistently re-experienced through memory, dreams, and experiential and emotional flashbacks. There is intense psychologic distress with exposure to symbols or aspects of the stress event (e.g., anniversaries). There are signs of avoidance of stimuli associated with the stress, numbing of general responsiveness, and symptoms of increased arousal (e.g., difficult sleep, irritability, hypervigilance, exaggerated startle response).

A history of physical, emotional, or sexual abuse is an important stress event with potential for long-term maladaptive consequences, including intensification of pain and subsequent disability. In the physical therapy setting, past abuse may yield a "touch-me-not" intolerance to the necessary physical handling of the patient. Dysfunctional posture may exist. For example, one such patient had a persistently elevated shoulder, having been constantly struck there. An involuted, kyphotic, slumped posture has been associated with recurrent sexual abuse. There may be an unexplainable, particularly midline or bilateral, undue soft tissue tension resistant to treatment. Thus, a component of psychophysiologic pain syndrome would be present. A passive, fragile (weak ego) personality may be noted.

Most pain psychologists consider an abuse history sufficient grounds for referral for further assessment and treatment. This need is enhanced when the patient admits that issues related to the abuse have not been fully "processed" by subsequent counseling.

CHEMICAL DEPENDENCY

Substance abuse is one of our major public health problems and has a direct impact on the practice of physical therapy. The chemically dependent pain patient will not be able to cooperate fully with therapy procedures, particularly offsite self-treatment techniques. This makes the patient more dependent on procedures administered by the therapist and prolongs recovery. Capacity to cope with pain stress issues is impaired. Psychophysiologic pain syndromes may

---

The CAGE Questionnaire

1. Have you ever felt you should cut down on your drinking or drug use?
2. Have people annoyed you by criticizing your drinking or drug use?
3. Have you ever felt bad or guilty about your drinking or drug use?
4. Have you ever used a drug or had a drink first thing in the morning to steady your nerves or get rid of a hangover (eye-opener)?

---

appear. Some abused substances are biologically toxic and impair tissue healing, notably alcohol and dirty intravenously administered agents.

Pain intensity is often increased by substance abuse (even narcotics) and is diminished by detoxification and withdrawal. Failure to recognize chemical dependency and refer for appropriate treatment endangers patients and the people they interact with. Coexisting treatment of chemical dependency and mechanical dysfunction can be most efficient and useful in addressing the "whole" patient.

Several screening procedures have been designed to help identify chemical dependency. A particularly useful test is the CAGE questionnaire.[24] An adaptation of this test would be to expand the four questions to all illicit drugs. Two or three "yes" answers strongly suggest chemical dependency.

Additional evidence indicating chemical dependency would arise with (1) any confirmation by the patient to questioned use of illicit drugs; (2) current or even minimal use of alcohol or an illicit drug when there has been past chemical dependency treatment or in spite of having been advised by a physician against use; (3) heavy caffeine use (12 + cups caffeinated beverage per day); (4) undue anger, evasiveness, rationalization or defensiveness when asked about drug and alcohol use; and (5) undue fidgeting or shakiness on repeated clinical visits.

Several guidelines are useful to improve information gathering about chemical dependency. The clinician should begin with questions about the least socially threatening agents (caffeine, tobacco, over-the-counter analgesics) and then proceed with questions about alcohol, narcotic analgesics, and street drugs. Questions that require a "yes"-"no" response should be avoided. Also to be avoided is offering educational or advisory responses before the information-gathering process is finished and certainly any value judgments to response statements, such as surprise, disgust, or disapproval. The overt toxicity and consequent defenseless use of certain agents, such as cocaine and amphetamines, should be kept in mind. If asked, the clinician should state that his or her personal chemical use is not at issue. Vague answers (e.g., "I drink socially," or "rarely") should not be accepted as valid.

PSYCHOLOGICAL TESTING

This discussion reviews the currently useful validated tests of psychological functioning in the pain patient. Owing to the multidimensional nature of pain, psychological testing is organized according to three essential components: measurement of overt behaviors; measurement of cognitive, sensory, affective, and coping responses; and measurement of physiological variables. Most existing tests were developed by psychologists for interpretation by psychologists. The Pain Distress Scale presented at the end of this section is a quickly administered tool, designed to assist the physical therapist in deciding when to bring in a psychology consultant.

The reader is alerted to some important limitations of psychological testing. There is no objective test to prove that the pain complaint is psychogenic and not organic or mechanical in nature. The value of these tests is improved definition of the psychological aspects of patient functioning and the standardization and formalization of the normal psychological assessment process. There also is no test for psychiatric diagnosis. The diagnosis depends on a detailed interview, on neurologic and mental status examinations, on knowledge of DSM III-R diagnostic criteria, and often on recurrent assessments during psychiatric treatment.

Behavioral Assessment

Perhaps most useful to the clinician is an accurate and meaningful interpretation of pain behavior in the clinical setting. Indeed, this is routinely performed, in every social interaction, including that between patient and clinician. This informal everyday process is subject to the bias, prejudice, evoked emotion, and naivete of the observer. Accuracy requires formalized consistency in clinical activities and observation methodology.

Display of excessive or prominent pain behavior is thought to be an important prognostic indicator of invasive diagnostic and therapeutic procedures. The following methods are designed to measure behavioral dimensions of pain[25]:

Self-observation: The patient monitors and records such activities as medication use, physical activity, pain behaviors, and pain experience. Significant discrepancies among these measures have been reported, as well as between self-reported behavior data and direct observation.
Automated recording: This method is relatively complex and involves the use of such devices as pedometer, "uptime" clocks, and ambulatory recording of heart rate and skeletal muscle activity.
Direct observation: This method involves a trained observer staff and, preferably, a relatively standardized clinical environment or sequence of patient behaviors. (the latter is classically present in the physical therapy setting). The occurrence and frequency of pain behavior are monitored (e.g., rubbing, bracing, guarding, grimacing, sighing). Studies have shown moderate correlations with patient self-report measures of pain experience. Interrater and test-retest reliabilities are as high as .89 to .96.

The Pain Behavior Scale[26] is a direct observation technique that has been validated for outpatient use. Ten items are observed for frequency, and each is graded numerically, then added up for a final score of 0 to 10.

Formal pain behavior protocols have been correlated with measures of pain-related functional disability, depression, and self-reports of pain intensity.[27] Al-

---

Pain Behavior Scale

1. Vocal verbal complaints
   none = 0; occasional = $\frac{1}{2}$; frequent = 1
2. Vocal nonverbal complaints, including moans, groans, and gasps
   none = 0; occasional = $\frac{1}{2}$; frequent = 1
3. Time spent lying down during the day because of pain
   none = 0; 0–60 min = $\frac{1}{2}$; >60 min = 1
4. Facial grimaces
   none = 0; mild/infrequent = $\frac{1}{2}$; severe/frequent = 1
5. Standing posture
   normal = 0; mildly impaired = $\frac{1}{2}$; distorted = 1
6. Gait
   normal = 0; mild limp or impairment = $\frac{1}{2}$; severe limp or impairment = 1
7. "Body language" indicative of pain, including clutching and rubbing pain site
   none = 0; occasional = $\frac{1}{2}$; frequent = 1
8. Visible equipment use, including crutches, cane, brace, TENS, leaning on furniture
   none = 0; occasional = $\frac{1}{2}$; constant or dependent = 1
9. Stationary motion
   can stand/sit still = 0; occasional position shifts = $\frac{1}{2}$; constant moving to shift posture or position = 1
10. Analgesic medication
    none = 0; non-narcotic nonpsychogenic = $\frac{1}{2}$; medication abuse or demanding increased narcotic dosage = 1

---

though statistically significant, correlation coefficients (.25 to .58) show poor predictability of one measure by another. Although valid, assessed pain behavior must be viewed as valuable patient data in its own right that helps describe the overall clinical picture. Each clinician must ultimately determine the significance of these data to practice procedures and prognosis.

Somewhat different from assessment of pain behavior,

yet within the domain of self-report measures, is the Sickness Impact Profile (SIP).[28] The SIP provides a profile of patient functional disability in several areas including gross mobility, gait and self-care activities. This 136 item scale and a 24 item modification[29] of the SIP are well validated and have demonstrated sensitivity to change as patients progress.

Cognitive, Affective, Sensory, and Coping Responses

Minnesota Multiphasic Personality Inventory

The Minnesota Multiphasic Personality Inventory (MMPI) is the most frequently used instrument to assess general aspects of personality. Developed during the late 1930s and recently updated as the MMPI-2, there is voluminous literature applying this test to the scope of psychopathologies, stress syndromes, medical illnesses, and chronic pain. Included are many attempts to effectively differentiate "psychogenic" from "organic" pain by the use of MMPI. The reader is referred to alternative sources for a review of this controversial literature.[30]

The MMPI is a 566-item questionnaire scored and interpreted either by computer or by a specifically trained psychology consultant. Output scoring is by scales: scale 1, hypochondriasis; scale 2, depression; scale 3, conversion hysteria; scale 4, psychopathic deviate subscales: familial discord, authority problems, social imperturbability, social alienation, self-alienation; scale 5, masculinity-femininity; scale 6, paranoia; scale 7, psychasthenia (constructed on patients showing obsessive worries, compulsive rituals, or exaggerated fears); scale 8, schizophrenia; scale 9, hypomania (early manic stage of bipolar disorder); and scale 10, social introversion.

Additional scales are used to ensure validity and truthfulness. Beyond these basic scales, many subscales have been developed to assess specific, otherwise unaddressed, concerns. Combination scores have been proposed as significant. *Functional* pain has been claimed to be associated with the MMPI conversion V configuration (high scores on scales 1 and 3, low score

on 2). Elevation of all three scales is referred to as the *neurotic triad*.

Although the MMPI cannot diagnose the source of pain, to the psychologist there is immense value in defining personality variables important to pain-coping skills and chronic pain rehabilitation. Furthermore, in confirming a clinical diagnosis, the MMPI may justify the prescription of psychoactive medication.

Illness Behavior Questionnaire

The Illness Behavior Questionnaire (IBQ)[31] is a 62-item questionnaire that assesses abnormal illness behavior. Seven independent dimensions are produced: general hypochondriasis, conviction of disease, psychological versus somatic focus of disease, affective inhibition, affective disturbance, denial of life problems unrelated to pain, and irritability. Three normal and three abnormal score patterns are described.[32] In spite of design intent, it is unclear whether abnormal illness behavior or anxiety or distress features of chronic pain are actually being measured.

Millon Behavioral Health Inventory

The Millon Behavioral Health Inventory (MBHI)[33] is a 150-item questionnaire that must be purchased and computer scored. It was originally developed to evaluate psychological functioning in a wide variety of medical specifically not psychiatric patients. The generated interpretive report attempts to provide information regarding the patient's likely style of relating to health care personnel, problematic psychosocial attitudes and stressors, and similarity to patient with psychosomatic complications or poor response to medical intervention. Again, output is by specific scales of basic coping styles (introvertive, inhibited, cooperative, sociable, confident, forceful, respectful, or sensitive), psychogenic attitude (chronic tension, recent stress, premorbid pessimism, future despair, social alienation, and somatic anxiety), psychosomatic correlates, and prognostic index.

Symptom Checklist

The Symptom Checklist-90 (SCL)[34] is a 90-item questionnaire that is easily administered and scored. It measures nine major psychological disturbances: somatization, obsessive-compulsive, interpersonal sensitivity, depression, anxiety, hostility, phobic anxiety, paranoid ideation, and psychoticism. Three global measures of psychic distress are derived: somatic distress, cognitive distress, and distrust.

Beck Depression Inventory

The Beck Depression Inventory (BDI) is a single-page, easily administered questionnaire that must be purchased.* Questions pertaining to depression are answered according to a hierarchy of severity. Answer numbers are then totaled to a numerical score, with significant depression, in our experience, having a score greater than 13. This is a very useful test to help diagnose a complicating depression or significant pain distress.

Visual Analogue Scale

Measurement of pain intensity is easily accomplished by the visual analogue scale, a straight line with "no pain" on one end, and "unbearable pain" on the other. The patient indicates perceived pain intensity by placing a mark appropriately within that continuum. Numerical categorization may be added by dividing the continuum into 5 or 10 equal spaces. In my experience, patient insistence on scoring their pain intensity beyond the scope of the visual analogue scale has universally led to eventual admission to a chronic pain rehabilitation program. Pain categories (faint, mild, moderate, strong, very strong) may be added. Generally these scales strongly intercorrelate.

McGill Pain Questionnaire

The McGill Pain Questionnaire (MPQ) was developed to separately assess three interrelated but conceptually distinct components of pain: sensory-discriminative, motivational-affective, and cognitive-evaluative. This is done by arranging 20 categories of intensity ranked, pain descriptive words. The patient is told to simply circle no more than one appropriate word from each category. Scoring is based on number of words cho-

sen, or according to the sum of the rank values of chosen words from each of the pain dimensions. Good reliability, validity and sensitivity to change have been demonstrated for the MPQ. In addition to providing a deeper understanding of the pain experience, the data indicate the tendency to overdramatize or minimize pain perception and suffering.

Coping Strategies Questionnaire

The Coping Strategies Questionnaire (CSQ)[35] is a recently developed instrument that assesses the extent to which pain patients use six different cognitive coping strategies (e.g., diverting attention, reinterpreting pain sensations, praying or hoping), and two behavioral coping strategies (e.g., increasing activity level, increasing pain behavior) in response to pain. Because this test is recent, supportive literature is limited. Fortunately, the CSQ provides valuable insight into a critical aspect of pain rehabilitation.

West Haven-Yale Multidimensional Pain Inventory

The West Haven-Yale Multidimensional Pain Inventory (WHYMPI)[36] is a 52-item test that is easily administered and scored. This comprehensive inventory of several aspects of the subjective experience of chronic pain is theoretically based on a cognitive-behavioral perspective. It was designed to fill an existing void in the assessment of pain by examining the subjective, behavioral, and psychophysiologic components of pain. It has demonstrated good validity, reliability, and sensitivity to change. Part one of the WHYMPI evaluates five dimensions of the pain experience: perceived interference of pain in various areas of patient functioning, support and concern of significant others, pain severity, self-control, and negative mood. Part two assesses the response of significant others to communications of pain: perceived frequency of punishing, solicitous (enabling) responses, and distracting responses. Part three evaluates patient capacity to function in common daily activities: household chores, outdoor work, usual activities outside the home, and social activities.

Measurement of Physiologic Variables

Physiologic variables include assessments of EMG activity as a measure of existing states of local muscle

---

* The Beck Depression Inventory can be purchased from the Center for Cognitive Therapy, Room 602, 133 South 36th Street, Philadelphia, PA 19104.

Pain Distress Scale

1. Do you think you will ever get over your pain?

      yes   no

2. Do you feel you have had an adequate medical evaluation?

      yes   no

3. Do you feel depressed, or have you lost interest in most of your daily activities?

      no   yes

4. During the past 6 months, have you considered suicide?

      no   yes

5. How much caffeinated coffee do you drink per day?

      0–12 cups   12 + cups

6. Does alcohol relieve your pain or help you sleep?

      no   yes

7. Has anyone ever told you they were annoyed with your use of alcohol, pain killers, or street drugs?

      no   yes

8. Do you feel that your life is out of control?

      no   yes

9. Do you think you will ever be able to work again?

      yes   no

10. Has your pain made you excessively angry, irritable, or violent?

      no   yes

11. Do you think you are coping well enough with your pain?

      yes   no

12. Does worrying about pain and what you are going through keep you awake at night?

      no   yes

13. Do you fear your pain will inevitably get worse?

      no   yes

14. What best describes how much you have limited your activities because of pain? (circle one)

      little change, can do work around the house   some bad days of bedrest   stopped all activities

15. Do you think you are being victimized by your employer or by the insurance company?

      no   yes

16. Are you being abused now, or have you ever been abused in the past (physical, sexual, or emotional abuse)?

      no   yes

17. Have you experienced panic attacks or periods of desperation?

      no   yes

18. Do you need help from family members or others for dressing, bathing, or pain treatments?

      no   yes

19. Are you having difficulties getting along with spouse, family, or friends?

      no   yes

20. Have you ever been hospitalized for a mental illness?

      no   yes

spasm, of generalized muscle tension associated with stress (typically frontalis), and of reactivity of paraspinal musculature to stress induction. As yet, no specific valid diagnostic information is raised by this assessment measure. EMG biofeedback for treatment depends on such information.

Another physiologic variable is the measurement of myofascial trigger-point pressure sensitivity. A spring-loaded plunger, pressure algometer, is used. Reliable and valid measures of trigger-point sensitivity result, but there is poor correlation with patient reports of pain intensity.

PAIN DISTRESS SCALE

In an effort to assist the busy clinician, a questionnaire is presented that summarizes essential questions to ascertain a need for psychology consultation for the pain patient.

This questionnaire asks basic, close-ended questions

concerning depression (#3,4), chemical dependency (#5,6,7), anxiety (#12,17), adequacy of stress and pain-coping skills (#8,10,11,14,20), past or present abuse (#15,16), perceived prognosis (#1,2,9,13), and family functioning (#18,19). There is good indication to obtain psychology consultation if at least two answers fall on the right margin. Indeed, one such answer may be enough (e.g., recent suicide ideation). Answers in the center must be interpreted within the clinical context. Obviously, they have an impact on prognosis (e.g., perceived inadequate medical evaluation; perceived inevitable persistence of pain), but the need for further referral may rest on the patient's clinical progress or on answers to further questions evoked by test results.

CHRONIC PAIN SYNDROME AND CHRONIC PAIN REHABILITATION

Chronic pain syndrome is defined as disabling pain lasting longer than 6 months, for which there is no associated progressive or treatable abnormality found upon medical or biomechanical evaluation. Chronic pain syndrome is thus untreatable by medical, surgical, or physical therapy methods. To avoid confusion with problems of cancer pain, medical stability is deemed an integral component of chronic pain syndrome. Equally important is the secondary disability; this pain impairs normal family life, social interaction, vocation, and future planning. The syndrome may or may not be associated with significant psychopathology.

Identification of chronic pain syndrome is obviously enhanced by competent biomechanical assessment and treatment. Accurate diagnosis and prompt treatment are critical to this disabled population. Failure or delay exacerbates the severity and complexity of the syndrome and worsens the prognosis for success.

Treatment of chronic pain syndrome is an evolving field yet in its infancy. Distinct methodologies have been developed, but all center on multidisciplinary input. These include procedural pain clinics and behavioral and cognitive pain rehabilitation programs.

Procedural Pain Clinics

To avoid confusion, procedural pain clinics are distinguished from behavioral and cognitive pain rehabilitation programs. Typically, procedural clinics are anesthesiology, neurology, surgery specialty, and psychiatry based. They emphasize injection procedures, medication (including psychotropics), accupuncture, transcutaneous electrical nerve stimulation (TENS), physical therapy modalities, exercise and educational activities, and surgical evaluation and treatment. Technically they are contraindicated for chronic pain syndrome because their focus is the treatment of causative organic pathology or mechanical dysfunction, which is not present in chronic pain syndrome as defined. Patients who fail the procedural approach are theoretically eligible for behavioral or cognitive pain rehabilitation programs.

Behavioral Rehabilitation Programs

Behavioral rehabilitation programs view chronic pain as a set of behaviors positively reinforced over time by multiple rewards. Rewards include money (disability income) and relief from responsibility at home and at work. Family members inadvertently reinforce the "sick role" by a variety of activities, termed enabling behaviors, which are appropriate only to acute illness, and are antithetical to the rehabilitation of chronic disability.

The health care system adds to the problem. Professionals subtly reinforce pain behavior by being verbally attentive to pain complaints, physically handling the complaining patient, ordering dramatic tests, and providing socially acceptable rationalization for the pain (e.g., diagnoses of fibrositis and myofascial pain syndrome). Items are prescribed, such as canes and neck collars, that reinforce the medical rationale of pain behavior. Whether helpful or not, they are socially obvious indicators and justifiers of the "sick role." The ring of credibility that comes from degrees and certifications further convinces the patient that a genuine disability, and perhaps severe medical problem, exists. Manual clinicians may add to the problem by attempting to address pain instead of mechanical dysfunction.

The behavioral approach to chronic pain rehabilitation

views pain as a conditioned behavioral response.[37] Treatment seeks first to identify the specific pain behaviors and the specific reinforcers. The patient is then placed in a milieu in which pain behavior is purposely not reinforced and pain-free behavior is positively reinforced. Counseling educates the patient and family members about the nature of chronic pain behavior, avoidance of enabling, and reinforcement of pain-free behavior. Also during this time, the patient is typically engaged in general physical exercise and reactivation. Nonessential medications are withdrawn.

Behavioral rehabilitation is a powerful, proven therapeutic methodology that has no regard for source of pain and by default assumes the absence of disease and mechanical dysfunction. Typically, behavioral programs are expensive 4- to 8-week inpatient programs that require a sophisticated staff capable of recognizing specific behaviors and reinforcers. Consistency of response to patient complaints is essential. Follow-up outpatient counseling is critical to assist the behavioral transition back to home and community.

Cognitive Pain Rehabilitation Clinics

In an effort to improve generalization of the behavior modification to home and community environment, the cognitive approach to chronic pain rehabilitation was developed to supplement or replace behavioral methods.[38] The cognitive approach attempts to teach the patient that pain as an entity is separate from organic disease and can be successfully managed through rational means. The patient is taught about the physiology of pain. For example, the gate control theory of pain directly supports the concept that alternative neurologic input may block neural transmission of pain sense. The patient is then taught self-treatment methods of blocking pain. These include self-hypnosis training, relaxation therapy, accupressure, self-applied deep muscle (fibrocytic) massage, and appropriate biofeedback for pain control or relaxation.

Education cuts the pain-fear relationship by convincing the patient that the pain is not an indication of serious progressive disease. Counseling procedures accomplish several goals. Behavioral patterns are looked for that may add to the suffering and disability of chronic pain. Self-defeating behaviors are identified that both impair coping and further stress relationships. Pacing problems are seen as consistent attempts to physically overwork in spite of chronic pain, ensuring failure and adding to anxiety and stress when the body cannot keep up with self-imposed excessive demands. The impact of pain on specific, nontolerated components of vocational and social activities is assessed. Subtle changes may be recommended, as feasible, that permit the general activity without affecting goal attainment. This includes training in a focused goal setting.

Some of the cognitive techniques that a patient is taught to address pain include intensity reduction by visualizing the turning down of a "gain control" on their body. The patient may "reinterpret" the pain sensation as a neutral (not negative) perception, shift the location of the pain, or visualize reduction the total area that hurts. Alternatively, the pain may be dissociated or displaced by imaging being someplace else that is pleasant. The patient may change the focus of attention to a specific thought or a specific muscle contraction. Ultimately, instructed techniques may be made "automatic" by practice or suggestion.

Counseling is also involved with assessment of significant psychosocial stressors that amplify suffering and disability. Family dysfunction is evaluated and treated. Stress management skills are taught. The long-term effects of physical or sexual abuse during childhood or of parental chemical dependency are evaluated and treated. Substance abuse and chemical dependency are evaluated and treated.

Depression, which is very common in the chronic pain population, is assessed and treated. Usually antidepressant medication is used to ensure the immediate benefit of improved sleep. Nonessential medications are withdrawn. Physical reactivation occurs through a general exercise program, along with instruction in posture control and proper lifting biomechanics.

As with the behavioral approach to chronic pain management, caution is taken to avoid enabling attentiveness to pain complaints and behaviors. Pain-free behavior is encouraged, including cessation of reliance on a cane or other nonessential orthotic device. From the time of admission, the expectation is clearly communicated that pain can be effectively and independently managed by the patient. With the cognitive approach, concomitant treatment of mechanical dysfunction is not automatically viewed as enabling of pain and disability. Rather, mechanical normalization is viewed as a useful treatment objective to improve physical capabilities, whether or not any effect on pain symptoms is achieved. In contrast to the behavioral approach, behavior is not the clinical focus. Rather, rehabilitation and reactivation in spite of the existing pain become the focus.

An observation raised by review of the chronic pain rehabilitation process concerns the importance of nurturance. Short of significant psychopathology, ego weakness, poor self-esteem, and fear of reinjury seriously lessen the patient's resiliance to the diverse effects of injury. Mounting stresses that result from significant pain are incompletely and inefficiently resolved by the weak, immature, insecure personality. A parental function is thus applied by the chronic pain rehabilitation program. Expression of grief is facilitated. Anger is creatively directed. Fear is soothed by training in goal setting and reasoned problem solving. Effective life management is encouraged and reinforced. A healthy life-style is taught. The patient grows in strength and endurance by the exercise component of the pain program. This simple nurturance appears to be invaluable for certain injured patients.

The cognitive approach to rehabilitation is eclectic, involving a diversity of professionals. Such programs are often provided over a 2- to 4-week period, in an outpatient or residential setting. In distinct contrast to the behavioral approach, outpatients may do better than inpatients through easier generalization of learned concepts to the "real world." The less confining the program, however, the greater the need to monitor substance abuse. Postgraduate aftercare sessions facilitate the struggling patient's integration back to the social and familial norm.

Competence in manual technique offers unique and potent resources to chronic pain rehabilitation programs. Primary is the ability to diagnose biomechanical dysfunction efficiently and accurately as the cause of the pain syndrome. Diagnosis is the key to health care. Subsequent "hands-on" conservative and potentially enabling therapy is thus assigned specific, quantifiable outcome goals, independent of mere pain reduction. Also, at least partially resolved is the relationship of pain and physical work capacity of the injured worker.

Concomitant treatment of manual therapy and chronic pain rehabilitation introduces a contradiction that has the potential to sabotage or diminish the effect of either. This problem is avoided in three ways: (1) completing manual treatment before chronic pain rehabilitation, (2) distinguishing separate goals for manual treatment (mechanical normalization for improved work capacity) and chronic pain rehabilitation program (learning to cope with pain), and (3) applying limited components of the chronic pain rehabilitation program during manual treatment. For example, specific family counseling, chemical dependency treatment, medication for depression, and so forth, are provided during manual treatment. The choices depend on the needs of the individual.

Pain patients with chronic, untreated mechanical dysfunction may have acquired sufficient psychosocial stressors to require pretreatment by a chronic pain rehabilitation program before successful manual intervention. Such cases are refractory to medication; these patients are often too irritable (or "touch-me-not") to tolerate the positioning and handling of manual techniques or to carry out recommended exercises. The benefit of the sequential treatment is a realistic, calm patient who is tolerant of the minor physical discomfort of manual treatment and whose expectation of outcome mirrors the clinician's therapeutic goals. The difficult patient is thus made an ideal patient.

EVALUATIVE ALGORITHM

Figure 11-1 presents an algorithm that summarizes the evaluative process in screening for psychologic disorders. It is recommended that, at a minimum, several questions be asked from the Pain Distress Scale or on the basis of the problems listed earlier regarding the chronic pain patient, the signs of family dysfunction,

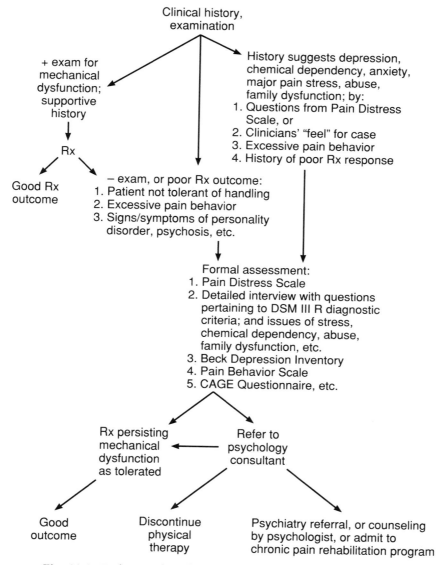

Fig. 11-1. Evaluative algorithm in screening for psychological disorders.

and the clinical markers of malingering. As previously stressed, biomechanical dysfunction supporting the symptom spectrum should be appropriately treated. However if treatment is hampered by, or if the clinical history indicates significant concern for psychopathology, there is a need for further, more formalized, assessment. This assessment better defines the "whole" of the situation and provides a formal rationale for subsequent specialty referral.

SUMMARY

The preceding sections have reviewed screening for psychological disorders, with a specific focus on the pain patient. This has included a discussion of definitions of pain, and how pain affects the patient and the family. Psychiatric disorders, personality disorders, and affective disorders, as well as their interaction with pain were covered. Issues of stress, abuse, and chemical dependency were reviewed. Useful psychological testing tools were introduced, particularly the Pain Distress Scale. Chronic pain syndrome and its rehabilitation were discussed to provide a framework for how physical symptoms are therapeutically addressed from a psychological perspective.

PATIENT CASE HISTORY

History

A. S. is a 36-year-old healthy female nurse who developed work-related, immediate-onset low back pain while lifting a patient. She sought immediate medical attention that diagnosed sacroiliac joint mechanical dysfunction. The problem was treated by manipulation, with good results. However, the problem reoccurred frequently from resumption of lifting activity. She quit work to pursue further education directed toward a more sedentary occupation.

Several months later, she presented in moderate distress. Without trauma, she had experienced exacerbation of severe, sharp pain in the sacroiliac region, with pain spreading into the entire left side of her body, including the hemicranium. There was associated lightheadedness, dizziness, visual blurring, and photophobia.

Objective Examination

Physical examination revealed a sweeping functional scoliosis throughout the spine, severe pubic and sacral torsion, marked tightness of regional abdominal fascia, and tightness of the chest wall, neck, and cranium. Segmental mechanical restrictions were limited to the upper cervical spine, T7 and L3.

Assessment and Outcome

Muscle energy manipulation, deep slow stretch techniques, and high-velocity thrust were administered with good results. Subsequent eval-uation and treatment occurred every 2 weeks over the next 8 months. Typically, she would have the expected 1 to 2 days of symptom aggravation, followed by only a few days of significant relief. Severe pain would then recur, varying in location and attendant disability. The fascial restrictions of the abdomen and chest wall, the cranial restrictions, and the pelvic dysfunctions continued to recur in spite of detailed reassessments and competent manipulative intervention, as demonstrated by short-term normalization of biomechanics.

Eventually, significant psychosocial stressors were uncovered. At age 13, she had experienced a near-drowning. She revealed that she was a single mother of two, divorced from an alcoholic spouse who had physically abused her. Her 13-year-old daughter had recently attempted suicide. In stoic fashion, no efforts had ever been made to discuss these issues with others or to resolve psychological effects through competent counseling. The next two clinic visits led to further introspection and progressive openness to expression of feelings; eventually, she was able to weep. She was referred to, and indeed read, several books on near-death experiences and family dysfunction.

Dramatic improvement was seen during subsequent biomechanical examinations. Manipulative techniques were now more easily accomplished. The fascia loosened up. She was finally able to advance to strengthening and conditioning exercise. Over the following year, there were infrequent recurrences associated with changes in physical demand and with the psychological stress of her academic activities. One suggestion from this case history is that significant psychosocial stress may mediate mechanical dysfunction through regional fascial restriction.

REFERENCES

1. Fields HL, Abram SE, Budd K et al: Core curriculum for professional education in pain. p. 8. International Association for the Study of Pain. Publications, Seattle, 1991

2. Sternbach RA: Psychologist's role in the diagnosis and treatment of pain patients. In Barber J, Adrian C (eds): Psychological Approaches to the Management of Pain. Brunner Mazel, New York, 1982

3. France RD, Krishnan KR, Houpt JL et al: Personality and chronic pain. p. 76. In France RD, Krishnan KR (eds): Chronic Pain. American Psychiatric Press, Washington, DC, 1988

4. Loeser JD: Perspectives on pain. In Proceedings from the First World Conference on Clinical Pharmacology and Therapeutics. Macmillan, London, 1980

5. Beecher HK: Measurement of Subjective Responses. Oxford University Press, London, 1959

6. Fordyce WE: Pain and suffering. A reappraisal. Psychol 43(4):276, 1988

7. Roy R: A problem centered family systems approach in treating chronic pain. p. 113. In Holzman AD, Turk DC (eds): Pain Management. Pergamon Press, New York, 1986

8. Talbott JA, Hales RE, Yudofsky SC et al: American Psychiatric Press Textbook of Psychiatry. p. 357. American Psychiatric Press, Washington, DC, 1988

9. Horowitz MJ: Stress and the mechanisms of defense. p. 39. In Goldman HH (ed): General Psychiatry. 2nd Ed. Appleton & Lange, E. Norwalk, CT, 1987

10. American Psychiatric Association: Diagnostic and Statistical Manual of Mental Disorders. 3rd Ed. Rev. Ed. American Psychiatric Press, Washington, DC, 1987

11. Engel GE: "Psychogenic" pain and the pain prone patient. Am J Med 16:899, 1959

12. Miller L: Neuropsychologic concepts of somatoform disorders. Int J Psychiatry Med 14:31, 1984

13. Katon W, Kleinman A, Rosen G: Depression and somatization: A review. Parts 1 and 2. Am J Med 72:127, 241, 1982

14. Krishnan KR, France RD, Davidson J: Depression as a psychopathological disorder in chronic pain. p. 196. In France RD, Krishnan KR (eds): Chronic Pain. American Psychiatric Press, Washington, DC, 1988

15. Hendler N: Depression caused by chronic pain. J Clin Psychiatry 45(3):30, 1984

16. Yudofsky SC: Conditions not attributable to a mental disorder. p. 1862. In Kaplan HI, Sadock BJ (eds): Comprehensive Textbook of Psychiatry. 4th Ed. Williams & Wilkins, Baltimore, 1985

17. Waring EM, Weisz GM, Bailey SI et al: Predictive factors in the treatment of low back pain by surgical intervention. p. 939. In Bonica JJ, Albe-Fessard D (eds): Advances in Pain Research and Therapy. Raven Press, New York, 1976

18. Blumetti AE, Luciano MM: Psychological predictors of success or failure of surgical intervention for intractable back pain. p. 323. In Bonica JJ, Albe-Fessard D (eds): Advances in Pain Research and Therapy. Raven Press, New York, 1976

19. Caldwell AB, Chase C: Diagnosis and treatment of personality factors in chronic low back pain. Clin Orthop 129:141, 1977

20. Frymoyer JW, Rosen JC, Clements J et al: Psychological factors in low back pain disability. Clin Orthop 195:178, 1985

21. Selye H: Stress without distress. p. 11. In Garfield CA (ed): Stress and Survival. CV Mosby, St. Louis, 1979

22. Appelbaum SH: Stress Management for Health Care Professionals. Aspen Press, Rockville, MD, 1981

23. Lazarus RS: A cognitive analysis of biofeedback control. p. 69. In Prokop CK, Bradley LA (eds): Medical Psychology. Academic Press, San Diego, 1981

24. Mayfield D, Mcleod G, Hall P et al: The CAGE questionnaire: validation of a new alcoholism screening instrument. Am J Psychiatry 131:1121, 1974

25. Feuerstein M, Greenwald M, Gamache MP, et al: The Pain Behavior Scale: Modification and validation for outpatient use. J Psychopathol Behav Assess 7:301, 1985

26. Richards JS, Nepomuceno C, Riles M, et al: Assessing pain behavior: The UAB Pain Behavior Scale. Pain 14:393, 1982

27. Romano JM, Syrjala KL, Levy RL, et al: Overt pain behaviors: Relationship to patient functioning and treatment outcome. Behav Ther 19:191, 1988

28. Bergner M, Bobbitt RA, Carter WB, et al: The Sickness Impact Profile. Med Care 19:787, 1981

29. Deyo RA: Comparative validity of the sickness impact profile and shorter scales for functional assessment in low back pain. Spine 11:951, 1986

30. Bradley LA, Anderson KO, Young LD, et al: Psychological testing. p. 573. In Tollison CD (ed): Handbook of Chronic Pain Management. Williams & Wilkins, Baltimore, 1989

31. Pilowsky I, Spence ND: Patterns of illness behavior in patients with intractable pain. J Psychosomat Res 19:279, 1975

32. Pilowsky I, Spence ND: Illness behavior syndromes associated with intractable pain. Pain 2:61, 1976

33. Millon T, Green C, Meagher R: Millon Behavioral Health Inventory Manual. 3rd Ed. National Computer Systems, Minneapolis, 1982

34. Shutty MS, DeGood DE, Schwartz DP: Psychological dimensions of distress in chronic pain patients: A factor analytic study of symptom checklist—90 responses. J Consult Clin Psychol 54:836, 1986

35. Rosenstiel AK, Keefe FJ: The use of coping strategies in chronic low back pain patients. Pain 17:33, 1983
36. Kerns RD, Turk DC, Rudy TE: The West Haven–Yale Multidimensional Pain Inventory. Pain 23:345, 1985
37. Roberts AH: The operant approach to the management of pain and exess disability. p. 10. In Holzman AD, Turk DC (eds): Pain Management. Pergamon Press, New York, 1986
38. Holzman AD, Turk DC, Kerns RD: The cognitive behavioral approach to the management of chronic pain. p. 31. In Holzman AD, Turk DC (eds): Pain Management. Pergamon Press, New York, 1986

SUGGESTED READINGS

Bradley LA, Anderson KO, Young LD, et al: Psychological testing. In Tollison CD (ed): Handbook of Chronic Pain Management. Williams & Wilkins, Baltimore, 1989

Goldman HH (ed): Review of General Psychiatry. 2nd Ed. Appleton & Lange, E. Norwalk, CT, 1987

Merskey H: Psychiatry and chronic pain. Can J Psychiatry 34:329, 1989

Turk DC, Rudy TE: Assessment of cognitive factors in chronic pain: A worthwhile enterprise? J Consult Clin Psychol 54:760, 1986

12

Clinical Pharmacology for the Physical Therapist

STEPHEN D. CAIN, B.A., B.S., PHARM.D.
STEVEN C. JANOS, M.S., P.T.

In almost every health care setting, physical therapists deal with patients who are taking some sort of medication. It may be a prescription drug or something as simple as aspirin. In either case, the medication may have enough of an impact on the patient's condition that it affects the clinical presentation or course of treatment. For example, up to 90 percent of ambulatory elderly patients take at least one medication, and most take two or more. As the role of the physical therapist continues to change and we see a greater percentage of patients as the entry point into the health care system, we take on a greater responsibility for a more holistic understanding of our patients.

The purpose of this chapter is to present drug classifications used in physical therapy-related patients, a listing and description of individual medications used for common pathologic processes, and side effects that may occur with their usage. This chapter is also designed to give the therapist clinical information that will be useful during the initial patient examination, treatment, and reassessment process.

Additional information for physical therapists concerning drugs, their actions, and possible side effects can be obtained from several sources. The most commonly used is the Physicians' Desk Reference (PDR). These are usually plentiful but may contain more detailed information than the therapist might need. Drug Use Education Tips (DUET) is a package published by the American Academy of Family Physicians. It was de-

signed as an easily readable manual for both the health care practitioner and the patient.

The principle of patient education, particularly in the area of information concerning medications, is no longer a debatable philosophy but has been established as a vital component of medical care. We have turned from the consideration of "the need to know" to the establishment of a "right to know" as an integral part of patient care. The DUET manual is a simple, convenient, yet informative way to assist patients toward a better understanding of the medications they may be taking. Patients who have questions about their prescriptions can be given a photocopy of the appropriate page from the DUET package.

CLINICAL EXAMINATION

The initial examination is when the physical therapist first obtains background information on the nature and state of the patient's condition. During the subjective review of symptoms, the therapist should inquire whether the patient is currently, or has in the past, taken medications for the problem. It can be helpful to have the patient fill out a pre-examination questionnaire relative to the medical history. It is useful to send these questionnaires to patients before they arrive for their first physical therapy visit, to give them time to fill in the specific names and dosages of medications they are taking (Fig. 12-1). The following list of questions can be used to screen for medications during the examination.

Subjective Examination Medication Screening

1. What medications (all) are currently being taken (prescription and nonprescription?)
2. What is the dosage of each medication?
3. How often is each medication being taken? (Include times of day.)
4. When was medication prescribed and by whom?
5. When did the patient begin taking each medication?
6. For what purpose was the medication prescribed?
7. Does the medication appear to be beneficial/helping?
8. Do there appear to be any side effects related to taking the medication?
9. Has the medication been taken in the past? If so, what was the effect?
10. When does the medication prescription run out?

This information helps in several ways. It assists in the overall determination of the severity of the patient's problem or pain tolerance level, or both. Are the symptoms so bad that medications are not apparently helping, or does the patient complain of high levels of pain, yet takes no medication, even when it is indicated?

The first question is to check with patients for all medications they are currently taking. Patients often will not volunteer information about drugs they do not believe are related to the physical therapy problem. It is important to be as specific as possible with patients in getting the correct name of each drug. If they are not sure, the therapist may review the names of various common medications given for this type of problem with the patient or ask the patient to bring the medication to therapy at the next visit. The therapist may feel the need to call the physician's office for further information. If it is not obvious, patients should be asked why they have been placed on these particular medications. Patients should know what each drug is used for. Often they are not sure why they are taking the drugs, which can lead to improper usage. This is especially true of patients who have either multiple problems or chronic conditions.

Occasionally patients will not offer correct historical information, even upon direct questioning. In many of these cases, a good basic knowledge of drug classifications and further questioning will help ascertain all the facts. For example, a patient reports initially that she has not had any surgical procedures in the past yet, when questioned about medications, reports that she is currently taking an estrogen/progesterone supplement. When asked why, she states that she underwent a hysterectomy several years before.

Another patient denies that he has any current medical problems or had any previous surgeries or hospitalizations. When asked about medication, he relates that he is taking lithium, which is an antidepressant medication. Upon further questioning, he admits to recently having been hospitalized for depression. This could be important information to the treating therapist and may have a bearing on the overall treatment course.

We also need to know, if possible, how much of each medication is being taken, how often, and at what time of day. For example, a patient states that he no longer takes his anti-inflammatory medication because it upsets his stomach, a common side effect. Upon further questioning, it is learned that he takes an 800-mg tablet of ibuprofen daily, on an empty stomach. The physician alters the medication to 200-mg tablets qid and makes sure the patient understands that he is to take it with meals. Soon afterward, the patient reports a marked improvement in his condition.

Upon initial examination, it may be important to ascertain from patients when they first started taking their medication. Many times patients state that their medication is not helping the condition, but upon further questioning, you find that they have only been taking it for 1 to 2 days. Some medications work immediately, but many take several days or longer.

PHYSICAL THERAPY

To facilitate the evaluation process during your first visit, please complete this questionnaire and give it to your physical therapist at your first visit. Your cooperation is greatly
appreciated.

NAME: _____   SOCIAL SECURITY #: _____

AGE: _____ Presently working?   Yes   No   Date last worked: _____

Occupation/type of work : _____

Leisure activities: _____

1. List any physician, dentist, osteopath, physical therapist, or chiropractor you have

   seen for your present condition.

2. List all general medical problems for which you have received treatment.

3. Describe any history of joint/muscle problems and treatment you may have received.

4. List all surgeries and hospitalizations you have had and their dates.

5. List all medications you are currently taking.

6. Have you taken steroids (cortisone, Prednisone)?   Yes   No

   If so, describe the condition for which they were prescribed.

Fig. 12-1. Physical therapy questionnaire.

After finding out what medications are being taken, the physical therapist must determine their effectiveness. More often than not, patients can tell whether it has had a beneficial effect or not. Occasionally, the therapist may have to help patients relate their medications not only to pain levels but to function, in order to determine their overall response.

It is often important to find out when medications were prescribed, when the prescription runs out, and by what physician(s). In today's world of specialized medicine, many times patients are taking several medications prescribed by different physicians for different problems. The therapist's role may also be one of a medication screener. If the patient has seen several physicians for the same problem, it is not uncommon to find that each has prescribed a different medication. For those who claim to be currently taking three different nonsteroidal anti-inflammatory drugs (NSAIDs) at the same time for the same problem, it can probably be correctly assumed that this should not be the case; a call to either the referring or primary physician, or both, is in order.

It may also be important to determine whether patients have been on the present medication before and what the results were. Did it alleviate symptoms earlier and not now? This may be a sign that either the patient is developing a tolerance to the drug or, if the problem is the same, the condition is now worse.

Most patients, when asked a general question such as "Are you presently taking any medication?," will respond with the names of prescription drugs only. It is then the examiner's task to ask about over-the-counter (OTC) medications. This may run the gamut from aspirin to sedatives, laxatives, tonics, nerve pills, vitamins, or birth control pills. It may also be important to ask the patients whether they are using any other recreational drugs or alcohol and about their caffeine or nicotine use (see Ch. 11 concerning the investigation of substance abuse). All these substances can affect the neuromuscular system and the patient's perception of pain or function.

This would also be the time to check out possible side effects of any of these medications (see Appendix I). Side effects are most often dose related. Most of this material may have been covered in the review of system questioning, but many times a drug-related side effect is not severe enough for the patient to volunteer information, and it is helpful to ask specific questions, depending on the particular medications being taken and common untoward effects.

About 10 to 20 percent of hospitalized patients and 2 to 5 percent of outpatients in whom adverse effects develop will be taking medications. This frequency varies greatly depending on the drug administered, the patient population treated, and the definitions of adverse effects.

Adverse drug reactions may be classified into those caused by excessive intended pharmacologic effects and those caused by unintended actions. Adverse effects from excessive intended pharmacologic affects are all dose dependent. For example, hypoglycemia may be caused by excessive doses of insulin and hypotension by excessive doses of antihypertensive agents.

Adverse effects caused by unintended actions of the drug may be categorized into those attributable to the physical and chemical properties of the drug, the direct cytotoxic effect of the drug, the induction of an abnormal immune response, and inherited enzyme defects. Most adverse drug reactions occur soon after administration and are dose related. The potential side effects of the different medications commonly prescribed are covered in more detail later in this chapter.

Again, most of this information is collected during the initial interview of the patient. Certain questions need to be asked of the patient concerning medications later during the course of treatment. If symptoms are changing, the therapist needs to check subjectively whether or not the patient is continuing on the medication. Is it more or less frequent? Is the dosage the same, or has it been changed? In some cases, one of the first signs of improvement may be a decreasing need for medication during the day. If medications do not seem to be helping the condition after a period of treatment, it may be important for the referring/primary physician to have this information. It is also more likely that patients will develop side effects to certain medications the longer they are on them, and this should be followed by questioning at subsequent visits.

As physical therapists, we quite often deal with patients whose primary complaint is one of pain and, although they are hurting, the connotation of a pain killer is not a good one to many people. This may lead to refusal to take the prescribed medication. This can sometimes interfere with the overall management of the patient's condition. For example, it is not unusual for a patients given a prescription for an anti-inflammatory medication not to take it because their understanding is that it has been prescribed for pain only. Many times a simple explanation of the role of the prescribed medication will alleviate the patient fears, improve their understanding of treatment, and allow for a better treatment course.

Patients will also at times alter their medication as it

relates to their pain before coming to therapy. If their prescribed medication has a profound beneficial effect on their condition, they may decide on their own either to take it just before physical therapy (for better tolerance of the therapy) or not to take it just before therapy (so that the therapist can really see what their condition is like at its worst). These do not have to necessarily be good or bad events but either way, the therapist should be aware of the situation for further insight into the nature of the patient's condition.

Certain medications and conditions should be brought to the physical therapist's attention, such as conditions of angina and diabetes mellitus and their usual prescribed medications.

The therapist should ask patients about medical conditions as well as medications that are being taken. If a patient is taking nitroglycerin for his heart problem and attacks of angina, the drug should be close at hand during the evaluation and/or treatment session. This is also true for the diabetic patient who may be taking insulin or oral supplementation for his condition. In this situation, some type of quick sugar replacement should be readily available for the patient.

PAIN AND INFLAMMATION

Drugs are widely used to treat pain and inflammation in physical therapy patients. Nonsteroidal anti-inflammatory drugs (NSAIDs), including salicylates, and certain corticosteroids are useful for treating both pain and inflammation. Opiate-like drugs are useful for treating pain, and skeletal muscle relaxants are useful for treating pain as a result of muscle spasm.

Salicylates

Salicylates are the most widely used nonsteroidal anti-inflammatory agent (NSAFA) employed. In the United States, consumption of the salicylate aspirin is on the order of 100 tablets for every man, woman, and child per year. Salicylates can be divided into two groups: those that are acetylated (aspirin) and those that are not. The acetylated portion of the molecule accounts for the differing properties between aspirin and other salicylates (Table 12-1). Both the acetyl and salicylate portion of the molecule account for the pain-relieving, anti-inflammatory, and fever-reducing properties of aspirin. In addition, the acetyl portion of the aspirin molecule confers antiplatelet clotting properties. The pain-relieving, anti-inflammatory, and fever-reducing properties of the nonacetylated salicylate are due only to the salicylate portion of the molecule, and there is no acetyl portion to confer antiplatelet clotting activity. Thus, aspirin has an additional mechanism of action not found on the nonacetylated salicylates.

Mechanism of Action

Precise mechanisms of action for the salicylates have not been clearly established. Aspirin has been found to irreversibly acetylate (and thereby inhibit) the enzyme responsible for prostaglandin synthesis in various tissues. The nonacetylated salicylates do not, but still cause a reduction in prostaglandin synthesis. In-

Table 12-1. Salicylates

Formulation	Example	Advantage	Disadvantage
Acetylated (Aspirin)			
Effervescent	Alka-Seltzer	Fast acting	1 g sodium per 640 mg
Buffered	Bufferin	Fast acting	
Uncoated	Generic	Fast-acting analgesic effect; onset within 30 min; peak effect 1–3 hr; duration of effect 3–6	GI side effects
Enteric-coated	Ecotrin	Prolonged onset of action	GI side effects
Nonacetylated			
Sodium salicylate	Generic		4.0 MEQ sodium
Magnesium salicylate[a]	Doan's pills		Contains magnesium
Magnesium-choline salicylate[a]	Trilisate	Liquid, tablet available	Contains magnesium
Salsalate[a]	Disalcid	bid dosing	

[a] Prescription drug.

hibition of the enzyme may be reversible for the non-acetylated salicylates.

Salicylates provide mild to moderate pain relief by inhibiting synthesis of prostaglandins that sensitize peripheral pain receptors to various stimuli. Salicylates may act centrally as well by decreasing production of prostaglandins at the level of the hypothalamus.

In much larger doses, salicylates produce an anti-inflammatory effect, useful in treating rheumatoid and nonrheumatoid inflammatory conditions. Although additional mechanisms of action for anti-inflammatory activity have been proposed, prostaglandin inhibition appears to play a major role. The fever-reducing properties of salicylates appear to result from prostaglandin inhibition in the portion of the hypothalamus that controls body temperature. Other mechanisms of action may be involved, however.

Aspirin inhibits platelet aggregation by inhibiting the enzyme responsible for converting arachidonic acid to thromboxane, a substance that promotes platelet aggregation. Nonacetylated salicylates do not inhibit this enzyme, hence are not useful in preventing the formation of thrombi on patients at risk of stroke or myocardial infarct.

Aspirin appears to be somewhat more potent than non-acetylated salicylates in relieving pain and reducing fever. By contrast, the nonacetylated salicylates are equivalent to aspirin in anti-inflammatory potency and thus are useful in treating inflammatory conditions that cannot be treated with aspirin (i.e., patients who are allergic or intolerant to aspirin). The equivalent anti-inflammatory efficacy of the nonacetylated salicylates with aspirin suggests that irreversible inhibition of prostaglandin synthesis is not as important, or merely one of many mechanisms in producing an anti-inflammatory effect.

Side Effects

Adverse side effects to the salicylates (especially aspirin) mainly involve the gastrointestinal (GI) tract. Two to 10 percent of those taking analgesic doses (less than 3 to 6 g/day) and 10 to 30 percent of those taking larger doses suffer symptomatic disturbances (e.g., dyspepsia, heartburn, epigastric distress, nausea, occasional vomiting, abdominal pain) GI effects can be minimized by taking salicylates with food, antacids, or a large glass of water (240 ml).

About 70 percent of patients taking analgesic doses of uncoated aspirin lose 2 to 8 ml of blood daily as a result of a direct irritant effect on the gastric mucosa. As many as 15 percent lose 10 ml or more. There appears to be no correlation between such occult (usually painless) bleeding and symptomatic GI distress. In a few cases, blood loss can be substantial (e.g., 500 ml); in other cases (those on long-term therapy), iron deficiency can result. Such blood loss is not reduced by taking aspirin with food or commercially available buffered preparations. Enteric-coated aspirin tablets, nonacetylated salicylates that usually produce little or no blood loss, may be a useful alternative in such cases.

A third major GI side effect of salicylates (especially aspirin) is damage to the GI mucosa, ranging from mild inflammation to major ulceration. A direct effect has been implicated but can also occur with rectal or intravenous administration. Such damage can occur with or without either symptoms or bleeding. Enteric-coated tablets have been shown to reduce the incidence of such aspirin-induced erosions; buffered tablets have not.

Since salicylates may aggravate GI bleeding, those with a history of GI bleeding or erosions should avoid them. Patients should avoid combining aspirin with alcohol, since the combination increases the risk of GI bleeding and ulceration. Patients should probably avoid using aspirin within 8 to 10 hours of heavy alcohol ingestion.

Other adverse reactions associated with the salicylates are a sensitivity reaction characterized chiefly by bronchospasm in predisposed patients, as well as tinnitus. Although extremely rare, death has occurred within minutes after ingestion of as little as one or two 5-gr tablets. Patients with the aspirin triad of asthma, nasal polyps, and aspirin allergy appear to be especially susceptible. No prostaglandin synthesis inhibitor such as NSAIAs or the preservative sodium benzoate or tar-

Table 12-2. Comparison of Acetylated Salicylates (Aspirin) and Nonacetylated Salicylates

Aspirin	Nonacetylated Salicylates
Blocks platelet aggregation	No effect on platelet aggregation
High incidence of occult gastrointestinal bleeding	Little or no gastrointestinal blood loss
Can induce bronchospasm	Little cross-sensitivity in aspirin-sensitive patients

Table 12-3. Nonsteroidal Anti-inflammatory Drugs

Drug[a]	Usual Dosage (mg)	Indications
Diflunisal (Dolobid)	250–500 8–12 h	R (I)
Fenoprofen (Nalfon)	300–600 tid–qid	RIP
Flurbiprofen (Ansaid)	50–100 bid–tid	R (I)
Diclofenac (Voltaren)	24–40 bid–qid	R (I)
Ibuprofen (Motrin)	400–800 tid–qid	RIP
Indomethacin (Indocin)	250–500 bid–qid	R (I)
Ketoprofen (Orudis)	50–75 tid–qid	RIP
Meclofenamate (Meclomen)	50–100 tid–qid	R (I)
Mefenamic acid (Ponstel)	250 q6h PRN	PI
Naproxen (naproxen sodium) (Naprosyn; Anaprox)	250–500 bid (275–550)	RIP
Phenylbutazone (Butazolidin)	100 qid	R
Piroxicam (Feldene)	10–20 qid–bid	R
Sulindac (Clinoril)	150–200 bid	R (I)
Tolmetin (Tolectin)	200–400 tid–qid	R (I)

Abbreviations: P, pain; R, rheumatoid osteoarthritis, arthritis; I, nonrheumatic inflammation; ( ), unapproved indications.
[a] Brand names are given in parentheses.

trazine dye should be administered to these patients. By contrast, it appears that the nonacetylated salicylates may be given cautiously (Table 12-2).

Tinnitus is a ringing or high-pitched buzzing sensation in the head. This side effect is usually observed with either large dosages or long-term use of salicylates, or both. It usually occurs only at dosages employed to treat rheumatoid conditions and in fact is occasionally used by clinicians as a therapeutic end point. Tinnitus and hearing loss that can also occur at higher dosages of salicylates are usually completely reversible. Permanent hearing loss has rarely been reported.

Contraindications

Patients whose kidneys are highly dependent on vasodilator prostaglandins should avoid aspirin and NSAIDs. These patients include those with congestive heart failure and liver or renal disease.

Salicylates should be avoided in the last trimester of pregnancy because of an increased risk of adverse hematologic effects in both the mother and neonate, as well as complications in delivery.

Nonsteroidal Antiinflammatory Drugs

Fourteen NSAIAs are available in the United States that are not salicylates (Table 12-3). Some agents have Food and Drug Administration (FDA)-approved indications for treatment of rheumatic diseases, such as rheumatoid arthritis and osteoarthritis. Other agents have approved indications for treatment of pain or non-

rheumatic inflammatory conditions, such as bursitis and tendinitis. Other approved indications for these agents are gout, vascular headache, and dysmenorrhea. One agent, naproxen (Naprosyn, Anaprox), has FDA-approved indications for the treatment of all these conditions. In other cases, although FDA approval may be lacking, many of these agents are used to treat one or more of these conditions.

Despite the diversity of approved and unapproved indications for these agents, all are considered equally efficacious in treating pain and inflammation. Selection of an agent, then, depends on such considerations as cost, convenience, side effect profile, patient tolerance, and the clinical experience of the physician. Some agents are considered too toxic to be used as a first-time agent (e.g., phenylbutazone, indomethacin).

Other agents offer the advantage of once-a-day or twice-a-day dosing (e.g., piroxicam, naproxen). Several agents are available as inexpensive generic compounds (e.g., ibuprofen, indomethacin).

Mechanism of Action

The NSAIDs have a mechanism of action that resembles that of the salicylates. Both block the enzyme responsible for converting arachidonic acid to various prostaglandins and thromboxanes (Fig. 12-2). Such a mechanism of action may account for the similar analgesic, anti-inflammatory, and anti-pyretic properties of these two classes of drugs, as well as their similar side effect profile. Unlike aspirin, however, the effect of NSAIDs on platelet aggregation is reversible upon discontinuation of the agent. Other mechanisms of action may be responsible for the anti-inflammatory and analgesic activity of NSAIDs, although inhibition of prostaglandin synthesis appears to play a major role.

Indications

Twelve of the 14 NSAIDs available in the United States are approved by the FDA for treatment of rheumatic diseases and rheumatoid disorders account for the primary use of these agents. These agents are generally used as an alterative for patients who cannot tolerate the large doses of salicylates required to treat rheumatoid conditions, although NSAIDs can cause similar side effects. Rheumatoid conditions for which NSAIDs are employed include rheumatoid arthritis, osteoarthritis, and ankylosing spondylitis.

Six NSAIDs have FDA approval for treating mild to moderate pain (e.g., musculoskeletal, postoperative, postpartum, visceral pain associated with cancer). Other agents may work just as well. All are believed to act by inhibiting the synthesis of prostaglandins that sensitize peripheral pain receptors. These agents may act centrally as well. Furthermore, their anti-inflam-

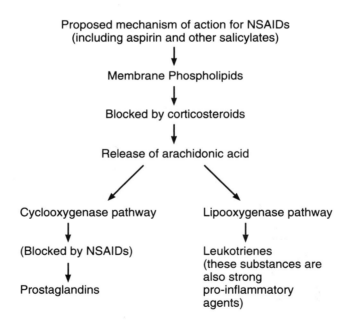

Fig. 12-2. NSAIDs block the cyclooxygenase pathway for membrane arachidonic acid. Potent mediators of pain and inflammation are not produced or are antagonized, accounting for their analgesic and anti-inflammatory effect. Corticosteroids that block production of mediators from both pathways are consequently more potent and inflammatory agents.

matory effect may also contribute to their analgesic effect.

Although only six NSAIDs have FDA approval for treating nonrheumatic inflammation, almost all agents have been employed to treat these conditions, which include bursitis, tendinitis, athletic injuries, pericarditis, and synovitis. Both the analgesic and the anti-inflammatory activities of the agents account for the clinical value in treating these conditions.

Side Effects

Like the salicylates, the major side effects of NSAIDs involve the GI tract. GI pain, heartburn, and nausea are particularly common with estimates as high as 30 percent in some cases. Constipation, diarrhea, and vomiting are other side effects that often occur with these agents. In order to minimize these side effects, it is recommended that they be taken with meals, milk, or antacids, but it should also be noted that such administration reduces both their rate and extent of absorption, possibly diminishing their therapeutic efficacy. The onset of analgesic action of these agents occurs sooner if taken 30 minutes before, or 2 hours after meals with at least 8 ounces of water.

Gastrointestinal irritation leading to bleeding, hemorrhage, and perforation of ulcers has been associated with these agents. Patients with a history of upper GI disease should be monitored closely if given these agents, since fatalities have resulted in such cases.

A second major class of side effects associated with NSAIDs involve the central nervous system (CNS). Dizziness and drowsiness often occur among these agents with a reported frequency of 3 to 9 percent. Mild to moderate headache also often occurs, with a reported frequency of 3 to 9 percent.

Indomethacin is particularly significant in causing headaches, with estimates of 25 to 50 percent in some cases. Headaches are often severe and occur especially in the morning.

Another frequent adverse reaction to these agents is skin rash or itching, with a reported frequency of 3 to 9 percent among many agents. Although this allergic reaction is rarely anaphylactic, it warrants medical attention. Patients allergic to aspirin or other NSAIDs should not be administered any NSAID, since cross-sensitivity occurs among these agents. Precautions regarding use of salicylates apply to NSAIDs as well.

Contraindications

Patients should be advised not to combine NSAIDs with alcohol, since the combination increases the risk of GI bleeding or ulceration. Nor should NSAIDs be combined with salicylates or other NSAIDs, as the combination does not offer any increase in therapeutic benefits but does increase the risk of GI irritation and bleeding. Prolonged used of acetaminophen (e.g., Tylenol) and NSAIDs increases the risk of adverse renal effects and should be avoided. Caution should be exercised if confusion, diarrhea, dizziness, drowsiness, ocular disturbances, or signs and symptoms of an allergic reaction occur in a patient taking these agents.

Acetaminophen

Acetaminophen is widely employed as both an analgesic and antipyretic by itself and in combination with other agents. It is devoid of anti-inflammatory activity and cannot suppress inflammation in sprains, strains, or rheumatoid conditions. Acetaminophen appears to block prostaglandin synthesis in the CNS with only minimal activity peripherally, in contrast to the salicylates and other NSAIDs. Like the latter two classes of drugs, acetaminophen is useful in treating mild and moderate pain and for reducing fever. In normal doses, acetaminophen is safe and relatively free of side effects and accounts in part for its widespread popularity in both over-the-counter and prescription drug products. In an overdose situation, acetaminophen is extremely toxic and can cause rapidly fatal liver failure.

Corticosteroids

Another class of drugs occasionally used to treat inflammatory conditions unresponsive to NSAIDs are the corticosteroids, so named because many are synthetized in the adrenal cortex in humans. (Corticosteroids are to be distinguished from anabolic steroids that are occasionally abused by some athletes in order to increase muscle mass and to enhance their athletic performance.) Corticosteroids are usually divided into two types, on the basis of their predominant activity. Mineralocorticoids have primary effects on sodium retention and potassium excretion and are primarily used in physiologic doses as replacement therapy in certain disorders, such as Addison's disease. These agents have no value in treating inflammatory conditions. Glucocorticoids are the second major type of corticosteroids; in pharmacologic (i.e., large) doses, they have powerful anti-inflammatory effects (Table 12-4). These agents are generally the ones referred to when discussing corticosteroids and are the ones discussed here. Nevertheless, it should be kept in mind that the distinction between these two types of corticosteroids is not complete; some glucocorticoids have mineralocorticoid (sodium-retaining) activity as well (e.g., hydrocortisone, prednisone).

Mechanism of Action

Corticosteroids work through several mechanisms in achieved an anti-inflammatory responses.

Mechanisms of Anti-inflammatory Activity of Glucocorticoids

1. Stabilizing leukocyte lysosomal membranes
2. Preventing release of destructive acid hydrolases from leukocytes
3. Inhibiting macrophage accumulation in inflamed areas
4. Reducing leukocyte adhesion to capillary endothelium
5. Reducing capillary wall permeability and edema formation
6. Decreasing complement components
7. Antagonizing histamine activity and release of kinin from substrates
8. Reducing fibroblast proliferation of collagen deposition
9. Other possible mechanisms as yet unknown

By inhibiting the inflammatory process at the cellular level, these agents suppress the symptoms of inflam-

Table 12-4. Equivalent Doses of Glucocorticoids

Action	Dose (mg)
Short acting (8–12 h)	
Cortisone	25
Hydrocortisone	20
Intermediate acting (12–36 h)	
Methylprednisolone	4
Prednisone	5
Prednisolone	5
Triamcinolone	4
Long acting (36–72 h)	
β-Methasone	0.6
Dexamethasone	0.75

mation (e.g., heat, redness, tenderness). These agents do not treat the cause of the inflammation and are not considered curative agents. When these agents are used for short periods of time, even massive dosages are unlikely to produce adverse effects. By contrast, long-term use of these agents is associated with a number of adverse effects.

Side Effects

Prolonged use of large doses of gluocorticosteroids may cause decreased secretion of endogenous corticosteroids through negative feedback on the pituitary. These patients may not secrete sufficient corticosteroids in response to stress and, if they are withdrawn abruptly, may show signs and symptoms of adrenal insufficiency (as little as 15 mg prednisone daily beyond 1 or 2 months can cause such suppression). In order to avoid such problems, glucocorticoids should be slowly withdrawn in patients who are discontinuing long-term use of large dosages of these agents.

Another adverse effect of prolonged use of these agents (e.g., prednisone 10 mg/day for years) is the development of osteoporosis, especially in geriatric or debilitated patients. The osteoporosis occurs mainly in the vertebral column and pelvic girdle. Often such osteoporotic changes are asymptomatic until a bone is fractured.

Steroid diabetes is another potential adverse effect of prolonged use of these agents. Glucocorticoids can either precipitate diabetes mellitus in predisposed patients or aggravate the condition in patients who already have it. Hypercortism, a cushingoid state, may also result from long-term use of these agents, manifesting as moon facies with a buffalo hump.

Other adverse effects associated with the use of glucocorticoids are increased susceptibility to, and masking of, infection, sodium retention, and potassium loss, GI side effects (e.g., nausea, vomiting, diarrhea, constipation, peptic ulcer formation), mind-altering effects ranging from mild euphoria to frank psychosis, and a wide variety of other adverse effects.

In spite of these side effects, short-term use of these agents (e.g., Medrol dospak) is unlikely to produce harmful effects. In order to minimize adverse effects, these agents should be taken immediately before, during, or immediately after meals, or with food or milk. If prolonged use of glucocorticoids is required, they should be administered every other day in the morning and eventually reduced and (preferably) discontinued.

Opioids

For more severe pain, a second class of analgesics are used in place of the salicylates and NSAIAs: the opioids (Table 12-5). The opioids include naturally occurring compounds from the opium poppy, such as morphine and codeine, as well as semisynthetic modifications of these substances, such as hydromorphone (Dilaudid) and oxycodone (Percodan, Percocet). A third class of opioids include completely synthetic substances that resemble morphine in activity, such as meperidine (Demorol), methadone, and, to a lesser extent, propoxyphene (Darvon) and pentacozine (Talwin). All these opioids own their analgesic (and other pharmacologic) activity to an interaction with opioid receptors existing in different areas throughout the CNS.

Mechanism of Action

Several different kinds of opioid receptors have been discovered. Actions at these receptors account for the analgesic and other effects of the opioids (Table 12-6). Morphine has strong affinity for MU-1 and MU-2 receptors, accounting for its analgesic, euphoric, and other effects. Pentazocine has an affinity for κ- and σ-receptors, thus accounting for its analgesic and "psychotomimetic" effects. Codeine has a weaker affinity for MU-1 and MU-2 receptors than does morphine and thus has weaker analgesic efficacy.

It is proposed that analgesia is achieved when either endogenous opioids (endorphins) or exogenous

Table 12-5. Oral Opioid Analgesics

Class	Usual Dosage (mg)	Side Effects
Codeine	15–60 q3–6h (usually prescribed in combination formulation Tylenol #3)	Constipation, drowsiness
Hydrocodone	5–10 q4–6h	Drowsiness, dizziness, increased sweating, flushing of the face
Hydromorphone (Dilaudid)	2 q3–6h	Drowsiness, dizziness, loss of appetite
Meperidine	50–150 q3–4h	Constipation, dizziness, drowsiness, increased sweating, flushing of the face, nausea, vomiting
Morphine	10–30 q4h (initial); dose must be individualized	As with meperidine
Oxycodone	5 q3–6h (usually prescribed in combination formulation (e.g., Percodan, Percocet)	Dizziness, drowsiness, nausea, vomiting
Pentazocine (Talwin)	50 q3–4h	Drowsiness, false sense of well-being, nausea, vomiting
Propoxyphene (often prescribed in combination formulation, e.g., Darvocet)	65 q4h	Dizziness, drowsiness, nausea, vomiting

Table 12-6. Characteristics of Opioid Receptors

Receptors	Agonist	Effect
μ_1	Morphine	Analgesia
μ_2	Morphine	Euphoria, respiratory depression, physical dependence, constipation
κ	Nalbuphine	Analgesia, sedation
σ	Pentazocine	Dysphoria, hallucinations, tachycardia, hypertension

opioids (e.g., morphine) bind to receptors that block the transmission of pain impulses within the CNS. Both the perception and the emotional response to pain are altered with this binding. Other neurotransmitters believed to be involved in modulating the transmission of pain impulses are serotonin and norepinephrine. Antidepressants that increase the concentration of these two neurotransmitters have been used as adjunctive analgesics in post-herpetic neuralgia and vascular headaches (e.g., amitriptyline).

Indications

Opioids such as morphine are indicated for the treatment of severe pain. For moderate to severe pain, all other opioid analgesics, with the exception of codeine and propoxyphene, are indicated. For mild to moderate pain, codeine and propoxyphene are indicated.

Oral Opioids

Codeine is the most commonly prescribed oral opioid analgesic in a formulation with either acetominophen or aspirin (e.g., Tylenol #3, Empirin #3). Formulations designated #4 contain 1 gr or 60 mg of codeine, #3 a half-grain or 30 mg, #2 a quarter-grain or 15 mg; #1 formulations are rarely prescribed. The combination of a peripherally acting analgesic (e.g., aspirin) with an opioid analgesic makes therapeutic sense. Pain relief is achieved with two mechanisms of action instead of one. The results of controlled studies have shown that the analgesic effects of each component are additive.

In the doses usually prescribed for the treatment of mild to moderate pain, the side effects of codeine are minor; constipation and drowsiness occur most fre-quently. When larger doses are employed (e.g., treatment of severe pain), codeine produces side effects similar to those associated with morphine, including respiratory depression. Increasing the oral dose beyond the therapeutic limit of 200 mg increases the incidence of side effects without an increase in analgesia.

Two semisynthetic analogues of codeine are hydrocodone and oxycodone. Both are usually prescribed in combination with a nonopioid analgesic for the same reason as codeine. Hydrocodone is combined with acetaminophen in Vicodin and oxycodone is combined with aspirin or acetaminophen in Percodan or Percocet, respectively. Oxycodone has a slightly greater dependence liability than codeine and is included in Schedule 11 of the Controlled Substances Act. Oxycodone is actually equivalent to morphine in analgesic potency. To limit abuse in the United States, it is combined with aspirin or acetaminophen in a very small amount (4.5 to 5 mg). Both hydrocodone and oxycodene share side effects similar to that of codeine.

Although commonly prescribed (especially in combination with acetaminophen or aspirin for the same reason as codeine) propoxyphene 65 mg was shown in one study to be no more effective than 325 to 650 mg of codeine. Propoxyphene on a milligram basis is only one-half as potent as codeine. Although its dependence liability may be less than that of codeine, its potential for causing life-threatening toxicity has led to its inclusion in Schedule IV of the Controlled Substances Act.

Pentazocine is an opioid that has both analgesic and weak narcotic antagonist properties. It blocks activity at receptors to which morphine binds but stimulates activity at κ-receptors (to produce analgesic) and at σ-receptors (to produce psychomimetic and cardiovascular effects). Pentazocine is effective at relieving moderate pain, but its high incidence of side effects limit its clinical value. Approximately 10 percent of patients will experience psychomimetic side effects such as dysphoria, nightmares, feelings of depersonalization, and, most commonly, visual hallucinations. Nausea, vomiting, and dizziness occur as frequently as the other strong opioids. The other formulation of pentazocine contains naloxone to antagonize the euphoric effects of pentazocine when the tablet is illicitly solubilized and injected intravenously. Evidence suggests that abuse of this drug persists. Pentazocine is included in Schedule IV of the Controlled Substances Act.

Skeletal Muscle Relaxants

A second major class of agents often used as an adjunct to physical therapy are the skeletal muscle relaxants. These agents are used to treat muscle spasms that occur as a result of injury at localized regions of the human body. There are two kinds of skeletal muscle relaxants: direct-acting agents that block the effects of the neurotransmitter at the level of the neuromuscular junction, and centrally acting agents. The direct-acting agents are usually administered intravenously as an adjunct to general anesthesia during surgery and are not discussed here. Centrally acting agents are usually administered orally and probably achieve most of their muscle relaxant effect through their general CNS depressant (sedative) properties. Three other skeletal muscle relaxants used in treating spasticity as a result of spinal cord injuries or other neurologic disorders, such as multiple sclerosis or cerebral palsy, are caclofen, dantrolene, and the anxiolytic diazepam.

Five major centrally acting skeletal muscle relaxants are available in the United States (Table 12-7). Chlorphenesin and metaxalone are also available but are rarely used.

Side Effects

All centrally acting skeletal muscle relaxants have drowsiness as a major side effect, with cyclobenzaprine particularly notable. Cyclobenzaprine is structurally similar to tricyclic antidepressants and may have side effects similar to those associated with these agents, such as dry mouth, blurred vision, and increased heart rare. A metabolite of carisoprodol includes meprobamate, a once popular antianxiety agent associated with some abuse potential; this agent should be used with caution in patients who have a history of drug abuse. Orphenadrine shares anticholinergic properties with cyclobenzaprine and should not be administered to patients with glaucoma, prostatic hypertrophy, or cardiac arrhythmias. All these agents are metabolized by the liver and excreted by the kidneys and should be used with caution in patients who have any impairment in these organs. Chlorzoxazone may color urine orange or reddish-purple, and methocarbanol black, brown, or green, especially if allowed to stand.

Baclofen, Diazepam, and Dantrolene

Three other drugs used to treat spasms in neurologic disorders such as spinal cord injury, multiple sclerosis, and cerebral palsy are baclofen, diazepam, and dantrolene. Baclofen is structurally related to a neurotransmitter that blocks conduction of impulses in the spinal cord and may act through this mechanism. Tran-

Table 12-7. Skeletal Muscle Relaxants (Central-Acting)

Drug[a]	Usual Dose (mg)	Adverse Reactions
Carisoprodol (Soma)	350 qid	Dizziness, drowsiness, GI disturbances
Chlorzoxazone (Paraflex; plus acetaminophen, Parafon Forte)	250–750 tid–qid	GI disturbances, drowsiness, dizziness
Cyclobenzaprine (Flexaril)	10 bid–qid	Drowsiness, dry mouth, dizziness
Methocarbamol (Robaxin)	Initially 1–5 qid 2–3 days, then 750 q4h to 1.5 tid	Lightheadedness, dizziness, drowsiness, nausea, uticaria
Orphenadrine (Norflex SR; Disipal)	100 bid, 50 tid	Dry mouth, weakness, dizziness

[a] Brand names are given in parentheses.

sient drowsiness is the most common side effect of this agent, occurring in 20 to 25 percent of patients. Psychiatric disturbances, such as hallucinations, excitation, confusion, depression, and anxiety, can occur, especially in patients with these preexisting disorders and in the elderly. Abrupt withdrawal of this agent has precipitated hallucinations, seizures, and increased spasticity in some patients.

Diazepam in an antianxiety agent that enhances the activity of the same inhibitory transmitter by which baclofen is believed to act. Diazepam acts on receptors both in the spinal cord and in the brain and, because of its activity at the latter site, is commonly used as an antianxiety agent and as a sedative. Drowsiness is a major side effect of diazepam, as it is with other benzodiazepenes. Nevertheless, it is a useful muscle relaxant both in chronic neurologic disorders and in acute localized self-limited traumatic disorders.

One agent not indicated for muscle spasms that is related to musculoskeletal trauma is dantrolene. Dantrolene is used orally to treat spasms occurring in neurologic disorders such as multiple sclerosis, cerebral palsy, and spinal cord injury. It is believed to act by blocking the intracellular release of calcium needed for contraction of skeletal muscle fibers. Such activity also accounts for its major side effect of muscle weakness which may result in slurring of speech, drooling, difficulty in swallowing, choking, and enuresis. Since dantrolene may cause severe liver toxicity, liver function should be monitored. Dantrolene is also contraindicated in patients with a history of liver disease.

OTHER MEDICAL CONDITIONS AND DRUG THERAPIES

Physical therapy patients not only receive drugs specific for pain and inflammation but, like the general population, receive drugs specific for other medical conditions as well. Examples include chronic cardiovascular diseases, such as hypertension and congestive heart failure, or certain psychiatric disorders, such as anxiety, depression, or schizophrenia. An understanding of the action and side effects of the drugs used to treat these medical conditions will prepare physical

therapists to evaluate the progress of the therapy they are administering, as well as detect any problems associated with such drug therapy. The concluding portion of this chapter presents a discussion of drug therapies employed to treat common cardiovascular disorders, such as hypertension, congestive heart failure, and angina; psychiatric disorders, such as anxiety, depression, and schizophrenia; neurologic disorders, such as epilepsy; and common medical conditions, such as peptic ulcer disease and asthma.

Cardiovascular Diseases

Hypertension

Hypertension is the most common chronic medical condition, with a prevalence rate of 20 percent among whites and 30 percent among blacks in the United States (in the over 65-year-old population, these rates are 40 percent and 50 percent, respectively). Hypertension has been defined as a systolic blood pressure greater than 140 mmHg or a diastolic blood pressure greater than 90 mmHg, or both. Since blood pressure can vary episodically, three measurements and a thorough medical evaluation should be made before the diagnosis of hypertension is made. Once diagnosed, hypertension should be treated, as it is a major cause of heart failure, kidney failure, stroke, and death.

Management of hypertension has undergone considerable change since 1973, when the National Heart, Lung, and Blood Institute issued their first guidelines. Several new agents have since been introduced that have made obsolete the first-time use of some of the earlier agents.

In 1988 the Joint National Committee on Detection, Evaluation, and Treatment of High Blood Pressure issued its latest recommendations on treating hypertension (JNC IV). In contrast to previous reports, greater emphasis is placed on the use of nonpharmacologic means to control hypertension, such as weight control and sodium, fat, and alcohol restrictions. If these approaches fail after 3 to 6 months (which occurs in 75 percent of cases), pharmacologic means are recommended. Reflecting the availability of new agents introduced in the 1980, JNC IV has recommended four classes of drugs as first-line therapy for hypertension:

Table 12-8. First-Line Therapy for Hypertension

Class/Example[a]	Usual Dose for Treating Hypertension
Diuretics	
Thiazide	
Hydrochlorothiazide	25–50 mg qd
Loop	
Furosemide (Lasix)	40 mg qd
Potassium sparing (triamterene combined with hydrochlorothiazide) in Dyazide and Maxzide	bid, qd
β-Blockers	
Acebutolol (Sectral)	200 mg bid
Atenolol (Tenormin)	50 mg qd
Betaxolol (Kerlone)	10 mg qd
Carteolol (Cartrol)	2.5–5 mg qd
Labetalol (Trondate, Normodyne)	200 mg bid
Metoprolol (Lopressor)	50 mg bid
Nadolol (Corgard)	40–80 mg qd
Penbutolol (Levatol)	20 mg qd
Pindolol (Visken)	5 mg bid
Propranolol (Inderal)	120–240 mg/day in individual doses
Timolol (Blocadren)	10 mg bid
ACE inhibitors	
Captopril (Capoten)	25–50 mg bid, tid
Enalapril (Vasotec)	10–40 mg qd in divided doses
Lisinopril (Prinivil, Zestril)	10–40 mg qd
Ramipril (Altace)	2.5–20 mg qd in individual doses
Calcium-channel blockers (useful for treating hypertension)	
Diltizem (Cardiem SR)	60–120 mg bid
Nifedipine (Procardia XL)	30–60 mg qd
Nicardipine (Cardene)	20–40 mg tid
Verapamil (Isoptin SR)	240 mg qd

[a] Brand names are given in parentheses.

diuretics, β-blockers, angiotensin-converting enzyme inhibitors, and calcium-channel blockers (see Table 12-8). Selection of one drug over another should be individualized and should take into consideration the special features of that drug that make it useful for that patient. Older patients seem to respond better to diuretics than do younger patients. Whites appear to respond better to β-blockers than blacks. β-blockers would not be a drug of choice for patients with diabetes, asthma, or peripheral vascular disease.

Diuretics

Diuretics reduce blood pressure initially by causing sodium and water loss. In the long run, diuretics reduce peripheral vascular resistance by a still unknown mechanism. Diuretics such as hydrochlorothiazide are inexpensive, convenient (once-a-day dosing), and effective for a large number of patients, especially in the elderly and among blacks; 40 to 70 percent of all hypertensive patients attain adequate control of their blood pressure with diuretics alone.

Diuretics can also cause potassium loss, which may be manifested by symptoms of muscle weakness, fatigue, and muscle cramps. A more serious, but fortunately rare, consequence of diuretic-induced hypokalemia is ventricular irritability, which may lead to ventricular ectopy or sudden death. Attempts to avoid hypokalemia include supplementation of potassium and/or reduction of sodium in the diet and the use of potassium-sparing diuretics along with or in combination with a potassium-depleting diuretic. Dyazide (hydrochlorothiazide/triamterene) and Maxzide are popular combination diuretics.

Other adverse reactions to both thiazide and loop diuretics (e.g., furosemide) include increases in both serum uric acid concentration (which may manifest itself in gouty arthritis) and serum glucose concentration (which may precipitate the onset of diabetes in certain patients).

β-Blockers

An alternative first-line class of drugs useful in treating hypertension are the β-adrenergic blocking agents, or β-blockers. β-Blockers are as effective as diuretics in lowering blood pressure, and most can be given in once-a-day or twice-a-day dosing. Although several mechanisms have been proposed for the activity of these agents, none has been consistently associated with a reduction in blood pressure.

Although 11 oral β-blockers are available in the United States, clinical differences among them appear nonexistent. Several agents are promoted as cardioselective, that is, β-receptors in the heart are blocked, whereas β-receptors in the lungs, kidneys, and arterioles are spared. Such cardioselectivity is not absolute, however, and at higher doses bronchospasm and arteriolar constriction can occur. Other agents are promoted as being less likely to penetrate the CNS, with less likelihood of causing CNS side effects, such as fatigue and insomnia. Good clinical data substantiating these claims have not been forthcoming.

Adverse side effects of β-blockers result from blockade of β-receptors and include bradycardia, bronchospasm, wheezing, fatigue, decreased exercise tolerance, insomnia, sexual dysfunction, shortness of breath, claudication, weakness, and cold extremities. β-Blockers should not be given to patients with pulmonary disease, peripheral vascular disease, diabetes, or congestive heart failure, as these conditions may be exacerbated by these agents. Patients predisposed to ischemic myocardial events should be tapered off β-blockers, as abrupt discontinuation may result in myocardial infarction or death.

ACE Inhibitors

An alternative first-line class of agents useful for treating hypertension are the angiotensin-converting enzyme (ACE) inhibitors. These agents block the enzyme responsible for converting angiotensin I to the extremely potent vasoconstrictive angiotensin II, a substance that also stimulates aldosterone secretion and sodium and water retention. Blockade of this enzyme also prevents the breakdown of the potent vasodilatory substance bradykinin. The end result of ACE inhibition is a reduction in peripheral vascular resistance.

Four ACE inhibitors are available in the United States. At the low doses used to treat hypertension, they are relatively free of adverse side effects. Eleven percent of patients receiving captopril (Capoten) develop a transient skin rash, and 6 percent a reversible loss of taste or a taste disturbance. The most worrisome side effect of ACE inhibitors has been neutropenia, agranulocytosis, and proteinuria. Fortunately, this side effect occurs rarely (in less than 1 percent of cases) and is most often associated with captopril. Enalapril (Vasotec) has been reported to cause primarily fatigue and headache; all ACE inhibitors have been associated with the development of a dry hacking cough, with an incidence as high as 15 percent. Despite these side effects and their relative expense, ACE inhibitors are becoming popular antihypertensive agents. They are also markedly effective and extremely popular in the treatment of congestive heart failure.

Calcium-Channel Blockers

The fourth class of first-line drugs useful in treating hypertension are the calcium-channel blockers. Calcium-channel blockers block the influx of calcium into the smooth muscle cells lining arteriolar walls, so that these muscle cells are unable to contract and produce vasoconstriction. Calcium-channel blockers also block the influx of calcium into cardiac muscle cells, thereby blocking contraction of cardiac muscle cells. The sites and intensity of action of the seven calcium-channel blockers available in the United States vary. Bepridil is a recently introduced calcium-channel blocker that, because of its toxicity, is reserved for treating angina in patients who are nonresponsive or intolerant to other antianginal agents. Verapamil and diltiazem have a more pronounced effect on cardiac contractility and are often used to treat cardiac disorders such as angina and arrhythmias. Nifedipine and nicardipine are potent peripheral vasodilators that may cause a reflex increase in heart rate and contractility. Nimodipine is a potent peripheral vasodilator with an affinity for cerebral vessels that makes it useful for treating acute stroke victims. Calcium-channel blockers are effective in treating mild to moderate hypertension, and FDA approval is available for verapamil, nicardipine, and sustained-release diltiazem and nifedipine.

The side effects of the various calcium-channel blockers reflect their mechanism of action. Verapamil and iltiazem are more likely to cause cardiac abnormalies, such as bradycardia, atrioventricular (AV) block, nd congestive heart failure. Both agents can also cause norexia, nausea, peripheral edema, and hypotension. Constipation occurs with verapamil, sometimes severe nough to necessitate surgery for fecal impaction.

ide effects related to the peripheral vasodilating properties of the vasodilating calcium-channel blockrs include headache, flushing, dizziness, ankle dema, hypotension, nausea, and tachycardia. Reflex achycardia is usually not a problem with long-term se, except in patients with ischemic heart disease. Other side effects often subside with continued use of hese agents.

Despite their high cost, calcium-channel blockers are becoming popular agents for treating hypertension, cardiac arrhythmias, angina, and other medical conditions (e.g., migraines).

Many other agents are available to treat hypertension, although none is considered a first-line choice. If an additional agent is needed (and 70 percent of patients will require one), an alternative first-line agent is usually selected. Other antihypertensive agents include those that act centrally to decrease sympathetic outflow (methyldopa, guanabenz, guanfacine) and/or peripherally (clonidine), direct-acting arterial vasodilators (hydralazine, minoxidil), and peripheral indirect-acting vasodilators (prazosin, terazosin). All are effective antihypertensive agents, but their noticeable side effect profile has substantially limited their clinical value.

Congestive Heart Failure

Congestive heart failure (CHF) has rapidly become one of the most important health problems in the United States. An estimated four million Americans have chronic CHF, and its incidence more than doubles each decade from age 45 to 75. CHF is the most common discharge diagnosis for patients over 65 years of age and is the most prevalent cause of death in hospitalized patients.

CHF results from a failure of the heart to pump blood to meet the body's needs. In normal patients, approx-

Table 12-9. Symptoms Associated with Heart Failure

Left-Sided Failure	Right-Sided Failure
Cardiomegaly	Anorexia
Cough	Abdominal discomfort
Dyspnea on exertion	Hepatojugular reflex
Paroxysmal nocturnal orthopnea	Jugular venous distention
Pleural effusions	Nocturia
Tachypnea	Edema
Wheezing	Weight gain

imately 60 percent of the blood presented to the ventricles is ejected during contraction. In CHF patients, the figure is 10 to 20 percent. Several factors may account for this reduced ejection fraction: (1) too much blood presented to the ventricles (preload); (2) too much pressure working against the ventricles (e.g., hypertension (afterload); or (3) a damaged myocardium, most commonly as a result of coronary artery disease. Hypertension is a major factor in CHF, and cardiac disease is the primary cause.

As a result of decreased perfusion to the kidneys, renin is released, angiotensin is formed, and sodium and water retention occurs. If the right ventricle is failing, fluid backs up in the veins, manifesting symptoms of right-sided failure. If the left ventricle is failing, fluid backs up into the lungs, manifesting symptoms of left-sided failure (Table 12-9). CHF patients often show symptoms of both left-sided and right-sided failure. The goal of therapy in these patients is to abolish their disabling symptoms and improve their quality of life. In spite of aggressive pharmacologic treatment, the outcome for CHF patients is poor. In the Framingham study, 60 percent of men and 40 percent of women died within 5 years of the diagnosis of CHF.

Diuretics

The first class of drugs usually employed after sodium restriction fails to control the volume overload is the diuretics. Thiazide diuretics (e.g., hydrochlorothiazide) are good first choices for mobilizing fluid; if these agents fail, the more potent loop diuretics are employed (fuorsemide, bumetanide). Since the loop diuretics cause significant potassium loss, potassium levels should be followed, particularly because many CHF patients are also on digoxin, and low potassium levels predispose to serious digoxin toxicity. NSAIAs also interact with diuretics and interfere with their effectiveness. The side effects of diuretics are discussed under therapy for hypertension.

Digitalis Preparations

Digitalis preparations are often used when diuretics alone fail to arrest the symptoms of CHF. Digitalis inhibits the enzyme responsible for exchanging intracellular sodium for extracellular potassium, thus freeing up more sodium to be exchanged with calcium. Calcium enhances cardiac contractility, increasing both the force and rate of contraction. Digitalis also slows the ventricular rate of contraction, allowing more time for the ventricles to fill and thus increase cardiac output.

Digoxin is the most commonly prescribed digitalis preparation. It has one of the lowest therapeutic indices of any drug on the market. Its therapeutic serum level is approximately 1 to 2 ng/ml. Toxic symptoms may appear when levels exceed 2.5 ng/ml. It is estimated that approximately 20 percent of patients develop signs of toxicity while on digitalis, that rhythmic disturbances occur in up to 80 to 90 percent of digitalis toxic patients, and that up to 18 percent of these patients may die from these arrhythmias. Almost all known arrhythmias can occur with digoxin toxicity.

Noncardiac signs of digitalis toxicity include those relating to the GI tract and CNS. Noncardiac signs do not always precede cardiac signs of digitalis toxicity, and arrhythmias may present as the only toxic sign. For this reason, patients must be closely followed on digitalis preparations. Given the modest benefits attributed to digoxin and its considerable toxicity, some clinicians have elected to use vasodilators instead of digoxin as their second choice of treatment for CHF.

Vasodilators

Vasodilators are generally reserved for treatment if both diuretics and digoxin have failed in managing CHF. Vasodilators can be of three types: those that dilate arterial vessels (reduce afterload), those that dilate venous vessels (decrease preload), and those that do both. Calcium-channel blockers and hydralazine are examples of afterload reducers. Various forms of nitrates are available for preload reduction. ACE inhib-

Table 12-10. Drug Treatment for Congestive Heart Failure

Class	Side Effect
Diuretics	
Thiazide (HCTZ, chlorthalidone)	Weakness, fatigue, muscle cramps, GI symptoms, sexual dysfunction
Loop (furosemide, bumetaldine)	
Potassium-sparing (triamterene, amiloride)	
Digoxin	Cardiac (50% of adverse reactions) includes PVCs, ventricular tachycardia, AV dissociation, accelerated nodal rhythm, atrial tachycardia with block, AV block
	Gastrointestinal system (25% of adverse reactions) includes anorexia, nausea, vomiting
	Central nerve system (25% of adverse reactions) includes blurred/yellow vision, headaches, weakness, apathy, psychosis
Unloading agents	
Preload reducing (venous dilators)	Headache, flushing, dizziness, hypotension
Nitrates, topical, oral nitroglycerin, isosorbide	
Afterloading reducing (arterial dilators)	Headaches, flushing, nausea, vomiting, fluid retension, lupus-like syndrome
Hydralazine	
Calcium-channel blockers	Dizziness, lightheadedness, headache, edema, weakness, constipation with verapamil
Nifedipine, Nicardipene, Diltiazem, Verapamil	
Balanced vasodilators	Hypotension, rash, taste disturbances
ACE inhibitors	

Abbreviations: AV, atrioventricular; GI, gastrointestinal; PVCs, preventricular contractions.

itors and prazocin are examples of mixed or "balanced" vasodilators (Table 12-10).

There are certain drugs that are often overlooked causes or exacerbators of CHF. Cardiac drugs such as arrhythmic agents, β-blockers, and several calcium-channel blockers decrease cardiac contractility and cardiac output. Even topically applied β-blocking drugs (Timolol) have been implicated. NSAIAs also cause or exacerbate CHF as a result of sodium and water retention (some agents have increased blood volume by 50 percent in some cases). Salicylates, androgens, estrogens, and medicinals high in sodium also increase volume overload, thus producing the symptoms of CHF.

Angina

Coronary heart disease is the leading cause of death in the United States (30 percent of all deaths). It is often first manifested as symptoms of angina. These symptoms, such as substernal chest pain that sometimes radiates to the left arm, shoulder, or jaw, occur when cardiac work and myocardial oxygen demand exceed the ability of the coronary arteries to supply adequate oxygen. Myocardial oxygen demand depends on heart rate, myocardial contractility, degree of ventricular filling, and the force against which the ventricles must work to eject blood. Drugs that decrease any of these factors will reduce myocardial oxygen demand.

A major determinant of myocardial oxygen supply is the extent of coronal artery obstruction by atherosclerotic plaques. When obstruction of these arteries exceeds the 70 percent range, symptoms of angina begin to appear. Pharmacologic agents have been introduced on the market in an effort to lower serum cholesterol, a substance that appears to be a major component of these atherosclerotic plaques.

Three classes of drugs are used to correct the imbalance between myocardial oxygen supply and demand in angina patients. Nitrates cause smooth muscle relaxation of both the venous and, to a lesser extent, the arterial system. By reducing both the amount of blood the ventricle has to eject (because of its venous pooling) and the force against which it has to be ejected (because of its arterial dilation), nitrates reduce oxygen demand, therefore reducing symptoms. Nitrates are available in many forms (Table 12-11). Many are used prophylactically and a few to treat acute episodes.

β-Blockers decrease myocardial oxygen demand by decreasing heart rate, contractility, and blood pressure. β-Blockers complement the activity of nitrates by limiting the latter's reflex increase in heart rate. Nitrates offset the increase in left ventricular size induced by β-blockers. As mentioned under Hypertension, β-blockers should be gradually tapered if they are to be discontinued in patients with myocardial ischemia. Otherwise acute myocardial infarction and sudden cardiac death may result (i.e., β-blocker withdrawal syndrome).

The third class of agents used to treat angina are the calcium-channel blockers. Calcium-channel blockers differ in their ability to produce peripheral vasodilation (and the force against which the ventricles must work), decrease contractility, or slow conduction across the AV node. The overall effect will depend on which agent is used; the net result will be a reduction in cardiac work and myocardial oxygen demand. Calcium-channel blockers are particularly useful in treating angina resulting from vasospasms of the large coronary arteries. Patients with heart failure or cardiac condition disorders (e.g., bradycardia) should not be

Table 12-11. Nitrate Products

Drug	Strength	Example	Initial Dose
Isosorbide nitrate			
Sublingual	2.5, 5, 10 mg	Sorbitrate, Isordil	2.5–5 mg
Chewable	5, 10 mg	Sorbitrate, Isordil	
Oral tablets	5, 10, 20, 30, 40 mg	Sorbitrate, Isordil	5–20 mg qid
Oral (sustained-release capsules, tablets)	40 mg	Sorbitrate SA, Isordil Tembids	40 mg q8–12h
Nitroglycerin			
Sublingual	0.15, 0.3, 0.4, 0.6 mg	Nitrostat	0.3 mg
Translingual spray	0.4 mg/metered dose	Nitrolingual	0.4 mg
Transmucosal buccal controlled-release tablets	1, 2, 3 mg	Nitrogard	1 mg
Sustained-release tablets/capsules	2.5, 2.6, 6.5, 9 mg	Nitrobid	2.5 mg tid
Transdermal patches	2.5, 5., 7.5, 10, 15 mg	NitroDur II, Transderm-nitro	1 patch
Topical	2% in a lanolin-petroleum base	Nitroglycerin	½ inch

Table 12-12. Drugs Used in Hyperlipidemia

Drug[a]	Dosage	Side Effects
Cholestyramine (Questran)	4 g tid initially, 4 g qid to 6×/d maintenance	Constipation, abdominal pain, heartburn, flatulence, nausea
Colestipol (Colestid)	15–30 g QD given bid–qid	Constipation, nausea, flatulence
Niacin	0.25 g tid, increasing to 2.5 g tid w/meals	Flushing, uticaria, anorexia, hyperglycemia, peptic ulceration, jaundice, hyperurecemia
Probucol (Lorelco)	500 mg bid with meals	Diarrhea, flatulence, nausea
Gemlibrozil (Lopid)	600 mg bid	Hyperglycemia, nausea dizziness, skin rash
Lovastatin (Mevacor)	5–40 mg bid	Headache, insomnia

[a] Brand names are given in parentheses.

given calcium-channel blockers because of the negative effects of these agents on cardiac contractility.

Another attempt at reducing the risk of developing angina has been to combine drugs with diet in an attempt to lower plasma cholesterol. A 15 percent decrease in cholesterol levels has been associated with a 30 percent reduction in the risk of developing coronary heart disease. If diet modification and other non-pharmacologic measures (e.g., weight control, smoking cessation, exercise) fail, drug therapy with one of the cholesterol-lowering drugs may be appropriate (Table 12-12).

Arrhythmias

Antiarrhythmic agents are used to treat and prevent abnormalities in the rate and rhythm of heart contractions that may impair the ability of the heart to function efficiently as a pump. Antiarrhythmic agents have been classified by Vaughn Williams into four types on the basis of their effects on the electrophysiologic properties of cardiac cells. Class I agents are local anesthetics that depress the initial phase of a cardiac cells generation of an electrical impulse. Class II agents are β-blockers that slow down the sinus rate,

depress contractility, and slow down the conduction of impulses between the atria and the ventricles. Class III agents markedly prolong the period during which a cardiac cell cannot be restimulated. Class IV agents are calcium-channel blockers that slow activity calcium-dependent cells on the SA and AV nodes. Selection of an antiarrhythmic agent depends on both the pathology of the arrhythmia and the effects of the drug, both of which are highly variable. Selection of an individual agent is thus largely empirical. See Table 12-13 for a list of these antiarrhythmic agents.

Quinidine is the most widely used oral Class I agent and is used for treating both supraventricular and ventricular arrhythmias. Quinidine is used orally to prevent the progression of ventricular tachycardia into serious ventricular arrhythmias that can lead to sudden cardiac death. GI effects occur often (30 percent) with quinidine (nausea, vomiting, diarrhea); resulting in discontinuation of therapy in up to 10 percent of patients. A sustained-release product taken with meals minimizes these effects, as well as substitution of a different salt of quinidine. Symptoms of *cinchonism* (e.g., tinnitus, blurred vision, headache), as well as serious arrhythmias and hypotension (quinidine syncope), can occur if blood levels are exceeded.

Table 12-13. Oral Antiarrhythmic Agents

Group	Example[a]	Usage Dosage
IA	Quinidine	200–300 mg tid–qid
	Procainamide	50 mg/kg/day in divided doses q6h
	Disopyramide (Norpace)	400–800 mg qd in divided doses
IB	Tocainide (Tonocard)	1,200–1,800 mg in divided doses tid
	Mexiletine (Mexitil)	200–300 mg q8h
IC	Encainide (Enkaid)	25–50 mg tid
	Flecainide (Tambocor)	100 mg q12h
II	Propranolol	10–30 mg tid–qid
III	Amiodarone (Cordarone)	(Maintenance dose) 400 mg qd
IV	Verapamil	240–320 mg in divided doses (for arterial fibrillation) 240–480 mg in divided doses (for PSVT)

[a] Brand names are given in parentheses.

Procainamide is an alternative oral Class I agent with effects on the heart very similar to those with quinidine. GI effects occur less frequently with procainamide, as does the development of serious arrhythmias. Up to 30 percent of patients treated chronically with procainamide may develop a syndrome resembling systemic lupus erythamatosus (e.g., fever, rash, myalgia, arthritis) that resolves upon discontinuing the agent.

A third oral Class I agent reserved for patients unable to tolerate or respond to quinidine or procainamide is disopyramide. Disopyramide frequently produces anticholinergic symptoms, such as dry mouth (40 percent), blurred vision (28 percent), urinary retention (10 to 20 percent), and constipation (30 percent). Disopyramide has a potent depressant effect on cardiac contractility that can lead to heart failure.

Two oral formulations similar to lidocaine are tocainide and mexiletine. Both are considered equivalent in treating and preventing ventricular arrhythmias. Side effects are similar with each agent and are mainly gastrointestinal (30 to 40 percent) and neurologic (10 to 20 percent).

Encainide and flecainide are two Class I agents reserved for serious arrhythmias that are unresponsive to other agents because of their ability to cause serious arrhythmias themselves (pro-arrhythmic effect).

β-Blockers block the effects of catecholamine-induced increases in cardiac contractility and heart rate. Patients with increased circulating levels of catecholamines (e.g., myocardial patients) often benefit from β-blockers, and β-blockers alone have been proved to reduce the risk of sudden cardiac death in these patients. For side effects of β-blockers, see the discussion on hypotension.

Amiodarone is an orally available Class III agent useful for treating both supraventricular and ventricular arrhythmias. Its toxicity is such that it is reserved only for life-threatening arrhythmias unresponsive to other agents.

Class IV antiarrhythmic agents include the calcium-channel blockers verapamil (the only FDA-approved

antiarrhythmic calcium-channel blocker) and diltiazem. Both are effective in treating supraventricular arrhythmias because of their depressant effect on the SA node. By delaying conduction through the AV node, calcium-channel blockers reduce the fast ventricular rate in atrial fibrillation and flutter and abolish tachyarrhythmias in paroxysmal supraventricular tachycardia. For side effects on calcium-channel blockers, see the discussion of hypotension.

Psychotrophic Drugs

Benzodiazepines

Benzodiazepines are among the most widely used class of drugs in the world. In the United States, 5 percent of all prescriptions filled are for a benzodiazepine. Of the 13 benzodiazepines available in the United States, eight are approved by the FDA, primarily for the treatment of anxiety, three for insomnia (Table 12-14). Such labeled indications do not reflect pharmacologic differences between these agents, but

Table 12-14. Benzodiazapines

Drug[a]	Usual Daily Dosage (mg)
Agents Used in Treatment of Generalized Anxiety Disorder	
Alprazolam (Xanax)	0.25–0.5 tid
Chlordiazeposide (Librium)	5–10 tid–qid
Clorazepate (Tranxene)	15–60 individual dose
Diazepam (Valium)	2–10 bid–qid
Halzepam (Paxipam)	20–40 tid–qid
Lorazepam (Ativan)	1 mg bid–tid
Oxazepam (Serax)	10–15 tid–qid
Pruzepam (Centrax)	20–60 individual doses
Agents Used in Treatment of Insomnia	
Flurazepam (Dalmane)	15–30 hs
Temazepam (Restoril)	15–30 mg hs
Triazolam (Halcion)	0.125–0.25 hs

[a] Brand names are given in parentheses.

rather marketing strategies of the manufacturers; the sedative flurazapam has anxiolytic properties, the anxiolytic diazepam is widely used as a sedative.

Benzodiazepines have anxiolytic, sedative, anticonvulsant, and muscle relaxant properties. These actions occur as a result of an enhancement of the effects of a major inhibitory neurotransmitter in the CNS, γ-aminobutyric acid (GABA). GABA is the most important inhibitory neurotransmitter in the CNS and is involved in nerve transmission of nearly one-third of brain impulses. Although pharmacologically similar, benzodiazepines differ in their approved indications and their pharmacokinetic properties. Selection of an agent for anxiety or sedation will depend on the onset and duration of the desired agent.

Anti-depressants

Depression severe enough to warrant medical attention is fairly common in our society, with a lifetime prevalence estimated to be about 15 percent (10 percent in males, 20 percent in females). Depression is highly amendable to drug treatment (80 to 90 percent success rate with careful monitoring). Unfortunately, one study indicates only one in 10 depressed patients receives adequate doses of antidepressants. Conservative estimates associate 16,000 suicides annually in the United States with depressive disorders.

Three classes of drugs are available for treating unipolar depression: traditional TCAs, newer antidepressants such as fluoxetine and trazadone, and monoamine oxidase inhibitors (MAOIs). All three classes are considered efficacious in treating depression; some of the newer agents have a more favorable side effect profile than that of the older agents, and the MAOIs may be more effective in treating depression with atypical symptoms.

Mechanism of Action

The proposed mechanism of action of antidepressants has recently undergone revision. Originally it was proposed that a deficiency of the neurotransmitters norepinephrine and serotonin on the synapses of the CNS accounted for the depressive state. By blocking their uptake, it was proposed that antidepressants increased their concentration, and thus neurotransmission. Since antidepressant activity often lags several weeks after this blockade, and since certain other antidepressants do not produce such blockade, it was subsequently proposed that changes in receptor sensitivity to these neurotransmitters (observed with long-term use of antidepressant therapy) accounted for the antidepressant activity of these agents. The recently proposed dysregulation hypothesis suggests that antidepressants correct the dysregulation of neuronal firing associated with the depressive state by allowing more norepinephrine to be released per impulse, with more effective neurotransmission.

Tricyclic Antidepressants

The TCAs are the oldest and most commonly used antidepressants. These agents commonly produce anticholinergic, neurologic, and cardiovascular adverse reactions. Anticholinergic effects occur most frequently and include dry mouth, blurred vision, constipation, and urinary hesitancy. Occasionally, more severe reactions, such as urinary retention, paralytic ileus, and acute glaucoma, also occur. Elderly patients are susceptible to a central anticholinergic syndrome characterized by confusion, disorientation, delusions, and hallucinations.

Sedation is the most common neurologic effect, with some agents less likely to cause this effect than others (Table 12-15). These agents also lower the seizure threshold. Seizures have occurred in patients started on antidepressants.

The most common serious side effects associated with TCAs are cardiovascular with a quinidine-like effect on cardiac condition. In patients with pre-existing defects in cardiac conduction and in overdoses, fatal arrhythmias can occur. Postural hypotension is another cardiovascular effect of the TCAs that often occurs early in therapy, and especially in the elderly. Certain TCAs are more likely to produce this effect than others.

Tricyclic antidepressants are extremely dangerous drugs when taken in overdose. In the United States they follow alcohol, sedatives, and narcotics in causing death due to drug overdosing.

Table 12-15. Comparison of Antidepressants

Drug[a]	Daily Dosage Range (mg)	Side Effect Frequency	
		Sedative	Anti-cholinergic
Tricyclic Agents			
Amitriptyline (Elavil)	75–300	VH	VH
Clomipramine (Anafranil)	250 maximum	H	H
Doxepin (Sinequan)	75–300	H	M
Desipramine (Norpramin)	75–300	S	S
Imipramine (Tofranil)	75–300	M	M
Nortriptyline (Pamelor)	50–200	M	M
Protriptyline (Vivactil)	15–60	S	H
Trimipramine (Surmontil)	75–300	H	M
Newer Agents			
Maprotiline (Ludiomil)	150–300	M	M
Amoxapine (Ascendin)	100–600	M	H
Trazadone (Desyrel)	50–600	M	S
Fluoxetine (Prozac)	20–80	None	S
Bupropion (Weelbutrin)	225–450	M	M

Abbreviations: VH, very high; H, high; M, moderate; S, slight.
[a] Brand names are given in parentheses.

Newer Antidepressants

The newer antidepressants include amoxapine, maprotiline, trazodone, bupropion, and fluoxetine. Overall, their clinical effectiveness is equivalent to that of the TCAs, although their side effect profiles often differ. Amoxapine is a derivative of the antipsychotic loxapine and shares many of the adverse side effects associated with the antipsychotic agents (see under Antipsychotic Agents in this chapter), in addition to those of traditional TCAs. Maprotiline shares side effects similar to those of TCAs, with a greater incidence of seizures in an overdose situation. Trazodone causes less anticholinergic and cardiac conduction side effects than do the TCAs but is similar to several TCAs in causing sedation and postural hypotension. Two newer antidepressants that have minimal anticholinergic and cardiovascular side effects are bupropion and fluoxetine. Both agents are more likely to have a stimulant, rather than a depressant, effect on the CNS, with occasional occurrences of anxiety and insomnia.

Monoamine Oxidase Inhibitors

A third class of antidepressants useful in patients refractory to, or intolerant of, other classes of antidepressants are the MAOIs. These agents are also useful in patients with atypical depression or in those with certain phobic disorders. Postural hypotension, sexual dysfunction (e.g., delayed ejaculation and inhibition of orgasm), and weight gain are common adverse side effects of MAOIs. Weight gain is related to a craving for carbohydrates and is sometimes indicative of a therapeutic response.

A rare but potentially fatal adverse reaction of MAOIs is hypertensive crisis, which occurs when these agents are taken concurrently with certain foods or drugs, especially those high in tyramine (Table 12-16).

Lithium

An agent useful in treating bipolar disorder (manic-depressive illness) is lithium. Bipolar patients experience periods of mood elevation that alternate with normal mood states. Depression often (but not always) occurs in these patients. Lithium is 60 to 80 percent effective in aborting acute episodes of mania after 1 to 2 weeks of treatment and is 80 percent effective in preventing recurrences of such episodes. According to one theory, lithium acts either by enhancing the uptake or by reducing the release of neurotransmitters in the synaptic cleft throughout the CNS, or by both.

Table 12-16. Food and OTC Drugs to Be Avoided by Patients on MAOI

Aged, matured cheeses (e.g., cheddar, camembert)

Smoked or pickled meats, fishes (e.g., herring, sausages)

Yeast extracts (Brewer's yeast)

Red wines (e.g., Chianti, burgundy, sherry)

Cold, hayfever, or weight-reduction preparations containing:
  Phenylpropranolamine
  Ephedrine
  Phenylephrine
  Pseudoephedrine

Abbreviations: MAOI, monoamine oxidase inhibitor; OTC, over-the-counter.

Side effects of lithium involve the GI tract, the CNS, and the kidneys. During initial therapy, up to 30 percent of patients will experience GI side effects, such as nausea, vomiting, diarrhea, and anorexia. If these side effects reappear during therapy, excessive lithium levels should be suspected.

Lithium often produces CNS and neuromuscular effects, including muscle weakness (30 percent of patients) and a fine hand tremor (50 percent of patients). These effects occur at therapeutic doses but usually subside with continued use. Four percent of patients continue to have an action tremor that can be managed by lowering the dose of lithium or using β-blockers. Neurologic symptoms, such as coarse tremors, stuttering, myoclonic jerking, and seizures, occur with lithium toxicity.

Fifty percent of patients begun on lithium therapy experience a diabetes insipidus-like syndrome characterized by a mild polyuria and polydipsia caused by an inhibition of antidiuretic hormone in the kidney. Dosage reduction or the use of sustained released tablets diminishes these effects. Other side effects of lithium include hypothyroidism, weight gain, cardiac conduction effects, and dermatologic reactions.

Neuroleptic Agents

A class of drugs taken by physical therapy patients with a diagnosis of schizophrenia are neuroleptic agents, otherwise known as antipsychotic agents or major tranquilizers. Neuroleptic agents diminish the outward symptoms of schizophrenia; they do not cure the disorder, and often patients have to be on these drugs for life. Neuroleptic agents appear to act by inhibiting the neurotransmitter dopamine in various portions of the brain. The agent clozapine (Clozaril), however, appears to act by a different mechanism. Neuroleptic agents can be divided into two types: low potency and high potency (Table 12-17). Low-potency agents such as chlorpromazine (Thorazine) and thioridazine (Mellaril) are associated with a high incidence of sedation, orthostatic hypotension, and anticholinergic side effects (e.g., dry mouth, urinary retention, constipation). High-potency agents such as haloperidol (Haldol) and fluphenazine (Prolixin) generally lack these side effects but, in contrast to the low-potency agents, have

Table 12-17. Comparison of Neuroleptic Agents

Drug	Usual Oral Dosage Range (mg)	Frequency of Side Effects			
		*	**	***	****
Low potency					
Chlorpromazine (Thorazine)	200–1,200	H	H	H	M
Thioridazine (Mellaril)	150–800	H	L	H	VH
Clozapine (Clozaril)	300–450	H	H	M	L
High potency					
Ioxapine (Loxitane)	20–250	M	M	M	H
Perphenazine (Trilafon)	16–64	M	M	M	H
Trifluoperazine (Stelazine)	10–60	M	M	M	H
Thiothixene (Navane)	10–80	M	M	M	H
Molindone (Moban)	20–225	M	M	M	H
Fluphenazine (Prolixin)	5–60	M	M	M	VH
Haloperidol (Haldol)	10–100	L	L	L	VH

Abbreviations: *, sedation; **, anticholinergic; ***, orthostatic hypotension; ****, acute extrapyramidal effects. VH, very high; H, high; M, moderate; L, low.

a high incidence of extrapyramidal reactions as a result of their dopamine-blocking properties in the substantia nigra of the brain (Table 12-18). Three of these common reactions occur early in therapy (Table 12-19) and are often controlled with anticholinergic agents such as benztropine (Cogentin), antihistamines such as diphenhydramine (Benadryl), or dopamine-enhancing agents such as amantadine (Symmetrel). These reactions are by and large reversible. Tardive dyskinesia, the fourth extrapyramidal reaction, usually occurs months to years after therapy has started and is often irreversible. There is no effective treatment for tardive dyskinesia; thus, it is imperative that neuroleptic agents be used only to treat psychosis in the smallest effective dose for the shortest period of time. Daily use of haloperidol as a minor tranquilizer is not an acceptable use of the drug.

Medical attention is warranted if patients develop abnormal tongue or finger movements while on neuroleptic agents. Often tardive dyskinesia develops

Table 12-18. Side Effects of Neuroleptic Agents

Anticholinergic
    Dry mouth
    Constipation
    Nasal dryness
    Dry skin
    Urinary hesitancy/retention
    Tachycardia
    Blurred vision
    Inhibition of ejaculation

Extrapyramidal
    Acute dystonias
        Oculogyric crisis
        Trismus
        Opisthotonus
        Torticollis
    Akathisia
        Subjective desire to be in constant motion
    Pseudoparkinsonism
        Pill-rolling movements of hands
        Slowing of body movements
        Masklike facies
        Cogwheeling of extremities
        Stiffness
        Stopped, shuffling gait
        Postural instability
        Festinating gait
        Salivary drooling
    Tardive dyskinesia

Sedation

Orthostatic hypotension

Table 12-19. Extrapyramidal Reactions Associated with Neuroleptic Agents

Reversible
    Acute dystonias (e.g., torticollis, retrocollis, opisthotonos, oculogyric crisis, laryngospasm)
    Akathisia (subjective desire to be in constant motion, manifested by patient's constant pacing or inability to sit still
    Parkinsonism (e.g., shuffling gait, difficulty with starting-and-stopping movement, bradykinesia, muscular rigidity, masked facies, tremor, postural instability, drooling)

Possibly irreversible
    Tardive dyskinesia—manifesting often as abnormal movements of the face (e.g., tremor of upper lip—rabbit syndrome, tongue protrusion, fly-catching syndrome), buccal (pressing of tongue, bon-bon sign), neck (retrocollis, torticollis), trunk (axial hyperkinesia, athetoid movements), extremities (chorea of hands or toes, athetosis, ballistic movements), grunting, vocalizations, and other symptoms

slowly with mild tongue movements. Later, manifestations of the reaction include lip smacking, puckering, sucking lip movements, jaw movements, protrusion of the tongue (flycatcher tongue), and difficulty swallowing. Blinking, grimacing, and arching of the eyebrows also often occur. In severe cases, these involuntary movements of the reaction can involve the extremities, causing choreiform and other abnormal movements.

Epilepsy

Epilepsy is estimated to affect 0.05 to 1 percent of the general population. Physical therapists will occasionally encounter these patients in their practice. Although there are more than 30 different types of seizures, four major types predominate in this disorder. Partial seizures, both simple and complex, and generalized tonic-clonic (formerly known as grand mal) respond to four different types of antiepileptic drugs (AEDS). Absence seizures (formerly known as petit mal) respond to an agent that is ineffective for the other seizures, as well as to an agent that is effective for all the others.

Antiepileptic drugs control the manifestations of epilepsy; they do not cure the disorder. Nevertheless, after a seizure-free interval, many patients can be slowly taken off these agents. AEDs act either by increasing the seizure threshold through a decrease in brain cell excitability or by limiting the spread of seizure discharge in the brain (through a slowing down of nerve cell electrical transmission). Some agents appear to stimulate an inhibitory pathway by increasing the brain concentration of GABA, an inhibitory neurotransmitter.

In the United States, five primary AEDs are available to treat these four major seizure disorders. One of them, phenytoin (Dilantin) has been among the top 25 most prescribed drugs for years. Another agent, valproate (Depakene, Depakote) is the most prescribed AED in Europe, partly because of its effectiveness in treating all major seizure disorders. A third agent, carbamazepine (Tegretol) was originally introduced on the market for the treatment of trigeminal neuralgia but is gaining increased popularity because of its effectiveness and relatively low toxicity in treating most major adult seizure disorders. A fourth agent, ethosuximide, is useful only for treating absence seizures that commonly affect children. Phenobarbital and primidone (Mysoline) are the fifth type of AED available and are considered together because prinidone is in part metabolized to phenobarbitol (see Table 12-20 for a list of AEDs).

Peptic Ulcer Disease

An estimated 15 to 20 percent of all Americans will develop peptic ulcer disease in their lifetime. The most frequently occurring ulcers are duodenal and gastric, and many physical therapy patients will be taking agents either to treat or to prevent recurrence of these ulcers. Other physical therapy patients will be taking a class of these agents (the H_2 antagonists) as treatment for gastroesophageal reflux disease.

Antacids have traditionally been the mainstay of therapy for the treatment of peptic ulcer disease but, because of their often unacceptable side effects (e.g., 27 percent incidence of diarrhea) and inconvenience (multidose per day regimen), they have been replaced by the H_2 antagonists and by sucralfate. H_2 antagonists act by binding to H_2 receptors on the parietal cell of the GI tract, blocking the release of gastric acid by these cells. In the United States four H_2 antagonists are

available, most of which have FDA-approved indications for treatment and maintenance of duodenal ulcer, as well as treatment of benign gastric ulcer. Nizatidine does not have FDA approval for treating the latter condition and ranitidine, unlike the other three, has FDA approval for treating gastroesophageal reflux disease (Table 12-21). Nevertheless, all four agents are probably equally efficacious in treating these conditions.

In treating peptic ulcer disease, any of these agents can be administered as a single nighttime dose, when acid secretion is highest. Food does not interfere with the absorption of these agents, so they may be taken without regard to meals. Antacids, however, interfere with absorption and should be taken 30 minutes to 1 hour apart from these agents.

H_2 antagonists are relatively free of adverse side effects. The overall incidence of adverse effects with cimetidine is 4 to 5 percent, mostly affecting the GI tract (2.1 percent) and CNS (1.2 percent). In elderly patients and in patients with kidney and liver dysfunction, more severe CNS adverse effects have occasionally been reported (e.g., confusion, agitation, hallucinations); in patients on high-dose long-term therapy with the agent, gynecomastia has developed.

Ranitidine is similar to cimetidine in its side effect

Table 12-20. Comparison of AEDs

Drug[a]	Dosage Range (mg)	Type Seizures Useful for	Side Effects
Ethosuximide (Zarontin)	250–500 qd	Absence	GI (e.g., nausea, vomiting) CNS (e.g., ataxia, drowsiness)
Phenytoin (Dilantin)	300–400 qd	Generalized tonic-clonic; simple and complex partial	CNS (e.g., nystagmus, ataxia) GI (e.g., nausea, vomiting) Gingival hyperplasia
Phenobarbital	50–100 bid–tid	Generalized tonic-clonic; simple and complex partial	CNS (e.g., drowsiness, lethargy)
Primidone (Mysoline)	125–500 tid–qid	Generalized tonic-clonic; simple and complex partial	CNS (e.g., ataxia, drowsiness) GI (e.g., nausea, vomiting)
Carbamazepine (Tegretol)	400–1,200 qd bid dosing	Generalized tonic-clonic; simple and complex partial	CNS (e.g., dizziness, drowsiness) GI (e.g., nausea, vomiting)
Valproic acid (Depakene, Depacote)	Maximum recommended dosage: 60 mg/kg/day	Absence, generalized tonic-clonic; simple and complex partial	GI (nausea, vomiting) CNS (drowsiness)

[a] Brand names are given in parentheses.
Abbreviations: CNS, central nervous system; GI, gastrointestinal.

Table 12-21. Dosing Guidelines for H$_2$-Antagonists

Drug[a]	Active Duodenal Ulcer (mg)	Healed Duodenal Ulcer (mg)	Active Benign Ulcer (mg)	Gastroesophageal Reflux (mg)
Cimetidine (Tagamet)	800 hs or 300 qid	400 hs	800 hs or 300 qid	Not currently indicated
Ranitidine (Zantac)	300 hs or 150 bid	150 hs	150 bid	150 bid
Famotidine (Pepcid)	40 hs or 20 bid	20 hs	40 hs	Not currently indicated
Nizatidine (Axid)	300 hs or 150 bid	150 hs	Not currently indicated	Not currently indicated

[a] Brand names are given in parentheses.

profile but, unlike cimetidine, does not cause gynecomastia. In addition, ranitidene does not appear to interact with the liver metabolism of drugs in the manner exhibited by cimetidine. Famotidine and nizatidine are relatively new H$_2$ antagonists. Little information is available on the side effect profile of these drugs. There is no reason to believe that their side effect profile will differ remarkably from that of the other agents. Famotidine causes muscle cramps, headaches, and constipation in up to 2 percent of patients.

Sucralfate is an aluminum salt of sulfated sucrose that forms a gel when exposed to the acid medium of the stomach. This gel serves to coat the ulcer and prevent backdiffusion of acid. Since sucralfate is not absorbable, side effects are rare (constipation in 2 percent; nausea, metallic taste, dry mouth in less than 1 percent). Drugs should not be coadministered with sucralfate, since binding with the agent may occur.

Oral Contraceptive Agents

Many physical therapy patients are taking oral contraceptive agents (OCAs); thus, it is important for the physical therapist to be familiar with how these agents work and what their minor and major adverse effects are. OCAs are available in two formulations: combination products containing both an estrogen and a progestin, and a product containing only a progestin, often known as the *minipill*. Combination products have undergone substantial changes since the first was introduced on the market in the United States in 1960. This product contained 200 mg of the progestin and 5,000 µg of the estrogen. Today's triphasic products

contain varying amounts of the progestin, all less than 1 mg and varying amounts of the estrogens, usually 30 to 40 µg. Reducing the amount of hormones in the agents has not reduced their effectiveness as contraceptive agents but has substantially reduced the incidence of adverse side effects.

Estrogens act as contraceptives by exerting a negative feedback effect in the female monthly cycle. The net result is suppression of ovulation and inhibition of implantation of a fertilized ovum. Progestins also exert a negative feedback effect on the monthly cycle, suppressing ovulation and creating an environment in the uterus that is harmful for implantation. When taken properly, oral contraceptives are extremely effective; the last observed failure rate for combination oral contraceptives is 0.5 percent; for progestin-only products, the lowest observed failure rate is 1 percent.

Side Effects

Most of the side effects of OCAs are dose related. The introduction of lower-dose agents has reduced the incidence of these side effects. Nausea is the most common adverse effect of OCAs; it can be minimized by taking the agent at bedtime. Taking the agent at bedtime can also reduce the risk of chloasma or facial hyperpigmentation that develops and can be exacerbated by exposure to sunlight when estrogen levels are high. Such symptoms as headache and breast tenderness are also helped by bedtime dosing. These effects, as well as the improvement in acne, are secondary effects of the estrogen component in combination formulations. Other CNS effects associated with oral contraceptives are dizziness, mental depression, lethargy, and decreased libido.

Cardiovascular effects are the most serious adverse effect of OCAs. Women using OCAs are to two to four times greater risk of the development of superficial or deep venous thrombosis and pulmonary embolism than are nonusers. Myocardial infarctions and strokes have also occurred more often in users than in nonusers, although most studies involved users of the older higher-estrogen-containing formulation. The risk of hypertension is also higher in users of older formulations of OCAs. It is infrequently encountered with the use of the newer agents. Lastly, there is an increased risk of subarachnoid hemorrhage in users of oral contraceptive users, particularly those who are hypertensive and who smoke.

Many of the cardiovascular risks associated with the estrogenic component of oral contraceptives can be avoided with the use of the progestin-only agent, or the minipill. In addition to being useful for nursing mothers (progestin is usually not present in breast milk), progestin-only pills avoid the estrogen-causing side effects, such as nausea, fluid retention, breast tenderness, headaches, chloasma, hypertension, and corneal edemas. Minipills, however, are less effective than combination products and must be taken every day. Irregular menses occur frequently, with some women having as few as two menstrual periods annually.

Patients on OCAs should memorize the mnemonic ACHES, the five early danger signs for patients on the pill, and should alert their physician if any of these symptoms appear.

Indications

Besides contraception, estrogens and progestins are often used to treat symptoms that some women experience during menopause. Approximately 75 to 85 percent of all women in their climacteric years will experience hot flushes (or hot flashes), characterized by a feeling of warmth in the chest, neck, and facial areas, often with visible red flushing. Other symptoms that may occur include headaches, dizziness, palpitations, nausea, vomiting, diaphoresis, and night sweats. Some women develop changes in the vagina that cause

---

Aches: Early Danger Signs of the Minipill

Abdominal pain (severe): may be sign of gallbladder disease, hepatic adenoma, pancreatitis, or blood clot

Chest pain (severe): may be indicative of a pulmonary embolism or myocardial infarction

Headache (severe): may be a sign of stroke or migraine headache

Eye problems, including blurred vision, flashing lights, or blindness, may be indications of hypertension or stroke

Severe leg pain, especially in the calves or thighs: may be indicative of venous thromboembolism

---

discomfort, especially during and after intercourse (atrophic vaginitis). Both symptoms are associated with declining estrogen levels and are responsive to estrogen therapy.

Estrogen products indicated for these two conditions include oral, transdermal, and topical formulations. Oral products, such as conjugated estrogens (Premarin) and transdermal estradiol (Estradiol), are usually administered cyclically (e.g., 3 out of 4 weeks), to avoid overstimulation of the uterus. Estradiol patches have the convenience of twice-weekly application. For atrophic vaginitis, the topical cream should be applied daily for 1 to 3 months, then intermittently, for relief of symptoms. In order to prevent overgrowth of the lining of the uterus (endometrium), progestins (e.g., medroxyproesterone, Provera) are often administered with estrogens for 10 days each month.

Another approved indication of estrogens is in the prevention of osteoporosis in postmenopausal women. Taking estrogens seems to slow down the bone loss that occurs in some postmenopausal women. A common schedule is 0.625 of conjugated estrogens administered daily for 3 out of 4 weeks.

Side Effects

Prolonged postmenopausal use of estrogens has been associated with an increased risk of the development of endometrial cancer. The coadministration of pro gestins during the last 10 days of the cycle has been shown to reduce the risk; nevertheless, any sign of vaginal bleeding warrants medical attention, as such bleeding could be an early sign of endometrial cancer. Postmenopausal use of estrogens has also been associated with an increased risk of gallbladder disease requiring surgery. These risks are explained more fully in the information sheets that pharmacists are obligated to dispense to patients with their prescriptions for estrogens and progestins.

Other side effects of estrogens include nausea, vomiting, weight gain, breast tenderness, and breast enlargement. The use of estrogens alone is associated with a dose-related risk of uterine bleeding; the addition of a progestin may increase this risk but also normalizes the bleeding pattern and reduces breakthrough bleeding. Progestins themselves may cause breakthrough bleeding, spotting, changes in menstrual flow, edema, weight gain or loss, mental depression, and many other side effects.

Asthma

Asthma is a chronic inflammatory condition of the airways that affects an estimated 10 million Americans. In contrast to other treatable diseases, the number of deaths caused by asthma appears to be increasing. Previously the focus of therapy for this disease was on its bronchoconstrictive component and on bronchodilating agents. New appreciation for the inflammatory component of the disease has led to an emphasis on the use of anti-inflammatory agents as prophylactic therapy, particularly the (inhaled) topical corticosteroids.

Although the mode of action of the inhaled corticosteroids is uncertain, these agents appear to act at various stages of the inflammatory process in asthma. Several formulations of inhaled corticosteroids are available in the United States (Table 12-22); all appear equally effective and in many cases can be given in twice-daily dosing. Occasionally, patients will require orally administered corticosteroids. The same precautions apply as in their chronic use in other inflammatory conditions (see under Corticosteroids). A somewhat less effective inhaled anti-inflammatory

agent is cromolyn sodium. It is particularly useful in children because of its negligible side effects.

For patients experiencing only occasional symptoms of wheezing, coughing, or difficulty in breathing, symptomatic treatment with an inhaled bronchodilator may be sufficient. Patients experiencing these symptoms in response to exercise may also benefit from prophylactic use of these agents. The largest category of inhaled bronchodilators are the β-agonists (antagonists?). All appear equally efficacious, and all are associated with minimal adverse side effects (Table 12-22).

An alternative, somewhat less effective, inhaled bronchodilating agent is the anticholinergic ipatropium bromide. Patients with chronic obstructive pulmonary disease may benefit more from the marginal improvement in bronchodilation provided by ipatropium.

An orally administered bronchodilatory agent that is widely used is theophylline. Theophylline is associated with several adverse side effects and interactions that may regulate its use to a third-line agent in the future. Although the bronchodilating activity of theophylline is weak, some patients benefit from its use. Theophylline is not effective as an inhalant and must be given by either the oral or intravenous route.

Diabetes

Of the 12 million Americans with diabetes, 10 percent are insulin dependent. The other 90 percent can usually be managed with diet, exercise, and oral hypoglycemic agents, although many of these patients require insulin as well. Insulin is available in three different strengths in the United States (U40, U100, U500) and in three different forms (short acting, intermediate acting, and long action) (Table 12-23). Human insulin produced through biosynthesis (recombinated DNA) or semisynthesis is probably less immunogenic than that obtained from beef or pork sources.

The goal of insulin therapy is to maintain normal blood glucose concentrations so as to avoid either hypoglycemic reactions (blood glucose less than 50 to 60 mg/dl) or symptoms of hyperglycemia (e.g., polyuria, pol-

Table 12-22. Antiasthmatic Agents

	Dosage	Dosage Range (Prophylaxis)
Anti-inflammatory agents		
Corticosteroid aerosols		
Beclomethasone (Beclovent, Vanceril)	2–3 puffs tid–qid	Throat irritation, hoarseness, dysphonia, coughing
Flunisolide (Aerobid)	2 puffs bid	
Triamcinolne (Azmacort)	2 puffs tid–qid	
Cromolyn sodium (Intal)	2 puffs qid	Rare
Bronchodilating agents		
Albuterol (Proventil, Ventolin)	2 puffs q4–6h	Rare with β_2-agonist inhalers
β_2-agonists (inhalers)		
Terbutaline (Brethaire)	2 puffs q4–6h	
Bitolterol (Tornalate)	2 puffs q8h	
Pirbuterol (Maxair)	2 puffs q4–6h	
β_2-agonists (oral)		
Albuterol (Proventil, Ventolin)	2–4 mg 16–8h	Tremor, tachycardia, palpitations
Terbutaline (Brethine)		
Anticholinergic agents (inhaler)		
Ipatropium (Atrovent)	2 puffs qid	Dryness of oropharynx, cough
Xanthine theophylline (Theo-Dur, Slo-phyllin)	Dosage must be individualized; maximum 900 mg qd in divided doses	Nausea, vomiting, palpitations, tachycardia, headache

ydipsia, fatigue). Studies are under way to determine whether insulin therapy will prevent or delay the complications of diabetes.

Insulin reactions occur when blood glucose levels are too low. These reactions usually appear suddenly and are most frequently caused by poor timing or by skipping meals, by extra exercise without additional food, and by the accidental administration of too much insulin. Symptoms include shakiness, nervousness, sweating, dizziness, tingling, irritability, and hunger. Insulin reactions should be treated immediately with a fast-acting carbohydrate (e.g., 5 ounces of regular soda such as Coke, 8 Lifesavers, 6 jelly beans) and by stopping all activity and resting for 10 to 15 minutes. Left untreated, insulin reactions can lead to convulsions and unconsciousness. In these cases, glucagon

should be administered or the patient should be taken promptly to the emergency department.

Any stress on the body, such as illness (e.g., common cold, flu), infection, injury, or emotional stress, can cause the release of several hormones that oppose the action of insulin. This state of insulin resistance cause the body to turn to body fat for an energy source. The subsequent formation of ketones combined with high blood glucose levels can lead to ketoacidosis, and possibly diabetic coma and death. Diabetic patients must be attentive to any illness or other situation associated with severe stress to the body. Any signs of dehydration or symptoms of ketoacidosis, such as nausea, stomach pain, vomiting, chest pain, rapid shallow breathing and difficulty staying awake, warrant immediate medical attention, as death would otherwise result.

For non-insulin-dependent diabetics, five oral hypo

Table 12-23. Comparison of Insulin Preparation

Insulin	Onset (hr)	Duration of Activity (hr)	Example
Short-acting			
Regular	$\frac{1}{2}$–1	5–7	Regular Iletin I, Novolix R, Humulin R
Semilente	1–2	12–16	Senilente
Intermediate-acting			
NPH	1–2	24	NPH, Humulin N, Novolin N
Lente	1–3	24	Lente, Humulin L, Novolin L
Long-acting			
PZ1	6–8	36	PZ1
Ultralente	6	36	Ultralente, Humulin U

glycemic agents are available for use after diet and exercise have failed to control high glucose levels (Table 12-24). These agents appear to make tissue cells more responsible to the hypoglycemic activity of the depressed levels of insulin in these patients. Duration of action and side effect profile account for the major differences among these agents. Tolbutamide (Orinase) is the shortest-acting sulfonylurea and must be dosed two or three times a day. Several of the other short-acting agents can be dosed once a day, with the exception of chlorpropamide. Side effects of the sulfonylureas are infrequent and mild. GI, dermatologic, and hypoglycemic reactions account for most of the adverse reactions. GI disturbances can generally be relieved by taking the agent at mealtime. Chlorpropamide causes a facial flushing reaction when alcohol

Table 12-24. Sulfonylureas Used to Control Blood Glucose

Drug[a]	Daily Dosage Range
Acetohexamide (Dymelor)	250 mg–1.5 g
Chlorpropamide (Diabense)	100 mg–250 mg
Tolazamide (Tolinase)	100 mg–3.0 g divided dose
Glipizide[b] (Glucotrol)	2.5–40 mg
Glyburide[b] (Diabeta, Micronase)	1.25–20 mg

[a] Brand names are given in parentheses.
[b] New agent.

is ingested in one-third of chloropramide-treated patients. Other adverse reactions to chlorpropamide include water retention and, because of its long duration of action, occasionally prolonged hypoglycemia.

CONCLUSION

Drug therapy often plays a role in the conservative care of patients seen by physical therapists. It may be a means to an end, as in an acutely inflamed joint and NSAIDs, or it may be "the cure," as in the case of diabetes mellitus and insulin. Medications may affect patients in many different ways and may therefore influence the therapist's examination findings, as well as the patient's response to treatment. These drugs (prescription and OTC) may resolve some symptoms while precipitating new ones (side effects). They are another variable to be considered in the puzzle of patient examination and treatment. Their role, actions, and side effects must be understood for all the "pieces" to fit. To be ignorant of the role played by drugs in the care of our patients can only handicap the clinician in being able to evaluate, treat, and manage patients to the best of our ability.

PATIENT CASE HISTORY 1

A 54-year-old woman is seen with the diagnosis of spondylolisthesis and a primary complaint of low back pain. Early in her treatment course, she was placed on Darvocet (opioid) for pain. Within several days, she was noted to have a flare-up of psoriasis on the arms and ankles, and upon questioning, a recent case of diarrhea. This information was passed on to the physician and the medication was discontinued. She was later placed on Motrin (NSAID). As physical therapy treatment progressed, she improved both subjectively and objectively, with her only complaint being an inability to sleep through the night, waking at about 3:00 A.M. with low back discomfort. She had been taking her evening dose of medication with dinner at approximately 5:00 P.M. When this was moved back to 9:00 P.M. with a snack, her final complaint of pain at night resolved.

PATIENT CASE HISTORY 2

A 48-year-old woman was seen with her primary complaint of right-sided low back and thigh pain, and a diagnosis of degenerative disc disease of the lumbar spine. Besides her mechanical lower back problem, it was noted upon initial examination that she was having respiratory problems as well. She stated that she had a history of respiratory infections. After her second physical therapy treatment, she returned several days later for her third visit and stated that all low back and leg symptoms were nearly gone. The initial thought was that this was secondary to therapy, but upon further questioning, she had recently started a course of prednisone (corticosteroid) for her respiratory problems.

PATIENT CASE HISTORY 3

A 42-year-old woman was seen for primary complaint of right shoulder pain. Upon questioning, it is learned from the patient that she has similar pain at the left shoulder, neck, and lower back, as well as a recent insidious onset of left knee pain and swelling. When questioned about medications, she stated that she takes only Tylenol (acetaminophen). The review of systems reveals a history of gastritis, easily irritated by aspirin or NSAIAs. After initial clinical examination, the patient was referred by physical therapy to a rheumatologist who was able to allay the patient's fears about medication for her condition and he placed her on a *controlled* trial of NSAIDs. In conjunction with physical therapy, all symptoms were soon alleviated without gastric upset.

Appendix 12-1

Review of Systems: Side Effects/ subjective complaints (in order of most common occurrence)

1. Gastrointestinal distress (dyspepsia, heartburn, nausea, vomiting, abdominal pain, constipation, diarrhea, bleeding)
   A. Salicylates
   B. NSAIDs
   C. Opioids
   D. Corticosteroids
   E. β-blockers
   F. Calcium-channel blockers
   G. Skeletal muscle relaxants
   H. Diuretics
   I. ACE inhibitors
   J. Digoxin
   K. Nitrates
   L. Cholesterol-lowering agents
   M. Antiarrhythmic agents
   N. Antidepressants (TCAs and MAOIs, lithium)
   O. Neuroleptics
   P. Antiepileptic Agents
   Q. OCAs (oral contraceptive agents)
   R. Estrogens and progestins
   S. Theophylline

2. Pulmonary (bronchospasm, shortness of breath, respiratory depression)
   A. Salicylates
   B. NSAIDs
   C. Opioids
   D. β-blockers
   E. ACE inhibitors

3. Central nervous system (dizziness, drowsiness, insomnia, headaches, hallucinations, confusion, anxiety, depression, muscle weakness)
   A. NSAIDs
   B. Skeletal muscle relaxants
   C. Opioids
   D. Corticosteroids
   E. β-blockers
   F. Calcium-channel blockers
   G. Nitrates
   H. ACE inhibitors
   I. Digoxin
   J. Antianxiety Agents
   K. Antidepressants (TCAs and MAOIs)
   L. Neuroleptics
   M. Antiepileptic agents
   N. OCAs
   O. Estrogens and progestins

4. Dermatologic (skin rash, itching, flushing of face)
   A. NSAIDs
   B. Corticosteroids
   C. β-blockers
   D. Opioids
   E. Calcium-channel blockers
   F. ACE inhibitors
   G. Nitrates
   H. Cholesterol-lowering agents
   I. Antiarrhythmic agents
   J. MAOIs and lithium
   K. OCAs
   L. Estrogens and progestins
   M. Antiepileptics

5. Musculoskeletal (weakness, fatigue, cramps, arthritis, decreased exercise tolerance, osteoporosis)
   A. Corticosteroids
   B. β-blockers
   C. Calcium-channel blockers
   D. ACE inhibitors
   E. Diuretics
   F. Digoxin
   G. Antianxiety agents
   H. Antiepileptic agents
   I. Antidepressants
   J. Neuroleptic agents

6. Cardiac (bradycardia, ventricular irritability, AV block, CHF, PVCs, ventricular tachycardia)
   A. Opioids
   B. Diuretics
   C. β-blockers
   D. Calcium-channel blockers
   E. Digoxin
   F. Antiarrhythmic agents
   G. TCAs
   H. Neuroleptics
   I. Oral antiasthmatic agents

7. Vascular (claudication, hypotension, peripheral edema, cold extremities)
   A. NSAIDs
   B. Corticosteroids
   C. Diuretics
   D. β-blockers
   E. Calcium-channel blockers
   F. ACE inhibitors
   G. Nitrates
   H. Antidepressants (TCAs and MAOIs)
   I. Neuroleptics
   J. OCAs
   K. Estrogens and progestins

8. Genitourinary (sexual dysfunction, urinary retention, urinary incontinence)
   A. Opioids
   B. Diuretics
   C. β-blockers
   D. Antiarrhythmic agents
   E. Antidepressants (TCAs and MAOIs)
   F. Neuroleptics
   G. OCAs
   H. Estrogens and progestins

9. HEENT (tinnitus, loss of taste, headache, lightheadedness, dizziness)
   A. Salicylates
   B. NSAIDs
   C. Opioids
   D. Skeletal muscle relaxants
   E. β blockers
   F. Nitrates
   G. Calcium-channel blockers
   H. ACE inhibitors
   I. Digoxin
   J. Antiarrhytmic agents
   K. Antianxiety agents
   L. Antidepressants (TCAs and MAOIs)
   M. Antiepileptic agents

Abbreviations: ACE, angiotensin-converting enzyme; MAOIs, monoamine oxidase inhibitors; NSAIDs, nonsteroid anti-inflammatory agents; NSAIDs, nonsteroid anti-inflammatory drugs; TCAs, tricyclic antidepressants.

13

Radiologic Assessment of the Musculoskeletal System

ROBERT D. KARL, JR., M.D.
JILL A. FLOBERG, P.T.

IMAGING ASSESSMENT IN PHYSICAL DIAGNOSIS

Diagnostic imaging supports, clarifies, and acts to confirm the findings from the physical therapist's history and neuromusculoskeletal physical examination. The intent of this chapter is to introduce physical therapists to the various imaging modalities available in current medical practice and to emphasize the use of imaging studies in the diagnosis and evaluation of the conditions more commonly encountered by physical therapists.

Before any imaging studies are considered, the emphasis must be on a complete history and physical and neurologic examinations. In current practice models, most physical therapy patients are seen by other health care practitioners before their referral to the physical therapist. In this practice model, the referring provider is responsible for arriving at the correct diagnosis before requesting physical therapy treatment. Increasingly, therapists receive referrals requesting evaluation and treatment, frequently without diagnostic information Physical therapists are also treating patients who do not have a referral from another health care practitioner. In this evolving practice model, physical therapists must take more complete patient histories, perform more complete physical and neurologic examinations, and decide which laboratory and radiologic tests, if any, are necessary to confirm the working clinical diagnosis before therapy is instituted. Equally important is the necessity to exclude pathologic and traumatic conditions that are not amenable to physical therapy.

This introduction is an overview of imaging studies normally used to assess the clinical problems encountered in daily practice. The major diagnostic imaging modalities, including their strengths and weaknesses, are highlighted. This discussion is followed by a description of anatomic regions, with suggestions for the most appropriate choices of imaging procedures for various clinical presentations.

Imaging assessment of the elbow, wrist, and hand is not included. These complex regions are undergoing rapid changes in imaging assessment algorithms and require a greater allotment of space than is available here. This chapter integrates an appropriate discussion of the cost-effectiveness of the various diagnostic imaging techniques, which is being ever more closely monitored by the various governmental and third-party agencies at all levels. Examples of imaging studies are presented to help the physical therapist put diagnostic imaging into a clinical perspective.

IMAGING MODALITIES AND BASIC CONCEPTS

Conventional Radiography

The production of x-rays occurs when a tungsten target (the anode) is bombarded with a beam of electrons. The resulting interaction of the tungsten and the electrons produces radiant energy that has a wavelength shorter than that of visible light. When Professor Wilhelm Konrad Roentgen, a physicist at the University of Würzburg, first observed the effects of this previously unknown energy, he named them "x-rays" after the mathematical symbol "x" for the unknown. These energy waves, or x-rays, have the ability to penetrate body tissues. In x-ray imaging, differential absorption, known as *attenuation*, of the beam of x-rays by body tissues of different electron densities is the source of the different contrasts identified on an x-ray film. Greater absorption by a tissue results in fewer x-rays reaching and exposing the film, producing a brighter image on the film. The relatively dense bony structures absorb the most x-rays and appear bright or white on the x-ray film. By contrast, the least dense tissue (air) absorbs the fewest number of x-rays and appears black on the x-ray image. Soft tissues are primarily water density, intermediate between bone and air, and appear gray on the film.

Viewing x-ray films, or radiographs, is a mental exercise in three-dimensional image reconstruction. A radiograph is a two-dimensional representation of a three-dimensional structure, much as a landscape painter presents a three-dimensional scene on canvas. Unlike the artist's painting, however, a radiograph represents the superimposed or composite image of internal body structures. Therefore, when viewing an x-ray image, the observer must think in three-dimensional layers.

When the x-ray beam passes through the body from front to back the film is named an anteroposterior (AP) film. Conversely, if the x-ray beam passes from back to front, the film is termed a posteroanterior (PA) film. In order to assist in the three-dimensional image thought process, a second radiographic exposure of the body part should be obtained at a 90-degree angle to the first view. This is termed the lateral view. Additional views are also frequently obtained to demonstrate anatomic structures to the best advantage. These additional views are described in the appropriate sections below. Just as the artist's skills increase with practice, the ability to recreate an anatomically correct three-dimensional image mentally from radiographs also improves with practice.

Conventional films or radiographs are widely used in the assessment of musculoskeletal problems. Radiographic examinations are readily available, relatively inexpensive, and excellent for the initial screening of primary skeletal pathology. They are the initial imaging study of choice in trauma for detecting fractures. They are also useful for detecting unstable injuries with the use of flexion, extension, and stress views obtained with force applied manually to the joint under evaluation, in order to determine ligamentous or other structural instability. Routine films are the initial screening study for most chronic conditions, readily detecting the range of pathology from congenital abnormalities to degenerative arthritis.

The radiographic examination is limited in its ability to detect subtle fractures in complex joints or in dense body structures and is very limited in its ability to assess soft tissue changes. Static radiographic images of complex and dynamic structures can only indirectly hint at underlying biomechanical abnormalities.

The radiographic examination is also limited in its ability to detect the presence of metastatic tumor in bone. Bone has a limited ability to respond to metastatic disease. The radiographic appearance of bone involved by metastatic tumor reflects the balance between bone production (osteoblastic activity) and bone destruction (osteolysis).[1] When osteoblastic activity predominates, the resulting lesion appears more dense or sclerotic than normal bone, the most common appearance with prostatic cancer. Conversely, when bone destruction is the predominant activity, less bone is present, and the lesion appears less dense than normal bone, or lytic, the most common appearance with lung and breast cancer. Conventional radiographs are relatively insensitive for the detection of metastatic disease in bone because almost 50 percent of the bone must be destroyed before the lesion can be visualized radiographically. Therefore, for the detection of metastatic disease, skeletal imaging with nuclear medicine is the most effective means of detecting early bony involvement, because this modality images metabolic activity.

Finally, with radiographic studies, there is concern about patient exposure to ionizing radiation. Although a minor consideration when filming a foot using proper equipment and technique, it is a more serious concern when the examination is of the lumbar spine or pelvis, where there will be significant gonadal exposure to radiation. Modern techniques and sensitive (high-speed) films have helped reduce gonadal exposure. Judicious decisions about the appropriateness and value of radiographic examinations will serve to reduce radiation exposure further.

Computed Tomography

A computed tomographic (CT) scan is produced through the use of x-rays passing through the body, as are conventional radiographs. In a CT scan, the x-rays are produced by an x-ray tube that rapidly rotates around the patient. Instead of producing a direct image on film, the x-ray beam passing through the body is measured by an electronic detector. A computer uses the data from the detector in order to reconstruct an image of the internal organs of the body, first on a television monitor and then subsequently printed on film.

Each axial image produced is a cross-sectional slice of the body, much like lifting a single slice of bread from a loaf. The entire series of axial images is used to reconstruct a three-dimensional image of the body, similar to repackaging the individual slices of bread to make the whole loaf. The result is an image of the inside of the body with exquisite anatomic detail that cannot be achieved with conventional radiographs.

A CT scan is effective because it images both the muscular and skeletal systems simultaneously. It yields superb cross-sectional anatomy and has excellent tissue contrast resolution. While conventional films have the ability to discriminate tissue density differences of about 5 percent, CT can distinguish density differences of about 1 percent, permitting differentiation of adjacent soft tissues. CT is also particularly valuable in detecting and characterizing skeletal abnormalities, especially in the spine, pelvis, and extremity joints, where complex articular relationships are present.

A CT scanner uses x-rays and exposes the patient to radiation, but the exposure is kept to a minimum through the use of a pencil-thin or collimated x-ray beam. Like a radiograph examination, a CT scan, is noninvasive. For most patients, a CT scan is a comfortable procedure. CT scanning is a valuable tool in assessing the musculoskeletal system, is widely available, and is a cost-effective method for evaluating many of the conditions commonly seen in physical therapy practices.

Magnetic Resonance Imaging

In less than a decade, magnetic resonance imaging (MRI) has gone from an exotic new technology to the imaging method of choice for most lesions of the central nervous system (CNS). Although still viewed as primarily a neurologic imaging modality, MRI has also proved very useful in assessing the musculoskeletal system.[2,3] Already the second diagnostic study of choice for the knee after the initial radiographs, MRI may also assume a similar position as the second study of choice for the other extremity joints.[4,5]

Advances in diagnosis using musculoskeletal MRI are possible because of the superb soft tissue contrast available with this imaging technique. Conventional radiographs are superior for visualizing cortical bone and assessing stability after trauma with flexion, extension, or stress views. Whereas CT provides superior cross-sectional anatomic definition, MRI, with its exquisite soft tissue contrast, permits complete assessment of the surrounding extraosseous structures (cartilage, tendons, ligaments, muscles) and intraosseous marrow.[6] Although MRI does not detect direct cortical bony injury, its sensitivity in detecting abnormal amounts of blood and water (edema) in the underlying marrow has led to an evolving role for MRI in the detection of occult trauma.

MRI has become the study of choice for demonstrating soft tissue tumors,[7–10] tumor infiltration of adjacent vascular and soft tissue structures, the intramedullary extent of tumor,[11] and the detection of recurrent tumor after therapy.[12]

MRI requires a new approach in thinking[13] and image interpretation because it is based on physical principles that are different from those of x-rays, γ-rays, or ultrasound. All medical imaging studies depend on physical interactions between energy photons (packets of energy) and body tissues. CT and radiographic images are based on the differential absorption of energy by body tissues of varying electron density and on the detection of the remaining transmitted energy by receptors on the opposite side of the body (the film or CT detector). By contrast, magnetic resonance products images by means of magnetic fields and radio waves and depends on the proton (not electron) density of the body tissues.

MRI relies on the behavior of protons (the nuclei of hydrogen atoms) to align with the axis of a strong magnetic field when placed within that magnetic field. When these protons absorb an applied radio wave energy from the transmitter of the MRI unit, they temporarily lose the initial alignment. As the hydrogen atoms realign, they transmit a faint radio signal. This signal is detected and amplified by the MRI unit and fed into a computer that plots the origin and intensity of the signal and presents this information in the form of an image. Different tissues contain varying amounts of water. Water has the highest concentration of hydrogen atoms; therefore, tissues with differing water content absorb and emit radio signal energy at different intensities. The stronger the signal, the brighter the image. It is this varying signal intensity that permits differentiation and characterization of normal and abnormal tissues. In simplest terms, the MRI unit can be thought of as a sophisticated radio transmitter and receiver operating in a magnetic field,[14] and the MRI can be thought of as an image of water distribution within the body.

Additional terms used in MRI are T1 and T2. These tissue-specific time constants refer to the rate of proton realignment with the external magnetic field after excitation by radio wave energy (T1) and the rate of decay of the transverse magnetization over time (T2). These tissue-specific time characteristics are important because they allow contrast differentiation between tissues. For example, fat has a very short T1 and produces a bright signal, whereas tumors have a relatively long T1 and appear dark on the MRI. Cortical bone has a relative paucity of free water protons and is represented as a signal void on MRI.

MRI is generally considered safe according to the National Institutes of Health (NIH).[15] There have been no published reports of harmful effects from the electromagnetic field per se.[16] The most important risk is that from ferromagnetic objects becoming ferromagnetic projectiles in the strong magnetic field and from ferromagnetic objects within the body, such as aneurysm clips, intraocular foreign bodies, or shrapnel becoming dislodged. Patients with cardiac pacemakers or neurostimulators should not undergo MRI examinations because of the risk of damage or deactivation of the device.

The limitations of MRI currently appear confined to the inability to visualize cortical bone, the relative length of time required to complete the study (usually 40 minutes for a complete examination of a joint, longer for the spine), patient claustrophobia, and the considerable expense of the examination. Currently there is limited availability of facilities with sufficient capacity to satisfy the demand for neurologic, let alone musculoskeletal, MRI. However, as MRI becomes more widely available, it will be routinely used in the diagnosis of musculoskeletal pathology.

Nuclear Skeletal Imaging

Nuclear imaging of the skeletal system, also referred to as skeletal scintigraphy, or more simply as bone scan, involves the use of trace (safe) amounts of radioactive materials to study the physiology and metabolism of the body. Skeletal imaging is successful because bone is a vascular, living, dynamically active tissue and not just a rigid framework supporting the soft tissue structures. A metabolically active lesion in bone, whether caused by tumor, inflammation, or trauma, concentrates the radioactive material to a greater degree than normal bone and appears more "intense" on the nuclear medicine images. It is generally accepted that approximately one-half of the bone must be destroyed before the changes can be noted radiographically. Therefore, because nuclear skeletal imaging is so sensitive, it will frequently reveal the presence of disease before it can be detected clinically and before routine radiographs demonstrate abnormalities. Nuclear medicine procedures are safe, easy to perform, and comfortable for the patient. Except for a single intravenous injection of a very small amount of liquid (about 1 to 2 ml), these procedures are noninvasive.

The traditional role of nuclear skeletal imaging has been in the detection of metastatic disease. However, newer techniques, newer radiopharmaceuticals, and advances in instrumentation (cameras and computers) during the past decade have greatly increased the specificity and anatomic resolution of nuclear imaging studies. These advances have expanded the role of radioisotopic imaging to include the evaluation of traumatic and sports-related injuries.[17,18] As physical therapists become aware of the expanded capabilities of this imaging modality, it will become a frequently used tool in the evaluation of a wide variety of both traumatic and nontraumatic conditions and for the differentiation of soft tissue from skeletal pathology.

Technetium skeletal imaging (the bone scan) is the most frequently requested nuclear medicine examination for the evaluation of musculoskeletal disorders. Technetium (Tc 99m) is a short-lived radioisotope with a half-life of approximately 6 hours. The carrier compounds to which the technetium radioisotope is tagged are diphosphonates, usually methylene diphosphonate (MDP). These compounds are rapidly cleared from the bloodstream and are concentrated in the skeleton. As the isotope undergoes radioactive decay, it emits a γ-ray with an energy of 140 keV. This energy makes Tc 99m an ideal agent for imaging with the currently available high-resolution gamma cameras.

The bone scan is both a sensitive and effective method of screening for potential skeletal pathology. However, because bone scanning images metabolism and not anatomy, its high sensitivity, that is, the ability to detect the presence of disease in a symptomatic patient, comes at the expense of lowered specificity, the ability to exclude the presence of disease in a normal patient. Because it is acutely sensitive to the earliest changes in metabolic activity, any process that affects bone, such as changes in blood supply, trauma, tumors, infections, or degenerative changes, will demonstrate an abnormality on the scan. Additional studies will usually be necessary to define the underlying abnormality further.

Routine Tc 99m skeletal images are obtained 3 to 4 hours after the administration of the radiopharmaceutical. The usual views consist of anterior and/or posterior images of the affected part. Oblique and lateral images are also often obtained.

Although less common, the physical therapist may see the results of gallium and indium studies performed to detect inflammatory conditions such as postoperative infections, infections in the intervertebral discs, joint infections, and infections of bone associated with foot ulcers in diabetic patients.

Gallium 67 is a radioisotope that is very sensitive for inflammatory lesions in the skeleton. It is most often used in the evaluation of osteomyelitis and is available in most nuclear medicine laboratories. Indium 111-labeled white blood cells (WBCs) are also very effective in the diagnosis of infection. However, because this test requires a complex technique to prepare the compound for injection, it is a relatively expensive study and is not routinely available.

All the radiopharmaceuticals used, whether technetium, gallium, or indium, are administered in the smallest amounts possible to minimize the radiation dose to the patient. This may amount to a radiation exposure that is less than that of a radiographic examination of the lumbar spine.

Bone scanning is a technique that is widely available and rapidly performed without complex patient preparation. It has a high degree of accuracy and reproducibility. Bone scanning is useful for imaging in all age groups and is almost totally without adverse reactions. It can be readily and safely repeated for serial follow-up of management and response to therapy. Bone scanning with technetium-tagged diphosphonates is readily available in any nuclear medicine department and is relatively low in cost.

Ultrasound

Diagnostic ultrasound is commonly used in modern medical practice to evaluate a wide variety of conditions from heart disease to early pregnancy. Ultrasound is a safe and effective means of visualizing the body's internal structures. Instead of ionizing radiation, like radiography and CT, ultrasound uses very high-frequency sound waves to create images of the internal organs. A transducer sends these high-energy sound waves into the body and "listens" for their return as they are reflected off internal tissues. A computer analyzes the location and intensity of the reflected sound and creates a picture of the interior of the body, which is subsequently photographed.

Although diagnostic ultrasound is used frequently in general medical diagnosis, it is used infrequently in the detection of musculoskeletal pathology. Diagnostic ultrasound does have the ability to distinguish solid from cystic soft tissue masses and is used to direct needle aspirations of soft tissue masses. Its usefulness in musculoskeletal imaging is limited because the sound waves are unable to penetrate bone. Still, ultrasound examination is valuable in assessing the popliteal fossa and in differentiating between a Baker's cyst and other causes of popliteal swelling, such as a popliteal artery aneurysm. In skilled hands, it has proved useful in assessing the rotator cuff muscles for evaluation of shoulder impingement syndrome. However, with the current advances in musculoskeletal imaging attained by CT and MRI, even these limited uses of ultrasound are being supplanted. Thus, with the exception of the assessment of the popliteal fossa and in characterizing certain soft tissue masses, diagnostic ultrasound is not a major imaging tool for the musculoskeletal system.

CERVICAL SPINE

Because of its complex anatomy, the cervical spine requires a variety of diagnostic studies for assessment, since no one single method may be adequate to answer completely the clinical questions encountered in patient evaluation. Radiographs, CT scans, MRI, nuclear medicine studies, and myelography are all applicable imaging studies for the cervical spine.

Trauma

The physical therapist is rarely involved in diagnosing acute trauma, with the exception of athletic events, where the physical therapist may be present but is not ultimately responsible beyond initial first aid for patient management. It is critical that the patient with suspected spine injuries be immobilized until the radiographic study has excluded spinal injury.[19] The determination of the full extent of the injury may require additional evaluation by CT, myelography or MRI.

Routine radiographs are the most effective primary screening method for detecting the presence of significant cervical spine injuries.[20] The lateral film is the most important study and permits visualization of 90 percent of significant injuries.[21] In the traumatized patient, the initial assessment of the cervical spine is with a cross-table lateral film. This view can be obtained with the patient's head and neck stabilized and permits detection of obvious fractures and abnormalities of alignment. The examination is completed with the addition of AP and odontoid views. If no unstable fracture is identified on the initial examination, flexion and extension lateral views may be obtained to assess soft tissue injury and instability. Additional information may be obtained with CT scanning, which is excellent for assessing complex cervical spine fractures and localizing bone fragments.[22–24]

MRI has also been evaluated for its use in assessing the extent of injury in cervical spine trauma.[25,26] MRI is superior to CT and conventional films in identifying spinal cord injury, acutely herniated intervertebral discs, and epidural hematomas.[27] An additional asset of MRI is the ability to perform multiplanar three-dimensional imaging in the axial, sagittal, and coronal planes. The unique insight provided with MRI in spinal cord injuries is invaluable for neurologically compromised or high-risk patients.[28,29]

Nontrauma

A more common scenario for the physical therapist is the assessment of the nontraumatized patient with either neck pain or radiculopathy, or both. The standard cervical spine radiographic series consists of an AP film, a lateral film, bilateral oblique views to visualize the neuroforamina, and an odontoid view to assess the atlantoaxial articular relationship.[30]

In addition to the assessment of alignment, routine

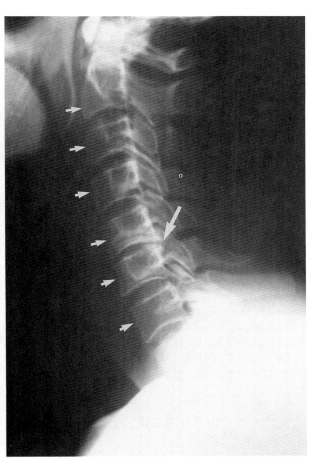

Fig. 13-1. This 41-year-old man complained of chronic cervical and right arm pain. Lateral film from his cervical spine radiographic examination reveals a normal anterior line of alignment (arrowheads). There is narrowing of the C5–C6 intervertebral disc with posterior osteophytes (arrow). An oblique view (not shown) revealed encroachment of the right C5–C6 neuroforamen by the osteophytes.

films are excellent for identifying vertebral anatomy. This includes narrowing of the intervertebral disc (Fig. 13-1), degenerative arthritis of the articulating facets, and neuroforaminal narrowing.

As visualized on the lateral view, there should be a gently curving line connecting the anterior vertebral margins—the prevertebral line of alignment. A parallel curving line connects the posterior margins of the vertebral bodies, the posterior vertebral line of alignment, which defines the anterior margin of the spinal canal. In addition, a gradually curving line should connect the bases of the spinous processes, the spinolaminar line of alignment, which defines the posterior margin of the spinal canal.

Further information about alignment and stability can be obtained with flexion and extension views. These are particularly useful for assessing atlantoaxial subluxation. Normally, the transverse ligament maintains the correct anatomic relationship between the odontoid process (dens) of C2 (the axis) and the anterior arch of C1 (the atlas). The normal distance in adults is 1 to 2 mm and up to 5 mm in children, who have greater ligamentous laxity. In trauma or in inflammatory processes, this ligament may be stretched or torn. Atlantoaxial subluxation is the most common abnormal finding in the cervical spine in patients with rheumatoid arthritis.[31] The result is an increased distance between the posterior margin of the anterior arch of C1 and the anterior margin of the odontoid process identified on flexion views. The consequence of atlantoaxial subluxation is compression of the anterior surface of the spinal cord by the posterior margin of the odontoid process with flexion.

Additional imaging of the cervical spine has previously been directed toward assessment of bony anatomic detail with CT scanning and assessment of cord or nerve root impingement with myelography. While CT scans provide superb definition of the bony anatomy of the cervical spine,[32] they fail to delineate neural and soft tissues. In addition, CT scans frequently failed to adequately assess the C6–C7–T1 levels because of beam-hardening artifacts caused by the patients scapulae and humeri.

Although CT during the 1970s significantly increased the ability to assess the bony anatomy of the cervical spine, MRI during the 1980s has revolutionized the detection and definitive diagnosis of degenerative diseases of the cervical spine in a noninvasive manner and on an outpatient basis. Routine cervical spine films, including oblique views, are still necessary to assess the bony anatomy of the cervical spine and to detect neuroforaminal encroachment by osteophytes, a relative blind spot for MRI.[33] CT scanning is still used to assess complex cervical spine fractures. However,

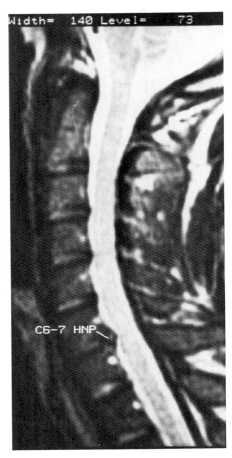

Fig. 13-2. This 29-year-old man sustained a cervical injury in a fall. Initial radiographs of his cervical spine were normal. He continued to complain of pain radiating into the right arm. Physical examination revealed decreased triceps strength on the right. An MRI scan was obtained. The T2-weighted sagittal image reveals a disc herniation at the C6–C7 level with anterior impression on the cervical cord. Axial MR images (not shown) revealed the disc herniation to impinge upon the right C7 nerve root. (Courtesy of Leonard Sisk, MD.)

MRI has now replaced myelography and CT with myelograph (the CT myelogram) as the second study of choice for the evaluation of most cervical spine pathology.

The excellent soft tissue contrast of MRI permits exquisite visualization of the contents of the spinal canal (Fig. 13-2), including the epidural space, the cervical cord, the nerve roots, the disc margins, and the cerebrospinal fluid (CSF) without the attendant risks and discomfort of the invasive cervical myelogram. The ability of MRI to assess the cord as well as the nerve roots in suspected cases of radiculopathy is considered essential.[34,35] Approximately 12 percent of patients with the clinical diagnosis of cervical spondylolysis will have myelopathy or radiculopathy from another cause.[36] The detection of intramedullary pathology, while present in a minority of cases, will significantly alter the diagnosis and treatment.

Although CT myelography with intrathecal contrast still provides the best anatomic assessment of the epidural space, MRI is noninvasive, provides almost the same quality of detail of the epidural space, provides more information about the spinal cord, and is more cost-effective. Furthermore, through the development of new imaging techniques with intravenous paramagnetic contrast agents and newer fast scanning techniques, coupled with improvements in both the hardware and software (resulting in improved signal-to-noise ratios), MRI has essentially replaced CT and myelography in cervical spine imaging.

THORACIC SPINE

The thoracic spine as such has little individual representation in the literature. Although much less studied from the musculoskeletal perspective, thoracic spine complaints find their way to the physical therapist with regularity if not frequency.

Trauma

The rib cage provides relative stability for the thoracic spine. Thus, most injuries involve the lower thoracic spine, particularly at the thoracolumbar level. Mechanisms of injury include hyperflexion with resultant anterior wedging of the vertebral bodies, axial loading with resultant burst fractures, and, less commonly, hyperextension and shearing injuries. Compression fractures caused by acute flexion are the most common thoracic spine injuries.

Thoracic spine injuries are frequently associated with

tracheobronchial and cardiovascular injuries, hemothorax, pneumothorax, and diaphragmatic tears. As with other spinal trauma, the goal is to provide stabilization while other associated life-threatening injuries are being treated.[19]

Nontraumatic Thoracic Pain

Scoliosis and compression fractures secondary to osteoporosis are the most common musculoskeletal problems of the thoracic region presenting to the physical therapist. Other abnormalities include congenital anomalies; metastatic disease affecting the vertebral bodies with collapse or destruction of the pedicles; and changes in the intervertebral disc, including degenerative disease, Scheuermann's deformity,[37] and infections.

Radiographic assessment is the first imaging study of choice in the evaluation of patients with thoracic pain. Plain radiographs provide important diagnostic information regarding vertebral alignment, congenital anomalies, skeletal changes caused by tumor and fracture, and the status of the intervertebral disc. The routine radiographic assessment of the thoracic spine consists of AP and lateral views. These views are more valuable for assessing vertebral alignment if performed with the patient in the erect position. The upper thoracic vertebrae are frequently obscured by the superimposition of the shoulder girdles. Additional coned views with the patient very slightly obliqued are necessary to visualize the upper thoracic segments.

Radionuclide imaging is used to determine multiplicity and extent of lesions. CT provides information about tumor matrix and the extent of bone destruction. MRI is useful in the evaluation of intracanalicular and paraspinous extension of lesions.

Scoliosis

Scoliosis is defined as one or more lateral abnormalities of the spinal curve, often associated with abnormal rotations and increased kyphosis and lordosis. Although the most common cause of scoliosis is not precisely known and is labeled idiopathic, there is a strong familial association, and most scoliosis probably occurs through genetic transmission. Idiopathic scoliosis accounts for approximately 80 percent of cases of scoliosis and is diagnosed by excluding the other causes of scoliosis.[38] This is in contrast to congenital scoliosis, probably not of genetic origin, which is attributable to the presence of an underlying structural bony abnormality. Scoliosis may also be due to neuromuscular conditions, neurofibromatosis, trauma, and tumors. Radiographic assessment is valuable for assessing the presence of underlying bony abnormalities and for quantitating and following the spinal curve(s).

Evaluation of scoliosis as part of student physical screening has become a common practice in many of the school systems in more than one-half of the states. These screening programs based on physical examination have led to an increased number of radiographic examinations of the spine.[39] After the initial screening examination, subsequent follow-up examinations in scoliotic patients frequently include radiographs with each visit, often at 3- to 6-month intervals, until skeletal maturity is reached.

Females, ranging in age from 9 to 14 years, comprise approximately two-thirds of the screened population requiring additional evaluation.[40] Developing breast tissue is particularly sensitive to the carcinogenic effects of radiation.[41] In these female patients undergoing multiple examinations, cumulative doses to the breasts of more than 10 cGy have been reported,[42] a potentially significant dose. To protect the breast tissue of adolescent girls from excess exposure to radiation during these radiographic examinations additional precautions are necessary. These techniques include fast film and screen combinations known as "rare earth" systems, compensating wedge filters that remove unnecessary radiation from the thoracic area, breast shields, and the PA position. When combined, these methods can reduce exposure to the breast by a factor of 12 or more.[39,40,42]

Osteoporosis

In the elderly population, therapists must be alert to the possibility of patients presenting with back pain caused by collapse of vertebrae weakened by osteoporosis. Osteoporosis is a generalized term referring to a state of decreased mass of normally mineralized bone. Of the many conditions that cause osteoporosis, the most common is postmenopausal bone loss. If the bone density becomes so low that the skeleton cannot support the normal activities of daily life, pathologic fractures occur, most commonly of the vertebral bodies and proximal femurs. Major contributing factors include inadequate nutrition, inadequate hormonal regulation, inactivity, and heredity.

Accurate detection and quantitation of bone mineral content, if readily available, would be integral to the management of osteoporosis and other metabolic bone diseases. Routine radiographs are of little benefit in the early detection of bone loss. Unfortunately, up to 50 percent of the bone mass must be lost by the time radiographic changes can be identified. Therefore, when routine radiographs demonstrate the washed-out appearance characteristic of osteoporosis, the disease is beyond the early stages. Although not beneficial in quantifying osteoporosis, routine radiographs are valuable in assessing the complications of osteoporosis, primarily the collapse of one or more vertebrae.

Several methods for the quantitative assessment of osteoporosis exist, but a persistent lack of precision among these techniques has prevented incorporation of bone mineral analysis into the usual diagnostic armamentarium.[43] Single-photon absorptiometry (SPA), using a single-energy γ-ray, measures bone mineral content of the distal radius and os calcis. However, these measurements do not correlate well with the mineral content of the proximal femur or spine, the most important fracture sites in osteopenic states.[44] Dual-photon absorptiometry (DPA), using two γ-rays of differing energies, measures cortical and trabecular bone in both the hip and spine. However, it has poor spatial resolution, and extensive time is required to complete and analyze the examination.[45] Quantitative computed tomography (QCT) yields high spatial resolution and is the best predictor of vertebral compression fractures. However, it is limited in the assessment of femoral mineral content by software requirements; requires very expensive equipment, which is usually in demand for other studies; and involves high radiation doses.[46] Dual-energy radiographic absorptiometry (DRA), currently limited in availability, offers excellent resolution, greater speed, increased precision, and long-term reproducibility. This technique, using x-ray beams of alternate energies, may become a useful tool for the evaluation and long-term follow-up of patients at risk of osteoporosis.[47]

Neoplasm

Middle-aged and older patients commonly present with complaints of chronic and/or increasing back pain. Degenerative arthritis is a common condition in this age group, as is metastatic disease, which may frequently present before the primary malignancy is diagnosed. Therapists must be cognizant of the concurrent presentation of these two conditions and choose appropriate clinical and imaging assessments to differentiate between them.

Metastases are the most common neoplasms of bone. Lung, breast, genitourinary, and gastrointestinal primary tumors account for approximately 80 percent of skeletal metastases.[48] Seventy percent of skeletal metastases in women are due to cancer of the breast, and in men 60 percent are due to prostate cancer. Dissemination from the primary tumor is usually through the bloodstream to the bone marrow in those skeletal regions engaged in active hematopoiesis (i.e., the spine, pelvis, and ribs).[49] As these skeletal regions have the greatest blood supply, the axial skeleton is the most likely site for metastatic disease. By contrast, it is uncommon for metastases to present distal to the elbow and knee.

Metastases frequently involve the pedicles of the vertebrae and are the major cause of the "missing" pedicle attributable to bone destruction (Fig. 13-3A). These patients frequently present with the clinical complaint of localized pain. Pathologic fractures may be visualized in up to 15 percent of cases.

In most cases, however, routine radiographs are insensitive for the detection of metastatic disease and will usually reveal only arthritic changes or may even be normal.[50] Those patients whose medical history and pain pattern suggest that the symptoms could be due to a systemic process, and whose initial radiographs

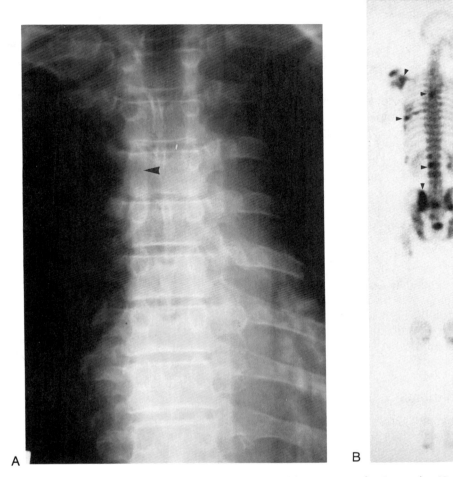

A   B

Fig. 13-3. This 42-year-old heavy smoker complained of mid-thoracic pain for 3 months. He was referred for physical therapy. Radiographs of the thoracic spine had not previously been obtained but were requested after the therapist's evaluation. **(A)** The AP film of the thoracic spine reveals absence of the right pedicle of the fourth thoracic vertebra (arrowhead). A chest radiograph (not shown) revealed a mass in the left lung that was subsequently proved to be bronchogenic carcinoma. The patient was referred to an oncologist who ordered a total-body bone scan. **(B)** The posterior image reveals multiple abnormal areas of increased uptake in the spine, ribs, left shoulder, and pelvis (arrowheads) representing metastases.

are not diagnostic should have a whole-body radio-nuclide bone scan to detect occult disease and to measure the extent of the disease (Fig. 13-3B).

Detection of metastases on bone scans is frequently the first indication of the presence of an underlying primary tumor. Radionuclide skeletal imaging is the most effective means of detecting skeletal metastases,

with a sensitivity of more than 95 percent for localizing skeletal metastases.[51] It is imperative to obtain an early diagnosis of metastatic disease in high-stress or weight-bearing areas. Early diagnosis permits timely intervention with internal stabilization and/or radiation therapy to prevent the development of pathological fractures.[52] Mechanical back pain caused by disc and facet disease does not usually result in altered bone metabolism, and the radionuclide scans will be negative. A positive scan almost always indicates underlying bone pathology.

LUMBAR SPINE

The presentation of a patient with back pain is a daily occurrence in the physical therapist's practice. To diagnose the etiology of the pain in these patients is a greater clinical challenge[53] than to diagnose the etiology of pain in the peripheral joints, because the spine is much less accessible to direct clinical examination. Before assessing these patients, there must be a solid understanding of the common pathologies and abnormalities that present as low back pain. As a result of the difficulty in clinically determining the etiology of a patient's back pain, a variety of radiographic studies have become available to assist in the evaluation of these patients. These studies include conventional radiography, CT scanning, MRI, myelography, and discography. The selection of the most appropriate imaging study is best determined after assessing the results from a thorough history and physical and neurologic examination.

Trauma

CT, plain radiographs, and, rarely, myelography are currently used in the diagnosis of acute spinal trauma. Conventional radiographs are frequently adequate for the assessment of lumbar spine injuries.[54] After the initial radiographic assessment, if additional anatomic information is necessary, CT is more definitive[22] in assessing the extent of the fractures and the potential complications of bony fragments compromising the spinal canal.

MRI has recently been added to the armamentarium available to assess the spine in the traumatized patient. After the patient is stable, MRI can be used to assess the status of the spinal canal visualizing retropulsed fragments, acute disc herniations, and cord edema.

Acute Lumbar Pain

In evaluating the patient with acute nontraumatic lumbar or lumbosacral pain, there are significant medicolegal concerns about what, if any, imaging tests to order.[55] In most cases, radiographs are not needed unless symptoms fail to improve within 6 weeks after a trial of conservative therapy, particularly in patients under the age of 40. However inappropriate,[56] many clinicians and even many patients insist on obtaining lumbar spine radiographs at the initial evaluation for back pain. Daffner[57] reviewed Nachemson's study[58] and estimated that 7 million lumbar spine radiographic examinations are performed yearly, at a cost of $500 million (1986). Routine lumbar spine radiographs have a relatively low yield in the detection of significant disease in the patient with acute nontraumatic back pain[59] and represent a significant radiation dose to the gonads.

It has been common practice to obtain a radiograph in patients with acute back pain, to exclude major pathology such as neoplasm, infection, trauma, or spondyloarthropathy. However, by obtaining a careful history, the therapist will usually identify the presence of chronic or progressive symptoms in patients with these pathologic conditions. This group of patients should actually be classified as having chronic, not acute, back pain.

Therefore, lumbar spine films should be obtained only rarely in the acutely symptomatic patient with no history of acute external trauma. Most of these patients have ligamentous or muscle strain caused by overuse or misuse, which will respond to conservative treatment.

When nontraumatic back pain does not respond to conservative measures, radiographic studies are appropriate. Routine radiographs of the lumbar spine consist of an AP film and a lateral film. Frequently the examination will also include a spot film centered at the L5–S1 junction, for greater anatomic detail at this level. This examination is frequently performed with the patient erect, to emphasize vertebral alignment in the weight-bearing position. Although not recommended because of the low diagnostic yield and greatly increased gonadal radiation exposure,[60] both oblique views of the lumbar spine are often considered part of the routine radiographic examination.

Routine radiographs, particularly if obtained with the patient erect, are excellent for the detection of align-

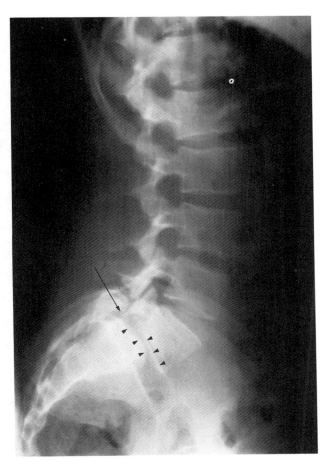

Fig. 13-4. This 25-year-old soccer player complained of chronic and increasing back pain made worse with running or prolonged standing. A standing lateral radiograph of the lumbar spine reveals a grade II spondylolisthesis of L5 on S1 (arrowheads) caused by a bilateral L5 spondylolysis (arrow).

ment abnormalities. These include scoliosis, spondylolisthesis (forward slippage) (Fig. 13-4) and retrolisthesis (reverse slippage). Underlying conditions detectable on plain radiographs that can produce these alignment abnormalities include congenital vertebral anomalies, transitional lumbosacral vertebrae with unilateral sacralization, degenerative disc disease, and spondylolysis (a defect in the posterior supporting elements of the vertebrae). Routine radiographs are also useful in detecting the presence of compression or other types of fractures, of lytic or destructive lesions

of the spine, and of osteoarthritis of the facet joints and in assessing the presence and extent of spondyloarthropathies such as ankylosing spondylitis.

Flexion and extension views may also be obtained to determine the presence of abnormal mobility of the vertebrae. The most common cause of abnormal movement of the vertebrae is a defect in the posterior bony neural arch (the pars interarticularis), termed *spondylolysis*. Although this defect may be visualized on AP or lateral radiographs, oblique projections are sometimes necessary to confirm its presence.

The second most common cause of instability is a combination of degenerative changes of the articulating facets[61] and narrowing of the intervertebral disc, known as *spondylosis*.[62] These abnormalities can produce not only abnormal movement of the vertebrae but may also result in abnormalities of alignment known as *spondylolisthesis* and *retrolisthesis*. Either with or without associated neurologic defects, lumbar spondylosis, spondylolisthesis, and retrolisthesis are significant causes of low back pain.

Chronic Pain, Neurologic Deficits, the HNP, and Spinal Stenosis

Before a discussion of appropriate secondary imaging techniques for the lumbar spine is presented, a brief review of common causes of protracted low back pain is integral to understanding the principles of imaging selection.[53,63]

In patients presenting with chronic low back pain, with or without radicular symptoms, muscle weakness, and sensory loss, the frequent clinical diagnosis is either disc herniation or spinal stenosis, or both. Disc herniation can occur either suddenly as the result of acute overload or gradually as the result of aging. With the normal aging process, there is a gradual loss of the water content of the nucleus pulposus and a concomitant gradual loss of height of the disc.[64] This process is accompanied by weakening and stretching of the outer fibers of the annulus fibrosis. This diffuse circumferential widening of the disc is termed a bulging annulus fibrosis. This is a normal process of aging and is usually not symptomatic. The weakened annulus may permit focal herniation of the central nucleus pulposus into the spinal canal (HNP).[64,65] If the herniated nuclear material is still contained within the annulus, the condition is termed *disc prolapse*. If there is a tear in the outer annular fibers permitting escape of nuclear material, it is termed *disc extrusion*. The herniated disc material may further extend through the posterior longitudinal ligament and migrate within the spinal canal.

Clinically, it is impossible to differentiate between a symptomatic diffusely bulging disc and a symptomatic focal herniation (HNP), whether attributable to prolapse or extrusion.[65] If a nerve root is not impinged, the patient will usually remain asymptomatic. Disc herniation occurs most commonly at the L4–L5 and L5–S1 levels, because these are the levels of maximum lumbar movement.

Spinal stenosis, also a frequent cause of back pain, is a general term, including both congenital and acquired (degenerative) conditions that lead to narrowing of the spinal canal, the lateral recesses, and the neuroforamen.[66] This encroachment results in nerve root entrapment and compression. Patients present with low back pain or buttock pain, frequently exacerbated with standing or walking, and often relieved by lying down or sitting and bending forward.[67] The clinical diagnosis is not obvious, and adjacent disc disease may occur concurrently, further confusing the clinical assessment.

Acquired stenosis is more common than congenital stenosis. Acquired spinal stenosis is narrowing of the spinal canal as a consequence of bony or soft tissue changes. These include degenerative changes of the posterior articulating facets with secondary osteophyte formation, inward buckling of the ligamentum flavum, commonly and incorrectly referred to as "hypertrophy" of the ligamentum flavum, and impingement on the canal by the bulging annulus fibrosis of a degenerated disc.[68,69]

Congenital stenosis can occur in conditions such as achondroplasia, in which the spinal canal is narrowed as a result of anatomic abnormalities. Usually, however, there is no known underlying cause and no specific hereditary pattern, and it occurs equally in both sexes.

Routine radiographs are not useful for the detection of herniation of the nucleus pulposus (HNP) and are of only very limited value for the detection and evaluation of spinal stenosis. They are useful only to exclude other causes of back pain, such as tumor, spondylolisthesis, and compression fracture.

The imaging modality of choice for the detection of an HNP and for the assessment of spinal stenosis is CT (Fig. 13-5). CT provides an anatomic visualization of the spine that cannot be achieved with conventional radiographs. Before the advent of CT, myelography was the diagnostic tool of choice for the assessment of lumbar disc disease. CT can evaluate the more common posterolateral and posterior disc herniations with accuracy equal to myelography.[71,72] In addition, CT is superior to myelography because of its ability to assess true lateral disc herniations (disc material protruding lateral to the neuroforamen), which are not visualized with myelography.[73] CT is valuable in detecting free

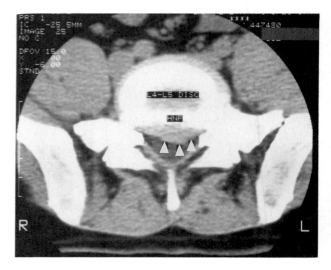

Fig. 13-5. This 28-year-old man was stacking heavy boxes when he experienced acute severe back pain radiating into his left leg. Neurologic examination suggested compression of the left L5 nerve root. A CT scan of the lumbar spine was requested. An axial CT image through the L4–L5 intervertebral disc level reveals a large posterior disc herniation (arrowheads) compressing the thecal sac and left L5 nerve root.

disc fragments in the spinal canal, which can migrate from the level of origin and present symptoms referable to another level.[74] CT can also visualize stenosis involving the neuroforamen and lateral recesses. The accuracy of CT imaging for HNP is superior to myelography, and its assessment of the bony structures of the spine is superior to that which can be obtained with MRI.

If there is discordance between the clinical symptoms and the CT findings, additional imaging with a contrast-enhanced CT can be obtained. This study is produced after the intrathecal administration of a small amount of nonionic iodinated contrast material. An MRI scan may also contribute increased sensitivity and serve to exclude other pathology, such as an epidural metastasis or a cauda equina tumor. MRI can clearly demonstrate the neural elements and any impingement on the thecal sac or nerve roots. Its sensitivity and noninvasiveness make it the preferred alternative to myelography.[75] With the availability of MRI for spinal imaging, there are now few indications for performing myelography. Discography is of dubious value and is seldom used unless performed in conjunction with chemonucleolysis.

The key to the best management of the patient with low back pain is the correlation of the history; physical and neurologic findings; the anatomic information available from radiographic, CT, and MRI studies; and the metabolic information available from the bone scan. Even with the advent of MRI, CT remains the most cost-effective method of correlating clinical symptoms and arriving at the diagnosis of HNP or spinal stenosis.

HIP AND PELVIS

Although often difficult to assess clinically as to the underlying etiology and site of pain, the hip and pelvis are regions that lend themselves well to evaluation with the multiple available imaging modalities. Particularly with the advent of MRI, evaluation of the hip can be relatively quickly and accurately completed.

The routine radiographic assessment of the pelvis consists of an AP film. This radiograph includes the iliac crests, the hips, and the proximal femurs to the level of the lesser trochanters, with the femurs in a neutral position. If the hips are of specific interest, a second AP radiograph of the pelvis with the hips flexed approximately 45 degrees and the femurs in abduction and external rotation ("frog leg lateral") is also obtained. Oblique views of the pelvis are necessary to assess the sacroiliac joints. A lateral radiograph of the pelvis is seldom obtained because overlapping skeletal structures obscure bony detail. Gonadal shielding should be used, to minimize radiation exposure.

Plain radiographs are excellent for the detection of osteoarthritis, fractures,[76] and other mechanical or structural abnormalities. However, for the detection of common pathologic conditions including metastatic disease and Paget's disease, nuclear medicine imaging, with its superior sensitivity, is the preferred study. Skeletal scintigraphy can easily detect the early metabolic changes associated with metastatic disease or Paget's disease,[77] an inflammatory disease of bone probably caused by a slow viral infection,[78,79] well before the radiographs become positive.

Osteoarthritis

Plain radiographs are excellent for the detection of osteoarthritis. Changes in the hip occur in the stressed or weight-bearing superolateral surfaces of the hip joint. Osteoarthritis is characterized radiographically by asymmetric joint space narrowing, irregularities of the adjacent articular surfaces, subchondral and juxta-articular cysts or erosions, increased density of adjacent articular surfaces (sclerosis), and marginal osteophytes.[80]

Osteonecrosis

Osteonecrosis (formerly termed avascular necrosis, ischemic necrosis, or aseptic necrosis) is a complex syndrome of clinical, radiographic, and histopathologic findings. The etiology is thought to be due to repeated trauma resulting in disruption of the blood supply, leading to death of bone cells and subsequent fragmentation.

Osteonecrosis of the hip, also known as Legg-Calvé-

Perthes disease, is a not uncommon clinical problem involving the hip. In post-traumatic osteonecrosis of the hip, the initial event is usually the result of a femoral head dislocation or fracture. True idiopathic osteonecrosis of the femoral head occurs in children, usually under the age of 10, and in men between the ages of 30 and 50.

The early clinical symptoms are nonspecific, usually consisting of focal pain, often increased with motion or weight bearing. Although early clinical signs and symptoms of osteonecrosis of the femoral head are not specific, early diagnosis is important. Treatment during the initial stages of the disease with surgical intervention may prevent or minimize subsequent deformities.

The initial diagnostic study of choice is a radiograph to exclude an obvious infection, tumor, or fracture. However, initial radiographs are usually normal and may remain so for many weeks. A radionuclide bone scan may be positive and has previously been the second study of choice in the detection of the metabolic changes associated with early osteonecrosis. Currently, MRI, with its high sensitivity for the detection of tissue changes and better spatial resolution, has superseded bone scanning as the method of choice

for evaluating suspected osteonecrosis of the radiographically normal hip[81,82] (Fig. 13-6).

With MRI, osteonecrosis appears as focal regions of low signal intensity in the marrow, indicating replacement of the marrow by edema, hemorrhage, and fibrous tissue.[83,84] The subchondral sclerosis, articular surface flattening, and collapse and bony fragmentation identified on conventional radiographs or CT scans are late changes that occur after the disease is well advanced and frequently beyond successful treatment.[85]

Trauma

Falls, particularly with a rotational component, are a frequent occurrence in the older population and represent a large percentage of inpatient physical therapy clients. In the outpatient population, the mechanism of the fall may be insufficient to produce a visible fracture or dislocation, but occult fractures of the femur or fractures of the acetabular rim are common. The patient presents with persistent hip pain or pain referred to the knee. The initial diagnostic evaluation is the plain radiograph. If the patient remains symptomatic, a bone scan may be performed to detect the increased metabolic activity associated with an occult

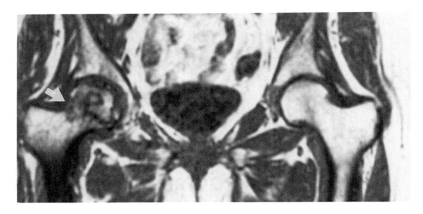

Fig. 13-6. This 65-year-old woman has been receiving high doses of steroids. She has been complaining of increasing right hip pain for the past 6 weeks. Routine radiographs of the hips were not conclusive, and an MRI scan was ordered. A coronal T1-weighted image of the hips reveals a large zone of decreased signal intensity in the right femoral head (arrowhead), consistent with marrow edema secondary to osteonecrosis. (Courtesy of Leonard Sisk, MD.)

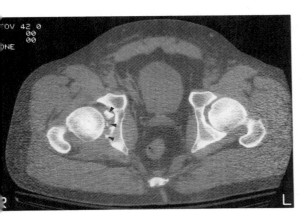

Fig. 13-7. This 30-year-old woman suffered a posterior dislocation of her right hip during a motor vehicle accident. After reduction, a CT scan was obtained revealing multiple intra-articular fragments (arrowheads). Surgery was necessary to remove the fragments before successful rehabilitation could be started.

fracture, or a CT scan may be performed to assess the bony anatomy.[86] CT delineates the precise extent of fractures, particularly acetabular fractures and complex fractures involving the articular surfaces. CT also detects associated joint abnormalities, such as osteochondral fractures and intra-articular loose bodies (Fig. 13-7). In patients with hip dislocations, MRI may be used to detect marrow edema associated with acetabular or femoral head compression fractures.

Stress Fractures

Patients engaging in vigorous physical activities may present with pain in the groin, hip, buttock, or thigh, all symptoms suggesting the clinical diagnosis of stress fracture. Stress fractures of the pubic rami are common in runners, particularly women, who overstride when matched with a taller running partner. Stress fractures of the femoral neck are also common. It is particularly critical to diagnose these femoral neck stress fractures early, in order to prevent the potentially catastrophic complications of a completed fracture.

Routine radiographs are the initial study of choice and may permit the diagnosis of stress fracture. Because these are very subtle fractures, however, the initial radiographs are frequently normal. If the initial examination is negative or nondiagnostic and the patient's symptoms persist, nuclear medicine imaging should be the next diagnostic examination.[17,18,87] While MRI may also visualize stress fractures before plain radiographs become positive,[5] nuclear medicine imaging, because of its sensitivity in detecting the early bony metabolic changes associated with overuse injuries, is still the second imaging modality of choice to detect early stress fractures in the hip and pelvis.

KNEE

The knee is one of the most frequently injured joints and often presents a diagnostic dilemma for the physical therapist. The knee is a vulnerable joint because it is exposed to both direct trauma and torsional stresses. Increasing participation in sports and fitness-related activities has resulted in greater numbers of knee injuries with both acute and chronic presentations that require evaluation. The clinical differentiation among bony, cartilaginous, and soft tissue injuries frequently cannot be specific. The application of correct rehabilitation strategies depends on accurate identification of the involved structures.

Current diagnostic imaging modalities for the knee include plain radiographs, bone scans, arthrography, CT, ultrasound, and MRI. Routine radiographs of the knee are the initial diagnostic study of choice.

The routine radiographic examination of the knee consists of AP, lateral, tangential patellar (sunrise), and open-joint projection (tunnel or notch) views. If the AP and lateral radiographs are performed with the patient in the erect weight-bearing position, valuable information is obtained regarding the degree of degenerative thinning of the articular cartilage, described as joint space narrowing. Additional oblique projections are occasionally useful in acute trauma for the clarification of possible fractures. Stress views are helpful to determine the presence of collateral ligament injuries. Occasionally, a repeat radiograph obtained after a delay of 10 to 14 days may be useful in demonstrating periosteal reaction and/or bone resorption at the margins of previously undetected fractures.

Diagnostic ultrasound is the study of choice for the rapid and least expensive means of evaluating the popliteal fossa for soft tissue masses and of evaluating the suprapatellar bursa. Radionuclide skeletal imaging is of value in detecting occult fractures, correlating clinical symptoms with radiographic changes in degenerative joint disease, identifying metastatic disease, and detecting the metabolic changes associated with osteonecrosis and osteochondritis dissecans. CT is useful for assessing the relationships of bony fragments in complex articular fractures. With sagittal and coronal reconstructions, CT is particularly useful for the preoperative assessment of depressed tibial plateau fractures.

Meniscal and Ligamentous Injuries

Everyone, regardless of fitness level or life-style, is at risk of meniscal injuries. The diagnosis is usually suggested by the clinical examination. Arthrography and arthroscopy were formerly used for further evaluation in patients with confusing clinical symptoms or when spasm and guarding made the clinical examination difficult.

While arthrography (Fig. 13-8), CT-arthrography,[88] and arthroscopy have all achieved an accuracy of 90 percent or greater in the evaluation of meniscal and ligamentous injuries, all are invasive studies. MRI is noninvasive and is able to produce high-quality images with high contrast and high resolution, without exposing the patient to ionizing radiation or surgery.[89,90]

Tissue characterization with MRI is superior to other imaging modalities. The ability of MRI to image ligaments, marrow, subchondral bone, and cartilage makes it ideal for assessing the knee because so many of the abnormalities involve a soft tissue component. With MRI, early soft tissue changes in patients with trauma, arthritis, and infection can be detected.[91,92]

The hallmark of meniscal abnormality on MRI is increased signal intensity within the meniscus. This increased signal intensity in meniscal tears is due to synovial fluid leaking into the torn meniscus. Within the meniscus, any signal intensity that communicates with

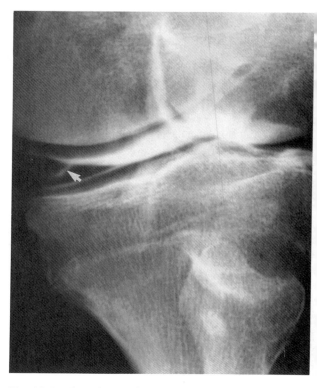

Fig. 13-8. This 24-year-old softball player "twisted his knee" sliding into second base. A conventional single-contrast arthrogram of the right knee reveals a tear of the superior surface of the medial meniscus (arrowhead).

an articular surface indicates a torn meniscus. This finding corresponds with meniscal tears with both a sensitivity and specificity of greater than 90 percent[93–95] (Fig. 13-9).

MRI is excellent in determining the presence, extent, and severity of injuries involving the collateral and cruciate ligaments of the knee.[96,97] Both the lateral collateral ligament and superficial fibers of the medial collateral ligament are extracapsular and therefore cannot be completely evaluated by either arthrography or arthroscopy.[98] In addition, the posterior cruciate ligament is not well seen on either arthroscopy or arthrography. The presence of injuries to these ligaments may affect the sequence of rehabilitation as well as the timing of reintroduction of activity.

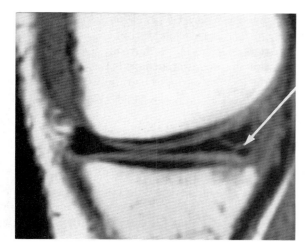

Fig. 13-9. This 30-year-old runner tripped and injured his right knee. A T2-weighted MRI scan revealed a tear of the anterior horn of the medial meniscus demonstrated by a linear zone of increased signal intensity extending to both the superior and inferior articular surfaces. (Courtesy of Leonard Sisk, MD.)

Osteochondral Fractures, Osteochondritis Dissecans, and Osteonecrosis

Osteochondritis dissecans, commonly of the medial femoral condyle, but also occurring in the lateral femoral condyle, patella, tibial plateaus, and talar dome of the ankle, may occur as the result of an undiagnosed osteochondral fracture or may be related to an overuse or stress syndrome. These injuries are a not uncommon sequelae of severe "sprains." The initial radiographs are normal. In the symptomatic patient with normal radiographs, radionuclide imaging can be of benefit in differentiating skeletal from associated soft tissue injuries and can localize the abnormality to the affected condyle. Subsequent conventional or CT images or arthrography may be necessary to confirm the diagnosis, identify bony fragments, and confirm the extent of cartilaginous fragmentation.

MRI has also proved especially useful in the detection of early osteonecrosis in the femoral condyle or tibial plateau and may be of value in the detection of early

osteochondritis dissecans, bone infarcts, meniscal and Baker's cysts, and occult fractures.[99]

Osgood-Schlatter Lesion

The Osgood-Schlatter lesion occurs as a result of repeated avulsions of the hyaline columnar cartilage of the apophyseal ossification center of the tibial tubercle.[100] It occurs predominantly in boys between the ages of 11 and 15 years, when the tibial tubercle is in the apophyseal stage.[101] There is frequently a history of increasing physical activity but seldom a history of a specific traumatic event. The diagnosis is made clinically. These patients present with painful swelling over the tibial tubercle. The tibial apophysis normally undergoes ossification from multiple centers. Since it is normally asymmetric, radiographs of the affected knee or comparison with the opposite knee seldom add to the clinical evaluation.[102]

Baker's Cyst

First described by Dr. William Baker, a nineteenth century surgeon, these "cysts" are a common cause of pain and swelling in the popliteal fossa. These popliteal "cysts" are not true cysts, but represent a communication between the knee joint and the gastrocnemio-semimembranosus bursa. There is usually an intra-articular abnormality, often traumatic internal derangement or a synovial inflammatory condition, such as rheumatoid arthritis, which produces an effusion. Fluid from the knee joint enters the bursa thru a one-way check-valve mechanism.

Rupture of a popliteal cyst or inflammation of or hemorrhage into the cyst can present with clinical symptoms that suggest deep venous thrombophlebitis. An enlarged cyst can also compress the popliteal vein, again producing the symptoms of thrombophlebitis.

Although arthrography and MRI can identify Baker's cysts, a noninvasive diagnostic ultrasound examination is the study of choice to evaluate swellings in the popliteal region. Ultrasound can identify a Baker's cyst and differentiate among other causes of popliteal swelling such as a popliteal artery aneurysm, venous thrombosis, a soft tissue tumor, or abscess. If indicated, percutaneous aspiration of the cyst can also be performed using ultrasonic guidance.

In the imaging assessment of the knee, routine radiographs remain the initial study of choice. Radionuclide bone scanning is currently the supplemental study of choice for the detection of occult fractures; CT scanning is the study of choice for the anatomic assessment of identified fractures. Arthrography is useful for evaluating cartilaginous fragments in the joint; arthroscopy is the modality of choice for evaluating chondromalacia of the patella. Ultrasound is the imaging modality of choice for popliteal masses; MRI is the imaging study of choice after the initial plain radiograph examination is completed. It is a noninvasive study with no morbidity that reveals the pathologic detail of meniscal and ligamentous injuries. Although MRI is not the procedure of choice for evaluating fractures, either acute or occult, this may change as experience is gained with MRI of trauma.[103–105]

FOOT AND ANKLE

Although anatomically distinct structures, each susceptible to specific injuries and pathologic conditions, the foot and ankle are grouped together for imaging purposes, because the same principles apply in their evaluation. The initial approach, as always, is a careful history and physical examination. After the initial examination, the first imaging modality to choose would be the plain radiographic examination of the symptomatic structure.[18]

Routine views of the ankle include AP, oblique, and lateral radiographs. Routine views of the foot also consist of three views: AP, oblique, and lateral. Routine radiographs are excellent for the detection of arthritis, calcaneal spurs, advanced stress fractures, and traumatic fractures and dislocations. They are occasionally useful for the detection of osteochondritis dissecans and tarsal coalitions. They are relatively insensitive for the detection of early stress fractures and for the more serious underlying pathology that would preclude treatment with physical therapy (e.g., osteomyelitis).

If the initial radiographic examination is abnormal, a CT examination may be necessary to define further the anatomic abnormality identified, such as a suspected tarsal coalition.[106] Normally, however, if the initial radiographic examination is not diagnostic and the patient remains symptomatic, a nuclear medicine bone scan is the next diagnostic imaging study of choice.[17,107]

Radionuclide skeletal imaging is superb in the early detection of occult or suspected fractures (Fig. 13-10A), early stress fractures, and early osteomyelitis.[108] A bone scan also aids in the differentiation of anatomic variants, such as accessory ossicles[109] from avulsion fractures when the initial radiographs are normal, or nondiagnostic or raise additional questions. Fractures can be detected by bone scanning within 24 to 48 hours of the traumatic event.[110] These fractures will demonstrate abnormally increased uptake of the radiopharmaceutical, in contrast to the normal uptake that occurs with anatomic variants. If the bone scan is normal, treatment can proceed with confidence, with the knowledge that a significant bony lesion is not present.[111] If, however, the bone scan is abnormal, further imaging is necessary, with either repeat radiographs or a CT scan (Fig. 13-10B), for a specific anatomic diagnosis.

CT has been applied to a broad range of diagnostic problems of the foot and ankle, including trauma, overuse injuries, tarsal coalitions, arthritis, and osteomyelitis. CT provides cross-sectional imaging of the foot and ankle to diagnose calcaneal fractures, subtalar coalitions, tarsal-metatarsal fractures, and dislocations and even primary soft tissue pathology and impingement syndromes.

MRI is just beginning to make inroads into foot and ankle evaluation.[112] It is not widely used, except for the assessment of skeletal and soft tissue neoplasms.

Stress Fractures

Stress fractures, usually occurring with unaccustomed or accelerated physical activity, develop gradually over a period of days to weeks. Persistent physical activity results in continuing bone resorption,[113] which in turn can led to a completed fracture and unnecessarily pro-

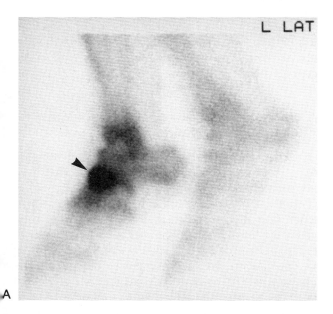

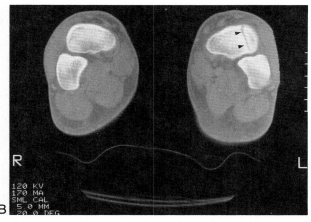

Fig. 13-10. This 19-year-old basketball player complained of persistent left foot pain since suffering a severe "sprain" during the final game of the season. Three sets of routine foot radiographs were normal. His symptoms did not improve with physical therapy. **(A)** A radionuclide bone scan requested after the third negative radiographic examination demonstrated intense abnormal uptake in the left tarsal navicular bone (arrowhead). **(B)** A CT scan was then obtained, revealing a fracture of the navicular (arrowheads), which subsequently progressed to nonunion and required internal fixation to achieve healing.

longed healing. The diagnosis of stress fractures is usually made clinically on the basis of the history and physical examination of a patient who is involved in increasing physical activity. Included in the differential diagnosis is tendinitis, arthritis, and other musculoskeletal disorders. The radiographic detectibility of a stress fracture at initial presentation is well below 50 percent.[14,114]

Skeletal scintigraphy has the ability to identify stress fractures weeks before the appearance of radiographic changes[115] and has a sensitivity approaching 100 percent.[116] The early detection of stress fractures permits prompt treatment, preventing progression of the fractures and the associated complications.[117,118] This is especially true with stress fractures of the midfoot,[119,120] which are particularly difficult to diagnose radiographically because of the complex and overlapping anatomy. Because isotopic scanning is so sensitive, multiple stress fractures will often be identified, even though only one site is symptomatic.

Osteonecrosis

When it occurs in the foot, osteonecrosis[121] usually involves the navicular bone and is referred to as Kohler's disease,[122] or the distal ends of the second and third metatarsals, known as Freiberg's infractions.[123] The initial clinical symptoms are nonspecific, usually consisting of focal pain that increases with motion or weight bearing. Early diagnosis and appropriate treatment are important to minimizing subsequent deformities. The initial radiographs are usually normal and remain so for up to 8 weeks. The radionuclide scan will usually be positive and will permit the correct diagnosis. Delayed radiographs may demonstrate increased sclerosis, fragmentation, or flattening of the involved articular surfaces.

Tarsal Coalition

Tarsal coalitions are frequent congenital abnormalities of the feet in which various bony, cartilaginous or fibrous unions between the tarsal bones may occur.[108] They are an important cause of foot and calf pain and of peroneal spastic flatfoot. The most common tarsal coalition is the calcaneonavicular, with the talocalcaneal or subtalar coalitions the second most common. Clinical symptoms often present after strenuous physical activity and are frequently thought to be due to stress fractures.[124] The first imaging study, after the clinical evaluation, should be the routine radiograph. While routine radiographs may reveal a bony calcaneonavicular coalition, they will often fail to visualize fibrous or cartilaginous unions. If these initial films are not diagnostic, radionuclide bone scanning will demonstrate focally increased uptake in the region of the coalition,[124] even if the coalition is fibrous or cartilaginous. With the abnormal radionuclide skeletal images as a guide, precise anatomic imaging with CT can complete the assessment of the painful foot condition. It is important to note that because of the complexity of the anatomic relationships, the imaging assessment of the foot and ankle commonly includes more than a single diagnostic modality.

SHOULDER

Shoulder pain and dysfunction are frequently encountered problems in the daily practice of the physical therapist. The mobility of this joint is critical to daily function; thus, dysfunction may be particularly disabling. Patients typically present with an inability to meet their work-required performance standards or to perform their daily activities.

The shoulder joint poses a unique challenge for imaging. This complex, highly mobile joint consists of the glenohumeral, acromioclavicular, scapulothoracic, and sternoclavicular joints. Radiographic evaluation with plain radiographs is an important initial diagnostic step after the clinical history and physical examination. Routine radiographs consist of two AP images with the humerus in external and internal rotation. Additional tangential, transthoracic, oblique, and axillary views are often performed after traumatic injuries. These plain radiographs are excellent for fractures and dislocations, are usually adequate for degenerative changes, and may demonstrate calcific deposits. Owing to the complex anatomy, plain radiographs are not generally sensitive or specific for other shoulder pathology. They are only occasionally diagnostic in the chronic impingement syndrome.

Plain radiographs not adequate for the common clinical problems of rotator cuff tears, injuries to the glenoid labrum, and other complications of trauma, biceps tendinitis, and rupture or intra-articular deposits.

Rotator Cuff Tears and the Shoulder Impingement Syndrome

Abnormalities of the rotator cuff are common, ranging from tendinitis to partial and complete tears. There are multiple etiologies[125] for rotator cuff pathology: age-related degeneration, failure from overuse, irritation from the chronic trauma of bony impingement, and acute trauma. It has been suggested that up to 95 percent of all rotator cuff lesions result from chronic impingement of the supraspinatus tendon against the undersurface of the coracoacromial arch.[126] This area of injury is called the critical zone, a poorly vascularized portion of the rotator cuff through which tears occur. Neer[126] classified the rotator cuff impingement injuries into three progressive stages. The initial stage, resulting from overuse, consists of reversible edema and hemorrhage of the supraspinatus tendon. Untreated, this progresses to the second stage of progressive inflammation leading to chronic fibrosis, finally progressing to the third stage of complete disruption. Early diagnosis and treatment are critical to prevent further progression of symptoms and improvement of function.

Clinically, the shoulder impingement syndrome consists of pain at the lateral margin of the shoulder. It is also referred to as rotator cuff tendinitis, subacromial bursitis, and supraspinatus tendinitis. The history and physical are frequently inadequate to pinpoint the cause of shoulder joint pain.[125,126]

Plain radiographs[127], arthrography,[128] and occasionally MRI[129] can be used to grade the acromial shape and can demonstrate a low-lying anterior acromion process that narrows the space between the anterior acromion and the humeral head. Early correct diagnosis is necessary because identification of the precise etiology leads to appropriate conservative treatment or surgical intervention. The plain radiographic findings of narrowing of the acromiohumeral distance occur late in the course of the disease. Therefore, because of the relative insensitivity of plain radiographs, additional imaging is frequently performed early in the evaluation of the painful shoulder. Positive contrast arthrography is the procedure of choice for the detection of complete and partial rotator cuff tears.[130]

Ultrasound imaging of the supraspinatus tendon has met with some success.[131] Although noninvasive, it requires a very high degree of skill from both the sonographer and sonologist that is not widely available. Until this technique is more readily available, it cannot be recommended as a routine imaging modality.

Advances in MRI contribute significantly to the assessment of shoulder pathology and are leading diagnostic imaging of the shoulder away from contrast arthrography and CT arthrotomography toward the use of MRI.[132–134] The anatomy and mobility of the shoulder

previously made MRI examination difficult. The early lack of appropriate surface coils resulted in suboptimal images, because of poor signal-to-noise ratios. Recent changes in technology have improved the sensitivity and specificity in MRI visualization of the tendons and articular cartilage.[135] However, positive contrast arthrography and CT arthrotomography[136] still remain the procedures of choice for diagnosing rotator cuff tears and labral and capsular abnormalities.

Trauma

Although the glenohumeral joint is one of the most mobile, it also one of the most unstable joints. After the initial evaluation and reduction of an apparently uncomplicated shoulder dislocation, it is common that patients will remain symptomatic or will suffer recurrent dislocations. Plain radiographic evaluation may

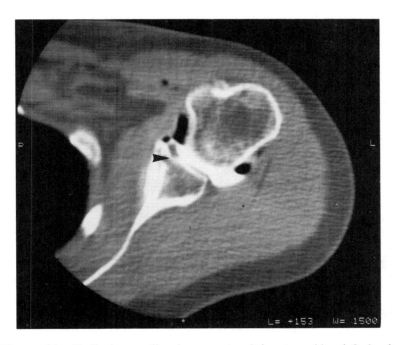

Fig. 13-11. This 32-year-old softball player suffered an anterior dislocation of her left shoulder in a collision with an opposing player. Successful reduction was accomplished, and postreduction radiographs revealed no fractures. She was referred to physical therapy for evaluation and treatment of persistent shoulder pain. When her symptoms did not improve, the consulting orthopaedist requested further evaluation with a CT-arthrotomogram. Axial CT imaging revealed a depressed fracture of the anteroinferior glenoid rim (Bankart fracture) and disruption of the anterior margin of the labrum (arrowhead). After arthroscopic surgery, rehabilitation was successful.

reveal normal bony structures but is inadequate to evaluate the glenoid labrum. Double-contrast CT arthrotomography (Fig. 13-11) is currently the study of choice for evaluating glenohumeral instability because of its ability to visualize the glenoid labrum and image capsular abnormalities.[137–140]

Calcific Tendinitis

In calcific tendonitis, calcific deposits form within the substance of the tendon and may remain clinically silent or be associated with chronic low-grade symptoms. These calcific deposits are usually detected with routine radiographs.

CONCLUSION

This chapter emphasizes an approach to diagnostic imaging for the physical therapist. Rather than analyze all possible traumatic, degenerative, or pathologic conditions of the musculoskeletal system, this chapter emphasizes an approach to the diagnosis and evaluation of the more common conditions encountered in daily practice.

Information is provided to help physical therapy clinicians make appropriate decisions about diagnostic imaging studies. While the typical practice model does not rely on the therapist to make the primary request for imaging studies, the therapist should review the patient's imaging studies and the reports that accompany them. Furthermore, the therapist is in an excellent position to collaborate with the referral source to select studies that aid in the accurate assessment of their patients' problems.

It cannot be stated strongly enough that before any imaging studies are considered, the emphasis must be on a complete history, physical assessment, and neurologic examination. Therapists must be constantly alert to patterns of findings that suggest problems not amenable to physical therapy treatment and make appropriate referrals. There is no need for "fishing expeditions" in diagnostic imaging. The physical therapist has a responsibility to collaborate with the imaging specialist before obtaining imaging studies. It is the radiologist's role to recommend the imaging modality that will answer the clinical question with the greatest degree of sensitivity and specificity. Greater communication of information among health care providers will ultimately lead to more accurate diagnoses, better patient care, and more focused therapy.

REFERENCES

1. Galasko CSB: Mechanisms of lytic and blastic metastatic disease of bone. Clin Orthop 169:20, 1982
2. Burk DL Jr, Dalinka MK, Scheibler ML, et al: Strategies for musculoskeletal magnetic resonance imaging. Radiol Clin North Am 26:653, 1988
3. Stoller DW: Musculoskeletal applications of magnetic resonance imaging. Appl Radiol 17:39, 1988
4. Edelman RR, Siegel JB: Advances in musculoskeletal MRI. MRI Decisions 5:27, 1988
5. Mandelbaum B: Optimizing sports medicine care with MRI. Diagn Imag 10:124, 1988
6. Moon KL Jr, Genant HK, Helms CA, et al: Musculoskeletal applications of nuclear magnetic resonance. Radiology 147:161, 1983
7. Wetzel LH, Levine E, Murphey MD: Comparison of MR imaging and CT in the evaluation of musculoskeletal masses. Radiographics 7:851, 1987
8. Kransdorf MJ, Jelinek JS, Moser RP Jr, et al: Soft-tissue masses: Diagnosis using MR imaging. AJR 153:541, 1989
9. Totty WG, Murphy WA, Lee JKT: Soft-tissue tumors: MR imaging. Radiology 160:135, 1986
10. Pettersson H, Gillespy T III, Hamlin DJ, et al: Primary musculoskeletal tumors: Examination with MR imaging compared with conventional modalities. Radiology 164:237, 1987
11. Vogler JB III, Murphy WA: Bone marrow imaging. Radiology 168:679, 1988
12. Vanel D, Lacombe MJ, Couanet D, et al: Musculoskeletal tumors: Follow-up with MR imaging after treatment with surgery and radiation therapy. Radiology 164:243, 1987
13. Sochurek H: Medicine's New Visions. Mack, Easton, PA, 1988
14. Winkler ML: The fundamentals of MRI: A primer for the referring physician. Curr Concept Magn Reson Imaging 1:3, 1988
15. National Institutes of Health Consensus Development Conference Statement on Magnetic Resonance Imaging, October, 1987
16. Shellock FG: Biological effects of MRI: A clean safety record so far. Diagn Imag 9:96, 1987

17. Holder LE, Matthews LS: The nuclear medicine physician and sports medicine. In Freeman LM, Weissman JS (eds): Nuclear Medicine Annual—1984. Raven Press, New York, 1984

18. Pavlov, H: Modern Imaging of the Athletic Injury. Postgrad Radiol 8:3, 1988

19. McCort JJ: Radiology's role in trauma evaluation. Postgrad Radiol 10:159, 1990

20. Harris JH, Edeiken J, Monroe B: The Radiology of Acute Cervical Spine Trauma. 2nd Ed. Williams & Wilkins, Baltimore, 1987

21. Berquist TH: Imaging of adult cervical spine trauma. Radiographics 8:667, 1988

22. Post MJ, Green BA, Quencer RM, et al: The value of computed tomography in spinal trauma. Spine 7:417, 1982

23. Pech P, Kilgore DP, Pojunas KW, Haughton VM: Cervical spinal fractures: CT detection. Radiology 157:117, 1985

24. Acheson MB, Livingston RR, Richardson ML, Stimac GK: High-resolution CT scanning in the evaluation of cervical spine fractures: Comparison with plain film examinations. AJR 148:1179, 1987

25. Hackney DB, Asato R, Joseph P, et al: Hemorrhage and edema in acute spinal cord compression. Demonstration by MR imaging. Radiology 161:387, 1986

26. Kulkarni MV, McArdle CB, Kopanicky D, et al: Acute spinal cord injury: MR imaging at 1.5T. Radiology 164:837, 1987

27. Chakeres DW, Flickinger F, Bresnahan JC, et al: MR imaging of acute spinal cord trauma. AJNR 8:5, 1987

28. Mirvis SE, Geisler FH, Jelinek JJ, et al: Acute cervical spine trauma: Evaluation with 1.5T MR imaging. Radiology 166:807, 1988

29. Kulkarni MV, Bondurant FJ, Rose SL, Narayana PA: 1.5 tesla magnetic resonance imaging of acute spinal trauma. Radiographics 8:1059, 1988

30. Christensen PC: Radiographic study of the normal spine. Radiol Clin North Am 15:133, 1977

31. Park WM, O'Neill M, McCall IW: The radiology of rheumatoid involvement of the cervical spine. Skel Radiol 4:1, 1979

32. Dorwart RH, LaMasters DL: Applications of computed tomographic scanning of the cervical spine. Orthop Clin North Am 16:381, 1985

33. Simon JE, Lukin RR: Diskogenic disease of the cervical spine. Semin Roentgenol 23:118, 1988

34. Masaryk TJ, Modic MT, Geisinger MA, et al: Cervical myelopathy: A comparison of magnetic resonance and myelography. J Comput Asst Tomogr 10:184, 1986

35. Teresi LM, Lufkin RB, Reicher MA, et al: Asymptomatic degererative disc disease and spondylosis of the cervical spine: MR imaging. Radiology 164:83, 1987

36. Crandell PH, Batzolorf U: Cervical spondylotic myelopathy. J Neurosurg 25:57, 1966

37. Alexander DJ: Scheuermann's disease. A traumatic spondylodystrophy? Skel Radiol 1:209, 1977

38. McAlister WH, Shackelford GD: Classification of spinal curvatures. Radiol Clin North Am 13:113, 1975

39. Educational program on exposure reduction in scoliosis radiography in full swing. Radiol Health Bull 19:1, 1985

40. Downey EF Jr, Butler P: Less radiation and better images: A new scoliosis radiography system. Milit Med 149, 526, 1984

41. Howe GR: Epidemiology of radiogenic breast cancer. In Boice JD Jr, Fraumeni JF Jr (eds): Radiation Carcinogenesis: Epidemiology and Biological Significance. Raven Press, New York, 1984

42. Protecting the breast during scoliosis radiography. FDA Drug Bull 5:1, 1985

43. Reinbold WD, Genant HK, Reiser UJ, et al: Bone mineral content in early-postmenopausal osteoporotic women: Comparison of measurements methods. Radiology 160:469, 1986

44. Riggs BL, Wahner HW, Dunn WL, et al: Differential changes in bone mineral density of the appendicular and axial skeleton with aging: Relationship to spinal osteoporosis. J Clin Invest 2:328, 1981

45. LeBlanc AD, Evans HJ, Marsh C, et al: Precision of dual photon absorptiometry measurements. J Nucl Med 27:1362, 1986

46. Firooznia H, Golimbu C, Farii M, Schwartz MS: Rate of spinal trabecular bone loss in normal perimenopausal women: CTR measurement. Radiology 161:735, 1986

47. Sartoris DJ, Resnick D: Dual-energy radiographic absorptiometry for bone densitometry: Current status and perspective. AJR 152:241, 1989

48. Resnick D, Sartoris DJ (eds): Bone Disease. 4th Ser., Test and Syllabus. American College of Radiology, Reston, VA, 1989

49. Springfield DS: Mechanisms of metastasis. Clin Orthop 169:15, 1982

50. Pagani JJ, Libshitz HI: Imaging bone metastases. Radiol Clin North Am 20:545, 1982

51. McNeil BJ: Value of bone scanning in neoplastic disease. Semin Nucl Med 14:277, 1984

52. Gainor BJ, Buchert P: Fracture healing in metastatic bone disease. Clin Orthop 178:297, 1983

53. Mooney V: The syndromes of low back disease. Orthop Clin North Am 14:505, 1983

54. Rogers LF: Radiology of Skeletal Trauma. 2nd Ed. Churchill Livingstone, New York, 1982

55. Gehweiler JA Jr, Daffner RH: Low back pain: the controversy of radiologic evaluation. AJR 140:109, 1983

56. Hall FM: Overutilization of radiological examinations. Radiology 120:443, 1980
57. Daffner RH: Radiographic evaluation of low back pain. Contemp Diagn Radiol 9:7:1, 1986
58. Nachemson AL: The lumbar spine: An orthopaedic challenge. Spine 1:59, 1976
59. Scavone JG, Latshaw RF, Rohrer GV: Use of lumber spine films. Statistical evaluation at a university teaching hospital. JAMA 246:1105, 1981
60. DeLuca SA, Rhea JT: Are routine oblique roentgenograms of the lumbar spine of value? J Bone Joint Surg 63A:846, 1981
61. Helbig T, Lee C: The lumbar facet syndrome. Spine 13:61, 1988
62. Epstein BS, Epstein JA, Jones MD: Degenerative spondylolisthesis with an intact neural arch. Radiology 15:275, 1977
63. Resnick D: Annual oration: Degenerative diseases of the vertebral column. Radiology 156:3, 1985
64. Lukin RR, Gaskill MF, Wiot JG: Lumbar herniated disk and related topics. Semin Roentgenol 23:100, 1988
65. Heiss JD, Tew JM Jr: Diskogenic diseases of the spine: Clinical aspects. Semin Roentgen 23:93, 1988
66. Dorwart RH, Vogler JB III, Helms CA: Spinal stenosis. Radiol Clin North Am 21:301, 1983
67. Paine K: Clinical features of lumbar spinal stenosis. Clin Orthop 118:77, 1976
68. Pleatman CW, Lukin RR: Lumbar spinal stenosis. Semin Roentgenol 23:106, 1988
69. Weisz GM, Lee P: Spinal canal stenosis. Concept of spinal reserve capacity: Radiologic measurements and clinical applications. Clin Orthop 179:134, 1983
70. Fries JW, Abodeely DA, Vijungco JG, et al: Computed tomography of herniated and extruded nucleus pulposus. J Comp Assist Tomogr 6:874, 1982
71. Raskin SP, Keating JW: Recognition of lumbar disc disease: Comparison of myelography and computed tomography. AJR 139:349, 1982
72. Haughton VM, Eldevik OP, Magnaes B, Amundsen P: A prospective comparison of computed tomography and myelography in the diagnosis of herniated lumbar disks. Radiology 142:103, 1982
73. Williams AL, Haughton VM, Daniels DL, Thornton RS: CT recognition of lateral lumbar disk herniation. AJR 139:345, 1982
74. Schipper J, Kardaun JWPF, Braakman R: Lumbar disk herniation: Diagnosis with CT or myelography? Radiology 165:227, 1987
75. Modic MT, Masaryk T, Boumphrey F, et al: Lumbar herniated disc disease and canal stenosis: Prospective evaluation by surface coil MR, CT, and myelography. AJR 147:757, 1986
76. Fernbach SK, Wilkinson RH: Avulsion injuries of the pelvis and proximal femur. AJR 137:581, 1981
77. Vellenga C, Pauwels EK, Bijvoet OL, et al: Untreated Paget disease of bone studied by scintigraphy. Radiology 153:799, 1984
78. Frame B, Marel GM: Paget disease: A review of current knowledge. Radiology 141:21, 1981
79. Singer FR, Mills BG: Evidence of a viral etiology of Paget's disease of bone. Clin Orthop 178:245, 1983
80. Forrester DM, Brown JC, Nesson JW: The Radiology of Joint Disease. WB Saunders, Philadelphia, 1978
81. Patten R, Shuman WP: MRI of Osteonecrosis. MRI Decis 4:2, 1990
82. Glickstein MF, Burk DL Jr, Schiebler ML, et al: Avascular necrosis versus other diseases of the hip: Sensitivity of MR imaging. Radiology 169:213, 1988
83. Mitcheli MD, Dundel HL, Steinberg ME, et al: Avascular necrosis of the hip: Comparison of MR, CT and scintigraphy. AJR 146:67, 1986
84. Mitchell RG, Rao VM, Dalinka MK, et al: Femoral head avascular necrosis: Correlation of MR imaging, radiographic staging, radionuclide imaging, and clinical finding. Radiology 162:709, 1987
85. Stansberry SD, Swischuck LE, Barr LL: Legg-Perthes disease: Incidence of the subchondral fracture. Appl Radiol 19:30, 1990
86. Ho C, Sartoris D: Modern assessment of hip fractures. Postgrad Rad 10:85, 1990
87. Zwas ST, Elkanovitch R, Frank G: Interpretation and classification of bone scintigraphic findings in stress fractures. J Nucl Med 28:452, 1987
88. Ghelman B: Meniscal tears of the knee: Evaluation by high-resolution CT combined with arthrography. Radiology 157:23, 1985
89. Tyrrell RL, Gluckert K, Pathrial M. et al: Fast three-dimensional MR imaging of the knee: Comparison with arthroscopy. Radiology 166:865, 1988
90. Reicher MA, Hartzman S, Duckwiler GR, et al: Meniscal injuries: Detection using MR imaging. Radiology 159:753, 1986
91. Crues JV, Morgan FW: Magnetic resonance imaging of the knee. Contemp Diagn Radiol 11:28;1, 1989
92. Bellon EM, Keith MW, Coleman PE: Magnetic resonance imaging of internal derangements of the knee. Radiographics 8:95, 1988
93. Crues JV, Mink J, Levy TL, et al: The accuracy of magnetic resonance imaging in the evaluation of meniscal tears of the knee: The first 144 cases. Radiology 164:445, 1987
94. Jackson DW, Jennings LD, Maywood RM. et al: Magnetic resonance imaging of the knee. Am J Sports Med 16:29, 1987
95. Stroller DW, Martin C, Crues JV, et al: MR imaging:

Pathologic correlation of meniscal tears. Radiology 163:731, 1987

96. Li DKB, Adams ME, McConkey S: Magnetic resonance imaging of the ligaments and menisci of the knee. Radiol Clin North Am 24:209, 1986

97. Mink JH, Levy TL, Crues JV: Tears of the anterior cruciate ligament and menisci of the knee: MRI imaging evaluation. Radiology 167:769, 1988

98. Lee JK, Yao L, Phelps CT, et al: Anterior cruciate ligament tears: MR imaging compared with arthroscopy and clinical tests. Radiology 166:861, 1988

99. Lee KR, Cos GG, Neff JR, et al: Cystic masses of the knee: arthrographic and CT evaluation. AJR 148:329, 1987

100. Ogden JA, Tross RB, Murphy MJ: Fractures of the tibial tuberosity in adolescents. J Bone Joint Surg 62A:205, 1980

101. Ogden JA, Southwick WO: Osgood-Schlatter's disease and tibial tuberosity development. Clin Orthop 116:180, 1976

102. Ozonoff MB. Pediatric Orthopedic Radiology. WB Saunders, Philadelphia, 1979

103. Yao L, Lee JK: Occult intraosseous fracture: Detection with MR imaging. Radiology 167:749, 1988

104. Lynch TC, Crues JV III, Morgan FW, et al: Bone abnormalities of the knee: Significance and prevalence at MR imaging. Radiology 171:761, 1979

105. Mink JH, Deutsch AL: Occult cartilage and bone injuries of the knee: Detection, classification and assessment with MR imaging. Radiology 170:823, 1989

106. Solomon M, Gilula L, Oloff L, et al: CT scanning of the foot and ankle: II. Clinical applications and review of the literature. AJR 146:1204, 1986

107. Maurice HD, Newman JF, Watt I: Bone scanning of the foot for unexplained pain. J Bone Joint Surg 69B:448, 1987

108. Karl RD, Hammes CS: Nuclear medicine imaging in podiatric disorders. Clin Podiatr Med Surg 5:909, 1988

109. Lawson JP, Ogden JA, Sella E, et al: The painful accessory navicular. Skel Radiol 12:250, 1984

110. Matin P: Bone scintigraphy in the diagnosis and management of traumatic injury. Semin Nucl Med 13:104, 1983

111. Matin P: Bone scanning of trauma and benign conditions. In Freeman LM, Weissman HS (eds): Nuclear Medicine Annual—1982. Raven Press, New York, 1982

112. Middleton WD, Macrander S, Lawson TL, et al: High resolution surface coil magnetic resonance imaging of the joints: Anatomic correlation. Radiographics 7:645, 1987

113. Wilson ES Jr, Catz FM: Stress fractures. An analysis of 250 consecutive cases. Radiology 92:481, 1969

114. Geslien GE, Thrall JH, Espinosa JL, et al: Early detection of stress fractures using 99m Tc-polyphosphate. Radiology 121:683, 1976

115. Norfray JF, Schlachter L, Kernahan WT, et al: Early confirmation of stress fractures in joggers. JAMA 243:1647, 1980

116. Pavlov H, Torg JS, Hersh A, Freiberger RH: The roentgen examination of runners' injuries. Radiographics 1:17, 1981

117. Torg JS, Pavlov J, Torg E: Overuse injuries in sports: The foot. Clin Podiatr Med Surg 4:939, 1987

118. McBryde AJ: Stress fractures in runners. Clin Sports Med 4:737, 1985

119. Pavlov H, Torg JS, Freiberger RH: Tarsal navicular stress fractures: Roentgen evaluation. Radiology 148:641, 1983

120. Goergen TG, Venn-Watson EA, Rossmand J, et al: Tarsal navicular stress fractures in runners. AJR 136:201, 1981

121. Graves J, Virtanen K: Osteochondrosis in athletes. Br J Sports Med 16:161, 1982

122. Brower AC: The osteochondroses. Orthop Clin North Am 14:99, 1983

123. Mandell GA, Harcke HT: Scintigraphic manifestations of infraction of the second metatarsal (Freiberg's disease). J Nucl Med 28:249, 1987

124. Goldman AB, Pavlov H, Schneider R: Radionuclide bone scanning in subtalar coalitions: Differential considerations. AJR 138:427, 1982

125. Keift GJ, Bloem JL, Rozing, PM, et al: Rotator cuff impingement syndrome. Radiology 166:211, 1988

126. Neer CS III: Impingement lesions. Clin Orthop 173:70, 1983

127. Bigliani LU, Morrison DS: The morphology of the acromion and its relationship to rotator cuff tears. Proceedings of the American Shoulder and Elbow Surgeons, New Orleans, 1986

128. Resnik CS, Deutsch AL, Resnick D, et al: Arthrotomography of the shoulder. Radiographics 4:963, 1984

129. Seeger LL, Gold RH, Bassett LW, et al: Shoulder impingement syndrome: MR findings in 53 shoulders. AJR 150:343, 1988

130. Goldman AB, Dines DM, Warren RF (eds): Shoulder Arthrography—Technique, Diagnosis and Clinical Correlation. Little, Brown, Boston, 1982

131. Mack LA, Matsen FA, Kilcoyne RF, et al: US evaluation of the rotator cuff. Radiology 157:205, 1985

132. Seeger LL, Ruszkowski JT, Bassett LW, et al: MR imaging of the normal shoulder: Anatomic correlation. AJR 148:83, 1987

133. Middleton WD, Kneeland JB, Carrera GF, et al: High-resolution MR imaging of the normal rotator cuff. AJR 148:559, 1987

134. Kneeland JB, Middleton WD, Carrera GF, et al: MR imaging of the shoulder: Diagnosis of rotator cuff tears. AJR 149:333, 1987

135. Zlatkin MB, Iannotti JP, Roberts MC, et al: Rotator cuff tears: Diagnostic performance of MR imaging. Radiology 172:223, 1989
136. Beltran J, Gray LT, Bools JC, et al: Rotator cuff lesions of the shoulder: Evaluation by direct sagittal CT arthrography. Radiology 160:161, 1986
137. Deutsch AL, Resnick D, Mink JH, et al: Computed and conventional arthrotomography of the glenohumeral joint: Normal anatomy and clinical experience. Radiology 153:603, 1984
138. Haynor DR, Shuman WP: Double contrast CT arthrography of the glenoid labrum and shoulder girdle. Radiographics 4:411, 1984
139. Shuman WP, Kilcoyne RF, Matsen FA, et al: Double-contrast computed tomography of the glenoid labrum. AJR 141:581, 1983
140. Rafii M, Firooznia H, Golimbu C, et al: CT arthrography of capsular structures of the shoulder. AJR 146:361, 1986

SUGGESTED READINGS

Jette A: Diagnosis and classification by physical therapists. Phys Ther 69:967, 1989

Lippert FG III, Teitz CC: Diagnosing Musculoskeletal Problems: A Practical Guide. Williams & Wilkins, Baltimore, 1987

Wood R: Footprints. Phys Ther 69:975, 1989

Wolf SL: Clinical Decision Making in Physical Therapy. FA Davis, Philadelphia, 1985

Appendix I
Examination: Review of Systems Summary

A. General health
1. Unexplained weight change
2. Fever, chills, sweats
3. Malaise
4. Weakness
5. Medical history (illness, surgery, medication)
6. Family medical history
7. History of smoking
8. Substance abuse

B. Skin
1. Color
2. Temperature
3. Texture
4. Dry/moist
5. Masses, lumps
6. Rash
7. Hair
8. Nails

C. Head
1. Headache
2. Head trauma
3. Dizziness
4. Lightheadedness
5. Visual: problems/changes
6. Nystagmus
7. History of glaucoma, cataracts
8. Hearing: problems/changes
9. Tinnitus
10. Vertigo
11. Ear discharge
12. History of ear infection, earache
13. Nosebleeds
14. Olfactory: problems/changes
15. Nasal congestion
16. History of hay fever, sinus trouble/infection
17. Condition of teeth
18. Condition of gums

19. Bleeding gums
20. Mouth sores
21. Sensory changes associated with taste
22. Difficulty with swallowing

D. Neck
1. Lumps in the neck
2. Swollen glands
3. Goiter
4. Pain and stiffness

E. Breasts
1. Date of last self-examination
2. Lumps, masses
3. Dimpling of tissue
4. Nipple discharge

F. Pulmonary system
1. Dyspnea
2. Wheezing
3. Stridor
4. Cough
5. Sputum
6. Hemoptysis
7. History of asthma, emphysema, pneumonia, tuberculosis, pleurisy, bronchitis

G. Cardiovascular system
1. Angina
2. Extremity intermittent claudication
3. Complaints of upper quarter pressure or tightness sensations
4. Pain associated with sweating
5. Palpitations
6. Dyspnea
7. Orthopnea
8. Fatigue
9. Syncope
10. History of heart trouble, high blood pressure, rheumatic fever, heart attack, heart murmur

H. Gastrointestinal system
  1. Difficulty with swallowing
  2. Heartburn, indigestion
  3. Specific food intolerance
  4. Nausea
  5. Vomiting
  6. Change in appetite
  7. Excessive belching or flatulence
  8. Bowel habits (frequency, stool caliber and color)
  9. History of liver, gallbladder, stomach problems, ulcers
I. Urinary system
  1. Urinary frequency, including nocturia
  2. Dysuria
  3. Hematuria
  4. Reduced caliber or force of urine stream
  5. Incontinence
  6. History of urinary, kidney infections
J. Genital reproductive system (male)
  1. Hernia
  2. Self-examination (sores, masses, lumps)
  3. Urethral discharge
  4. Pain with intercourse
  5. Sexual dysfunction
  6. History of venereal disease
K. Genital reproductive system (female)
  1. Hernia
  2. Change in menstruation (frequency and duration of cycle, dysmenorrhea, and amount of bleeding)
  3. Date of last period
  4. Menopause
  5. Vaginal discharge
  6. Self-examination (lumps, masses, sores)
  7. Number of pregnancies
  8. Number of deliveries
  9. Complications of pregnancy and delivery
  10. Pain with intercourse

  11. Sexual dysfunction
  12. Birth control methods
  13. History of venereal disease, infertility
L. Peripheral nervous system
  1. Numbness
  2. Paresthesias
  3. Weakness
  4. Radiating pain
  5. Seizures
  6. Syncope
  7. Tremors
M. Hematologic system
  1. Easy bruising
  2. Easy bleeding
  3. Anemia
N. Endocrine system
  1. Excessive thirst
  2. Excessive hunger
  3. Polyuria
  4. Excessive sweating
  5. Heat or cold intolerance
  6. Fatigue
  7. Weakness
  8. Paresthesia
  9. History of diabetes, thyroid trouble
O. Psychiatric
  1. Nervousness
  2. Tension
  3. History of depression, other psychological disorders.
  4. History of abuse (physical, emotional, sexual)

SUGGESTED READINGS

1. Bates B: A Guide to Physical Examination and History Taking. 4th Ed. JB Lippincott, Philadelphia, 1987
2. Malasanos L, Barkauska V, Stoltenberg-Allen K: Health Assessment. 4th Ed. CV Mosby, St. Louis, 1990

Appendix II
Glossary of Terms

Abscess: a focal collection of pus resulting from liquifactive necrosis of a tissue, usually caused by a pyogenic microorganism

Acetone: the simplistic ketone, formed by decarboxylation of acetoacetic acid and occurring in the blood and breath of persons with high concentrations of this acid in their blood

Acetylation: the introduction into a molecule of an acetyl group in replacement of a hydrogen atom

Acidosis: a disturbance of the acid-base state of the body toward the acid

Acinus: a rounded sac that opens into a small excretory duct in the terminal secretory portion of an exocrine gland

Acroparesthesia: paresthesia of the hands and feet

Acuity: sharpness, distinctness, acuteness

Adenohypophysis: the anterior lobe of the pituitary gland

Adenoma: a benign epithelial tumor of glandular structure; the cells may show evidence of glandular function, such as production of mucous and hormones

Adriamycin: a proprietary name for doxorubicin hydrochloride

Adventitia: the outermost layer of organs or structures that are not covered by a serous coat (e.g., the outermost layer of the three layers of an artery)

Agranuocytosis: the absence of granulocytes in the blood

Akathisia: the inability to sit down or remain seated because of motor restlessness and a sensation of muscular quivering that occurs as a side effect of neuroleptic drugs, especially phenothiazine; it is also an uncommon manifestation of Parkinson's disease

Akinesia: the inability to initiate movement

Amenorrhea: the absence of menstrual bleeding

Amyloid: starchlike

Amyloidosis: an incurable multisystemic disease process of uncertain etiology, characterized by the interstitial accumulation of amyloid fibriles; the affected tissues have a firm, waxy texture

Amyotrophy: muscular atrophy of neurogenic origin

Anabolic: denoting any substance that increases the rate of metabolism in a cell or organism

Analgesic: causing loss of sensitivity to pain without loss of consciousness

Anaphylaxis: an acute or exaggerated allergic response in a sensitized host following injection of or exposure to a foreign protein or other substance

Anasarca: severe edema involving the entire body, including marked swelling of subcutaneous tissues and the accumulation of fluid in serous cavities

Anemia: an abnormal decrease in the concentration of erythrocytes, hemoglobin, or hematocrit, which may result from decreased production, increased loss, or destruction of erythrocytes; often accompanied by characteristic signs and symptoms including pallor, asthenia, and dyspnea

Anesthesia: partial or complete loss of all forms of sensation, such as cold, heat, pain, or touch, attributable to a lesion of the nervous system; conventionally the term anesthesia is often used to identify loss of touch sensation, while analgesia is more often used to identify loss of pain sensibility

Aneurysm: a saccular or fusiform outpouching of a layer or layers of an arterial wall, usually found in the elderly and thought to arise from a systemic collagen synthetic or structural defect

Angina: severe sore throat with implied quality of choking

Angina Pectoris: a strangling sensation or heavy chest discomfort often radiating to the arms, especially the left, and usually precipitated by exertion; in current usage the term implies a cardiac ischemic origin

Angioma: a benign vascular tumor composed of blood or lymphatic vessels

Anhidrosis: a deficient production of sweat, also called *anaphoresis*

Ankylosis: stiffness or immobilization of a joint, resulting from injury, disease, or surgical intervention

Anorexia: a lack of appetite or desire for food

Anteflexion: a forward bend or curvature as in part of an organ, for example, a forward bending of the body of the uterus at its junction with the cervix

Anticholinergic: counteracting the action of acetylocholine, used especially with drugs that block conduction at cholinergic endings

Apnea: the absence or cessation of breathing

Arrhythmia: any variation from normal, regular rhythm, especially cardiac rhythm

Arthralgia: joint pain with objective findings of heat, redness, tenderness to touch, loss of motion, or swelling

Arthropathy: any joint disease

Ascites: the intraperitoneal accumulation of watery fluid in the nature of a transidate

Asthenia: a nonspecific symptom characterized by loss of energy and strength and a feeling of weakness; it usually accompanies chronic debilitating conditions such as infectious diseases and cancer

Ataxia: unsteadiness, incoordination, or disorganization of movements in the absence of paralysis

Atelectasis: a state of airlessness and hence reduced volume, especially of the lung

Atheroma: a disorder of arterial walls characterized by degenerative changes, deposition of the lipid, proliferation of smooth muscle cells, and fibrosis

Basal: pertaining to or situated adjacent to the base of a structure or organ

Benign: relatively mild, likely to have a favorable outcome; not malignant, not having the potential for metastasis; describes a neoplasm

Bradycardia: a slow heart rate, usually defined as less than 60 beats per minute in adults

Bronchiectasis: abnormal dilatation of bronchi

Bronchophony: the auscultatory sound of the voice characteristically heard over an area of consolidation in the lung

Bruit: an auscultatory sound of murmur, especially when arising from the heart or vessels

Bruxism: a grinding or gnashing of the teeth in sleep

Buccal: relating to or in the direction of the cheek; in dentistry, used especially to describe the surface of a tooth facing the cheek or lips

Carcinoma: a spreading sore, ulcer, or cancer

Causalgia: a specific syndrome of severe, peculiar, unpleasant, and burning pain, often associated with smooth, shiny skin in the affected area; there may also be hypersensitivity to touch and temperature, following an incomplete lesion of a peripheral nerve

Chloasma: moth patch; melandoderm or melasma characterized by the occurrence of extensive brown patches of irregular shape and size on the skin of the face and elsewhere

Cholecystic: of or relating to the gallbladder

Cholecystitis: inflammation of the gallbladder

Cholinergic: denoting a synapse, nerve terminal, or aggragate of neurons for which the principle neurotransmitter is acetylcholine

Chondrogenic: giving rise to or forming cartilage

Chorea: a form of involuntary movement marked by fine, disorganized, and random movements of the extremities, usually affecting the hands and feet and involving the proximal limb and trunk muscles to a lesser extent

Choreiform: resembling the movements of chorea

Chronotropism: an alteration in the rate of a recurring phenomenom; for example, an alteration in heart rate

Claudication: lameness or limping, often associated with pain; cramplike pain and weakness in muscles, most often those of the calf with consequent lameness

Clonus: a repetitive rhythmical contraction and relaxation such as that which may occur in one phase of a convulsion, the similar phenomenom induced at a joint by stretching a muscle in a spastic limb, or one showing hyperreflexia

Colic: relating to or associated with the colon, used primarily in anatomic terms; also, any of various conditions characterized by abdominal pain, especially paroxysmal pain occurring in a crescendo-decrescendo pattern, dependent upon visceral smooth muscle peristalsis

Constipation: the condition in which bowel movements are delayed or inadequate; undue retention of feces in the large intestine

Cyanosis: a bluish discoloration, particularly of the skin or mucous membranes, due to an excessive proportion of reduced hemoglobin in the blood, to stagnation of blood in capillaries of the skin or mucous membranes, or to the presence of methemoglobin, sulfhemoglobin, or other abnormal pigments

Cystitis: acute or chronic inflammation of the urinary bladder

Cystocele: a defect of the pelvic supporting structures causing a prolapse of the bladder into the vagina, clinically manifested by varying degrees of frequency, urgency, incontinence, dysuria, and mechanical discomfort

Cytotoxic: having the effect of poisoning or destroying cells, as a drug or infective organism

Dactylitis: inflammation or infection of a finger

Delirium: an organic brain syndrome characterized by clouding of consciousness, difficulty in sustaining attention, impaired orientation in memory, and perceptual disturbances leading to hallucinations

Dementia: a state in which there is a significant loss of intellectual capacity and cognitive functioning leading to impairment in social or occupational functioning, or both

Diaphoretic: an agent capable of inducing sweating

Diarrhea: abnormal fecal discharge characterized by frequent and/or watery stool

Diastole: the period of atrial and ventricular myocardial relaxation in the cardiac cycle

Diplopia: the seeing of a single object as double, usually resulting from misalignment of the two eyes, but sometimes due to optical faults such as variations of density and consequently of refractive index within the crystaline lens

Discoid: roughly disk shaped or characterized by disk-shaped lesions

Diuretic: inducing a state of increased urine flow

Diverticulum: a localized sac or pouch formed in the wall of a hollow viscus and opening into its lumen

Dysesthesia: abnormal spontaneous sensation, often with an unpleasant quality, for example, itching, pins-and-needles, burning, or sensation as of hot or cold water, or of an electric shock; these are symptoms of disease or dysfunction of sensory pathways

Dyskinesia: any abnormality of movement, such as incoordination, spasm, or irregular or ill-formed movements

Dysmenorrhea: painful menstruation; the colicky lower abdominal pain of ovulatory menstruation

Dyspareunia: coitus associated with recurrent, persistent genital pain

Dyspepsia: indigestion and upset stomach; a functional disturbance of the upper gastrointestinal tract characterized by abdominal discomfort, bloating, and, to a variable degree, nausea

Dysphagia: difficulty in swallowing; a sensation of food sticking in the esophagus

Dysphonia: abnormal phonation; an abnormal low-pitched, rough vocalization produced not by the vocal cords, but by the ventricular bands, often occurring when an attempt is made to disguise some underlying vocal cord disease

Dysphoria: a feeling of unpleasantness or discomfort

Dyspnea: shortness of breath; labored or difficult breathing; breathlessness

Dysrhythmia: disordered or abnormal rhythm

Dystonia: any abnormality of muscle tone

Dysuria: painful or difficult urination, generally caused by lower urinary tract disease such as cystitis, urethritis, urethral stricture, and prostatic disease

Ectopic: out of place, outside the usual range of locations or relationships, or abnormally exposed to view

Egophony: a vocal sound likened to the bleating of a goat, heard on auscultation of the chest over pleural effusion

Embolus: a thrombus formed within or a foreign material introduced into the vascular tree and carried by the blood stream to a site where it lodges and obstructs further flow of blood

Empyema: the accumulation of pus in a cavity, especially in the thoracic cavity

Endocrine: secreting into the bloodstream; describes a gland that delivers a substance into the circulation, causing that substance to have an affect at a remote site

Endogenous: originating within an organism or resulting from causes within the organism

Enteric: of or relating to the intestine, especially the small intestine; intended to be dissolved or digested in the intestine but not in the stomach; describes capsules and pill coatings that protect their contents from the action of gastric juice

Enthesitis: traumatic disease occurring at the insertion of muscles where recurring concentration of muscle stress provokes inflammation, with a strong tendency toward fibrosis and calcification

Enuresis: incontinence of urine with full bladder emptying, after the age at which bladder control should have been attained

Epigastrium: the wall of the abdomen above the naval

Epiphenomenon: an incidental event or symptom occurring as an accompaniment of a disease, but not essentially or typically with it

Erythema: an increased redness of the skin that is caused by capillary dilation

Exocrine: secreting in the direction of the body surface, usually through a duct

Exogenous: produced or otherwise originating outside the organism

Extroversion: a personality trait that orients one toward external events, other people, and social interactions rather than toward inner feelings or thoughts

Fibrillation: spontaneous contraction of single muscle fibers which can be recorded electromyographically and which is usually a manifestation of deneravation, with wallerian degeneration of at least some motor axons

Fugue: a condition in which the subject takes leave of his usual activities and wanders about; typically, the individual suffers from amnesia for the period he is absent from his usual activities

Functional: of or relating to a function; specifically, serving to contribute to the operation of a bodily function; having no known organic cause as in functional disorder

Goiter: any diffuse or nodular enlargement or swelling of the thyroid gland, often visible as a prominence in the lower anterior neck

Gynecology: the branch of medicine which devotes itself to the care and prevention of genital tract disorders in woman which for the most part is not concerned with pregnancy

Gynecomastia: enlargement of the male breast, occurring sometimes in mild form as a normal phenomenom of male puberty and as a sequela of various pathological conditions

Hemarthrosis: a hemorrhage into a joint

Hematochezia: the passage of bright red, easily identifiable blood from the anus, usually a sign of fresh bleeding distal to the ileocecal valve

Hematoma: a localized accumulation of blood in a tissue or space

Hematuria: excretion of urine containing blood either gross or microscopic

Hemianesthesia: loss of sensation on one side of the body

Hemoptysis: the expectoration of blood

Hemothorax: a collection of blood within the pleural cavity

Hepatic: of or relating to the liver

Hirsutism: the growth of hair in woman in the male sexual pattern

Hormone: any substance secreted by specialized cells in the endocrine glands, in clusters, or diffusely spread through the brain, lungs, and gastrointestinal tract; the substances act upon specific target tissues more or less remote from the site of secretion or upon the regulation of metabolic processes throughout the organism

Hydrocele: an accumulation of serous fluid in a body cavity, especially between the visceral and parietal layers of the tunica vaginalis in the scrotum

Hyperacusis: a condition in which sounds are perceived as unduly loud

Hyperalgesia: excessive sensitivity to painful stimuli

Hypercapnia: an elevated concentration of carbon dioxide in the blood

Hyperesthesia: exaggerated sensibility

Hyperparathyroidism: a condition resulting from excessive secretion of parathyroid hormone by the parathyroid glands

Hyperplasia: increase in the number of cells in a tissue or an organ with concomitant increase in the size of the structure involved

Hypertension: abnormally high tension or pressure; applied especially to the systemic arterial or pulmonary arterial blood pressure

Hyperthyroidism: excessive secretion of thyroxine and/or riiodothyronine from the thyroid gland, accompanied by increased rate of oxygen consumption, accelerated basal metabolic rate, thyroid enlargement, and systemic disturbances

Hypoesthesia: reduction in sensitivity

Hypokalemia: an abnormally low concentration of potassium in the blood or blood serum

Hypokinesia: a reduction in motor activity or in the range of motion of the body or limbs

Hyponychium: the part of the fingertip that extends from the distal end of the nail bed to the distal crease on the palmar aspect of the finger; it corresponds to the pulp of the finger

Hypoparathyroidism: a condition resulting from subnormal or absent secretion of parathyroid hormone by the parathyroid glands

Hypophysis: an unpaired, ovoid body that lies below the hypothalamus in the pituitary fossa of the sella turcica; the pituitary gland

Hypothyroidism: deficient hormone secretion by the thyroid gland or the condition resulting from it

Hypoxemia: reduced oxygen concentration in arterial blood

Impotence: a dysfunction in which the male is unable to perform the sexual act

Incontinence: absence of voluntary control of an expiratory function, especially defecation or urination

Infarct: a discreet, usually wedge-shaped area of ischemic coagulative necrosis caused by interruption of blood flow

Inotropic: affecting the force of speed of muscular contraction either by enhancing or inhibiting it

Intima: denoting an innermost layer

Introversion: the dynamic process in personality development by which the psychic energy of the individual is directed inwardly toward the self

Ischemia: inadequate blood flow to a part or organ

Jaundice: yellow discoloration of the skin and membranes, resulting from hyperbilirubinemia and subsequent deposition of bile pigment in the involved structure

Ketoacidosis: a metabolic acidosis associated with an accumulation of ketone bodies that are characteristic of uncontrolled diabetes mellitus

Leukorrhea: a gynecologic disorder characterized by an abnormal, whitish, nonbloody discharge from the genital tract

Libido: the energy of the sexual drive in Freud's psychoanalytic psychology; it is often used to include the energy of the aggressive drive as well

Lingula: a small structure or process shaped like or suggestive of a tongue

Lysis: any form of dissolution, particularly the breaking of membrane-bound structures such as cells

Malaise: a feeling of untoward weakness, lethargy, or discomfort as of impending illness

Malar: pertaining to the cheek

Malignant: tending to destroy, harm, or kill; as malignant tumor

Mania: a syndrome consisting of elated although unstable mood, hyperactivity, mental overactivity, and expressed garrulousness

Media: a middle layer

Melena: the passage of dark or blackish, tarlike stools stained with altered blood

Meningioma: a tumor of the cellular elements of the meninges; it is most often attached to the dura, especially where arachnoid villi are numerous

Menopause: the immediate postreproductive phase of a woman's life, when menstrual function ceases due to failure to form ovarian follicles and ova

Menorrhagia: excessive or prolonged menstruation

Metastasis: the transfer of a disease from one body site to another; said especially of cancers and infectious diseases

Metrorrhagia: uterine bleeding occurring at times other than the expected menses

Micturition: urination

Murmur: a prolonged or continuous auscultatory sound, particularly one deriving from the heart or cardiovascular system

Myalgia: pain in the muscles

Myelogenous: the development of bone marrow

Myeloma: a neoplastic proliferation of plasma cells, characterized by bone tumors and often complicated by pathological fractures

Myopathy: any disease of skeletal or voluntary muscle

Myxedema: the condition that accompanies severe hypothyroidism, characterized by yellowish pallor and nonpitting edema, especially in the face with scanty hair in the eyebrows, periorbital puffiness, and thick lips

Narcissism: the stage and development of object relationships that follow the autoerotic or sematogenic stage

Necrosis: the morphologic changes that follow cell death, characterized most frequently by nuclear changes

Neoplasm: a benign or malignant expanding lesion composed of proliferating cells; a tumor

Neurohypophysis: the posterior lobe of the pituitary gland

Neurosis: any of various functional disorders of behavior characterized by excessive anxiety, by behavior distorted by an exaggerated use of avoidance behaviors, or by other recognized mechanisms for defending against anxiety

Neutropenia: a decreased number of neutrophils in the circulating blood

Nidus: a focus of origin, such as a collection of bacteria in infections or the point of precipitation in calculus formation

Nociception: pain sense

Nociceptive: denoting responsiveness of sensitivity to noxious stimuli capable of eliciting pain

Nociperception: the recognition by the nervous system or an organism of a traumatic or hurtful stimulus

Nocturia: urination during normal sleeping hours

Nosology: the science of the systematic classification of diseases

Nystagmus: spontaneous, rapid, rhythmic movement of the eyes, occurring either on fixation or on occular movement, and often due to faulty supranuclear or internuclear innervation

Obstetrics: the field of medicine dealing with the care of women during pregnancy, labor, delivery, and the postpartum period

Occult: not readily apparent or detectable; hidden or disguised, as an infection, presence of blood, or a tumor

Oculogyric: describing, pertaining to, or producing spontaneous or sustained occular movements, usually in an upward direction as in Parkinsonism

Oligoarthritis: arthritis of a few joints

Onychia: an inflammation of the nail matrix, either following trauma or accompanying paronychia

Onycholysis: a separation of the nail plate from the nail bed

Opisthotonos: spasmodic contraction of the muscles of the neck and back with arching of the body; when severe, the subject may rest only on their head and heels

Orchitis: inflammation of the testes, manifested by swelling and tenderness and usually of infectious origin, as in tuberculosis, mumps, syphyllis, or certain fungal diseases

Organic: of or relating to an organ, structural in nature or origin as in organic defect

Orthopnea: shortness of breath experienced when lying down

Orthostatic: relating to the erect posture

Osteogenesis: the process by which bone tissue and the bones of the skeleton are formed, including all stages of bone formation, not just mineralization

Osteolysis: the resorption of bone, especially its mineralized component

Osteopenia: a reduction in bone mass that is caused by decreased osteoid formation and the presence of normal bone resorption; any decrease in bone density or mass below normal amounts

Osteoporosis: a reduction in the quantity and quality of bone by the loss of both bone marrow and protein content

Pallor: paleness due to lack of melanin or lack of blood in the skin

Palpitation: the sensation produced by rapid, forceful, or irregular beating of the heart

Papilloma: a benign tumor of skin, mucous membrane, and ducts, composed of epithelium covering a fibrous stalk

Paradoxical: possibly true, but appearing to contradict facts or confirmed opinion

Parenchyma: the characteristic or functional tissue or cells of a gland or an organ

Paresthesia: any sensation, such as pins-and-needles, burning, or prickling, that occurs spontaneously without external cause in disease or dysfunction of the central or peripheral nervous system

Paronychia: an inflammation of the proximal or lateral nail folds

Pericarditis: inflammation of the pericardium

Perineum: the diamond-shaped area superficial to the inferior pelvic aperature

Peristalsis: successive waves of contraction passing for shorter or longer distances along tubular muscular organs such as the alimentary tract

Phobia: pathologic fear, dread, avoidance, or abhorrence

Photophobia: an abnormal intolerance of light, usually due to inflammation of the iris and ciliary body

Pneumothorax: the presence of air in the pleural cavity

Polyarthritis: arthritis of multiple joints

Polydipsia: the drinking of water in abnormally large quantities

Polymyositis: an inflammatory autoimmune disorder of muscle, related to other disorders of the collagen or connective tissue group

Polyneuropathy: any systemic infection of the peripheral nerves of toxic, metabolic, or unknown etiology

Polyp: any mass of tissue that protrudes outward from a surface, usually an epithelium

Polyuria: the formation of urine in abnormally large volume, reflected by frequency and by volume of urination

Prognathism: the characteristic of having a projected jaw; an abnormally anterior anatomic position of the mandible

Proteinuria: urinary excretion of abnormal amounts of protein; normally, up to 150 mg of protein may be excreted per 24 hours

Psyche: the mind in contradistinction to the body

Psychogenic: of psychological or mental origin

Psychosis: a class of mental disorders that usually includes organic mental disorders, schizophrenias, major affect disorders, and certain paranoid states

Ptosis: the prolapse or downward displacement of an organ; commonly used to describe abnormal downward displacement of the upper eyelid which may result from paralysis of the third cranial nerve

Purpura: a focal hemorrhage into the skin

Pyelography: reontgenography of the renal pelvis after the use of a contrast agent

Pyelonephritis: inflammation of the renal pelvis and parenchyma due to bacterial infection

Pyogenic: able to cause formation of purulent lesions in tissues

Pyuria: the presence of an abnormal number of leukocytes or pus in the urine, reflecting urinary tract inflammation such as that resulting from infection

Rale: an abnormal sound heard on auscultation of the chest during breathing, especially one that is caused or seems to be caused by air passing through fluid in the airways

Rhonchus: an abnormal sound heard on auscultation of the lungs, ranging from a wheeze to a snoring sound and due to air passing through a partially obstructed or narrowed airway

Roentgenogram: radiograph

Roentgenography: a special radiologic technique that demonstrates, on film, the details of structures in a predetermined plane of tissue while blurring the detail of structures in other planes

Sarcoidosis: a disease of unknown cause characterized by noncaseating granulomas in many organs of the body; the most commonly involved tissues are those of the lungs, lymph nodes, and liver

Scintigraphy: a clinical diagnostic procedure consisting of an injection, usually intravenous, of a solution containing a radioactive agent with a specific affinity for an organ or tissue of interest, followed by the determination of the distribution of radioactivity

Sclerosis: a hardening of the interstitial connective tissue following damage to the parenchyma of an organ; hardening is due to increases in the amount of interstitial fibers connective tissue

Scotoma: a circumscribed area of blindness or reduced vision within the visual field

Sepsis: a syndrome resulting from overwhelming invasion of the circulation by pathogenic microorganisms or the toxins they produce

Septicemia: severe generalized infection resulting from hematogenous dissemination of pathogenic microorganisms and their toxins

Serotonin: a neurotransmittor with action on blood vessels; it also acts as a hormone and is formed by the decarboxilation of 5-hydroxytryptophan

Soma: all the body tissues except germ cells; the body as distinct from the mind or psyche

Somatic: relating to or involving the skeleton or skeletal muscle as distinct from the viscera of the body; also relating to or involving the body as distinct from the mind or psyche

Somulence: unnatural sleepiness or drowsiness

Souffle: a soft, blowing murmur, especially an extracardiac murmur

Spermatogenesis: a series of stages and cellular differentiations resulting in the formation of spermatozoa

Splenomegally: enlargement of the spleen

Spondylitis: an inflammation of one or more vertebrae

Spondylolisthesis: a forward displacement of one vertebrae upon the other, usually in the lower lumbar spine, due to either a traumatic or congenital weakness defect of the pars interarticularis

Spondylolysis: the breaking down of a vertebrae

Spondylosis: a noninflammatory disease of the spine, usually osteoarthritis and/or degenerative disk disease

Squama: a scale-like or thin plate-like structure

Stridor: a harsh, high-pitched noise on breathing, especially on inspiration, indicative of a degree of obstruction of the airway, especially of the larynx or trachea

Syncope: transient loss of consciousness due to generalized cerebral ischemia secondary to a global reduction in cerebral blood flow

Systole: the contraction phase of the atria or ventricles in a cardiac cycle

Tachycardia: a fast heart rate; term applied when adult heart rate exceeds 100 per minute

Tachypnea: rapid breathing

Tardive: characterized by lateness or delay; said especially of a condition with late-emerging signs and symptoms

Tetany: a syndrome marked by a state of neuromuscular hyperexcitability, which may cause reversable muscular contractures, particularly in the extremities

Thrombus: a semisolid aggregate of blood cells enmeshed in fibrin and clumps of platelets that results from the rapid conversion of fibrinogen to fibrin, especially within a blood vessel

Thyrotoxicosis: a condition resulting from hyperthyroidism due to any cause

Tinnitus: any form of adventitious noise arising within the ears or head and audible to the subject; the nature of the noise may be whistling, ringing, clicking, or pulsating, and in some instances may be audible to others

Tomography: a radiologic examination in which a thin, collimated x-ray beam rotates about the patient with registration of photon exist doses on detectors; the exit doses then undergo manipulation by computer to produce an image of the slice of tissue examined

Trismus: spasm or contracture of the masticatory muscles, making it difficult to open the mouth

Trophic: having to do with nutrition; pertaining to that which stimulates growth and development or stimulates increased activity; pertaining to nutritional changes in skin and other tissues that may follow impairment of a nerve supply

Tumor: an expanding lesion due to progressive, apparently uncontrolled proliferation of cells; a neoplasm

Tympany: a low pitched, drumlike sound produced by percussion over air-filled region, especially in the stomach and intestine or in the peritoneal and pleural cavities

Varix: a mass composed of enlarged and tortuous blood or lymphatic vessels

Vegetative: engaged in or relating to the process of nutrition or growth as distinct from reproduction; also, pertaining to involuntary bodily functions or to the autonomic nervous system

Vertigo: a hallucination of movement, especially of rotation, of the subject or of his or her surroundings

Vesicular: designating a soft auscultatory breath sound presumably originating in the pulmonary vesicles and generally characteristic of the normal lung

Wheeze: to emit a high-pitched, more or less musical nonvocal sound during breathing, usually audible subjectively and without auscultation; it is usually produced by bronchial, tracheal, or laryngeal constriction or obstruction

INDEX

60. *Plasmodium vivax* ring
61. *P. vivax* trophozoite
62. *P. vivax* trophozoites
63. *P. vivax* trophozoites
64. *P. vivax* trophozoites
65. *P. vivax* trophozoites, early schizont
66. *P. vivax* schizont
67. *P. vivax,* thick film
68. *P. vivax,* thick film
69. *P. malariae* band forms
70. *P. malariae* early schizont
71. *P. malariae* schizont
72. *P. malariae* gametocytes
73. *P. malariae,* thick film
74. *P. ovale* trophozoite
75. *P. ovale* trophozoite
76. *P. ovale trophozoite,* early schizont
77. *P. ovale* gametocytes
78. *P. falciparum* ring stages
79. *P. falciparum* ring stages
80. *P. falciparum* ring stages
81. *P. falciparum* ring stages
82. *P. falciparum* ring stages, schizont
83. *P. falciparum* early gametocyte
84. *P. falciparum* gametocyte
85. *P. falciparum,* thick film
86. *P. falciparum* in brain
87. *Plasmodium* exoerythrocytic stage
88. *Leishmania donovani* in liver

89. *Leishmania,* impression smear
90. *Trypanosoma gambiense*
91. *Trypanosoma cruzi*
92. *T. cruzi,* heart muscle
93. *Toxoplasma gondii* trophozoites
94. *T. gondii* cyst in brain
95. *T. gondii* cyst in liver
96. Toxoplasmal chorioretinitis
97. *T. gondii,* cat intestine
98. *T. gondii,* cat intestine
99. *Sarcocystis*
100. *Sarcocystis*
101. *Pneumocystis carinii*
102. *P. carinii*
103. *Opisthorchis sinensis* eggs
104. *O. sinensis* egg, trichrome
105. *Opisthorchis* in bile duct
106. *Fasciolopsis buski* egg
107. *Paragonimus westermani* egg
108. *P. westermani* egg
109. *Schistosoma mansoni* egg
110. *S. mansoni* egg, hatched
111. *S. mansoni* egg, trichrome
112. *S. mansoni* egg, rectal biopsy
113. schistosome egg, liver
114. schistosome egg, liver
115. *S. haematobium* eggs
116. *S. haematobium* egg
117. *S. haematobium* eggs, bladder wall
118. *S. japonicum* egg
119. *S. japonicum* eggs, rectal biopsy

Continued on back end sheet

MEDICAL
PARASITOLOGY

FOURTH EDITION

EDWARD K. MARKELL, Ph.D., M.D.

Department of Internal Medicine,
Kaiser-Permanente Medical Center,
Oakland, California;
Clinical Professor of Family,
Community and Preventive Medicine,
Stanford University School of Medicine,
Palo Alto, California

MARIETTA VOGE, M.A., Ph.D.

Professor of Microbiology and Immunology,
Department of Microbiology and Immunology,
University of California School of Medicine,
Los Angeles, California

W. B. SAUNDERS COMPANY • Philadelphia • London • Toronto

W. B. Saunders Company: West Washington Square
Philadelphia, PA 19105

1 St. Anne's Road
Eastbourne, East Sussex BN21 3UN, England

1 Goldthorne Avenue
Toronto, Ontario M8Z 5T9, Canada

Medical Parasitology   ISBN   0-7216-6083-5

Last digit is the print number: 9   8   7   6   5   4   3   2

Dedicated to the late

PROFESSOR HAROLD KIRBY

University of California, Berkeley,

Under whose guidance the authors received their professional training in parasitology

PREFACE

Proliferation of the already over-abundant medical literature requires justification. This edition of *Medical Parasitology* includes several disease entities described in the past few years, and attempts to bring up-to-date a discussion of treatment, including where practicable pediatric dosages. We have added more information on the distribution of parasitic infections and their prevalence. The distribution of these diseases is outlined in tabular form for the purpose of quick reference. A separate chapter is devoted to immunodiagnostic procedures for parasitic infections. Useful new laboratory diagnostic techniques have also been added.

We have attempted to improve the illustrations by the substitution of better figures in some cases, and the addition of a number of new ones. A revised and expanded filmstrip has been prepared for optional use. The photomicrographs comprising the filmstrip are also available as 35 mm. color slides.

The present edition rests on the foundation of its predecessors, and we wish to acknowledge the help of our colleagues who have advised us on this and previous editions: Drs. Larry Ash, William Balamuth, Gordon H. Ball, Ralph Barr, Paul Basch, John N. Belkin, Robert S. Bray, Jack K. Frenkel, Quentin Geiman, Robert C. Goldberg, William L. Hewitt, Marion W. Hood, John F. Kessel, David L. McVickar, and Jerrald Turner. In addition, Mrs. Patricia E. Quinn and Mrs. Ruby Kuritsubo have provided material for illustrations and constructive criticism for the chapter on techniques.

Many not named above have also contributed ideas and information, for which we are grateful. As usual, the staff of the W. B. Saunders Company was at all times kind, helpful, and considerate of our whims and shortcomings.

THE AUTHORS

One hundred eighty illustrations supplementing those in this book are reproduced in color on a set of 35 mm. slides or filmstrips, available from the publisher. Subjects of the individual frames are listed on the end sheets of this volume.

CONTENTS

1

Introduction

With the nearly simultaneous development of the antibiotic drugs DDT and other insecticides, and various new antiparasitic agents, it was for a time widely believed that the infectious diseases would for all practical purposes disappear from the clinical scene. That this has not happened is obvious. Bacterial resistance appeared early; alterations in the normal bacterial flora, sometimes combined with iatrogenic modifications of host resistance, have resulted in the appearance of numbers of organisms in unfamiliar pathogenic roles. DDT and other insecticides not only have failed to eliminate the vectors of malaria, filariasis, and other parasitic diseases, but have themselves brought on problems too well known to require mention here. The development of resistance to the synthetic antimalarials has been an ominous occurrence in recent years. The increased mobility of large segments of the population exposes them to a largely undiminished threat of parasitic infection, and the speed of transportation insures that many will return to their native shores before their infections become patent. For this reason it remains necessary that all physicians have some familiarity with the parasitic diseases, no matter how "exotic."

Modifications of the environment as typified by construction of the Aswan Dam and the Transamazon Highway in Brazil have brought about major increases in parasitic disease. Flooding of vast areas with the creation of Lake Nasser has resulted in new habitats for the snail hosts of schistosomiasis and a tremendous upsurge in incidence of that disease, brought in by infected construction workers. Building the Transamazon Highway necessitated the importation into the area of large numbers of susceptible laborers, causing them to be exposed to enzootic diseases of the area, notably leishmaniasis. It behooves us to consider the impact

1

of such projects upon the ecology before rather than after the damage is done.

With the ever-increasing pressure of a crowded medical curriculum, the time allocated to the study of protozoan, helminthic and arthropod parasites has been severely curtailed in many institutions. The same demands of an expanded technology have depleted the ranks of laboratory technologists with good training in the field of parasitology. The primary purpose of this book is to serve as a guide both to the clinical diagnosis and treatment and to the laboratory diagnosis of the protozoan and helminthic diseases of medical importance in this country, and to a lesser extent to the arthropods in relation to disease. We cannot limit ourselves to those organisms which are indigenous to this country or seen here with some frequency.

While intended primarily for the medical student and physician, it is hoped that this book will prove equally useful to the medical technologist and all others concerned with the laboratory identification of the animal parasites of man. The success of the cooperative diagnostic efforts of the physician and laboratory technologist depends upon a mutual appreciation of their several problems. In the chapters dealing with technical methods, the problems of the technologist are discussed; the physician will be better able to utilize his laboratory service if he understands them. The manner in which parasitic organisms are acquired, and how they produce disease in man, is perhaps of no direct importance to the technologist. Yet, a basic understanding of these matters should not only make the technologist's work more interesting, but also enable him to do it better and more efficiently.

A word of explanation should be given concerning the illustrations. They are largely original, and have been planned to emphasize points of diagnostic importance. The drawings which accompany the chapter on intestinal protozoa are all made at the same magnification, to facilitate a comparision of size ranges between different organisms, and within a single species. Structures not of importance from the standpoint of identification have been omitted from the majority of drawings, with the purpose of emphasizing those features to which especial attention should be paid. Nuclear structure is of great importance in the identification of many species of intestinal protozoa, but the variation which may be encountered is often a source of confusion. Drawings of nuclei alone, illustrative of the range of nuclear variation in the different species, have been included. These are not drawn to scale, but are all shown at the same size.

A series of transparencies has been prepared for supplemental use with this book. Its use is not mandatory, but it is hoped that they will help, particularly in situations where good laboratory reference materials are not readily available.

With reference to therapy for parasitic infections, it must always be borne in mind that any drug intended to disembarrass the host of his parasites does so on the basis of differential toxicity. That is to say that the antiparasitic agent is, hopefully, more toxic to parasite than to host. However, in some cases the margin is slim, and individual variation in host resistance may render it even slimmer. Frequently, toxic side effects are to be expected as the price of therapeutic effectiveness. It is to be hoped that, before treatment, the clinician will always ask himself whether the parasite is causing, or has a reasonable potential of causing, more trouble than may be anticipated from the treatment to be used. Treatment of certain parasitic diseases is changing almost as rapidly as that of the bacterial infections, and it is essential for the physician to keep abreast of the advances in this field. Review articles on this subject are seen occasionally in the medical journals, in such publications as the *Annual Review of Medicine, The Medical Letter on Drugs and Therapeutics,* and in the *Tropical Diseases Bulletin.* Under the title of "Current Concepts in Therapy," treatment of the parasitoses is considered from time to time in the *New England Journal of Medicine.*

A listing of some of the more important texts and monographs, written in English, is given at the end of this chapter. Some of the English language journals devoted to parasitology and tropical medicine are also listed. The *Tropical Diseases Bulletin* has already been mentioned. This monthly abstracting journal, published in England, is invaluable. It lists, under headings of the various etiological agents, the world-wide literature of tropical medicine, and publishes periodic summaries of work in certain fields as well as occasional comprehensive clinical reviews.

TEXTS AND MONOGRAPHS

Adams, A. R. D., and Maegraith, B. G. 1971. *Clinical Tropical Diseases.* 578 pp. Blackwell Scientific Publications, Oxford and Edinburgh.

Alicata, J. E., and Jindrak, K. 1970. *Angiostrongylosis in the Pacific and Southeast Asia.* 105 pp. Charles C Thomas, Springfield, Illinois.

Ash, J. E., and Spitz, S. 1945. *Pathology of Tropical Diseases; an Atlas.* 350 pp. W. B. Saunders Company, Philadelphia.

Brown, H. W. 1975. *Basic Clinical Parasitology.* 4th Ed. 355 pp. Appleton-Century-Crofts, New York.

Buxton, P. A. 1946. *The Louse.* 2nd Ed. 164 pp. Williams & Wilkins Co., Baltimore.

Ciba Foundation. 1974. *Parasites in the Immunized Host: Mechanisms of Survival.* Ciba Foundation Symposium 25 (new series). 280 pp. Associated Scientific Publishers, Amsterdam.

Ciba Foundation. 1974. *Trypanosomiasis and Leishmaniasis with Special Reference to Chagas' Disease.* Ciba Foundation Symposium 20. 353 pp. Associated Scientific Publishers, Amsterdam.

Faust, E. C., Beaver, P. C., and Jung, R. C. 1975. *Animal Agents and Vectors of Human Disease.* 4th Ed. 479 pp. Lea & Febiger, Philadelphia.

Frazier, C. A. 1969. *Insect Allergy: Allergic Reactions to Bites of Insects and Other Arthropods.* 493 pp. Warren H. Green, Inc., St. Louis, Missouri.

Garcia, L . S., and Ash, L. R. 1975. *Diagnostic Parasitology. Clinical Laboratory Manual.* 112 pp. C. V. Mosby Company, St. Louis, Missouri.

Garnham, P. C. C. 1966. *Malaria Parasites and Other Haemosporidia.* 1114 pp. Blackwell Scientific Publications, Oxford, England.

Gould, S. E. 1970. *Trichinosis in Man and Animals.* 540 pp. Charles C Thomas, Springfield, Illinois.

Heilesen, B. 1946. Studies on *Acarus scabiei* and scabies. Acta Dermato-Venereologica, *26* (Suppl. 14):1–370.

Hoogstraal, H., and Heyneman, D. 1969. Leishmaniasis in the Sudan Republic 30. Final epidemiologic report. Amer. J. Trop. Med. & Hyg. *18*:1091–1210.

Hunter, G. W., Swartzwelder, J. C., and Clyde, D. F. 1976. *Tropical Medicine.* 5th Ed. 900 pp. W. B. Saunders Company, Philadelphia.

International Encyclopedia of Pharmacology and Therapeutics; Section 64. 1973. *Chemotherapy of Helminthiases.* 537 pp. Pergamon Press, New York.

James, M. T., and Harwood, R. F. 1969. *Herms' Medical Entomology.* 6th Ed. 484 pp. Macmillan, New York.

Malek, E. A., and Cheng, T. C. 1974. *Medical and Economic Malacology.* 398 pp. Academic Press, New York.

Marcial-Rojas, R. A. (Ed.) 1971. *Pathology of protozoal and Helminthic Diseases with Clinical Correlation.* 1010 pp. Williams & Wilkins Co., Baltimore.

Mostofi, F. K., 1967. *Bilharziasis.* 357 pp. Springer-Verlag, New York.

Muller, R. 1975. *Worms and Disease. A Manual of Medical Helminthology.* 161 pp. William Heinemann, London.

Mulligan, C. H. W. (Ed.) 1970. *The African Trypanosomiases.* 950 pp. George Allen and Unwin Ltd., London.

Pinder, R. M. 1973. *Malaria, the Design, Use and Mode of Action of Chemotherapeutic Agents.* 316 pp. Scientechnica (Publishers) Ltd.

Roche, M., and Layrisse, M. 1966. The nature and causes of "hookworm anemia." Amer. J. Trop. Med. & Hyg., *15 (part 2)*:1–172.

Sadun, E. H., and Moon, A. P. 1972. *Basic Research in Malaria.* Vol. 39. 582 pp. Proc. Helm. Soc. Wash.

Scott, H. H. 1942. *A History of Tropical Medicine.* Vols. I and II. 1219 pp. Williams & Wilkins Co., Baltimore.

Šlais, J. 1970. *The Morphology and Pathogenicity of the Bladder Worms.* 144 pp. Dr. W. Junk N.V., the Hague.

Spencer, H., Dayan, A. D., Gibson, J. B., Huntsman, R. G., Hutt, M. S. R., Jenkins, G. C., Köberle, F., Maegraith, B. G., Salfelder, K. 1973. *Tropical Pathology.* 765 pp. Springer Verlag, New York.

Spencer, F. M., and Monroe, L. S. 1975. *The Color Atlas of Intestinal Parasites.* 158 pp. Charles C Thomas, Springfield, Illinois.

Steck, E. A. 1972. The Chemotherapy of Protozoan Diseases. Vols. 1–4. Walter Reed Army Institute of Research, Washington, D.C.

Wilcocks, C., and Manson-Bahr, P. E. 1972. *Manson's Tropical Diseases.* 17th Ed. 1164 pp. Williams & Wilkins Co., Baltimore.

SOME JOURNALS WHOLLY OR IN PART DEVOTED TO MEDICAL PARASITOLOGY AND TROPICAL MEDICINE

American Journal of Tropical Medicine and Hygiene
Annals of Tropical Medicine and Parasitology
Current Therapy
Journal of Parasitology
Journal of Tropical Medicine and Hygiene
Journal of Tropical Pediatrics
Parasitology
The Medical Letter
Transactions of the Royal Society of Tropical Medicine and Hygiene
Tropical Diseases Bulletin

2

Parasites, Parasitism and Host Relations

In view of the tremendous numbers and diversity of living things, and the varied circumstances of their existence, it is not surprising that they should obtain their nourishment in many different ways. These various methods have basic similarities, so that frequently it is difficult to draw a firm line between one method of nutrition and another. Many terms have been devised to describe the relationships which exist between different kinds of plants and animals, at the fundamental food-seeking or food-supplying level. These terms are not always used by everyone to denote the same thing, with the result that they may lead to confusion rather than clarity. We need not concern ourselves here with many terms which have been created to designate slight differences in relationship, and shall adopt somewhat rigid definitions of those which we do consider. However, it must be emphasized that any one organism may at different times exhibit different nutritional habits, or at the same time obtain its nutriment in more than one way. *If a definition is helpful in the understanding of a biological process, it is worthwhile, but it should never be allowed to channel or limit one's ideas.*

In a consideration of the major nutritional relationships between different species, we will limit ourselves to those involving different kinds of animals, with the understanding that much, but not all, of what is said may be extended to cover animal-plant interrelationships as well. Fundamentally, there are two different ways in which an animal may obtain food at the expense of other animals. It may attack another living animal, consuming part or all of its body for nourish-

5

ment, and in the process frequently but not necessarily killing it. This process is known as *predation;* the attacker is the predator and the victim the prey. Or an animal may derive its nutrition from already dead animals, either devouring those dead of natural causes or taking the leavings of a predator. Animals which subsist in this manner are known as *scavengers.* Some animals are pure predators, others pure scavengers, but many predators are not averse to an occasional bit of scavenging. Some animals always seek their food by their own efforts, or in association with others of their own species. This is the most conspicuous and perhaps the most common way in which animals go about obtaining food; it is this large group to which we commonly refer when we speak of scavengers and predators.

Other animals, still in essence predators or scavengers, have become so modified that they are unable to obtain food except in close association, either continuous or at intervals, with members of another species. This association of two species, perhaps primarily for food-getting on the part of one or both members of the group, is known as *symbiosis.** Symbiosis means literally "living together" and may also involve protection or other advantages to one or both partners. Different forms of symbiosis may be distinguished, on the basis of whether or not the association is detrimental to one of the two partners. *Commensalism,* from the Latin for "eating at the same table," denotes an association which is beneficial to one partner and at least not disadvantageous to the other. A specialized type of commensalism, known as *mutualism,* is seen where such associations are beneficial to both organisms. *Parasitism,* on the contrary, is a symbiotic relationship in which one animal, the host, is to some degree injured through the activities of the other animal, the parasite. Parasitism, like other forms of symbiosis, necessarily involves an intimate relationship between the two species, and it is this close and prolonged contact which differentiates parasitism from the predatory activities of many non-parasites.

Parasitism as a way of life may be the only possibility for a given organism, or it may be but one alternative. An organism which cannot survive in any other manner is called an *obligate parasite.* A *facultative parasite* is an organism which may exist in a free-living state, or as a commensal, and if opportunity presents itself may become parasitic. It is implicit in this term that the organism does not of necessity have to be a parasite at any stage of its existence. Some animals are obligatory parasites at one or more stages of their life cycles, but free-living at others. The term "temporary parasite" is sometimes applied to such animals. Parasites living within the host may be distinguished as *endo-*

---

*The definitions given here for symbiosis, commensalism and mutualism differ from those used by many authors. However, they conform to the recommendations of the Committee on Terminology of the American Society of Parasitologists.

parasites, while those which are found upon the surface of the body are called *ectoparasites*.

Small organisms, such as mosquitoes, which must periodically seek out other and larger forms on which to nourish themselves, have occasionally been called "intermittent parasites." This unhappy use of the term "parasite" comes from the assumption that a predator must be larger and stronger than its prey, whereas a parasite is small and weak. This generalization is certainly true of most predators and parasites, or at least of the most obvious ones. However, the essence of the parasitic relationship, which separates it from predation, is the protracted and intimate association between parasite and host. The association between the mosquito and its victim is neither prolonged nor intimate. Cameron (1956) refers to those blood-sucking arthropods which lead an independent existence except for occasional nutritional forays as micro-predators.

Many organisms customarily considered to be parasites are actually commensals. *Entamoeba coli* lives within the lumen of the intestine, subsists there upon the bacterial flora of the gut, and does its host no appreciable harm. This is a symbiotic relationship in which no advantage or disadvantage accrues to the host, whereas the ameba is supplied with food and protected from harm. Other cases are less definite. There is considerable controversy over the question of whether *Entamoeba histolytica* is at all times parasitic or if it can at times have a purely commensal relationship with its host.

Adaptations to Parasitism

The parasitic relationship probably evolved very early in the history of living organisms. We know little about how such relationships arose, but may hypothesize that we can see in the facultative parasite one possible initial step along the road to obligate parasitism. The possibility of the adaptation of a parasitic mode of existence may depend upon what is known as "pre-adaptation," or evolutionary changes which make possible existence in an environment otherwise unsuitable. Such pre-adaptive changes might be in the nature of increased resistance to the enzymatic activities of the host. Further physiological adaptations to parasitism might involve the loss of enzymes or enzyme systems which are then supplied by the host. Such losses may be expected to make a parasitic or at least symbiotic relationship obligatory.

Certain groups of parasites exhibit profound morphological adaptations to their way of life. As might be expected, these modifications are more striking in those groups which are wholly parasitic than in those containing both free-living and parasitic species. Organs not necessary to a parasitic existence are frequently lost. The only class of

Protozoa which contains nothing but parasitic forms is the Sporozoa. Members of this class have no locomotor organelles, although these structures are present in one form or another in all other classes of Protozoa, even in their parasitic representatives. Most of the free-living turbellarian flatworms are provided with a ciliated epidermis in the adult stage. Cilia are not found on the parasitic members of this group, or on the related, but strictly parasitic, trematodes and cestodes. A digestive tract, of moderate complexity in the turbellarians, is generally reduced in the trematodes and is absent in the cestodes. The reproductive system is very highly developed in the two latter groups; this seems a reflection of the difficulties inherent in transfer of these organisms to new hosts. Specialized attachment organs in the form of suckers and hooks have been developed in the parasitic flatworms. Body size may be greatly affected by the parasitic state. Although we think of parasites as small organisms, many of them are much larger than their free-living relatives. The majority of free-living turbellarians are under half a centimeter in length, and while some land planarians may reach a half meter, none approaches the length of 10 meters or more seen in some tapeworms. Most free-living nematodes barely attain naked-eye visibility as adults, but *Ascaris* can reach 35 cm. and *Dracunculus* as much as a meter in length.

Specialized mechanisms for effecting entrance into the body or tissues are seen in some parasites. *Entamoeba histolytica* elaborates a proteolytic enzyme which aids its penetration of the intestinal mucosa. No such enzyme has been found in the commensal *E. coli*. The cercarial stage in the life cycle of the blood fluke is able to penetrate through the skin of man to produce infection. This it does with the aid of penetration glands which produce an enzyme capable of digesting the skin. The embryo of *Hymenolepis nana*, before developing into a cysticercoid larva, penetrates an intestinal villus with the help of the six hooklets which it bears.

Increased reproductive capacity has been already mentioned as characterizing two parasitic groups in contrast to their free-living relatives. Most metazoan parasites exhibit such an increase, which in some cases involves larval stages as well as adults. The chances of a particular ovum successfully infecting a new host are usually very small, and if more than one host species is involved, the chance of successful completion of the cycle becomes still smaller. If a parasite is successful in infecting an intermediate host, it is obviously advantageous if the larval stage which develops there can multiply to produce many additional organisms, capable of infecting the definitive or a second intermediate host. Such a modification is seen in the trematodes and many of the cestodes, where a single ovum develops in the intermediate host into a larva which in turn produces many larvae of a more advanced kind.

Effects of Parasites upon the Host

A parasite, by definition, is an organism which to some degree injures its host. However, we have already found that many organisms which are loosely termed parasites are in reality commensals. Some may be at times truly parasitic and at other times commensal in their relationship to the host. In many instances it cannot be said with certainty whether or not an organism injures the host. Even if we can be fairly sure that some injury is produced, we may not be able to detect it. Thus a distinction is made between hookworm disease and hookworm infection, on the basis of the presence or absence of clinical symptoms. Overt symptoms of infection with this parasite may depend upon the number of worms present, upon the nutritional status of the host, or both.

Injury to the host may be brought about in a wide variety of ways. Some of these mechanisms are common to all parasites, even if this term is used in its broad sense to include bacteria, viruses and fungi. The most widespread type of injury is that brought about by interference with the vital processes of the host, through the action of secretions, excretions or other products of the parasite. Such interference is probably largely or exclusively on the level of the host enzyme systems. Parasites producing such effects may be in the tissues or organs of the host, in the blood stream, within the gastrointestinal tract, or may even be ectoparasitic. Invasion and destruction of host tissue may be distinguished from injury which does not involve gross physical damage, although both types of injury reflect biochemical changes brought about in the host tissue by the parasites. When the giant intestinal fluke, *Fasciolopsis buski*, is present in large numbers, absorption from the intestinal tract of its secretions and excretions may lead to severe toxicity. *Entamoeba histolytica* erodes the intestinal wall, destroying the tissues locally by means of a proteolytic enzyme. Malarial parasites invade and multiply in red blood cells, which are destroyed in the process. The helminth parasites, by virtue of their size, may damage the host in other ways impossible for the smaller parasites. In addition to its toxic effects, *Fasciolopsis buski* may produce severe local damage to the intestinal wall by means of its powerful suckers. *Ascaris* may perforate the bowel wall, cause intestinal obstruction if present in large numbers, and invade the appendix, bile duct or other organs. Some parasites exert their effects by depriving the host of essential substances. Thus hookworms suck blood, and by so doing may deprive the host of more iron than is replaced by his diet, and so bring about an anemia. The broad fish tapeworm, *Diphyllobothrium latum*, selectively removes vitamin B_{12} from the alimentary tract, producing a megaloblastic anemia in some infected persons.

Effects of the Host on the Parasite

The effects of the parasite on the host are more obvious than those which operate in the reverse direction, but the latter are nonetheless important. The genetic constitution of the host may profoundly influence the host-parasite relationship. It is now well known that there are racial variations in resistance to certain strains of *Plasmodium vivax*. There is also considerable evidence which suggests that possession of the sickle cell trait, an inherited characteristic, is also associated with increased resistance to infection with the malarial parasite, *P. falciparum*.

The diet or nutritional status of the host may be of major importance in determining the outcome of a parasitic infection (Frye, 1955). A high protein diet has been found to be unfavorable for the development of many intestinal protozoa, while a diet low in protein was shown by Elsdon-Dew (1953) to favor the appearance of symptoms of amebiasis and the complications of this disease. It has been shown that a carbohydrate-rich diet favors the development of certain tapeworms, and the presence of carbohydrate in the diet is known to be essential for some of these worms. The general nutritional status of the host may be of considerable importance both in determining whether or not a particular infection will be accompanied by symptoms and in influencing their severity if present. Major nutritional disturbances may influence resistance through their effects upon the immune mechanisms of the host.

While the fundamental immune processes are generally considered to be the same in infection with the animal parasites as in bacterial, viral and mycotic infections, the details are much better known for bacteria and viruses than for the larger forms. Every species of animal is naturally resistant to infection with many organisms which parasitize different species. As we have seen in the case of certain strains of malaria, resistance may also be a racial phenomenon. In some cases it has been possible to adapt parasites to hosts which they normally infect poorly, or not at all. This does not necessarily involve changes in the host's natural resistance, but rather changes in the parasite. Acquired immunity can be demonstrated in many parasitic diseases. This is generally found to be at a lower level than that produced by bacteria and viruses. Absolute immunity to reinfection, such as is generally seen following infection with smallpox, measles, whooping cough and a number of other viral and bacterial diseases, occurs but rarely following protozoal infections and probably never with helminth infections of man. Primary infection with *Leishmania* seems to confer a degree of immunity to reinfection. While many protozoal and helminthic infections confer no long-lasting immunity to reinfection, they do seem to stimulate resistance during the time that the parasites are still in the body. This resistance to hyperinfection is known as premunition. Premunition may be of great importance in endemic areas in limiting the extent of infection with plasmodia, hookworms and other parasites.

There is increasing evidence of the importance of the "secretions and excretions" of protozoa and helminths as antigenic substances stimulating host resistance. Work by Thillet and Chandler (1957) indicates that in *Trypanosoma lewisi* infections in rats the metabolic products of the parasites are more effective in producing immunity than the dead trypanosomes themselves. Various immunologic tests have been devised based on the ability of the serum of an infected host to precipitate the secretions or excretions of eggs, larvae or adults of a number of different helminths. Some of these will be discussed in Chapter 16.

Parasites and the Compromised Host

We have already alluded to the compromised host in reference to the relationship between nutritional status and the outcome of a parasitic infection. Surgery, transfusion, intubation and prolonged hospitalization are other ways in which the natural defenses of a patient may be compromised. The therapeutic armamentarium of the modern physician is also capable of compromising these defenses. Benefits to be derived from the use of corticosteroids and other immunosuppressive agents, and of the antimetabolites, must always be weighed against their effects upon the defenses of the patient. Among these parasites commonly infecting the therapeutically compromised host, *Pneumocystis carinii* (Ruskin and Remington, 1967; Hamlin, 1968) undoubtedly ranks first. Aggressive treatment of leukemia and other malignancies may pave the way for fatal toxoplasmic infection (Wertlake and Winter, 1965), and acute amebic colitis may follow the use of corticosteroids in presumed ulcerative colitis (Wruble et al., 1966; Fleischli, 1967).

Parasitic infection of tissues compromised by malignant involvement is typified by the report of primary gastric amebiasis in a case of reticulum cell sarcoma (McDonald and Moore, 1965) in which the resistant normal gastric mucosa was largely supplanted by tumor cells. There is also good evidence to suggest that certain helminth infections, notably strongyloidiasis and trichinosis, may flourish in the cortisone-treated (or otherwise immunologically compromised) host.

Life Cycles of Protozoa and Helminths

Many parasitic organisms have but a single host, being transferred from one individual to another of the same species either through direct physical contact, or by means of resistant or semiresistant forms able to survive a period outside or away from the host. *Entamoeba gingivalis,* a commensal organism which inhabits the mouth, has no cyst stage or other means of survival out of the host, and probably is transferred by direct contact. *Trichomonas hominis* likewise is unable to form cysts, but probably can survive for short periods outside the body so that direct contact is not necessary. Many protozoa and helminths have cyst stages or eggs which will survive for some period away from the host, and by means of which new hosts become infected.

Parasitic infections may be carried from one host to another by means of arthropod *vectors.* A vector may also be a host, if development of the parasite takes place within its body. If the arthropod is simply an instrument of passive transfer, we refer to it as a *mechanical vector.* If a fly, feeding on fecal matter containing cysts of *Entamoeba histolytica,* becomes contaminated with some of these cysts which it then transfers to food, it is acting as a mechanical vector of the ameba. When an anopheline mosquito sucks blood from a malarial patient, the parasites must develop in the mosquito before she is able to transmit the infection. In this instance the mosquito is both host and vector.

Some protozoa and many helminths have complex life cycles, with not one but two and sometimes more hosts. When more than one host species is necessary to the development of the parasite, that host in which sexual reproduction occurs is called the *definitive host.* The species in which larval stages of the parasites develop are called *intermediate hosts;* they are usually designated first and second intermediate hosts if there is more than one. Disconcerting as it may be to those with a strictly anthropocentric point of view, man is but the intermediate host of the malarial parasite, *Plasmodium,* which undergoes sexual reproduction in mosquitoes of the genus *Anopheles.* Many protozoa are asexual; if an arthropod host is required in the life cycle of an asexual parasite one may refer to its vertebrate and invertebrate hosts.

Important Groups of Animal Parasites

The animal parasites of man and most vertebrates are contained in five major subdivisions or phyla. These are the Protozoa, the Platyhelminthes or flatworms, the Nematoda or roundworms, the Acanthocephala or thorny-headed worms, and the Arthropoda, which include the insects, spiders, mites, ticks and so forth. With the exception of the Acanthocephala, all of these phyla contain both parasitic and free-living forms. Within each phylum only those groups which include species of medical importance will be discussed here. Animal phyla may be subdivided into classes and the latter into orders. Each order may again be divided into families containing one or more genera and species. Assignment to these categories is made largely on the basis of morphological characters; identification of any animal parasite requires some knowledge of its structure.

PHYLUM PROTOZOA. The Protozoa are essentially unicellular organisms of varied size and shape. All those parasitic in man are microscopic in size except for the ciliate *Balantidium* which is just large enough to be seen with the naked eye. Protozoa possess a great variety of specialized and intricate structures which function in nutrition or locomotion. These structures, which perform the functions associated with organs in multicellular animals, are called organelles. For various reasons including the complexity of organization and the fact that certain protozoa have more than one nucleus, some workers have suggested that these organisms should be considered as acellular. Important symbionts of man are found in four of the five classes of the phylum.

The Mastigophora or flagellates move by means of specialized structures known as flagella. A flagellum is a long thread-like extension of cytoplasm which functions as a means of propelling the organism. Flagella always arise from small intracytoplasmic granules known as blepharoplasts. The number and position of flagella vary a great deal in different species. In addition to the flagella, and often associated with them, one may observe a variety of structures which serve supportive and other functions and give a characteristic appearance to each species. A number of flagellates are blood parasites or inhabit the tissues, while others are found in the alimentary canal. Most of the latter forms are commensals, but one species, *Giardia lamblia,* is frequently pathogenic.

The class Sarcodina contains those forms which move by means of cytoplasmic protrusions called pseudopodia. It includes all free-living amebae, as well as those symbiotic in the intestinal tract and elsewhere in the body. Most of the amebae of man are commensals; one species, *Entamoeba histolytica,* is an important pathogen.

Members of the class Sporozoa are tissue parasites. While reproduction in the Mastigophora and Sarcodina is frequently asexual, Sporozoa have an involved life cycle with an alternation of sexual and asexual generations. Four species of *Plasmodium* are found primarily as blood parasites, and cause malaria; a species of *Isospora* is parasitic in the mucosa of the intestinal tract.

The class Ciliata contains a great variety of free-living and symbiotic species. Locomotion is accomplished by means of cilia, relatively short threads of cytoplasm arising from small basal granules. Cilia are structurally similar to flagella, but are usually shorter and more numerous. Some ciliates are multinucleate, while others contain but two nuclei; a large macronucleus and a small micronucleus. The only ciliate parasite of man is *Balantidium coli,* found in the intestinal tract. Although rare, it is important as it may produce severe intestinal symptoms.

PHYLUM PLATYHELMINTHES. The Platyhelminthes or flatworms are multicellular animals characterized by the possession of a flat, bilaterally symmetrical body. Most flatworms are hermaphroditic, having both male and female reproductive organs within the same individual. Adults may be less than 1 mm. long or they may reach a length of many meters. Most members of the phylum are symbionts living on or in the body of their hosts. Free-living species belong to the class Turbellaria, which also contains forms parasitic in lower animals. The classes Trematoda and Cestoda contain parasitic forms only.

The Trematoda or flukes are leaf shaped or elongate and slender organisms which possess attachment organs in the form of hooks or cup-shaped muscular depressions called suckers. A simple digestive tract is present. Of the three orders of the Trematoda, the order Digenea contains all the species parasitic in man. Members of this order have complex life histories with at least one intermediate molluscan host. Included in the digenetic trematodes of man are forms which parasitize the intestinal tract, the liver, the blood vessels and the lungs.

Members of the class Cestoda typically have an elongate, ribbonlike and segmented body which bears a specialized attachment organ, the scolex, anteriorly. A digestive tract is absent. Adult cestodes or tapeworms inhabit the small intestine. With the exception of *Hymenolepis nana*, cestodes require an intermediate host for larval development. Man may be host to either adult or larval stages, depending on the species of cestode.

PHYLUM NEMATODA. The Nematoda or roundworms are elongate cylindrical worms frequently attenuated at both ends. They possess a stiff cuticle which may be smooth or may be extended to form a variety of structures, particularly at the anterior and posterior ends. The sexes are separate, the male frequently being considerably smaller than the female. A well-developed digestive tract is present. While most nematodes are free living, a large number of species parasitize man, animals and plants. Intermediate hosts are necessary for the larval development of some forms. Parasites of man include intestinal and tissue-inhabiting species.

PHYLUM ACANTHOCEPHALA. The thorny-headed worms are all endoparasitic organisms having the anterior end of the body modified into a hook-bearing, retractible proboscis which serves in attachment. A digestive tract is absent. Sexes are separate and the males are usually smaller than the females. The life cycle requires an intermediate host. While thorny-headed worms are widely distributed among wild and domestic animals, only two species have been reported to occur in human beings.

PHYLUM ARTHROPODA. Arthropods are segmented and bilaterally symmetrical animals with a body enclosed in a stiff chitinous covering or exoskeleton and bearing paired, jointed appendages. The digestive system is well developed. Sexes are separate. The phylum is subdivided into a number of classes, many of which are of medical importance.

The class Crustacea contains primarily aquatic forms which breathe by means of gills. Included here are the crabs, shrimps, crayfish and the copepods. Certain of these serve as intermediate hosts of human parasites.

The class Chilopoda contains the centipedes, which are characterized by the possession of one pair of legs on each body segment. The first pair of appendages is modified as poison claws.

The Arachnida or spider-like animals possess a body divided into two parts, called the cephalothorax and abdomen. Adults have four pairs of legs. Included in this class are the scorpions, the spiders and the ticks and mites. Scorpions and spiders produce venom, which in some species may be extremely toxic. Certain ticks and mites may transmit disease.

The class Pentastomida contains only endoparasitic forms known as tongue worms or linguatulids. The name is derived from their body shape, which is elongate and in some species tongue-like. Other species have a ringed or annulated body. Linguatulids lack external appendages and possess two pairs of hooks near the mouth. Adults live in the respiratory tract of vertebrates. Encysted larval stages may occur in the lungs and other internal organs of man, primarily in tropical areas.

From a medical or economic point of view, the class Insecta includes by far the most important of the arthropods. Insects have a body divided into three distinct parts, head, thorax and abdomen, and possess three pairs of legs. Several orders of insects are worthy of special mention. The Anoplura, or sucking lice, are wingless dorso-ventrally compressed insects, among which are included the human lice. The order Heteroptera, or true bugs, includes the wingless bedbugs, as well as the more characteristic forms with wings. Two pairs of wings are seen in this group, and the first pair has thickened membranous bases. The cone-nose bugs, or reduviids, are important as vectors of South American trypanosomiasis. The Coleoptera, or beetles, also have two pairs of wings, but the anterior pair is thickened throughout. Certain grain beetles are intermediate hosts of tapeworms. The Hymenoptera include ants, bees, wasps and so forth. Bees and wasps are important because of the venom of their stings, and ants may serve as an intermediate host for one of the trematode parasites of man. The Siphonaptera, or fleas, are wingless and laterally compressed; in addition to their irritating bites, some fleas act as intermediate hosts of a species of tapeworm. The Diptera are insects with only one pair of true wings. This order includes several groups of medical importance, notably the mosquitoes, flies and gnats. Some larval flies are parasitic in man and animals, while mosquitoes and gnats transmit many different diseases.

The distribution of some of the important parasitic diseases of man is shown in Tables 1 to 5 below.

Table 1. Distribution of Selected Parasitic Diseases: The Americas

	North America	Mexico–Central America	Caribbean	Tropical South America	Temperate South America
Malaria	X*	X	Hispaniola	X	X
Leishmaniasis					
Cutaneous	0	X	0	X	0
Mucocutaneous	0	X	0	X	X
Visceral	0	X	0	X	X
Trypanosomiasis					
cruzi	X*	X	0	X	X
Schistosomiasis					
mansoni	0	0	X	X	X
Paragonimiasis	0	X	0	X	0
Diphyllobothriasis	X	0	0	0	X
Taeniasis solium	X*	X	0	X	0
Hydatid disease	X	X	0	X	X
Filariasis					
Bancroftian	0	X	X	X	0
Onchocerciasis	0	X	0	X	0

Key: X – Present
0 – Absent
*Sporadic occurrence

Table 2. Distribution of Selected Parasitic Diseases: Europe

	Northwest	Southwest	Central	Eastern	Mediterranean Littoral
Leishmaniasis					
Cutaneous	0	0	0	X	X
Visceral	0	0	0	0	X
Schistosomiasis					
haematobium	0	Portugal	0	0	0
Opisthorchiasis	0	0	X	X	0
Diphyllobothriasis	X	0	X	0	0
Hydatid disease	X	X	X	X	X

Key: X – Present
0 – Absent

Table 3. Distribution of Selected Parasitic Diseases: Africa

	North	West	Central	East	South
Malaria	X	X	X	X	X
Leishmaniasis					
Cutaneous	X	X	X	X	X
Visceral	X	X	X	X	X
Trypanosomiasis					
Gambian	0	X	X	0	0
Rhodesian	0	0	0	X	X
Schistosomiasis					
haematobium	X	X	X	X	X
mansoni	X	X	X	X	X
Paragonimiasis	X	X	X	0	0
Hydatid disease	X	X	0	X	0
Filariasis					
Bancroftian	X	X	X	X	0
Loiasis	0	X	X	X	0
Onchocerciasis	0	X	X	X	0

Key: X — Present   0 — Absent

Table 4. Distribution of Selected Parasitic Diseases: Asia

	Southwest	Central South	Southeast	East
Malaria	X	X	X	X
Leishmaniasis				
Cutaneous	X	X	0	0
Visceral	0	X	0	0
Schistosomiasis				
haematobium	X	India	0	0
mansoni	0	0	0	0
japonicum	0	0	X	X
Paragonimiasis	0	X	X	X
Opisthorchiasis/				
Clonorchiasis	0	X	X	X
Fasciolopsiasis	0	X	X	X
Diphyllobothriasis	0	0	0	X
Hydatid disease	X	0	X	0
Filariasis				
Bancroftian	0	X	X	X
Malayan	0	India	X	X?

Key: X — Present   0 — Absent

Table 5. Distribution of Selected Parasitic Diseases: Oceania

	Australia	New Guinea	South Pacific	Polynesia	West Pacific	Hawaii
Malaria	0	X	X	0	X	0
Paragonimiasis	0	0	X	X	0	0
Filariasis						
Bancroftian	X	X	X	X	X	0
Eosinophilic						
Meningitis	X	0	X	X	X	X

Key: X — Present   0 — Absent

Prevalence of Parasitic Infections

Estimates of the prevalence of parasitic diseases are at best extremely rough, as morbidity reporting is essentially nonexistent in many of the areas in which these diseases occur. The World Health Organization supplies the following estimates, as of 1975:

Amebiasis: 10 per cent of world population
Malaria: population at risk: 1,138,553,000
          population currently infected: 177,000,000
          annual deaths from malaria: 1,000,000
African trypanosomiasis: population at risk: 35,000,000
                          new cases per year: 10,000 or more
American trypanosomiasis: population at risk: 35,000,000
                          population currently infected:
                          10,000,000 or more
Schistosomiasis: more than 200,000,000 (includes combined cases)
          S. haematobium: approximately 100,000,000
          S. mansoni: approximately 60,000,000
          S. japonicum: approximately 100,000,000
Opisthorchiasis: 19,000,000
Paragonimiasis: 3,200,000
Fasciolopsiasis: 10,000,000
Filariasis: 250,000,000
Onchocerciasis: more than 20,000,000
Dracunculiasis: 50–80,000,000
Ascariasis: 650,000,000
Hookworm: 450,000,000
Trichuriasis: 350,000,000
Strongyloidiasis: 35,000,000
Trichostrongyliasis: 5,500,000
Cestodiases: 65,000,000

REFERENCES

Cameron, T. W. M. 1956. *Parasites and Parasitism.* 322 pp. John Wiley and Sons, Inc., New York.
Elsdon-Dew, R. 1953. The pathogenicity of *Entamoeba histolytica.* S. Afr. Med. J., *27:*504–506.
Fleischli, D. J. 1967. Chronic diarrhea. J.A.M.A., *199:*925–927.
Frye, W. W. 1955. Nutrition and intestinal parasitism. Ann. N.Y. Acad. Sci., *63:*175–185.
Hamlin, W. B. 1968. *Pneumocystis carinii.* J.A.M.A., *204:*173–174.
McDonald, H. G., and Moore, M. M. 1965. Primary gastric amebiasis superimposed on reticulum-cell sarcoma. J.A.M.A., *193:*971–972.
Ruskin, J., and Remington, J. S. 1967. The compromised host and infection. I. *Pneumocystis carinii* pneumonia. J.A.M.A., *202:*1070–1074.
Thillet, C. J., Jr., and Chandler, A. C. 1957. Immunization against *Trypanosoma lewisi* in rats by injection of metabolic products. Science, *125:*346–347.
Wertlake, P. T., and Winter, T. S. 1965. Fatal toxoplasma myocarditis in an adult patient with acute lymphocytic leukemia. New Eng. J. Med., *273:*438–440.
Wruble, L. D., Duckworth, J. K., Duke, D. D., and Rothschild, J. A. 1966. Toxic dilatation of the colon in a case of amebiasis. New Eng. J. Med., *275:*926–928.

3

Procedures in Examination of Stool Specimens

Many methods have been described for the examination of stool specimens; some of these are of general applicability, while others serve only limited purposes. Individual preference will at times dictate the particular method or methods to be employed, but success will be directly proportional to the user's familiarity with various methods of examination, so that he may choose those which will be most suitable for a particular specimen, or for detection of a particular type of parasite. For routine examination, it is best to employ certain standard techniques, so that one may become familiar with the advantages and limitations of each. Much time may be lost through use of a method for purposes for which it was never intended, and frequently identification of a parasite becomes very difficult or impossible unless the correct method of examination is employed.

Physical Characteristics of the Specimen

The consistency of a stool specimen, whether formed, mushy or liquid, is of great importance, giving an indication of the types of organisms which it may contain. Trophozoites of the intestinal protozoa are usually found in liquid or soft stools, almost never in fully formed ones. Protozoan cysts are rarely seen in liquid stools, unless these are the result of administration of a cathartic, in which case both trophic and cystic forms may be present. Cysts will usually be found in fully formed specimens. Helminth eggs may be found in either liquid or formed stools, but as the liquid stool is usually very dilute, they will often be difficult to detect in such specimens.

The surface of the entire specimen should be examined for macroscopic parasites. Frequently pinworms will be seen on the surface of a stool specimen, and tapeworm proglottids may likewise be found there or in the interior of the specimen. The stool should be broken up with applicator sticks to check for helminths. The presence of blood in the specimen is always of interest. If bright red blood is seen on the surface of formed stools, it is most frequently a sign of bleeding hemorrhoids; bloody mucus in loose or liquid specimens is highly suggestive of amebic ulcerations in the large intestine, though it may be due to other conditions. Patches of mucus, particularly if blood-tinged, on the surface of a specimen, should always be examined with care for trophic amebae. Occult blood in a stool is of no interest *per se* to the parasitologist; it may be a result of intestinal bleeding caused by parasitic organisms, but is more likely to be indicative of other gastrointestinal disorders.

The age of a specimen is of prime importance. Freshly passed specimens are essential for the detection of trophic amebae or flagellates. Therefore, it is well to insist that all liquid or soft stools be examined within one-half hour of the time of passage (*not* the time of arrival at the laboratory). If this is impossible, part of the specimen should be preserved within this time for subsequent examination. The immediate examination of fully formed stool specimens is not so important, but they should be kept under refrigeration if their examination must be delayed. Incubation of these specimens at 37°C. will result in more rapid death and disintegration of protozoan trophozoites and cysts, and promote maturation and hatching of hookworm eggs. Formed stools may be examined even when several days old, and are sometimes mailed to central laboratories for this purpose; this procedure is not recommended, and if they cannot be examined within three or four hours they should be preserved. Suitable preservation methods are discussed under the heading of "Preservation of Stool Specimens."

Containers for Collection of Stool Specimens

A tightly covered container of stout cardboard construction, preferably waxed, is recommended. Half-pint ice cream containers are very satisfactory. If sputum cups or other containers are used, it is essential that they be clean and free of soap or disinfectants. If possible, information as to time of passage of the specimen should be included with other pertinent data on the label.

Techniques of Stool Examination

Unfortunately, no single technique of stool examination will yield satisfactory results, as none of the methods is equally applicable to the detection of trophic protozoa, cysts and helminth eggs. For this reason, a combination of two or more techniques of examination is essential. The more useful of these methods are outlined below, with indications of their role in the detection of the various forms of parasites.

A. DIRECT WET FILM. This method is most useful for the detection of trophic forms of amebae and flagellates. It possesses the advantage of allowing the observer to study the motility of the organisms, which is often characteristic and of value in making a precise identification. Cysts of the various protozoa and helminth eggs may also be seen on wet film if they are present in large enough numbers; however, these forms may be concentrated by various means, and such methods of examination are more efficient for their detection.

In the preparation of a wet film, a small portion of feces is mixed with a drop of normal saline on a clean slide, a coverslip is placed on the preparation, and it is first examined unstained. It is best in making the wet film to take small amounts of material from several parts of the stool specimen. The film should not be too thick, or it will be very difficult to observe individual organisms. A convenient rule of thumb is to prepare the film just thin enough so that ordinary newsprint can easily be read through it. After the wet film has been thoroughly checked for trophic amebae and flagellates, under low power of the microscope and using a low intensity of illumination, an iodine stain may be prepared.

Iodine stains the cysts of amebae and other protozoa, revealing some details which cannot be seen in the unstained preparation. Trophozoites are rapidly killed, and sometimes unidentifiable after iodine staining; it should not be applied until after the specimen has been thoroughly examined in the unstained condition. Gram's iodine or Lugol's solution will give satisfactory results, but a modified D'Antoni's iodine solution is preferable. Preparation of stains and reagents is outlined in Chapter 17.

A separate iodine stain may be prepared by addition of a small drop of this reagent to a wet film of fecal material before it is covered, or the iodine may be added to the edge of the coverslip, so that it gradually diffuses into the saline mount. The latter technique has the double advantage of not requiring a separate preparation, and of staining the fecal material gradually, so that by searching the preparation one may find areas in which the intensity of stain is optimal. It should be borne in mind that a concentrate of the stool may also be stained with iodine and will reveal, in larger numbers, any organisms which may be seen on the iodine-stained direct examination. Organisms present in such small numbers that they may not be seen at all on direct examination may at times be detected with ease after concentration of the specimen.

A combined fixative, preservative and stain for direct examination has been described by Sapero and Lawless (1953). Lugol's iodine solution and Merthiolate are the staining agents, while formaldehyde solution is the fixative. This MIF stain will fix and stain both trophozoites and cysts; D'Antoni's stain is unsuitable for use with trophic amebae or flagellates, as it shrinks and distorts them. For use in direct examination, the three ingredients of the MIF stain must be combined daily, according to the proportions given in Chapter 17. A drop of freshly prepared stain and a drop of distilled water are placed on a slide and mixed, and a small quantity of feces is added as in the preparation of a saline film.

B. CONCENTRATION TECHNIQUES. Many concentration methods have been employed, all of which attempt the separation of protozoan cysts and helminth eggs from the bulk of fecal matter through differences in specific gravity. The described methods fall into two general classes: sedimentation and flotation techniques. With the various sedimentation methods, eggs and cysts which are heavier than the suspending liquid concentrate in the bottom of a tube. Flotation of eggs and cysts involves the use of a heavy liquid, to the surface of which the lighter parasites rise. One sedimentation technique and one flotation are recommended for general use. Various other methods are excellent for specialized purposes, but these two are of the widest applicability. The formalin-ether sedimentation technique of Ritchie (1948) is excellent for the concentration of both cysts and eggs, and possesses the added advantage that it may be applied to formalin-preserved specimens. None of the sedimentation methods results in as good a separation of fecal debris from the eggs and cysts as may be achieved by a flotation method; the one recommended is our own modification of the zinc-sulfate centrifugal flotation method of Faust. The zinc-sulfate flotation is also excellent for the recovery of protozoan cysts and most eggs, but it does not work well with trematode eggs or those of the broad fish tapeworm. Eggs of other types and protozoan cysts will be concentrated relatively free from fecal debris by this method.

The zinc-sulfate method is perhaps to be preferred for routine use, as it yields a cleaner concentrate. It, however, must be carried out with meticulous attention to detail. The laboratory worker should be familiar with both methods, details of which are given in Chapter 15. After concentration by either method the diagnostic material is transferred to a microscope slide and a drop of iodine added to stain any protozoan cysts which may be present. This will also stain the helminth eggs; although it is of no help in their identification, it does not render this more difficult. It is well to make a habit of examining completely every concentrated preparation with low power of the microscope. A little practice will make it possible to recognize even the smaller protozoan cysts at this magnification, though for specific identification high dry magnification may be necessary. Some persons attempt to use oil-immersion magnification with iodine-stained preparations, either of concentrates or direct films. This serves no useful purpose, as the structural differentiation produced by iodine staining is not sufficiently precise to be improved by increased magnification.

C. PERMANENT STAINED SLIDES. The direct wet film provides information about motility of the parasites, which may be of importance in identification. Iodine or MIF staining will increase the amount of detail which can be seen in most cysts, and concentration will of course reveal cysts and eggs when their numbers are small. At times, however, it is impossible to make an exact identification of certain protozoa on the basis of what is revealed by one or a combination of the preceding techniques. In such cases, the cytological detail revealed by one of the permanent staining methods may be essential for an accurate identification. It has been proved that a combination of the permanent stain, with direct examination and concentration of the stool, will reveal a significantly higher percentage of *Entamoeba histolytica* and other protozoan parasites than is detected when the two latter methods only are used. The routine use of a permanent stain is very highly recommended.

A small quantity of feces is transferred to a clean slide with an applicator stick. The material is then streaked out in a thin uniform film, as indicated in Figure 1. A little practice will enable one to produce films which are of the correct thickness. Generally, formed stools are of the proper consistency for making films, but if the specimen is particularly hard it may be necessary to add a small amount of saline to a portion of the stool. A liquid stool will sometimes fail to adhere to the slide; in such cases a thin layer of serum or of egg albumin, as used in mounting tissue sections, will increase adherence. It is essential in all staining techniques that the film be placed in fixative immediately after it is made; if it dries at any time, it will be useless.

Gomori's trichrome stain, originally intended for histological use, has been adapted by Wheatley (1951) for use in staining intestinal protozoa, and is the method most frequently used at the present. It is not generally realized that eggs of helminths can be identified in the trichrome-stained fecal film, but with a little experience it is possible to recognize the commoner ones (and some less common species) by this method. More precise cytological detail may be obtained with the use of iron hematoxylin, but this stain requires considerable technical com-

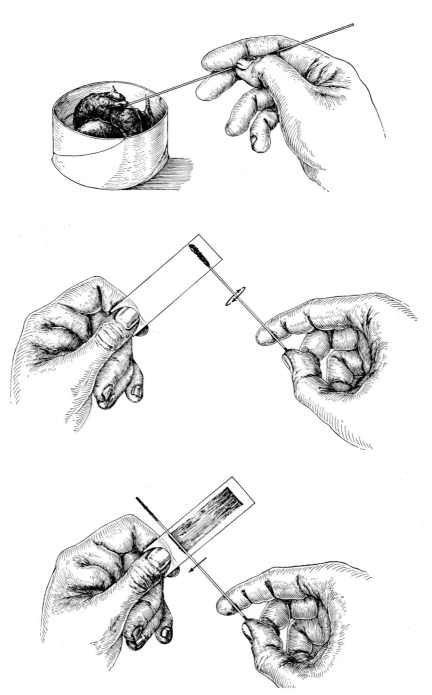

FIGURE 1. Preparation of fecal film for permanent staining.

petence, whereas the trichrome stain will give quite satisfactory results even in the hands of relatively inexperienced persons.

Lengthy staining procedures are often impractical in a small laboratory. The trichrome stain requires about forty-five minutes. A combination fixative and permanent stain requiring less than five minutes was introduced by Lawless (1953). The stain achieved by this method is inferior to trichrome, but it is adequate for diagnosis by well-trained personnel.

Number of Specimens to Be Examined

This is a subject over which the laboratory frequently has little or no control, yet it may at least have some influence in setting a normal number of stool examinations to be performed on a patient. The number to be done will also depend upon the purpose for which the examination is being made. If one is interested only in determining the presence or absence of helminth parasites, one or two examinations may be sufficient if concentration methods are used, as these methods are very efficient in detection of small numbers of eggs. On the other hand, Sawitz and Faust (1942) have stated that a single stool examination, even if a combination of techniques be used, will uncover somewhat under 50 per cent of *Entamoeba histolytica* infections, and that at least six examinations are necessary if over 90 per cent of positives are to be recognized. This is shown graphically in Figure 2. These percentages apply to normally passed stools only. Many authorities recommend the routine use of purged stools if one is searching for *Entamoeba histolytica*. There is little question that the proper use of purged specimens will increase the chances of finding parasites. On the other hand, purged specimens must be examined immediately, or they are worthless. If one has the facilities to collect and examine purged specimens immediately after they are passed, this procedure will probably increase the percentage of positive results. Unless one has such facilities it is probably best to examine only normally passed stools.

If purgation is to be used, castor and mineral oils should be avoided, as they will make examination of the specimen almost impossible. A saline purge of Epsom salts or Fleet's Phospho-Soda, is recommended. Parasites in the first bowel movement will probably be distorted; and the second and subsequent movements will be most likely to contain recognizable parasites.

Culture Methods

Many of the intestinal protozoa have now been successfully cultured, with the use of special techniques and different culture media

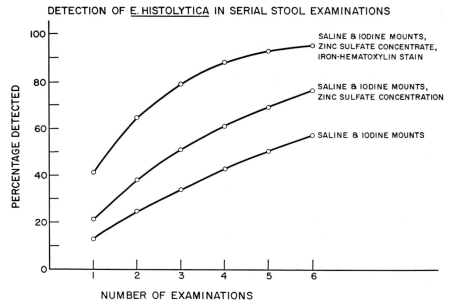

FIGURE 2.   Probability of detecting *Entamoeba histolytica* by successive stool examinations, using various methods. (Adapted from Sawitz and Faust, 1942.)

for almost every species. Cultivation of the non-pathogenic amebae, and of the flagellates, and *Balantidium* falls into the category of research procedures, requiring too much material and time to be of diagnostic usefulness.

Entamoeba histolytica can be cultivated on a variety of media, some of which may be purchased in the dehydrated form and prepared with a minimum of effort. Various authorities advocate the use of *E. histolytica* cultures in the diagnostic laboratory, as a screening procedure. Others suggest that cultures should be employed in every suspected case of amebiasis when the microscopic examination yields negative results. A third viewpoint is that expressed by certain workers who have determined the number of *E. histolytica* cysts which must be present per gram of feces to insure a high percentage of successful cultures. Results of these studies indicate that the number of cysts necessary for viable cultures is so large that they should be detectable by ordinary microscopic methods, and suggest that cultures are superfluous.

The success with which *E. histolytica* is cultivated will depend very largely upon familiarity with the techniques involved. For this reason, sporadic use of culture techniques is not recommended, and they should only be undertaken in laboratories where the number of specimens examined is sufficiently large to justify a considerable portion of time being spent on their maintenance and examination. Likewise, culture methods should never be used as a substitute for routine and thorough microscopic examination by the various methods outlined previously. Boeck and Drbohlav's L.E.S. medium and Cleveland and Collier's medium are solid media, with liquid overlays which contain serum or buffered saline. The latter medium is obtainable from the Difco Laboratories under the name of Bacto-Endamoeba medium. Balamuth's medium is a very satisfactory liquid culture medium, which is not difficult to prepare. Directions for the preparation of Balamuth's and the L.E.S. medium are given in Chapter 15.

Procedures for the isolation of *Strongyloides* and hookworm larvae, often referred to as culture methods, may be very useful in detecting low grade infections. These procedures are also described in Chapter 15.

Character of the Cellular Exudate in Amebic and Bacillary Dysentery

Much information can be obtained from the types of cellular elements found in wet mounts or permanent stained slides of a stool specimen. The character of the exudate is quite different in amebic and bacillary dysenteries, and while a diagnosis of amebic infection can never be made solely on the basis of an exudate of the amebic type, the presence of such an exudate should cause one to search even harder for the amebae. It must be remembered that mixed bacterial and amebic dysentery can occur, and the type of exudate considered characteristic of bacillary dysentery does not rule out the possible presence, or minimize the significance, of *Entamoeba histolytica*.

Because of the possibility of a mixed infection, or the presence of bacterial pathogens instead of animal parasites, it is important to subject stool specimens to the appropriate culture procedures for the isolation of enteric bacteria.

The characteristic microscopic pictures of the two types of infection are summarized by Kessel (1944) as follows:

Amebic Dysentery

1. Scantiness of cellular exudate, especially the polymorphonuclear element.

2. Preponderance of mononuclear leukocytes over polymorphonuclear leukocytes.

Bacillary Dysentery

1. Abundance of cellular exudate, mostly polymorphonuclear leukocytes.

2. Preponderance of polymorphonuclear leukocytes over mononuclear leukocytes, the "polys" exhibiting clear-cut ring nuclei. The macrophages sometimes contain red blood cells.

Amebic Dysentery	*Bacillary Dysentery*
3. Evidence of proteolytic digestion of the cells, beginning at the periphery and affecting the nucleus last.	3. Evidence of toxic necrosis of the cells, the degenerative changes occurring early in all parts of the cells, including the nucleus.
4. Charcot-Leyden crystals present in about 25 per cent of cases, usually in long-standing cases.	4. Charcot-Leyden crystals usually absent.
5. Red blood cells numerous, occurring in clumps or rouleaux.	5. Red blood cells numerous and scattered throughout.
6. Eosinophilic cells present, varying from 2 to 5 per cent.	6. Eosinophilic cells seldom or never present.
7. Epithelial cells numerous and apparently undamaged.	7. Epithelial cells common, generally bile-stained and disintegrated.
8. Bacteria motile and in large numbers.	8. Bacteria scarce.
9. *E. histolytica* present.	9. *E. histolytica* absent except in cases of mixed infection.

The exudate of ulcerative colitis (or of any other inflammatory bowel disease) can mimic that of either bacillary dysentery or amebiasis, as the cellular elements vary in number and type with the activity of the disease.

Preservation of Stool Specimens

At times, either because of the press of work in the laboratory, the distance a specimen must be transported or for other reasons, it is impossible to examine a specimen within the time limits which have been given. If a liquid or mushy specimen cannot be examined within half an hour, or a fully formed one within three or four hours, a portion of the specimen should be preserved for subsequent examination. MIF solution may be used for this purpose. The composition of the solution for this purpose is slightly different from that used for direct staining; both are given in Chapter 17. This solution will preserve the specimen for a period of some months, and at the same time stain it for examination. A permanent preparation cannot be made from MIF-preserved material, and identification must be made on the basis of detail revealed by Merthiolate and iodine staining.

If it is desired to preserve fecal material in such condition that permanent stains can be made from it, polyvinyl alcohol (PVA) fixative solution should be used. A small portion of stool is mixed with PVA solution, following the directions in Chapter 17; trichrome stains may be prepared from it at a later date. We have been unable to achieve consistent results in staining PVA-preserved material with the Lawless technique. PVA-preserved material retains excellent staining properties for about one month, after which time it gradually deteriorates. Many of the helminth eggs are distorted by fixation in PVA. If worm infection is suspected, it is well to preserve a portion of stool in MIF or in 10 per cent formalin. Formalin preservation lends itself very well to subsequent concentration by the formalin-ether sedimentation technique.

Key to the Helminth Eggs

a. Egg non-operculate, spherical or subspherical, containing a six-hooked embryo .... b
   Egg other than above .... e
b. Eggs separate c
   Eggs in packets of twelve or more .... *Dipylidium caninum*
c. Outer surface of egg consists of a thick radially striated capsule or embryophore .... *Taenia* sp.
   Outer surface of egg consists of very thin shell, separated from inner embryophore by gelatinous matrix .... d
d. Filamentous strands occupy space between embryophore and outer shell .... *Hymenolepis nana*
   No filamentous strands between embryophore and outer shell ... *H. diminuta*
e. Egg operculate .... f
   Egg non-operculate .... j
f. Egg less than 35 microns long .... *Opisthorchis* sp.
                                                                   or
                                                Heterophyes heterophyes
                                                                   or
                                                Metagonimus yokogawai
   Egg 38 microns or over .... g
g. Egg 38 to 45 microns in length .... *Dicrocoelium dendriticum*
   Egg over 60 microns in length .... h
h. Egg with shoulders into which operculum fits............*Paragonimus westermani*
   Egg without opercular shoulders.. i
i. Egg more than 85 microns long .... *Fasciolopsis buski*
                                                                   or
                                                Fasciola hepatica
                                                                   or
                                                Echinostoma sp.
   Egg less than 75 microns long .... *Diphyllobothrium latum*
j. Egg 75 microns or more in length, spined .... k
   Egg less than 75 microns long, not spined .... m
k. Spine terminal .... *Schistosoma haematobium*
   Spine lateral l
l. Lateral spine inconspicuous (perhaps absent) .... *S. japonicum*
   Lateral spine prominent .... *S. mansoni*
m. Egg with thick tuberculated capsule .... *Ascaris lumbricoides*
   Egg without thick tuberculated capsule .... n

Key to the Helminth Eggs (Continued)

n. Egg barrel shaped, with polar plugs .... o
   Egg not barrel shaped, without polar plugs .... p
o. Shell non-striated .... *Trichuris trichiura*
   Shell often striated .... *Capillaria* sp.
p. Egg flattened on one side .... *Enterobius vermicularis*
   Egg symmetrical .... q
q. Egg with large blue-green globules at poles........ *Heterodera marioni* (Fig. 110)
   Egg without polar globules .... r
r. Egg bluntly rounded at ends, 56 to 76 microns long .... hookworm
   Egg pointed at one or both ends, 73 to 95 microns long . *Trichostrongylus* sp.

REFERENCES

Kessel, J. F. 1944. *The Distinguishing Characteristics of the Intestinal Protozoa of Man. A Laboratory Syllabus.* 37 pp. Univ. of Southern California Press, Los Angeles.

Lawless, D. K. 1953. A rapid permanent-mount stain technic for the diagnosis of the intestinal protozoa. Amer. J. Trop. Med. & Hyg., 2:1137-1138.

Ritchie, L. S. 1948. An ether sedimentation technique for routine stool examinations. Bull. U.S. Army Med. Dept., 8:326.

Sapero, J. J., and Lawless, D. K. 1953. The "MIF" stain-preservative technic for the identification of intestinal protozoa. Amer. J. Trop. Med. & Hyg., 2:613-619.

Sawitz, W. G., and Faust, E. C. 1942. The probability of detecting intestinal protozoa by successive stool examinations. Amer. J. Trop. Med., 22:131-136.

Wheatley, W. B. 1951. A rapid staining procedure for intestinal amoebae and flagellates. Amer. J. Clin. Path., 21:990-993.

4

Examination of Blood and Other Tissues

The preparation of good blood films will depend to a large extent upon the cleanliness of microscope slides and coverglass employed. All glassware must be free of dust and oil. It is essential that both slides and coverslips be washed in alcohol and dried with a clean towel before a blood film is prepared. New slides should be used for the preparation of permanent stains; it is impossible to make uniform films on old scratched slides, and they cannot be thoroughly cleaned.

Examination of Fresh Blood

Microscopic examination of fresh blood is not undertaken routinely but is useful for the detection of two types of parasites. Trypanosomes and microfilariae may be easily recognized by their characteristic motility in fresh blood. For specific identification of these organisms a permanent stain is, however, essential. When fresh blood is to be examined it is important to make a sufficiently thin preparation so that the relatively small protozoan parasites are not masked by several layers of blood corpuscles. A small drop of blood is placed on a slide and covered with a coverglass to prevent clotting. If the preparation is too thick it may be diluted with normal saline. For the detection of trypanosomes, the high-dry objective with reduced illumination is most suitable. When searching for microfilariae, the low power of the microscope should be employed. Whip-like motions of microfilariae, and the rapid undulating and twisting movements of trypanosomes are usually seen before the precise shape of the organism is apparent. Organisms may quickly attract one's attention through their movements even when they are so few in number that long search may be required to reveal them in fixed preparations.

Permanent Preparations

Many methods have been described for the preparation and permanent staining of blood films. Only those most commonly employed in laboratory work will be discussed. It is important to bear in mind that correct initial handling of the blood is essential if good stains are to be obtained, regardless of the specific methods used. The necessity of absolute cleanliness of all equipment has been emphasized. It is preferable to use peripheral blood, from fingertip or ear lobe. The skin should be cleansed with alcohol before an incision is made, in order to remove all fatty substances, and the incision should be sufficiently deep so that blood flows freely. Blood which has been "milked" from the finger is mixed with tissue fluids which dilute the parasites, and make their detection more difficult. Films should be prepared as quickly as possible, to prevent clotting. If venous blood must be employed, a small amount of heparin or other anticoagulant must be added, but preparations made from such blood will usually show a considerable degree of distortion.

Both thin and thick films may be used for the identification of blood parasites. The advantages and disadvantages of each are discussed below.

The Thin Film

Thin blood films are used for the specific identification of malarial parasites, trypanosomes and microfilariae. It is essential that a thin film be, as the name indicates, really thin. A thin film should consist of *one* layer of evenly distributed blood cells. Since malaria parasites are intracellular, a piling up of red blood cells makes specific identification of these parasites difficult, if not impossible. Specific identification of blood parasites rests on their morphological characteristics. The chief advantage of a thin film is that it preserves the structure of the parasites with a minimum of distortion. If the film is too thick, the structural detail of individual parasites will not be observable.

There are several ways to make a thin blood film, and while the procedure to be adopted will vary with individual preference, the following is recommended. Place a small drop of blood near one end of a microscope slide, as shown in Figure 3, *A*. Raise the end of the slide farthest from the drop of blood by placing the end of the slide on your

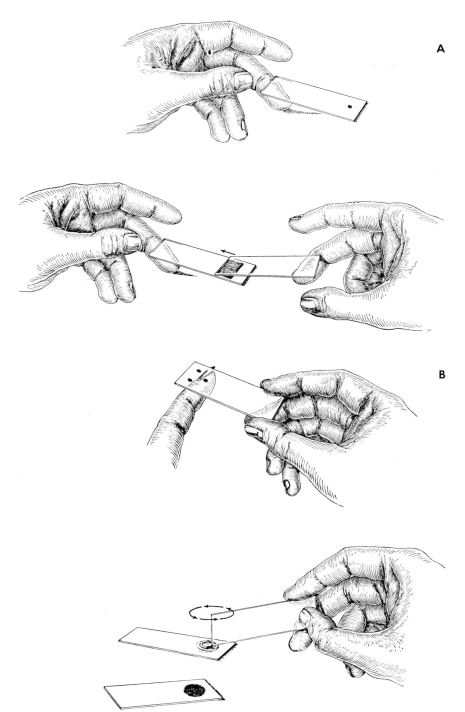

FIGURE 3. *A*, Preparation of a thin blood film. *B*, Preparation of a thick blood film.

finger, as your hand rests on a table or other steady surface. Take a second slide for a spreader, and rest one end of it against the first slide, and one end on the middle finger of the hand which is not supporting the first slide. Hold your hand so that the second slide makes an angle of approximately 30 degrees with the first; do not grasp either slide, but allow gravity to hold the two in contact. Draw back the supporting finger to move the slide back toward the drop of blood until the drop of blood touches the spreader and begins to run out toward the edges. Before the blood has a chance to reach the edges of the spreader, move the finger which supports it forward in an even quick motion, so that the drop is drawn out into a thin film. Ideally, this should not reach the edges of the slide, and should taper off into a "comet's tail" toward the end of the slide. After the film has been air-dried, it may be stained.

The stains commonly used are of two general types. One of these has the fixative incorporated in the staining solution so that fixation and staining of the dried film are accomplished simultaneously. An example is Wright's stain, in which methyl alcohol acts as a fixative. Wright's stain will give satisfactory results and requires but a short staining period. However, more precise detail is seen in slides prepared with Giemsa's stain. Since this stain does not contain a fixative, thin films must be fixed in absolute methyl alcohol and air-dried before they are placed in the staining solution. It is important to dry slides in a vertical position after removal from either fixative or stain. As soon as the stained films are dry, they may be examined under oil immersion of the microscope. Immersion oil may be placed directly on the uncovered blood film and, when no longer needed, carefully removed with lens paper. If magnifications lower than oil immersion are to be used, a coverglass should be placed over the film. Slides which one desires to keep for a permanent collection should always have the protection of a coverslip. It is best not to use Canada balsam as a mounting medium, as preparations so mounted tend to fade; the newer mounting media, such as Permount, are preferable.

Thick Blood Films

The thick film may also be used in identification of malaria parasites, trypanosomes and microfilariae. As a thick layer of blood is used in this method, many more parasites will be present in each field. Increased distortion of the parasites is a disadvantage of this method, but experience enables one to recognize them as readily as in the thin film.

To make a thick film, place three drops of blood, each of about the size which would be used to make a thin film, close together near one end of the slide. With one corner of another absolutely clean slide, stir the blood, mingling the three drops over an area 2 cm. in diameter, as shown in Figure 3, *B*. Continue stirring for at least one-half minute; this prevents the formation of fibrin strands, which otherwise tend to obscure the parasites. Allow the films to dry normally; do not heat, because this will fix the blood. After the films are thoroughly dry they must be laked to remove the hemoglobin. This can be done by immersion in buffer solution, prior to staining, or in the Giemsa stain itself. Thick films which cannot be stained immediately should be laked in buffer solution before storage, because removal of hemoglobin becomes increasingly difficult with time. When Giemsa's stain is used for thick films, the procedure is exactly the same as that employed with thin films, except that fixation in methyl alcohol is omitted. Staining times for thick and thin films are similar, but if separate preparations are made, different staining times may be required for optimal results. Thick and thin films may, however, be made on the same slide, and stained simultaneously with Giemsa. To accomplish this, the thin portion of the slide is fixed for one minute in methyl alcohol and then dried before staining.

Another method which may be used in the staining of thick films is that described by Field. It is very rapid and gives satisfactory, though not outstanding, results. The Field technique has been used extensively for survey purposes and when large numbers of slides must be prepared, but is not recommended for routine use.

Details of the composition of stains and of staining procedures are outlined in Chapter 17.

TISSUE IMPRESSIONS

The detection of intracellular parasites such as *Leishmania* and *Toxoplasma* is greatly facilitated by the examination of tissue impression smears stained with Giemsa's or Wright's stain. Fresh lymph nodes, liver biopsy material, or bone marrow is lightly impressed on a clean microscope slide; the film is allowed to dry at room temperature and is stained in the manner of a thin blood film. Whole cells, with organisms showing little if any distortion, may be clearly distinguished in such preparations. When dealing with lymph nodes or other fairly solid tissue, it is best to prepare the smear from a freshly cut surface. The remaining tissue can then be fixed for conventional pathologic procedures or be used as desired.

Silver Stain for Pneumocystis Carinii

Tissue impressions of lung biopsy material or smears of tracheal aspirate suspected to contain *Pneumocystis* should be stained using Grocott's method, which employs a methenamine-silver stain which clearly outlines *Pneumocystis* organisms (or various fungi) in black. The method, although relatively complex, may be found in most standard manuals on staining procedures such as the *Manual of Histologic Staining Methods of the Armed Forces Institute of Pathology* (Luna, 1968.)

REFERENCE

Luna, L. G. (Ed.) 1968. *Manual of Histologic Staining Techniques of the Armed Forces Institute of Pathology.* 3rd Ed. 258 pp. McGraw-Hill Book Co., New York.

5

Lumen-Dwelling Protozoa

We have chosen to consider together not only the intestinal proto-zoa of man but those found in the mouth, upper respiratory passages and urogenital tract. The list includes the parasites *Entamoeba histolytica, Giardia lamblia, Trichomonas vaginalis, Isospora belli,* and *Balantidium coli.* It also comprises a number of commensals, some species of questionable pathogenicity, and certain opportunistic pathogens or commensals. These organisms are generally of world-wide distribution, their prevalence in the population varying roughly with the level of sanitation.

THE AMEBAE

Four species of the genus *Entamoeba,* including the commensals *Entamoeba gingivalis, E. coli* and *E. hartmanni,* and the sometimes pathogenic *E. histolytica,* occur in man. *Entamoeba polecki,* a swine ameba, is seen occasionally as a human commensal. Other commensals are *Endolimax nana* and *Iodamoeba bütschlii.* Representatives of the normally free-living genera *Hartmannella, Acanthamoeba* and *Naegleria* have been isolated from the human nasopharyngeal cavity, central nervous system, eye and skin. As CNS invaders *Naegleria* may cause a fatal infection.

The Genus Entamoeba

Amebae of this genus, widely distributed in both vertebrate and invertebrate animals, are characterized by possession of a vesicular

37

nucleus with a comparatively small karyosome, located at or near its center, and with a varying number of peripheral chromatin granules attached to the nuclear membrane. Morphologic differences distinguish all the species except *Entamoeba histolytica* and *E. hartmanni*, which are separated primarily on the basis of size. During recent years there has been an increasing acceptance of the serologic and pathogenic differences between these two amebae. *E. hartmanni* was formerly known as the "small race" of *E. histolytica*.

Entamoeba histolytica

Increasing evidence suggests the existence of a number of strains or species of amebae, morphologically indistinguishable one from another but perhaps differing greatly in their pathogenic potential, that make up the species-complex now referred to as *Entamoeba histolytica*. Some of the serologic and biochemical means by which these amebae can be differentiated are presented later in this section. Unfortunately, there is as yet no practical laboratory method for such differentiation, and from a clinical standpoint we are forced to consider any ameba meeting the morphologic criteria for *E. histolytica* as being a potential pathogen.

Entamoeba histolytica inhabits primarily the large intestine where the trophozoites, or active forms, multiply in the mucosal crypts. The parasites may invade deeply into the wall of the intestine, feeding upon red blood cells and forming ulcers. Ulceration of the intestinal wall may give rise to amebic dysentery, or there may be fairly extensive damage without any clinical signs of disease. The invading amebae at times find their way into capillaries, to be transported via the blood stream to the liver or other organs where abscess formation may occur. Those amebae which enter the lumen of the gut find conditions less suitable for their continued existence in the trophic state. If intestinal motility is rapid, they may be passed out in liquid or semiformed stools while still trophozoites, but if motility is normal they will round up, extrude any ingested food, and enter the resistant cyst stage.

Living trophozoites of *Entamoeba histolytica* vary in size from about 12 to 60 microns in diameter; they average slightly over 20 microns. In preparations made from a freshly passed stool, trophozoites are usually actively motile. They move by means of pseudopodia, cytoplasmic protrusions which may be formed at any point on the surface of the organism. The pseudopodium is quickly thrust out, and may vary in form from short, blunt and broad to long and finger-like. The clear glass-like ectoplasm which forms the outer layer of the body of the ameba flows out to form the pseudopodium, which in this species is characteristically hyaline when first formed. The more granular endoplasm flows slowly into the pseudopodium as the ameba moves in the direction in which it was extruded. Motility is usually progressive and directional, rather than apparently aimless as in other amebae. The characteristic motility is only seen in freshly passed specimens. It may be enhanced by warming the slide by means of a thermostatically controlled "warm stage." A reasonably good substitute, and one which is less expensive, is the use of a copper coin, heated in the flame of a Bunsen burner and placed on the glass slide. It must be stressed that neither this expedient nor a warm stage will "revive" amebae which have been kept too long at room temperature.

Red blood cells may be ingested but are often not seen in chronic infections. The freshly ingested erythrocytes appear as very pale greenish refractile bodies lying in the cytoplasm of the ameba. While ingestion of red cells has been reported to occur in rare instances in other amebae, for all practical purposes it may be considered as confined to *Entamoeba histolytica.* The nucleus of the unstained trophozoite is usually not visible. Bacteria may at times be ingested by this ameba. They may also be seen in the cytoplasm if the ameba is degenerating. Death or degeneration of the parasites leads quickly to the formation of vacuoles in the cytoplasm — a Swiss cheese appearance—and such degenerate forms can never be identified with any accuracy. Similarly, even without such gross degenerative changes, if the amebae are kept too long at room temperature before fixation, the finer structures of the nucleus will undergo change. These structures, to be described below, are of great importance in specific identification of the amebae.

When seen properly fixed and stained with hematoxylin, trichrome or Lawless stain, details of nuclear structure may be observed. The nuclear membrane appears as a delicate but distinct line, on the inner surface of which is seen the peripheral chromatin, a layer of granules, characteristically uniform and small in size. In the center of the nucleus is a small mass of chromatin, the karyosome; between the karyosome and the peripheral chromatin the faintly stained fibrils of the linin network sometimes are seen. Typical nuclear structure, as described above, is depicted in most of the organisms showing in Figure 6. Some of the variations in morphology which may be encountered are shown in Figure 7. *It must be emphasized that, strictly speaking, there is no "characteristic" nuclear morphology for any species of Entamoeba.* While most will conform to type, some may present a nuclear structure more like that usually associated with a different species.

Ingested red blood cells will be stained according to the degree to which they have been digested by the ameba. When stained with hematoxylin (Figs. 4 and 5), the cytoplasm of the ameba is grayish, nuclear structures are an intense bluish-black, and freshly ingested erythrocytes are stained similarly; the red cells become progressively paler as they are digested. In a trichome stain, the cytoplasm is typically green,

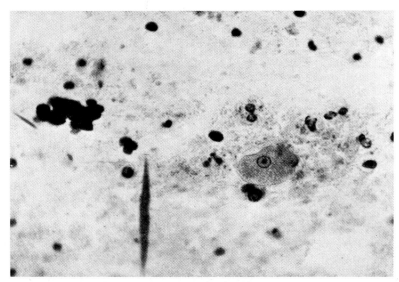

FIGURE 4. Trophozoite of *Entamoeba histolytica* stained with iron hematoxylin. Note Charcot-Leyden crystals and clumped red blood cells. (Courtesy of Hunter, G. W., Schwartzwelder, J. C., and Clyde, D. F. 1976. Tropical Medicine. 5th Ed. W. B. Saunders Company, Philadelphia.)

nuclear structures dark red, and freshly ingested erythrocytes may be cherry red or green in color; the cytoplasm of trichrome-stained amebae is occasionally a light pink, and sometimes green- and pink-staining forms will alternate in the same preparation. With the Lawless stain, all parts of the ameba and ingested materials stain with differing intensities of a dark blue color.

In preparation for the formation of the resistant cyst stage, trophozoites extrude all ingested material and assume a rounded form. This stage is referred to as the pre-cyst; it may be distinguished by its rounded single nucleus, absence of ingested material and lack of a cyst wall. However, nuclear morphology is often confusing at this stage, and it is best to rely upon either trophozoites or cysts for specific identification.

Cysts (Figs. 6 and 14) may be recognized by the presence of a hyaline cyst wall. They are usually spherical, but may be ovoidal or irregular in shape, and they vary from about 10 to 20 microns in diameter. In unstained preparations, the cyst wall is highly refractile. Cysts contain from one to four, or rarely more, nuclei. The nuclei may at times appear as small refractile spheres within the cytoplasm of the unstained cyst, but more often are not visible. Chromatoidal bars, so named because they stain with hematoxylin like the chromatin of the nucleus, are probably reserve food, used by the ameba while encysted. If present, these will be seen as rod-shaped clear areas in the cytoplasm. When stained with iodine (Fig. 29), the cytoplasm of the cyst will be a light yellowish-green to yellow-brown in color, the nuclear membrane and karyosome distinct and light brown. Chromatoidal bars do not stain, and appear as clear spaces in the cytoplasm. If the glycogen is present in vacuoles in the cytoplasm, it will stain a dark yellow-brown.

Stained with hematoxylin, trichrome or the Lawless stain, nuclear structure is similar to that seen in the trophozoites (Figs. 6, 7 and 14). The peripheral chromatin ring may appear to be thicker and less uniform in size. Some strains of *Entamoeba histolytica* consistently have eccentric karyosomes, and in some the peripheral chromatin, instead of appearing as a layer of spherical granules, forms thin plaques on the nuclear membrane. A third variant of nuclear structure is seen when all the peripheral chromatin is massed in crescentic fashion at one side of the nuclear membrane. One or more chromatoidal bars may be

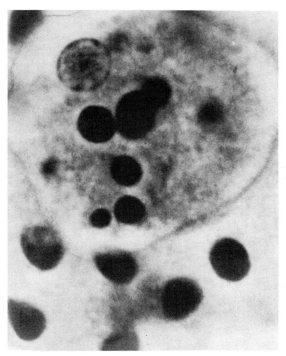

FIGURE 5. *Entamoeba histolytica* trophozoite. Note ingested red cells. (Trichrome stain.)

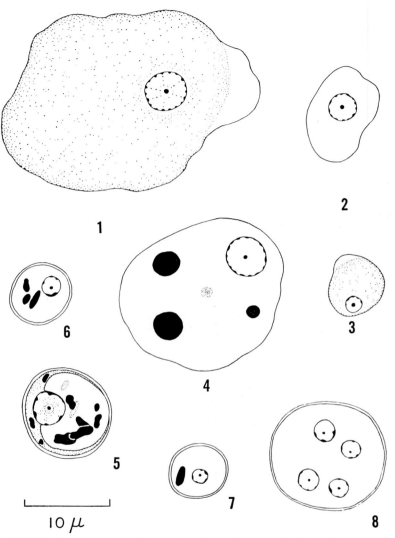

FIGURE 6. *Entamoeba histolytica:* 1, trophozoite with hyaline pseudopodium; 4, trophozoite containing red blood cells; 5, early cyst containing glycogen
mass and chromatoidals; 8, mature 4-nucleate cyst without chromatoidals. *E.
hartmanni:* 2, 3, trophozoites; 6, 7, uninucleate cysts. (2, 4, 6, 7 and 8 show diagnostic features only.)

found in the cytoplasm; they may attain a length only slightly less than
the diameter of the cyst, or may be considerably shorter. Occasionally,
especially in very young and usually uninucleate cysts, large numbers
of very small chromatoidal bars are seen, usually surrounding a glycogen vacuole. The chromatoidals generally appear in the form of elon-

gate bars with rounded or squared ends, but may occasionally be ovoid or cigar shaped. Chromatoidal bars of this characteristic morphology are considered as diagnostic of *E. histolytica* and *E. hartmanni*, but may occur also in *E. polecki* (Fig. 14). Chromatoidals are more frequently encountered in the one- and two-nucleate cysts, and a large proportion of mature four-nucleate cysts will not possess them. With hematoxylin the chromatoidals take the same bluish-black stain as the chromatin material of the nucleus, with trichrome they stain a bright red, and with Lawless stain they are a deep blue color.

In summary, the following characteristics are of value in the identification of *Entamoeba histolytica*:

I. Trophozoites, unstained.
SUGGESTIVE: (a) progressive motility, (b) hyaline pseudopodia, (c) no ingested bacteria, (d) nuclei not visible.
DIAGNOSTIC: ingestion of red blood cells.

II. Trophozoites, stained.
SUGGESTIVE: (a) clear differentiation of ectoplasm and endoplasm, (b) no ingested bacteria.

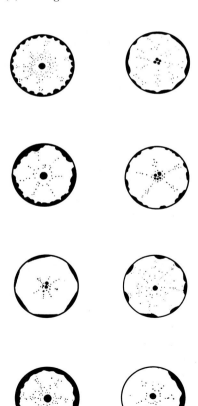

FIGURE 7. *Entamoeba histolytica.* Variations in nuclear structure. (Some original, others adapted from various sources.)

DIAGNOSTIC: (a) fine uniform granules of peripheral chromatin and small central karyosome in nucleus, (b) ingested red blood cells, (c) average size over 12 microns.

III. Cysts, unstained.

SUGGESTIVE: (a) four nuclei, (b) rod-like chromatoidals.

IV. Cysts, stained.

SUGGESTIVE: (a) maximum of four nuclei having both karyosome and peripheral chromatin, (b) diameter over 10 microns.

DIAGNOSTIC: (a) typical nuclear structure, (b) chromatoidal bars with rounded or squared ends, (c) diameter over 10 microns.

SYMPTOMATOLOGY AND PATHOGENESIS. The following clinical classification has been adapted from the WHO Report on Amebiasis (1969). Percentages given were not in that report and are rough approximations only:

   I. Asymptomatic infections (85-95 per cent of cases)
  II. Symptomatic infections
    A. Intestinal amebiasis
      1. Dysenteric
      2. Non-dysenteric colitis
    B. Extra-intestinal amebiasis
      1. Hepatic
        a. Acute non-suppurative
        b. Liver abscess (about 5 per cent of symptomatic patients)
      2. Pulmonary (about 0.25 per cent of symptomatic patients)
      3. Other extra-intestinal foci (very rare)

The symptomatology of amebiasis is far from clear-cut and of course depends in large measure upon the extent of tissue invasion, as well as whether the infection is confined to the intestinal tract or has spread to involve other organs. Intestinal amebiasis is the most common form of infection and is frequently asymptomatic. Certain patients with intestinal amebiasis have very vague and non-specific abdominal symptoms. Although these symptoms may improve or disappear after antiamebic therapy, they cannot specifically be related to the infection. Another group of patients, in this country usually the smallest, will have more definite symptoms, such as diarrhea or dysentery, abdominal pain and cramping, flatulence, anorexia, weight loss and chronic fatigue. Frequently all patients with symptomatic intestinal amebiasis are spoken of as having amebic dysentery. This term should be reserved for those patients who actually have dysentery, or blood and mucus in the stools. Amebic colitis is a term which can be used to denote any symptomatic intestinal infection.

It seems probable that strain differences as to virulence and, from time to time, differences in susceptibility of the host both play a part in determining whether or not tissue invasion takes place. At any rate, when *E. histolytica* succeeds in entry into the intestinal mucosa, this penetration is generally unaccompanied by inflammatory response. Since the local response is minimal, the constitutional response of the host is likewise. The amebae, secreting proteolytic enzymes, produce a necrosis of the surrounding tissues. From the crypts, amebae penetrate into the mucosa (Fig. 8). Most frequently the cecal area is involved, but the ascending colon and rectosigmoid and indeed any part of the colon may also be sites of primary invasion.

While the initial intestinal invasion may be accompanied by little local reaction, and often no recognizable symptoms, a diffuse inflammation, indistinguishable from the non-specific inflammatory lesion of other types of colitis, may be seen in sections of biopsies taken from patients with acute amebic colitis (Pittman et al., 1973). The diarrhea thus provoked may be mild, with only a few loose stools daily, perhaps alternating with periods of constipation. Even in patients with mild diarrhea, or normal stools, careful examination of the feces may reveal flecks of blood-tinged mucus, often containing numbers of motile *E. histolytica.* More acute cases may have a dozen or more explosive liquid

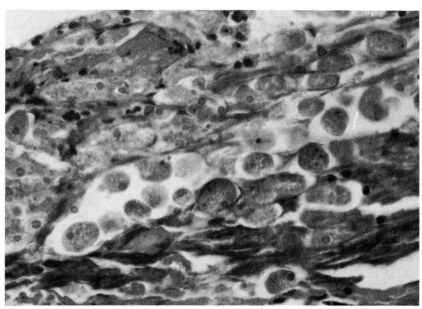

FIGURE 8. *Entamoeba histolytica* in ulcer of colon. (Photomicrograph by Zane Price.)

stools daily, containing much blood and mucus and perhaps accompanied by abdominal cramps. Tenesmus, or painful spasms of the anal sphincter, is a sign of rectal ulceration.

Amebae may penetrate through the muscularis mucosae into the submucosa (Fig. 8), where they spread out into classic "flask-shaped" ulcers and erode into blood vessels to give rise to the intraluminal bleeding characteristic of acute infections. If large numbers of ulcers are produced, they may coalesce by means of intercommunicating submucosal sinus passages. The undermined mucosa may remain fairly normal in appearance, or if the undermining is extensive and there is secondary bacterial infection, there may be necrosis and sloughing of large portions of the intestinal wall. Rarely, intestinal casts may appear in the stools.

Sigmoidoscopic examination may demonstrate an almost normal mucosal pattern, or one which is indistinguishable from ulcerative or granulomatous colitis. There may be scattered ulcerations up to a few millimeters in diameter, characterized by an erythematous border and yellowish center. In more advanced cases greater numbers of ulcers may be seen, ranging in size up to 10 or 12 millimeters in diameter, often with raised edges, but with normal appearing mucosa elsewhere. Presence of a grossly normal mucosa between the ulcers serves to differentiate amebic from bacillary dysentery on sigmoidoscopic examination, the entire mucosa being involved in bacillary dysentery. As the amebic infection progresses, coalescence of the ulcers may produce irregularly wandering ulcer trenches, sometimes with hairlike remnants of the more resistant supportive structures projecting from their bases ("Buffalo skin" or "Dyak hair" ulcers).

The characteristics of the amebic cellular exudate are helpful and are described on pages 27 and 28.

Abdominal examination may reveal tenderness of the cecum, transverse colon, or sigmoid. Some hepatic enlargement and tenderness may be evident, but this does not necessarily indicate amebic invasion of that organ. Fever is not characteristic of uncomplicated amebic colitis. A mild leukocytosis may be seen; this is probably a response to the secondary bacterial infection so frequently present. The white cell count seldom rises above 12,000; in bacillary dysentery the average may be not too much higher, but counts may reach 16,000 to 20,000. Even in moderately severe attacks of diarrhea or dysentery, spontaneous subsidence or alternation with periods of constipation is common.

Perforation of an amebic ulcer (Powell and Wilmot, 1966) is generally a dramatic event, accompanied by the usual signs of peritoneal irritation or infection. Surgical intervention in such cases, or in amebic appendicitis, may be unfortunate, as the infected gut is quite friable. A chronic granulomatous lesion, known as an ameboma, develops most frequently in the cecal or rectosigmoid regions. It may produce a "napkin-ring" constriction of the bowel wall, indistinguishable on x-ray from an annular carcinoma, or it may give rise to a characteristic conical configuration of the cecum (Fig. 9, *D*).

Hepatomegaly and tenderness may occur in amebic colitis without any evidence of hepatic infection. The hepatic enlargement is thought to be a toxic response to intestinal infection, unrelated to the local presence of amebae. A condition known as amebic hepatitis has been postulated, but if defined as a diffuse early stage of liver infection, without abscess formation, remains hypothetical. At any rate, it is clear that spread of the infection to the liver may occur in cases in which intestinal complaints never develop.

Hepatic infection is characterized by liver tenderness and enlargement, fever, weight loss, and sometimes a cough with evidence of pneumonitis involving the right lower lung field. The right leaf of the diaphragm may be elevated and fixed in position (Fig. 9, *A*). Multiplication of amebae in the liver may lead to the development of single or multiple abscesses, although the majority of amebae which reach the liver are probably destroyed there and do not produce abscesses. Single large abscesses (Fig. 9, *B*, *C*) may arise from the coalescence of multiple smaller ones. With abscess formation, hepatic pain becomes more severe and continuous; pain may also be referred to the right or left shoulder, depending upon the position of the abscess. There is a leukocytosis of 15,000 to 35,000 without a characteristic differential, fever, and night sweats. The fever tends to occur daily in the afternoon, reaching a peak of about 102° F. and accompanied or followed by profuse sweating. Liver scans (Fig. 10) reveal areas of non-visualization, most frequently single and in the right lobe, less often multiple or in other locations (Parmley et al., 1968). Gallium 67, which concentrates in tissues affected with many neoplastic and inflammatory diseases, does not seem to be taken up by amebic abscesses. Pritchard et al. (1974) suggest a combination of Gallium 67 scanning with ultrasonography as a diagnostic approach. The wall of the abscess cavity may be visualized by infusion of sodium diatrizoate (Hypaque), as used for intravenous pyelography, according to Chang et al. (1974). Liver function tests are of little value in the differential diagnosis of amebic abscess. Aspiration of an amebic abscess usually yields a thick reddish-brown fluid, which rarely contains amebae. Organisms are confined to the hepatic tissue of the abscess walls. Under these circumstances, diagnosis through response to therapy is not infrequently the only practical approach.

Erosion of a hepatic abscess through the diaphragm into the lung may lead to pulmonary amebiasis. Pleurisy, with or without effusion or pleural rub, or right lower lobe pneumonitis may signal a subdiaphragmatic abscess without actual rupture into the pleural space. With rupture into the pleural cavity, a characteristic x-ray picture may result

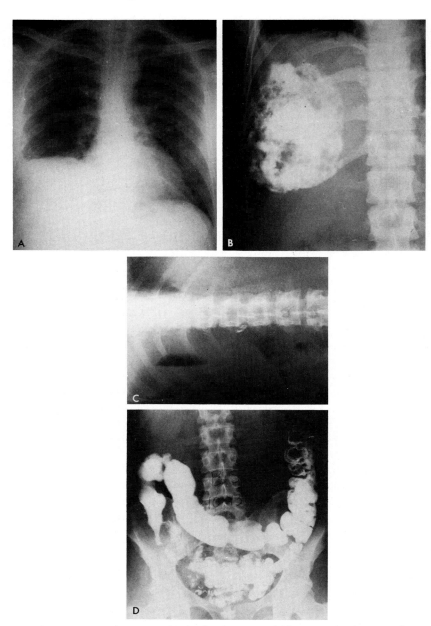

FIGURE 9. *A,* Elevation of right diaphragm and blunting of right costophrenic angle in amebic cyst of liver. *B,* Large amebic cyst of liver outlined by injection of contrast material. *C,* Amebic cyst of liver; note air in cyst cavity and fluid level after partial aspiration of contents. *D,* Amebiasis of the cecum; note funnel-shaped deformity seen on barium enema. (*A, B* and *C* courtesy of Dr. Jerrald Turner, Harbor General Hospital, Torrance, California.)

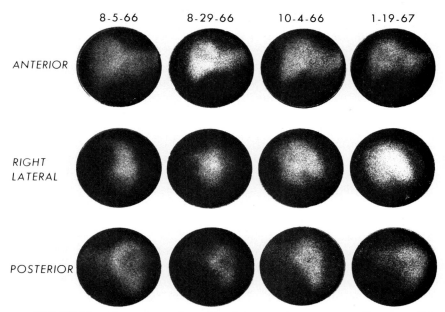

FIGURE 10. Hepatoscan of amebic abscess under treatment. (Courtesy of Dr. Paul Weber, Department of Clinical Pathology, San Francisco General Hospital, San Francisco.)

(Whittaker, 1973), with evidence of an effusion ascending the greater fissure, sometimes followed by rupture into the pleural space. If the abscess is localized in the left lobe of the liver, it may, of course, involve the left lung. If hepatic spread of the infection extends to involve a bronchus, amebae may be found in the sputum. Primary pulmonary amebasis, blood-borne from an intestinal focus rather than arising from a hepatic abscess, has been reported. Amebic abscesses of other organs, such as the brain, pericardium (MacLeod et al., 1966; Watson et al., 1972) and spleen, are uncommon. Signs of such infection are related to the organs involved. Amebic infection of the skin is rare but may produce extensive gangrenous ulcerations of the perineal tissues or affect the skin surrounding a colostomy or draining hepatic abscess. Vaginal or urethral infections have been reported. In all of these conditions, trophic amebae may be recovered from the affected tissues.

The standard methods of stool examination are outlined in Chapter 3. Amebae may often be found in specimens obtained by sigmoidoscopy. Material may be expressed from the ulcers by means of gentle pressure from a long-handled curette or loop and suspended in saline for microscopic examination. Serologic techniques (see Chapter 16) have been employed for many years in the diagnosis of amebiasis. Indirect hemagglutination, complement fixation and gel-diffusion tests are available. The IHA test is perhaps slightly more sensitive. All are more likely to be positive in extraintestinal or in invasive colonic amebiasis (Juniper et al., 1972). A skin test has also been developed, and will perhaps find its greatest usefulness in epidemiologic studies.

EPIDEMIOLOGY. The prevalence of amebic infection, as of most enteric diseases, varies with the level of sanitation and is generally higher in the tropics and subtropics than in temperate climates (Elsdon-Dew, 1968). Severity of the disease and the incidence of complications may likewise be greater in the tropics. In temperate climates, the majority of cases are usually asymptomatic, except in rare epidemic situations. While various factors may play a role in determining the severity of the infection, in one area in Africa Elsdon-Dew (1958) has found dietary deficiencies to play a crucial role, apparently in an indirect manner through their effect on the intestinal flora. In the United States amebiasis is commoner in rural reas and in lower socioeconomic groups. In any region it is more prevalent under crowded conditions, and it may reach epidemic proportions in orphanages, prisons and asylums (Sexton et al., 1974). Outside such settings, in the United States, Canada and Europe, the relatively few epidemic outbreaks can usually be traced to sewage contamination of drinking water. The prevalence of E. histolytica infection in the general population of the United States is probably between 1 and 5 per cent; a world-wide average incidence may be close to 10 per cent. An incidence of 50 to 80 per cent has been reported in some tropical and subtropical areas.

From an epidemiologic standpoint, it is important to differentiate between the acute, chronic and asymptomatic (or 'cyst-passer") stages of the infection. The acute case of amebic dysentery is of no significance in transmission of the disease, as trophozoites cannot long survive outside the body of the host. Trophozoites or cysts may be passed at different times by the patient who has a chronic infection, while the asymptomatic patient generally produces only cysts and is thus of utmost importance in the transmission of the disease. Cysts are relatively resistant, but are killed by drying, by temperatures over 55° C, and by superchlorination or the addition of iodine to drinking water. While contaminated water is in many areas a prime source of infection, food handlers may also play a role. The use of "night soil" for fertilizer and the contamination of foodstuffs by flies and possibly cockroaches are of epidemiologic importance in some areas.

A number of strains of amebae resembling Entamoeba histolytica are able to survive and multiply at room temperature (unlike E. histolytica) and have been isolated from human feces. The first such eurythermic ameba to be isolated and grown in culture is known as the "Laredo" strain. Laredo-type strains have an optimum growth temperature of 25 to 30° C. and can survive at temperatures from 0 to 41° C., whereas the classical *E. histolytica* has an optimum of 37° C and can survive a range of 20 to 43° C. Laredo amebae are able to grow in hypotonic media, have certain demonstrable serologic differences from *E. histolytica*, are of limited pathogenicity to experimental animals and probably non-pathogenic to man, and exhibit greater drug-resistance than classical strains of *E. histolytica*.

A very similar ameba, isolated from sewage plants in many parts of the world, has been named *Entamoeba moshkovskii*. This ameba has a wide temperature tolerance, multiplying at 10 to 37° C. It will grow in hypotonic media and is apparently non-pathogenic for laboratory animals. Like the classical *E. histolytica* and the Laredo-type strains, *E. moshkovskii* lacks nuclear DNA/histone, which is present in free-living protozoa. Biochemical characterization of the DNA of various strains of amebae shows clear-cut differences between *E. histolytica*, Laredo-like strains, and *E. moshkovskii*. Among the "classical" *E. histolytica* strains, two or more genotypically distinct species can be differentiated, while specific differences can also be demonstrated between the "Laredo" and "Huff" strains of temperature-tolerant amebae (Gelderman et al., 1971).

TREATMENT.   This varies with the clinical stage of the infection. For *asymptomatic intestinal amebiasis*, treatment may not be strictly necessary. However, it is perhaps imprudent to neglect such infections, which may either become symptomatic or provide a nidus for extra-intestinal spread. Methods of treatment of the asymptomatic case and of amebic colitis are essentially identical. The mainstays of treatment have been iodo-hydroxyquinolines such as diiodohydroxyquin (Diodoquin), and arsenicals like Carbarsone (p-carbamido-benzine arsonic acid). The iodides are contraindicated in severe liver damage; certain persons may manifest an idiosyncrasy to iodides or to arsenicals; hemorrhagic encephalopathy is a rare complication of the use of Carbarsone. The drugs may be used separately, or in combination. Our preference is for a combined course: diiodohydroxyquin 0.65 gm. three times daily before meals for 20 days, followed by a rest period of 10 days, after which Carbarsone 0.25 gm. is given three times daily for 10 days. Unfortunately, diiodohydroxyquin has been withdrawn from the market in the United States by its chief manufacturer, because of reports (Behrens, 1974) that it may cause the type of subacute myelo-optic atrophy associated with use of the related drug iodochlorhydroxyquin (Enterovioform). Diodoquin is still approved for use in amebiasis; the excellent British drug emetine bismuth iodide has never received approval of the Food and Drug Administration. The antibiotics, tetracycline 0.25 gm. four times daily for 5 days, or paromomycin (Humatin) 0.5 gm. three times daily for 7 days, are also used either alone or, more frequently, in combination with diiodohydroxyquin.

Metronidazole (Flagyl), 1-(β hydroxyethyl)-2-methyl-5 nitroimidazole, in doses approximating 750 mg. three times daily for five days, has been recommended (Powell et al., 1967) for treatment of *acute amebic dysentery*. Many authorities now extend the treatment period to ten days. Side effects of metronidazole treatment include nausea, diarrhea, parosmia and headache. Other side-effects are uncommon, and none is usually of such severity as to preclude use of the drug. The patient should be warned to abstain from alcohol during treatment with metronidazole. Reports of increased incidence of tumors in mice fed the drug from birth (Rustia and Shubik, 1972) are a cause for concern, but dosages employed clinically are not comparable.

Treatment failures do occur; the development of resistant strains may be a consequence of metronidazole treatment. The appearance of liver abscess following apparent successful treatment with metronidazole (Weber, 1971) has prompted the adjunctive use of the 4-aminoquinoline, chloroquine (Aralen). When used in addition to metronidazole or other amebacides in treatment of amebic colitis, 250 mg. twice daily for two to three weeks seems appropriate. Chloroquine may on occasion produce dermatitis, even of the severe exfoliative type. Ocular lesions were common with the prolonged high dosages formerly used in the treatment of rheumatoid arthritis and systemic lupus erythematosus but should not be seen with the dosage schedules outlined above. Other side-effects include tremulousness, irritability and insomnia.

Another very effective treatment for *acute amebic dysentery* is the alkaloid, emetine hydrochloride, administered by subcutaneous or intramuscular injection at the rate of 1 mg. per Kg. of body weight (maximum dose 65 mg.) daily. It should be given *only* until the acute dysentery is controlled, *or* for no longer than five days. If given in this manner, toxic symptoms are not likely to occur.

Signs and symptoms of emetine toxicity include EKG abnormalities, hypotension, tachycardia, dyspnea and precordial discomfort. The EKG changes (Fig. 11) may include T-wave abnormalities (the initial effect, usually the last to disappear as the tracing reverts to normal, is T-wave inversion in the precordial leads), Q-T, P-R, or QRS prolongation, or S-T depression. Microscopically one sees evidence of myocardial fiber destruction without inflammatory changes (Hurst and Logue, 1966).

Dehydroemetine* is less toxic than emetine, but should be administered with the same precautions. The usual dosage is 1.5 mg. per Kg. of body weight daily. Tincture of opium (paregoric) may be administered in conventional doses for symptomatic relief of cramping. Emetine is only effective against amebae in ulcers in the intestinal

---

*Available at present in the United States only from the Parasitic Disease Service, Center for Disease Control, U.S. Public Health Service, Atlanta, Ga. 30333.

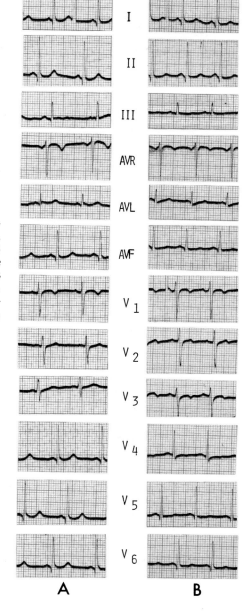

FIGURE 11. Electrocardiographic changes in emetine toxicity. *A,* Pretreatment. *B,* After emetine 65 mg. daily for 10 days. Note T-wave inversion or depression in leads V3–6. (Tracings courtesy of Dr. Alfred A. Bolomey, Kaiser-Permanente Medical Center, Oakland, California.)

mucosa, in hepatic abscesses or in other extra-intestinal locations. Control of the acute symptoms always should be followed by a course of treatment with one or more drugs effective against parasites in the intestinal lumen. This usually will be the same treatment regimen as used in mild or asymptomatic cases.

Metronidazole is generally considered to be effective in the treatment of *hepatic abscess*, especially because it simultaneously eliminates the intestinal infection. Although smaller amounts may sterilize the liver, doses recommended are those used in treatment of intestinal amebiasis. Some reports, such as those of Powell and Elsdon-Dew (1971), Stillman et al. (1974), and Datta et al. (1974), suggest that metronidazole, used alone, may not effect a cure in all cases. Emetine hydrochloride (1 mg. per Kg. of body weight, not to exceed a total of 65 mg. per day) or dehydroemetine (1.5 mg. per Kg. of body weight per day) may be given by intramuscular injection daily for ten days. The patient must be carefully observed during treatment for the signs and symptoms of emetine toxicity. If either of these drugs is used, it should probably be combined with chloroquine to prevent relapse. Chloroquine may be administered at the rate of 500 mg. twice daily for two days, and continued at 250 mg. two or three times daily for an additional 28 days. Tsai (1973) suggests, on the basis of extensive experience in Taiwan, a combination of emetine hydrochloride or dehydroemetine, 60 mg. intramuscularly daily for seven days, metronidazole 2.4 gm. daily (he employs a single daily oral dose) for ten days, and chloroquine 750 mg. daily for two days, followed by 500 mg. daily until clinical recovery.

Aspiration of amebic abscesses was at one time a routine procedure. With the advent of chloroquine and metronidazole therapy, this is no longer true. Smaller abscesses may be expected to resorb, and their disappearance can be monitored by the use of liver scans. Drainage of larger abscesses may be necessary under exceptional circumstances.

The use of Entero-vioform (iodochlorhydroxyquin) by tourists as a routine prophylaxis, or for treatment of diarrhea, is to be deplored as it is ineffective and has the potential of causing serious eye disease. The usual "traveler's diarrhea" is probably caused by toxigenic *Escherichia coli* (Gorbach et al., 1975) and is treated more effectively with tincture of opium or diphenoxylate hydrochloride (Lomotil). These drugs should not be used in patients suspected of having bacillary dysentery, as they can adversely affect the course of this infection.

Entamoeba hartmanni

Entamoeba hartmanni (Fig. 6) has now attained general acceptance as the name for the amebae formerly designated as "small race" *Entamoeba histolytica* (Neal, 1966). The confusion surrounding the relationship between the two forms is based on their morphologic similarity. The only clear-cut distinction between the two species is one of size. Arbitrarily, but generally satisfactorily, the two species can be separated by considering the upper limits of size of *E. hartmanni* trophozoites to be 12 microns, and of its cysts to be 10 microns. These measurements are likewise the lower limits of the size range of *E. histolytica*. Fortunately, most *E. hartmanni* will measure definitely below the dividing point, and most *E. histolytica* above it. If but a few 12-micron trophozoites or 10-micron cysts are seen, it may be impossible to make a specific identification.

Rounded trophozoites of *E. hartmanni* measure from 3 to nearly 12 microns in diameter; the cyst size range is from 4 to 10 microns. Nuclear structure shows the same variations seen in *E. histolytica*, and there is no consistent difference between the two species in nuclear-cytoplasmic ratio. The chromatoidal material assumes a similar rod- or cigar-like form in the two species. *E. hartmanni* ingests bacteria but not red blood cells.

Serologic differences between *E. hartmanni* and *E. histolytica* have been measured and are considerably greater than those noted between different strains of *E. histolytica*.

Studies of prevalence in which this ameba has been differentiated from *E. histolytica* indicate a roughly similar incidence and distribution for the two amebae. Although there have been reports to the contrary, many authorities consider *E. hartmanni* to be non-pathogenic and accordingly do not treat this infection.

In summary, the following characteristics are of value in the identification of *Entamoeba hartmanni*:

I. Trophozoites, unstained.	Not characteristic.
II. Trophozoites, stained.	DIAGNOSTIC: (a) nuclear structure similar to that of *E. histolytica*, (b) ingested bacteria, (c) diameter less than 12 microns.
III. Cysts, unstained.	SUGGESTIVE: (a) four nuclei, (b) rounded form.
IV. Cysts, stained.	DIAGNOSITIC: (a) typical nuclear structure, (b) chromatoidal bars with rounded or squared ends, (c) diameter less than 10 microns.

Entamoeba coli

This non-pathogenic ameba very closely resembles *Entamoeba histolytica;* the two species may be confused, leading either to superfluous treatment for a non-pathogenic parasite or to omission of appropriate therapy for a pathogen.

The trophozoites are about the same size as those of *E. histolytica*, varying from 15 to 50 microns in diameter; they perhaps average slightly larger than trophozoites of the pathogenic species. The cytoplasm is granular, frequently containing many vacuoles. Red blood cells are not ingested by this ameba except under most unusual circumstances. *E. coli* is sluggish in its movements in comparison to *E. histolytica.* Pseudopodia are short and blunt, never long and finger-like as they may be in *E. histolytica.* They are extruded slowly, are not hyaline, and there is no striking differentiation of the cytoplasm into ectoplasm and endoplasm. Motility is not progressive; the pseudopodia appear to function more in the ingestion of food than in production of directional movement. Bacteria are regularly seen in vacuoles in the cytoplasm.* The nucleus is usually easily discerned. A ring of refractile granules representing the peripheral chromatin encloses another eccentric refractile mass, the karyosome.

When stained, the nuclear morphology is more distinct (Fig. 12). Peripheral chromatin in *Entamoeba coli* is irregular both in size and in arrangement upon the nuclear membrane; it is definitely more abundant than is usual in *E. histolytica.* The karyosome is large, frequently irregular in shape, usually eccentric in position and is surrounded by a halo of unstained material. Granules of chromatin may be seen scattered between the karyosome and the peripheral chromatin, and sometimes a linin network is visible.

Precystic forms are seen, as in *E. histolytica,* but as in that species their morphology is not very distinctive, and identification should never be based upon examination of these forms alone, whether stained or unstained.

The cysts of *E. coli* (Figs. 12 and 14) overlap the size range of *E. histolytica,* being from 10 to nearly 35 microns in diameter; the average diameter is definitely greater than in cysts of the pathogenic species. The cyst wall is highly refractile, the cytoplasm granular in appearance; food vacuoles are absent. The nuclei are usually readily observed, and vary in number from one to eight. The eccentric position of the karyosome can frequently be distinguished, even in unstained amebae. Chromatoidal bodies are less commonly seen than in *E. histolytica,* but occasionally may be observed as clear thin lines or rods of refractile material in the cytoplasm.

With an iodine stain (Fig. 29), glycogen may be seen in the cysts of *Entamoeba coli;* often masses of this dark-staining material completely surround the nuclei, which are not, however, entirely obscured. While glycogen may occur in the cysts of *E. histolytica,* the perinuclear disposition of this material is more characteristic of *E. coli.* Eccentric karyosomes may be observed, especially in the uninucleate and binucleate

---

*This ameba seems to be omnivorous, ingesting in addition to bacteria other species of protozoans and even smaller members of its own species.

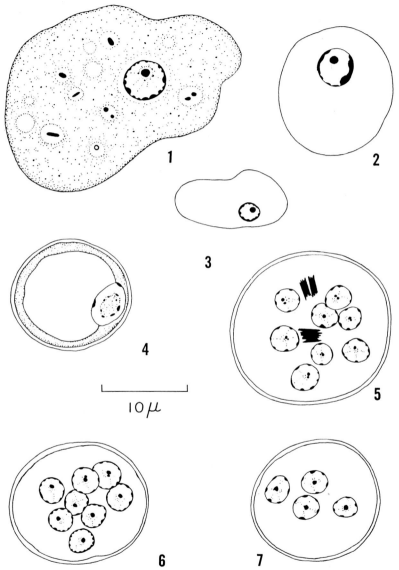

FIGURE 12. *Entamoeba coli: 1,* trophozoite with ingested bacteria and granular pseudopodium; *2, 3* trophozoites; *4,* early cyst with nucleus undergoing division, and containing glycogen mass; *5,* 8-nucleate cyst with chromatoidals; *6,* 8-nucleate cyst; *7,* 4-nucleate cyst. (*2, 3, 5, 6* and *7* show diagnostic features only.)

cysts, where their size is larger. Permanent stains bring out details of nuclear structure, which is similar to that of the trophozoites. Variants in nuclear structure are shown in Figure 13. From one to eight nuclei are ordinarily seen; rarely hypernucleate forms with sixteen or thirty-two nuclei are observed. The chromatoidals are seen to be composed of splinter-shaped or rarely ribbon- or thread-like bodies; heavier bodies with irregular ends are also frequently seen. The cytoplasm of *E. coli* cysts is very granular; areas occupied by glycogen before fixation are marked by empty spaces in the cytoplasm of the fixed and stained cysts.

In summary, the following characteristics are of value in the identification of *Entamoeba coli:*

I. Trophozoites, unstained.	SUGGESTIVE: (a) sluggish, nondirectional motility, (b) short, granular pseudopodia, (c) ingested bacteria, (d) visible nucleus.
II. Trophozoites, stained.	SUGGESTIVE: (a) granular cytoplasm without much differentiation into ectoplasm and endoplasm, (b) bacteria in food vacuoles.

FIGURE 13. Entamoeba coli. Variations in nuclear structure. (Some original, others adapted from various sources.)

	DIAGNOSTIC: nucleus with irregular clumps of peripheral chromatin; large, irregular, eccentric karyosome.

III. **Cysts,**
    unstained.

SUGGESTIVE: (a) eight nuclei, (b) glycogen mass surrounding nuclei (iodine stains).

IV. **Cysts, stained.**

SUGGESTIVE: maximum of eight nuclei, having karyosome and peripheral chromatin.

DIAGNOSTIC: (a) typical nuclear structure, (b) splinter-shaped or irregular chromatoidals.

Entamoeba polecki

First reported as an intestinal parasite of pigs and monkeys, *Entamoeba polecki* has been found occasionally in man. In parts of Papua–New Guinea it is apparently the most common intestinal ameba of man. *E. polecki* (Figs. 14 and 15) resembles *E. histolytica*, but can be differentiated from it with comparative ease. Culturally, and in its reaction to various therapeutic agents, it behaves somewhat differently from *E. histolytica*. Little is known about the pathogenicity of this species for man, although Lawless (1954) followed one human case for almost three years without any evidence that the organism caused disease. It is important that it be differentiated from *E. histolytica*, since it is not affected by many amebicidal drugs, to which the patient might otherwise needlessly be subjected.

Trophozoites of *E. polecki* resemble those of *E. coli* in their motility, in the granularity and degree of vacuolization of their cytoplasm and in the ingestion of bacteria. The nucleus is occasionally visible in the unstained trophozoite. Directional motility such as is seen in *Entamoeba histolytica* occurs only sporadically if at all; pseudopodia are usually formed slowly but occasionally may be thrust out in the explosive manner characteristic of *E. histolytica*. In stained preparations the nuclear structure appears somewhat intermediate between that of *E. histolytica* and *E. coli*. The karyosome is small in trophozoites, and usually central or nearly so in position. Normally compact, it is occasionally dispersed. The peripheral chromatin is generally seen in the form of fine granules evenly distributed on the nuclear membrane; sometimes larger granules are scattered among the smaller ones, or the peripheral chromatin may be massed at one or both poles.

The cyst stage of *E. polecki* is characterized by the possession of a single nucleus (Fig. 15). Very rarely it is binucleate, or quadrinucleate. Chromatoidal material resembling that seen in *E. histolytica* is formed in the cysts, and is often abundant. The ends of the chromatoidals are frequently angular and sometimes pointed, rather than regularly rounded or squared off as in *E. histolytica*. Thread-like chromatoidals

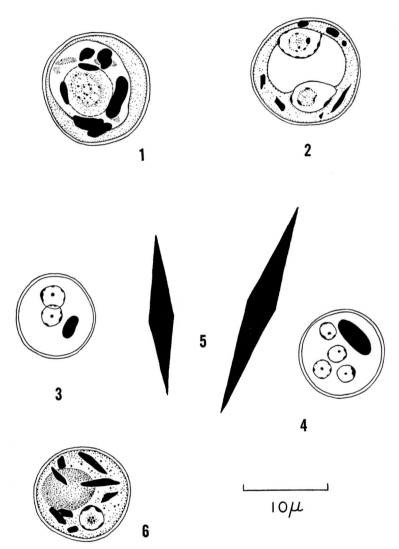

FIGURE 14. 1, 2, Early cysts of Entamoeba histolytica and E. coli respectively; both contain nuclei undergoing division; 3, 2-nucleate cyst of E. hartmanni with resting nuclei; 4, 4-nucleate cyst of E. hartmanni; 5, Charcot-Leyden crystals; 6, E. polecki cyst with inclusion mass and chromatoidals with angular and pointed ends. (3 and 4 show diagnostic features only.)

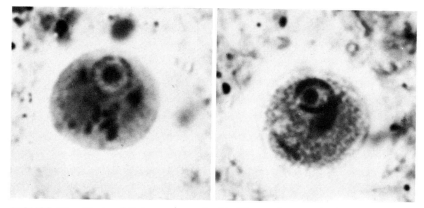

FIGURE 15.   Cysts of *Entamoeba polecki*. (Photomicrographs by Zane Price.)

have also been reported. Glycogen may be present and in addition approximately one half of the cysts contain an "inclusion mass," the nature of which is unknown. These masses are spherical or ovoidal in shape, without being sharply defined. In hematoxylin preparations, they are not dissolved as is glycogen, and they stain much more faintly than chromatoidal material.

Unstained cysts cannot be differentiated with any certainty from uninucleate cysts of the other two species of *Entamoeba*, though the presence in a formed stool of large uninucleate cysts, and absence of ones with greater numbers of nuclei, is suggestive. Iodine-stained cysts are likewise not distinctive. The inclusion mass does not take the dark stain characteristic of glycogen, and is not seen clearly. In permanently stained preparations, the karyosome is usually large and central in position. It may be spherical or stellate in shape, or it may consist of a group of small granules. A single minute central karyosome is sometimes observed. Peripheral chromatin appears evenly distributed, in the form of small spherical granules or flattened plaques, sometimes with interspersed irregular larger granules. As in the trophozoite, the chromatin may be massed at one or both poles. An inclusion mass, if present, will stain lightly but uniformly. Chromatoidals may be seen to exhibit the characteristic shape mentioned above.

In summary, the following characteristics are of value in the identification of *Entamoeba polecki:*

I. Trophozoites, unstained.	Not characteristic.
II. Trophozoites, stained.	SUGGESTIVE: (a) nucleus with minute central karyosome, with peripheral chromatin evenly distributed or massed at one or both poles, (b) ingested bacteria.

III. Cysts,   SUGGESTIVE: uniform uninuclear condition.
    unstained.

IV. Cysts, stained.   SUGGESTIVE: (a) uninucleate cysts, (b) large central karyosomes with evenly distributed peripheral chromatin or peripheral chromatin massed at one or both poles.

                                  DIAGNOSTIC: (a) inclusion masses, chromatoidal bars with angular or pointed ends.

Entamoeba gingivalis

Bearing a close morphological resemblance to *Entamoeba histolytica*, *E. gingivalis* (Fig. 16) is often found in pyorrheal pockets between the teeth and gums, and in the tonsillar crypts. It has been reported to multiply in bronchial mucus, and appear in the sputum, where it might be mistaken for *E. histolytica* from a pulmonary abscess. The cytoplasm of the ameba may contain bacteria and occasional red cells, but most frequently is filled with portions of ingested leukocytes. Nuclear fragments from the leukocytes will usually be recognizable in stained specimens, and will serve to identify the ameba, as *Entamoeba gingivalis* is the only species which will ingest these cells.

No cysts are formed by *E. gingivalis*.

These amebae are most frequently recovered from the mouths of patients suffering from pyorrhea alveolaris. Although numerous attempts have been made to implicate these organisms in the production of parodontal disease, it seems probable that they are most conspicuous under disease conditions simply because they find there a more suitable environment.

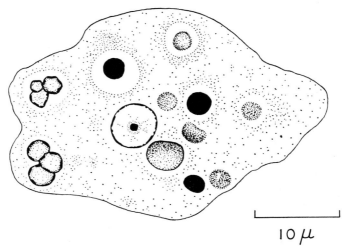

$10 \, \mu$

FIGURE 16.   *Entamoeba gingivalis.* Note ingested leukocytes.

Other Intestinal Amebae

It is generally not difficult to distinguish amebae belonging to the genus *Entamoeba* from other amebae occurring in the stool, even before a specific identification is possible. Trophozoites of the various species of *Entamoeba*, if we except *Entamoeba hartmanni*, are on the average larger than those of *Iodamoeba* or *Endolimax*, but differentiation on this basis alone should not be attempted. Cysts of *Entamoeba* are usually larger than those of *Endolimax* or *Iodamoeba*, although there is somewhat more of an overlap in size range. Cysts of all four species of *Entamoeba* are usually spherical; those of *Endolimax* may be spherical but tend more often to be ovoid, while *Iodamoeba* cysts are frequently irregular in shape. Nuclear structure in *Entamoeba* is quite different from that seen in the other genera, and affords a basis for immediate identification of this genus in stained preparations. Fundamentally, nuclear strucure in all four species of *Entamoeba* is the same; it is possible to distinguish a karyosome, and in addition a layer of peripheral chromatin which typically lies just under the nuclear membrane. Peripheral chromatin forming a distinct layer under the nuclear membrane is not regularly seen in the other two genera.

Like *Entamoeba histolytica*, which is cosmopolitan in distribution, *Iodamoeba bütschlii* and *Endolimax nana* have prevalence rates roughly paralleling those of the pathogenic species. *E. nana* is usually encountered with about the same frequency as *E. coli*; both are somewhat commoner than *E. histolytica*. *Iodamoeba* generally has prevalence rates somewhat similar to those of *E. histolytica* and *E. hartmanni*.

There is general agreement that these amebae are non-pathogenic and require no treatment.

Iodamoeba butschlii

This ameba (Figs. 17 and 18) receives its generic name from the characteristic glycogen vacuoles of the cyst stage (Fig. 17). These are so prominent that in iodine stains the cysts seem to contain little else. While glycogen vacuoles occur in other amebae, they are never as regular in outline nor as consistently present as in *Iodamoeba*. Large somewhat irregular glycogen masses are frequently seen in iodine stains of *Entamoeba coli* cysts; in mature cysts they often appear to surround the nuclei. In *Iodamoeba* cysts the single nucleus is seen at one side of the glycogen vacuole. Rarely, hypernucleate forms with two or three nuclei are reported.

Positive identification of unstained trophozoites is difficult. They vary in size from 4 to 20 microns in diameter, the majority being within the range of 9 to 14 microns. *Iodamoeba* is sluggishly progressive and

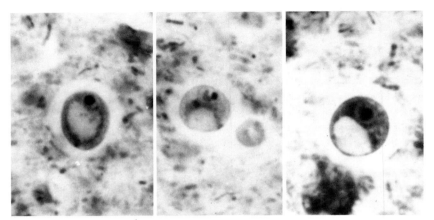

FIGURE 17.   Cysts of *Iodamoeba bütschlii*.

has hyaline pseudopodia. Bacteria may be seen scattered throughout the cytoplasm, and red blood cells are never ingested. The nucleus is usually not visible. Permanent stains will reveal the characteristic nuclear structure (Fig. 19). The nuclear membrane is delicate, and if it does not take the stain the karyosome will appear to be contained in a vacuole. The karyosome is large, more or less central in position, irregularly rounded, and is surrounded by a layer of small granules. The granules may lie closely applied to the karyosome, in which case they will not be visible unless staining and subsequent differentiation have been optimal. In other instances the small chromatin granules form a ring at varying distances from the karyosome, between it and the nuclear membrane.

Cysts range in diameter from 6 to 16 microns, with an average of about 9 or 10 microns. The unstained cyst is surrounded by a refractile wall. Instead of having the spherical or ovoid shape of most amebic cysts, the majority of cysts of *Iodamoeba* are irregular in outline, and there is much variation in shape. The glycogen vacuole is prominent even in the unstained cyst because of its refractility. The nucleus is seldom distinct in unstained cysts. When stained with iodine, the glycogen vacuole is a dark brown mass, often over half the diameter of the cyst (Fig. 29). The nuclear membrane and karyosome appear as highly refractile structures within the pale yellow cytoplasm. The procedures employed in staining with hematoxylin and other permanent stains dissolve glycogen, but the vacuole is nevertheless characteristic because of its size and clearly demarcated margins. The karyosome is usually quite eccentric, and may even be in contact with the nuclear membrane. The chromatin granules, which surrounded the karyosome

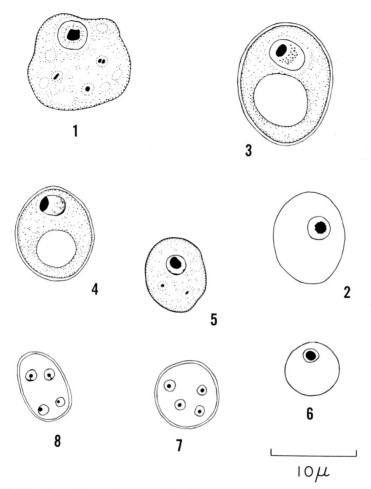

FIGURE 18. *1, 2, Iodamoeba bütschlii* trophozoites; *3, 4, I. bütschlii* cysts containing glycogen vacuoles; *5, 6, Endolimax nana trophozoites; 7, 8, E. nana cysts.* (2, 6, 7 and 8 show diagnostic features only.)

in the trophic stage, in the cyst usually form a crescentic aggregate between the karyosome and the nuclear membrane. In particularly well-stained specimens, linin fibrils may be seen running between the karyosome and the chromatin granules. Nuclei exhibiting this structure have been likened to a basket of flowers, with the karyosome forming the basket, the linin fibrils the stems, and the granules the blossoms. In other cysts the chromatin granules form a compact crescent closely applied to the nuclear membrane, or are disposed as in the trophozoite.

FIGURE 19. Iodamoeba bütschlii. Variations in nuclear structure.

In summary, the following characteristics are of value in the identification of *Iodamoeba bütschlii:*

I. Trophozoites, unstained.	Not characteristic.
II. Trophozoites, stained.	DIAGNOSTIC: nucleus with large central karyosome which is surrounded by a ring of small chromatin granules; or nuclear structure as in cyst.
III. Cysts, unstained.	SUGGESTIVE: (a) large refractile body in cytoplasm, (b) single nucleus.
IV. Cysts, stained.	DIAGNOSTIC: (a) basket nuclei or nuclei as in trophozoite, (b) large glycogen vacuole.

Endolimax nana

The most common of the smaller intestinal amebae, *Endolimax* (Figs. 18 and 20) is usually encountered with about the same frequency as

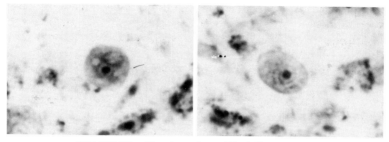

FIGURE 20.   Trophozoites of Endolimax nana.

Entamoeba coli. Both species are considerably commoner than are the other human amebae. The size range for both trophozoites and cysts is similar to that of *Entamoeba hartmanni*, with which they may be confused in the unstained condition.

Trophozoites range from 5 to 12 microns in diameter, with an average size close to 7 microns. Pseudopodia are blunt and hyaline; they are extruded rapidly as in *E. histolytica*, but fail to produce directional locomotion as seen in that species. Movement is sluggish and random. The cytoplasm contains food vacuoles with ingested bacteria. When stained, the characteristic nuclear structure (Fig. 21) becomes visible. The outstanding feature is a large karyosome, central or eccentric in position, and often irregular in outline (Fig. 20). Smaller extrakaryosomal chromatin granules are sometimes present. When the trichrome

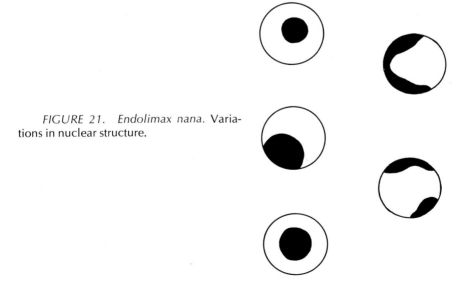

FIGURE 21.   *Endolimax nana*. Variations in nuclear structure.

stain is employed, the chromatin may at times be seen massed against the nuclear membrane, without formation of a distinct karyosome.

Cysts of *Endolimax* exhibit about the same size range as the trophozoites. They are most frequently ovoid, but sometimes spherical or subspherical in shape. A refractile cyst wall is present, which is particularly evident when concentrations are made by the zinc sulfate technique, and the cysts are stained with iodine. Zinc sulfate concentration results in a shrinkage of the cytoplasm of many of the cysts, which pull away from the cyst wall, leaving a clear space on one side of the organism, between the cytoplasm and the undistorted cyst wall. This effect is sometimes seen also in *Giardia*, but rarely in the other species of intestinal protozoa. In unstained cysts, little detail can be seen, and an iodine stain (Fig. 29) is seldom more rewarding. Occasionally, minute brown masses of glycogen may be seen in the cytoplasm of cysts stained with iodine. When stained with a permanent stain, the cysts are seen to possess one to four nuclei. Rare hypernucleate forms containing eight nuclei have been reported. A large karyosome, most frequently eccentric in position, characterizes the nucleus. Other chromatin granules and intranuclear fibrils have been reported, but are seldom seen in routine stains. While bacteria are of course not seen in cysts, granules of chromatoidal material which resemble them may be present.

In summary, the following characteristics are of value in the identification of *Endolimax nana:*

I. Trophozoites, unstained,	Not characteristic.
II. Trophozoites, stained.	DIAGNOSTIC: a nucleus with a large karyosome, generally with little or no peripheral chromatin.
III. Cysts, unstained.	SUGGESTIVE: ovoid shape.
IV. Cysts, stained.	SUGGESTIVE: ovoid shape. DIAGNOSTIC: presence of four nuclei with large karyosomes and little or no peripheral chromatin.

The Opportunistic Amebae

Several species of ordinarily free-living amebae have been found as human symbionts. In some instances, the association seems to be without pathological consequence, while in others it may result in devastating disease.

The free-living amebae comprise a large group, inhabiting fresh, brackish and salt water, moist soil, and decaying vegetation. Some are coprozoic. The taxonomy of this group has only recently been clarified (Page, 1967a,b), and the former confusion is reflected in many of the earlier case reports. The invasive potential of this group has been recognized since 1959; human infections were first reported in 1965. Much remains to be learned of the role of these amebae in disease production.

NAEGLERIA. This genus of ameboflagellates has an ameboid phase which alternates with one possessing two flagella. The forms found in the tissues are ameboid, and in the tissues are distinguished with difficulty from the two genera to be discussed next. In fact, while fatal intracerebral infections of this type are now thought to be caused primarily by *Naegleria*, amebae found in the earlier cases were erroneously identified, as belonging to the other two genera to be discussed.

Since the first reports by Fowler and Carter (1965) and Butt (1966) of primary amebic meningoencephalitis in Australia and America, a number of similar infections have been documented both in the United States and in Europe. Both epidemiologically and clinically, a characteristic pattern is seen. Most cases have occurred during the summer months in young persons who have within the preceding week swum or dived in fresh or brackish water. Both lakes and swimming pools have been apparent sources of the infection. The clinical course is dramatic. A day or so of prodromal symptoms of headache and fever is followed by the rapid onset of nausea and vomiting accompanied by the signs and symptoms of meningitis with involvement of the olfactory, frontal, temporal, and cerebellar areas. Olfactory lobe involvement is perhaps most characteristic; disturbances in the sense of smell or taste may be noted early in the course of the disease, but are not always seen. Patients often become irrational before lapsing into coma. Death occurs early; the entire clinical course seldom exceeds three to six days. There is serologic evidence that infection in man is caused by a single species, distinct from the non-pathogenic *Naegleria gruberi* isolated from soil (Visvesvara and Healy, 1975). The causative organism is now generally referred to (Carter, 1972) as *N. fowleri*.

Spinal puncture reveals a cloudy to frankly purulent or sanguino-purulent fluid usually under increased pressure. The cell count ranges from a few hundred to over 20,000 white blood cells, predominantly neutrophils, per cubic millimeter, and the failure to find bacteria in such a purulent spinal fluid should alert one to the possibility of amebic meningoencephalitis. Spinal fluid protein is generally, though not invariably, increased. Red blood cells are frequently present, and motile amebae may be found in unstained preparations of the spinal fluid. Their activity is enhanced by warming the slide and is characterized by the explosive formation of blunt pseudopodia, like those of *E. histolytica*, rather than the tapering projections seen on the pseudopodia of *Acanthamoeba*. Characteristically, these amebae do not stain well with the usual staining procedures. Iron haematoxylin stains of impression smears reveal a nucleus with a large karyosome which nearly extends to the delicate nuclear membrane. The nuclei can be distinguished in Wright's stain, and in hematoxylin and eosin stained tissues (Fig. 22). Red blood cells may be seen within the amebae.

On autopsy, an acute meningoencephalitis is seen; an exudate of neutrophils and monocytes is found in the subarachnoid space (Duma et al., 1969), and hemorrhage and an inflammatory exudate extend into the grey matter. Rounded amebae, 10 or 11 microns in diameter, are seen in the grey matter (Fig. 22), ahead of the advancing margin of hemorrhage or necrosis. They are particularly prominent in the Virchow-Robin spaces.

While neurologic symptoms predominate, other organ systems may be involved. Pulmonary edema seems not uncommon. Although apparent hematogenous spread of the infection has been demonstrated, the short course of the disease seems to make this of little clinical significance.

HARTMANNELLA AND ACANTHAMOEBA. The majority of the infections described above were first thought to be caused by amebae variously classified as *Hartmannella* or *Acanthamoeba*. These two closely related genera are similar in appearance to the ameboid stage of *Naegleria*, but have no flagellate stage. They belong to the family Hartmannellidae, and are generally referred to as hartmannellid amebae. *Hartmannella* probably does not produce infection in man, but *Acanthamoeba* may do so.

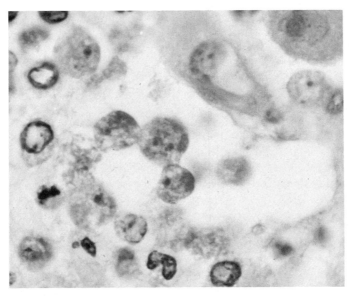

FIGURE 22. Naegleria in human brain. (Photomicrograph by Zane Price.)

Hartmannellids were first noted as contaminants in tissue cultures, and subsequently were found to produce lethal meningoencephalitis on nasal instillation into mice and other animals. *Hartmannella* has been reported as a transient member of the changing fauna and flora of the upper respiratory tract of man (Wang and Feldman, 1967), but it has not been noted to produce disease in that location. The possibility that these isolations represent inhaled cysts is raised by the studies of Kingston and Warhurst (1969), who demonstrated these and other free-living amebae in random air samples, collected by means of a slit-sampler. *Acanthamoeba* has been isolated from the central nervous system in a small number of cases, most but not all of which have been non-fatal (Bhagwandeen et al., 1975). *Acanthamoeba* has also been reported to cause a progressive corneal ulceration, leading to blindness (Nagington et al., 1974), and chronic granulomatous infections of the skin (Spencer, 1973). In such infections, characteristic cysts may at times be found in the tissues. Cysts are never seen in the tissues in *Naegleria* infections.

Various culture media have been advocated for isolation and identification of the opportunistic amebae from human tissues. The simplest involves the use of non-nutrient agar plates, to which live bacteria of the *coli-aerogenes* groups are added. Inoculated onto such a medium (see Chapter 15), the amebae will multiply; the flagellate form of *Naegleria* may be readily induced by the addition of sterile water.

TREATMENT. Although experimental *Acanthamoeba* infections respond to sulfadiazine, human cases of amebic meningoencephalitis (in all likelihood caused by *Naegleria*, however) have been unaffected by this drug. Other medications which have seemed ineffective include penicillin, ampicillin, tetracycline, erythromycin, chloramphenicol, emetine, chloroquine, and metronidazole. Carter (1969) has investigated the *in vitro* effectiveness of various drugs against *Naegleria*. Amphotericin B, effective in vitro, is the only one for which there is evidence of clinical effectiveness. It was administered intravenously at the rate of 1 mg. per Kg. of body weight daily, with intrathecal administration of 0.1 mg. on alternate days, to a patient who subsequently recovered (Carter, 1972).

THE FLAGELLATES

There are four common species of intestinal flagellates, *Giardia lamblia, Chilomastix mesnili, Trichomonas hominis* and *Dientamoeba fragilis.* In addition, two small flagellates, *Enteromonas hominis* and *Retortamonas intestinalis,* are sometimes encountered. There is no evidence that any of these organisms other than *Giardia* and *Dientamoeba* can cause disease. A pathogenic trichomonad, *T. vaginalis,* occurs in the urogenital tract, and the commensal *T. tenax* is found in the mouth.

The flagellates other than *Dientamoeba* are readily recognized as such by their characteristic rapid motility, and the three larger species can usually be identified in the unstained saline mount. Trichrome stain is generally preferable to iron hematoxylin for the staining of flagellates. The intracytoplasmic fibrillar structures of these organisms, often of diagnostic importance, are much better brought out by trichrome than by any but the most careful hematoxylin staining.

Giardia lamblia

Trophozoites of *Giardia* are found in the upper part of the small intestine, where they live closely applied to the mucosa. They may penetrate down into the secretory tubules of the mucosa, and are found at times in the gallbladder and in biliary drainage. The anterior portion of the ventral surface of the organism is modified to form a "sucking disk," which is considered to serve for attachment of the organism, and which, in relation to its size, may produce a considerable degree of mechanical irritation to the tissues.

Giardia is one of the most easily recognized intestinal protozoa. The trophozoite is bilaterally symmetrical, each structure being paired (Fig. 23). Like *Dientamoeba*, it possesses two nuclei in the trophic form. Body length ranges from 9 to 21 microns and body width from 5 to 15 microns. Motility is somewhat erratic, with a slow oscillation about the long axis. This type of motility has been likened to the motion of a falling leaf. The organism is roughly pear-shaped when seen in surface view, having a broad anterior and a very much attenuated posterior end. *Giardia* trophozoites have four pairs of flagella: anterior, lateral, ventral and posterior in position. Two nuclei lie in the area of the sucking disk in the anterior portion of the body. Two curved rods are seen posterior to the sucking disk. These rods are known as median bodies. The sucking disk is bordered by the curved intracytoplasmic portions of the anterior flagella, the axonemes. Axonemes of the caudal pair of flagella are straight, closely approximated, and run parallel to each other dividing the body into two halves throughout most of its length. The nuclei are spherical or ovoid and contain a large, usually central, karyosome. There is no peripheral chromatin.

In unstained trophozoites the characteristic body shape and motility may be observed, and some of the flagella can usually be seen. In preparations stained with any of the permanent stains, the most readily observable features are body shape, nuclei, axonemes and the median bodies.

The cysts are ovoid and measure 8 to 14 microns in length by 7 to 10 microns in width. While some of the nuclei or median bodies may

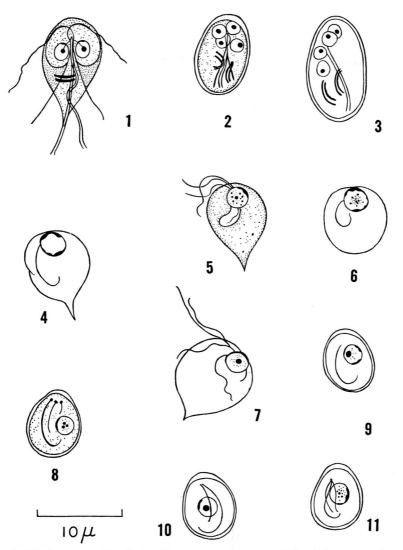

FIGURE 23. 1, *Giardia lamblia* trophozoite; 2, 3, *G. lamblia* cysts; 4, 5, 6, 7, *Chilomastix mesnili* trophozoites showing variation in structural detail which may be seen in permanent preparations; 8, 9, 10, 11, *C. mesnili* cysts. (3, 4, 6, 7, 9, 10 and 11 show diagnostic features only.)

occasionally be detected in living specimens, the addition of D'Antoni's iodine will usually reveal these structures. In permanent stains of cysts one observes four prominent nuclei and four median bodies, as well as twice the number of intracytoplasmic flagellar structures seen in the trophozoite all dispersed in a seemingly helter-skelter fashion. The cyst wall is smooth and colorless and is usually well set off from the cytoplasm owing to shrinkage of the latter at the time of fixation. When stained with trichrome, *Giardia* cysts may appear in varying shades of green or red, or the internal structures may be reddish-brown against a green background.

Giardia does not appear consistently in the stools of all patients. Danziger and Lopez (1975) describe three patterns of excretion: high, with parasites present in nearly all stools; low, with small numbers of parasites present in only about 40 per cent of stool specimens; and a mixed pattern with one to three weeks of a high excretion rate alternating with a shorter period of low excretion. With this in mind, it is well to collect specimens at intervals some days apart, if initially they are negative.

In summary, the following characteristics are of value in the identification of *Giardia lamblia:*

I. Trophozoites, unstained.	SUGGESTIVE: (a) progressive, "falling leaf" motility, (b) pear-shaped body with attenuated posterior end.
II. Trophozoites, stained.	DIAGNOSTIC: (a) nuclei in the area of a sucking disk, (b) the two median bodies posterior to the sucking disk, (c) typical arrangement of axonemes.
III. Cysts, unstained.	SUGGESTIVE: (a) ovoid body shape, numerous refractile threads in cytoplasm.
IV. Cysts, stained.	DIAGNOSTIC: (a) four nuclei, (b) four median bodies, (c) jumble of axonemes.

PATHOGENESIS. Long considered non-pathogenic and often found in completely asymptomatic individuals, there is now abundant evidence for the pathogenic potential of *Giardia.* Children are more frequently affected than adults, although all ages may exhibit symptoms ranging from mild diarrhea, flatulence, anorexia, cramp-like abdominal pains and epigastric tenderness to steatorrhea and a full-blown malabsorption syndrome. Like celiac disease in children, and its adult counterpart, non-tropical sprue, severe giardiasis may be marked by the production of copious light-colored fatty stools, hypoproteinemia with hypogammaglobulinemia, folic acid and fat-soluble vitamin deficiencies, and changes in the architecture of the intestinal villi. In sprue and celiac disease, a gluten-free diet effects a cure, while in giardiasis, administration of quinacrine will do the same. Achlorhydria may predispose to symptomatic giardial infections, as may hypogammaglobulinemia, or a relative deficiency in secretory IgA in the small bowel even in the presence of normal serum immunoglobulin levels. Lactose intolerance, apparently precipitated by *Giardia* infection, may persist after eradication of the parasites (Wolfe, 1975).

Biopsy of the jejunum (Hoskins et al., 1967) reveals in some patients shortening and blunting of the villi, reduction in height of the columnar epithelial cells of the mucosa, and hypercellularity of the lamina propria. In others with as severe symptoms, a fairly normal villus architecture is seen. Using the same technique of jejunal biopsy, but with special stains (Chapter 15), Brandborg et al. (1967) have demonstrated mucosal invasion by *Giardia*, and penetration into mucosal cells has been demonstrated by electron micrography (Morecki and Parker, 1967). It is by no means clear what relationship mucosal or cellular invasion by the parasite bears to the pathophysiology of giardial infection. X-rays of the affected small bowel show a picture characteristic of malabsorptive states, with mucosal edema and segmentation of the barium (Fig. 24).

EPIDEMIOLOGY. *Giardia* is world wide in distribution. In the United States, its prevalence ranges from about 1.5 per cent to 20 per cent; it is affected by much the same socioeconomic factors which influence the distribution of *E. histolytica*. Although it is not usually seen in epidemic outbreaks, one such outbreak was described from Aspen, Colorado, during the 1965-66 ski season (Moore et al., 1969); it was traced to contamination of well water by sewage leaking from defective pipes. Outbreaks elsewhere in this country have also been traced to drinking water (Morbid. and Mortal. Weekly Report, Oct. 31, 1975), as have those affecting travellers to Leningrad in recent years (Schultz, 1975). Giardiasis should be considered in the differential diagnosis of any "traveller's diarrhea" (Babb et al., 1971).

TREATMENT. Quinacrine hydrochloride, an acridine dye, is effective in the treatment of giardiasis and, in the dosage necessary for eradication of this parasite (0.1 gm. three times daily after meals for five days), seldom causes side effects in adults. Rare central nervous stimulation is seen, and psychotic episodes have been reported, especially in children. An occasional patient will develop nausea, but this is usually well controlled with prochlorperazine (Compazine). Metronidazole (Flagyl), 0.25 gm. three times daily for five days, is likewise effective and less toxic to children than quinacrine. The total daily dosage for children is as follows:

under 2 years	—	125 mg.
2 to 4 years	—	250 mg.
4 to 8 years	—	375 mg.
8 to 12 years	—	500 mg.

Chilomastix mesnili

As far as is known, *Chilomastix* is not pathogenic to man. It must, however, be differentiated from *Giardia* and from the other flagellates

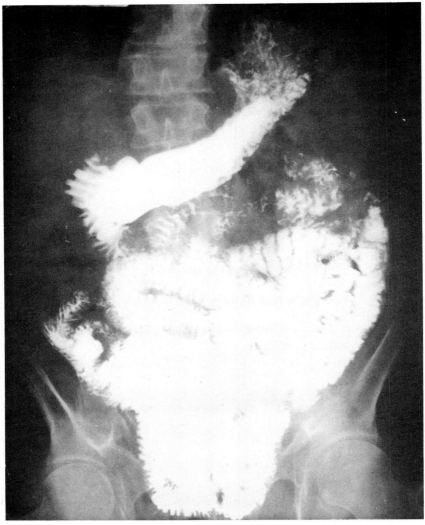

FIGURE 24. X-ray of small bowel in patient with giardial malabsorption syndrome. Note thickened walls and prominence of transverse folds of jejunum.

occasionally seen in stool specimens. The trophozoites of *Chilomastix* (Fig. 23) are elongate, tapering toward the posterior end. They measure 10 to 20 microns in length. At the anterior, broad end of the body are three flagella by means of which the animal moves in a directional manner. In fresh specimens one readily distinguishes the flagella and a groove running in a spiral manner along the length of the body. The stained trophozoites are characterized by a single nucleus near the origin of the anterior flagella, the cytostome, or oral depression, bordered by cytostomal fibrils, and a short flagellum which is directed posteriorly within the cytostomal area. The most prominent of the cytostomal fibrils, curving posteriorly around the cytostome, resembles a shepherd's crook. The three flagella seldom take a distinct stain. Nuclear chromatin may appear in the form of granules; in addition, it may form plaques applied to the nuclear membrane. A small, central or eccentric karyosome may at times be observed.

Cysts of *Chilomastix* are from 6 to 10 microns long, their width being somewhat less. At the anterior pole of the cyst is a nipple-like protuberance giving this stage a characteristic lemon shape not seen in any of the other intestinal protozoa. In stained preparations a single, large nucleus may be distinguished with the chromatin frequently condensed to appear as a large central karyosome. The curved cytostomal fibrils are usually quite prominent, and may even be apparent in iodine stained preparations (Fig. 21); in specimens particularly well stained with hematoxylin, the recurrent flagellum may be seen between the cytoplasm and the cyst wall at the anterior end of the organism.

In summary, the following characteristics are of value in the identification of *Chilomastix mesnili:*

I. **Trophozoites, unstained.**	DIAGNOSTIC: (a) anterior flagella, (b) a spiral groove.
II. **Trophozoites, stained.**	DIAGNOSTIC: (a) single anterior nucleus, (b) cytostome with curved shepherd's crook fibril, (c) no costa or undulating membrane (see *Trichomonas*).
III. **Cysts, unstained.**	DIAGNOSTIC: protuberance at one end of cyst (lemon shape).
IV. **Cysts, stained.**	DIAGNOSTIC: (a) body shape, as above, (b) single, large nucleus, (c) curved cytostomal fibril.

Trichomonas hominis

There is little evidence that *Trichomonas hominis* is pathogenic for man. It is, however, indicative of direct fecal contamination, as it does not form cysts. Living trophozoites are 7 to 15 microns long; they move about very rapidly, with a jerky and non-directional motion, and are difficult to observe until slowed down. *T. hominis* (Fig. 25) has four anterior flagella. In addition to the anterior flagella, a recurrent flagellum arises anteriorly and parallels the body, running to the posterior end. It forms the outer edge of the undulating membrane, a thin sheet of protoplasm which joins the body along a line marked by the presence of a curved thin rod called the costa. The costa is about the same length as the un-

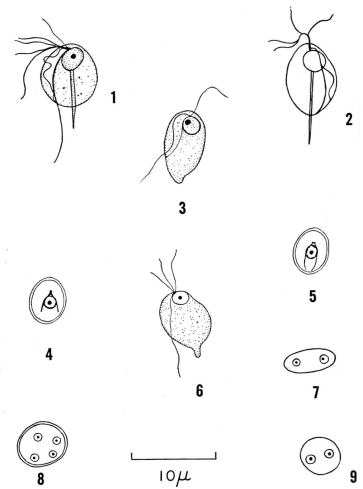

FIGURE 25.   1, 2, Trichomonas hominis; 3, Retortamonas intestinalis trophozoite; 4, 5, R. intestinalis cysts; 6, Enteromonas hominis trophozoite; 7, 8, 9, E.
hominis cysts. (2, 4, 5, 7, 8 and 9 show diagnostic features only.)

dulating membrane, and as it stains well is an important diagnostic character. The recurrent flagellum, which forms the outer edge of the undulating membrane, projects posterior to the body as a free flagellum.
The undulating membrane imparts a rotatory motion to the organism,
while the anterior flagella serve for propulsion. The single nucleus is
situated at the anterior end of the body, close to the origin of the anterior flagella. Its chromatin is unevenly distributed, and a small karyosome may be observed. A slender rod, the axostyle, extends through the

body from the anterior to the posterior end. It is sharply pointed, and protrudes beyond the posterior end of the body in a prominent manner.

In living trophozoites, the wave-like motion of the undulating membrane may be observed when the organisms are moving slowly or are at rest. The activity of the anterior flagella may be distinguished even if the individual flagella cannot be seen. The posteriorly protruding axostyle may be seen even when other structures are not distinguishable, and is diagnostic.

Identification of the stained organisms is more difficult than that of living material. In a routine iron hematoxylin preparation, the flagella and undulating membrane do not stain well. However, the single nucleus at the anterior end, and the costa, are diagnostic. No other intestinal protozoon possesses the latter structure. The costa stains intensely with iron hematoxylin, but careful focusing is needed to demonstrate it. The trichrome stain is superior to hematoxylin to bring out the flagella and axostyle.

In summary, the following characteristics are of value in the identification of *Trichomonas hominis:*

I. Trophozoites, unstained.	DIAGNOSTIC: (a) an undulating membrane, (b) an axostyle protruding through the posterior part of the body.
II. Trophozoites, stained.	DIAGNOSTIC: (a) the costa, (b) the axostyle.

Trichomonas vaginalis

Closely related to *Trichomonas hominis,* yet morphologically and physiologically distinct from it, is *T. vaginalis* (Fig. 26). The usual size range of this parasite is apparently from 5 to 15 microns, but it may reach a length of 30 microns. In general appearance these flagellates are very similar to *T. hominis,* from which they differ in having a short undulating membrane, extending only about half the distance to the posterior end of the body, with no free flagellum.

While it is possible to distinguish *T. vaginalis* from *T. hominis* on morphological grounds, this is not a practical necessity since the two organisms are quite site-specific. Numerous attempts have been made to introduce *Trichomonas hominis* into the vagina, but without success. When *T. vaginalis* is similarly introduced, a high percentage of successful infections results. Therefore, a specific identification may be made on the basis of finding a trichomonad in the vaginal secretions. A jerky, non-directional motility characterizes this species, as it does *T. hominis,* and if the organisms are observed under the high dry power of the microscope, when they have become sufficiently slowed down, the undulating membrane will be clearly visible.

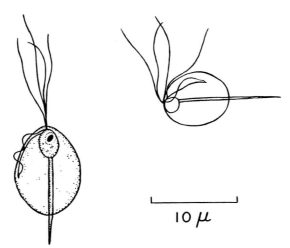

FIGURE 26.   *Trichomonas vaginalis,* as seen in permanently stained preparation.

PATHOLOGY.   Vaginal discharge is the most common complaint associated with vaginal trichomoniasis. The discharge is frequently profuse, and often associated with burning, itching or chafing. When viewed through a speculum, the vaginal mucosa is sometimes diffusely hyperemic, with bright-red punctate lesions, sometimes only patchily hyperemic, and not infrequently normal in appearance. Frequency of urination and dysuria are the commonest associated symptoms, and urethral involvement will be found in a large proportion of cases. Cystitis may occur in a small per cent of cases. A possible relationship between this infection and cervical carcinoma has been suggested.

Infection in males is frequently asymptomatic, but more severe symptoms are likely to be seen in cases where the infection involves the prostate and seminal vesicles, or higher parts of the urogenital tract. A thin discharge, frequently containing trichomonads, may be observed, with dysuria and nocturia. The prostate may be enlarged and tender, and there is sometimes associated epididymitis.

DIAGNOSIS.   Diagnosis is by demonstration of the trichomonads, most commonly in wet film preparations although staining procedures may be employed. Specimens for examination may best be obtained through a vaginal speculum, using a cotton-tipped applicator stick. If the applicator is placed for a short time in a tube containing a small quantity of 5 per cent glucose in normal saline before examination, the organisms are less likely to be rounded up and motionless under the microscope. Examination of urethral discharge in the female may yield positive results when no organisms can be found in the vaginal discharge. In the male, the diagnosis is made by examination of urethral discharge, prostatic secretions or centrifuged urine. Culture methods may be employed, and will sometimes increase the percentage of positive identifications. A culture method is given in Chapter 15.

TREATMENT. Metronidazole (Flagyl), in doses of 0.25 gm. three times daily for ten days is still generally effective in vaginal trichomoniasis; as the infection can be transmitted by sexual intercourse, treatment of the male should be considered in recurrences. Suggested dosage in the male is 0.25 gm. twice daily for ten days. Resistance to the drug has been reported from a number of areas (De Carneri, 1971). Metronidazole also might be effective in cases of non-specific urethritis in which *Trichomonas vaginalis* can be demonstrated.

Trichomonas tenax

Trichomonas tenax, which has also been called *T. buccalis*, resembles more closely *T. vaginalis* than *T. hominis*. It is a small organism, averaging only 6 to 10 microns in length. Like *E. gingivalis*, it occurs most frequently in pyorrheal pockets and tonsillar crypts, and is sometimes aspirated to set up a transitory bronchial or pulmonary infection.

The only treatment necessary is that directed at the underlying condition, if any.

Dientamoeba fragilis

Until recently *Dientamoeba* was considered by most parasitologists to be an ameba, albeit unique among the intestinal amebae in its binucleate condition, and the absence of a cyst stage. Despite the lack of flagella, various protozoologists (including Professor Harold Kirby, Jr., to whom this book is dedicated) have recognized its flagellate affinities. It remained for electron microscope studies (Camp et al., 1974) to confirm the flagellate relationships of this organism, which is classified among the trichomonads (Honigberg, 1974).

Despite its specific name, *Dientamoeba fragilis* (Fig. 27) is a rather resistant organism. Trophozoites may sometimes survive periods of some hours in the stool specimen after passage. *Dientamoeba* has been

 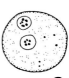

FIGURE 27. 1, 2, Dientamoeba fragilis, 1- and 2- nucleate trophozoites.

1   2

associated with diarrhea, nausea, vomiting and rather non-specific abdominal complaints. It is known to live in mucosal crypts of the large intestine, and has been seen to ingest red blood cells. It does not normally take in red cells even if they are present in some numbers in the stool, and apparently never invades the tissues.

Diagnosis of dientamoebal diarrhea should always be one of exclusion, entertained only after other likely causes have been eliminated. Under these circumstances, a therapeutic trial of one of the amebicidal drugs, such as diiodohydroxyquin (Diodoquin), may be employed in the dosage used for *E. histolytica* infections.

While the specific name of *D. fragilis* may seem inappropriate, its generic name is not, as the majority of organisms are binucleate. The binucleate form is considered to be in an arrested telophase, and in optimally stained specimens an extranuclear spindle can be seen extending between the two nuclei. Frequently as large a number as 80 per cent of them are seen in the binucleate form, although at times the percentage may be considerably lower. Occasional forms are seen with three or four nuclei.

Dientamoeba varies from 3 microns to as much as 18 microns in diameter, but is generally seen within the range of 7 to 12 microns. Pseudopodia are hyaline, broad and leaf-like in appearance, with characteristic serrated margins. Motility is progressive, and organisms are quite active in freshly passed stools but round up quickly upon cooling. Unstained, they are inconspicuous, especially if rounded and motionless. Vacuoles containing ingested bacteria may be seen scattered through the cytoplasm; nuclei are not visible in the living trophozoite. When stained, *Dientamoeba* is identified on the basis of a high percentage of binucleate forms, and the typical nuclear structure (Fig. 28). The nuclear membrane is delicate, and there is no peripheral chromatin. In the center of the nucleus lies a large mass, composed of from four to eight separate chromatin granules, usually arranged in a symmetrical manner. With good iron hematoxylin stains, the separate granules are readily observed. Trichrome and Lawless stains are less likely to reveal the separate granules of chromatin. Mononucleate forms may be confused with *Endolimax nana* if the individual chromatin granules are not obvious, but binucleate forms will be recognized without difficulty.

In summary, the following characteristics are of value in the identification of *Dientamoeba fragilis:*

I. Trophozoites, unstained.	Not characteristic.
II. Trophozoites, stained.	DIAGNOSTIC: (a) high percentage of binucleate trophozoites, (b) nuclei without peripheral chromatin and with four to eight chromatin granules in a central mass.

FIGURE 28. *Dientamoeba fragilis.* Variations in nuclear structure.

Enteromonas hominis

The small flagellate *Enteromonas* (Fig. 25) is encountered but rarely. Trophozoites are 4 to 10 microns in length. The body is broadly oval anteriorly, and tends to be somewhat attenuated posteriorly. There are three anterior flagella, by means of which the organisms move in a rapid, jerky fashion. The fourth flagellum adheres in part to the body, and is directed posteriorly. In living specimens little can be observed other than the general body shape, anterior flagellar movement and the trailing flagellum. In stained preparations, the single nucleus is seen near the anterior end. There is a distinct nuclear membrane, and a large central karyosome.

Cysts are inconspicuous, usually ellipsoid in shape and measure 6 to 8 microns in length. In fresh specimens they are very likely to be mistaken for yeasts. Stained cysts may be seen to possess from one to four nuclei, generally with a predominance of the binucleate condition. Cyst nuclei have the same structure as those of the trophozoites. Cysts of *Enteromonas* are of about the same shape as those of *Endolimax nana,* the nuclei of the two organisms are not dissimilar, and while *Enteromonas* is on the average distinctly smaller than *Endolimax,* the size ranges of cysts of the two species overlap. A predominance of binucleate cysts, of small size, is highly suggestive of *Enteromonas.*

In summary, the following characteristics are of value in the identification of *Enteromonas hominis:*

I. Trophozoites, unstained.	DIAGNOSTIC: (a) anterior flagella, (b) trailing flagellum but no undulating membrane.
II. Trophozoites, stained.	SUGGESTIVE: (a) absence of costa, axostyle or cytostomal fibrils, (b) single nucleus with large central karyosome, (c) small size.
III. Cysts, unstained.	Not characteristic.
IV. Cysts, stained.	SUGGESTIVE: (a) oval shape, (b) one to four nuclei, with predominance of binucleate forms, (c) small size.

Retortamonas intestinalis

Retortamonas (Fig. 25), also known by the generic name of *Embadomonas,* is not frequently seen. The trophozoites are ovoid or tear-shaped, and move rapidly by means of two anterior flagella. Body length ranges from 4 to 10 microns. A cytostome at one side of the body extends from near the anterior end about half the length of the organism. It is difficult to identify the unstained trophozoites but is sometimes possible to see the two anterior flagella and cytostome. In stained preparations, a relatively large nucleus is seen at the anterior end. The nucleus contains a small compact central karyosome; there is a layer of fine chromatin granules on the nuclear membrane. A fibril borders the cytostome. This fibril does not have the shepherd's crook curve characteristic of *Chilomastix.*

The pear-shaped cysts are 4 to 7 microns long, and up to 5 microns wide. They contain a single relatively large nucleus, frequently near the center of the cyst. Two fibrils extend from the nuclear region to the attenuated end of the cyst. This fibrillar arrangement, suggesting a bird's beak, is quite characteristic. Unstained, they are difficult or impossible to identify.

In summary, the following characteristics are of value in the identification of *Retortamonas intestinalis:*

I. Trophozoites, unstained.	DIAGNOSTIC: (a) a cytostome, (b) two anterior flagella only, (c) small size.
II. Trophozoites, stained.	DIAGNOSTIC: (a) large nucleus with small central karyosome, fine granules of peripheral chromatin, (b) cytostomal fibril (not in form of a shepherd's crook), (c) small size.
III. Cysts, unstained.	Not characteristic.

IV. Cysts, stained.   SUGGESTIVE: (a) pear shape, (b) small size.
DIAGNOSTIC: bird beak fibrillar arrangement seen in small, pear-shaped cysts.

The appearance of the more common protozoa discussed above, and of *Blastocystis hominis,* when stained with iodine, is illustrated in Figure 29.

THE CILIATES

Balantidium coli is the only member of its class to parasitize man. Cosmopolitan in its distribution, *Balantidium* is rare in most areas, although epidemic outbreaks are occasionally seen (Walter et al., 1973). A morphologically identical organism occurs in hogs, and epidemic outbreaks in man may follow its successful transfer from porcine to human hosts. The organisms inhabit the large intestine, cecum and terminal ileum. They are chiefly lumen dwellers, subsisting on bacteria, but may penetrate the intestinal mucosa to cause ulceration (Fig. 30).

Trophozoites of *Balantidium* (Fig. 31) have been reported to attain a length of 200 microns. According to Sargeaunt (1971), two size ranges are consistently seen. The smaller organisms average 42 to 60 microns long by 30 to 40 microns in width, while the larger range from 90 to 120 microns by 60 to 80 microns. Conjugation occurs only between "large" and "small" individuals, never between two of the same size range. The body shape is ovoid, somewhat flattened on one side. A funnel-shaped cytostome opens on the flattened side near the anterior end. The body is covered with cilia, which are especially long and stout near the cytostome. Unstained, the organisms are readily recognized because of their size and ciliary covering. Stained, the characteristic two nuclei of a ciliate may be observed. The larger nucleus, or macronucleus, situated near the middle of the body, may be spherical, ellipsoid, elongate, curved or kidney shaped. The micronucleus is spherical and quite small, and lies quite close to the macronucleus. Both nuclei stain intensely with the ordinary stains. Food vacuoles and contractile vacuoles may be seen in the cytoplasm.

The spherical or ellipsoid cysts are about 50 to 75 microns in length. There is a thick refractile cyst wall, within which the organism may be seen. In some specimens, newly encysted, the cilia are still present and the organisms may be seen slowly rotating. After a longer period of encystment, the cilia disappear. In stained specimens the macronucleus can usually be seen within the cyst wall, but other structures are usually not observed.

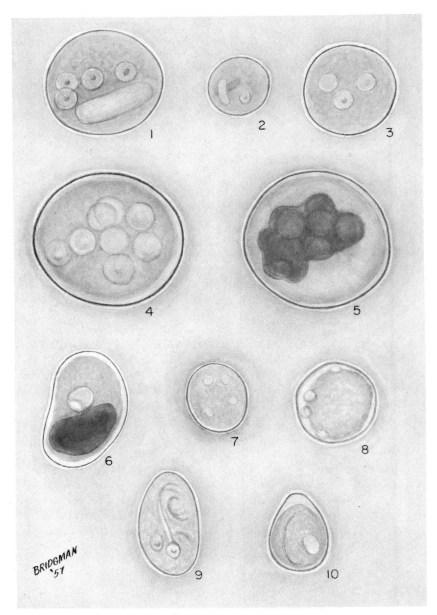

FIGURE 29. Cysts of intestinal protozoa and the yeast *Blastocystis* stained with iodine. *1, 3, Entamoeba hisolytica; 2, E. hartmanni; 4, Entamoeba coli; 5, E. coli* with glycogen mass obscuring nuclei; *6, Iodamoeba bütschlii; 7, Endolimax nana; 8, Blastocystis hominis; 9, Giardia lamblia; 10, Chilomastix mesnili.*

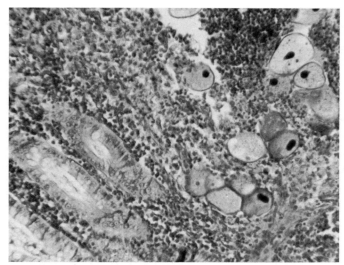

FIGURE 30. *Balantidium coli,* parasites in intestinal ulcer. (Photomicrograph by Zane Price.)

In summary, the following characteristics are of value in the identification of *Balantidium coli:*

I. Trophozoites, unstained.	DIAGNOSTIC: ciliary covering.
II. Trophozoites, stained.	DIAGNOSTIC: possession of macronucleus and micronucleus.
III. Cysts, unstained.	DIAGNOSTIC: cyst containing ciliated organism.
IV. Cysts, stained.	DIAGNOSTIC: possession of macronucleus and micronucleus.

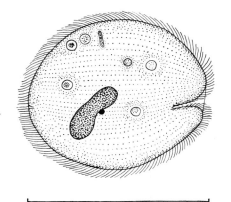

FIGURE 31. *Balantidium coli* trophozoite, stained specimen.

50 μ

In the United States balantidiasis is sometimes encountered in epidemic form in mental hospitals, but is almost unknown in the general population.

Balantidium produces the enzyme hyaluronidase, which presumably facilitates its tissue invasion. Many patients are symptomless carriers of the infection; clinical balantidiasis may simulate closely a severe amebic dysentery, or there may be only mild colitis and diarrhea. Extra-intestinal spread to the mesenteric nodes, liver, pleura, lungs and urogenital tract has been reported but is most uncommon. Oxytetracycline (Terramycin), 0.5 gm. three times daily for 10 days, or diiodohydroxyquin 0.65 gm. three times daily for 20 days, is usually effective in treatment of this parasite.

THE SPOROZOANS

The intestinal sporozoa of man include *Isospora belli* and one or more species of *Sarcocystis*. Their recently recognized relative, *Toxoplasma gondii*, is an intestinal parasite of the cat but, as far as is known, not of man. These parasites demonstrate the classic sporozoan alteration of asexual or schizogonic and sexual or sporogonic cycles.

Isospora

Belonging to the order Coccidia, *Isospora* is closely related to members of the genus *Eimeria*, which cause disease in various domestic animals, to the ubiquitous *Toxoplasma,* and to *Sarcocystis*. While the life cycle of *Isospora* is not fully known, much can be deduced by analogy with related genera. *Isospora* is a parasite of the epithelial cells of the intestine, in which it may undergo repeated asexual development, with consequent destruction of the surface layer of considerable portions of the intestine. The parasites have been found by small bowel biopsy (Brandborg et al., 1970). In addition to asexual stages which serve to spread the infection within the bowel wall, sexual stages occur, and these culminate in oöcysts passed in the feces.

Three species of *Isospora* have been recognized as human parasites. One of these, *I. natalensis*, has been reported but twice, and will not be discussed further. The organisms formerly known as *I. hominis* are no longer considered to belong to this genus at all, but to represent sexual stages of two species of *Sarcocystis, S. fusiformis* from cattle and *S. miescheriana* from swine (Rommel and Heydorn, 1972). *Isospora belli* is a valid species, and probably infects only man.

Isospora belli

As redescribed by Elsdon-Dew and Freedman (1953), *I. belli* is characterized by release of immature oöcysts from the intestinal wall, so that in this species all stages in development of the oöcyst occur in the stool. Immature oöcysts are ellipsoid or at times spindle shaped, with blunt ends. They average 30 microns in length by 12 in width. Contained in the immature oöcyst is a spherical mass of protoplasm, which soon divides to form two sporoblasts. The sporoblasts, still within the oöcyst, in turn develop heavy cyst walls and are known as sporocysts. Within each sporocyst, four curved sausage-shaped sporozoites develop (Fig. 32). All stages, from immature oöcysts containing nothing but an undivided mass of protoplasm to those containing fully developed sporocysts and sporozoites, may be seen in the feces. If in an immature condition when first passed, they will mature within four to five days to form sporozoites. The sporocysts are rarely seen broken out of the oöcysts, but measure approximately 11 by 9 microns.

Isospora oöcysts may be seen on direct examination of the stool, or may be detected in concentrates. They concentrate well with the zinc sulfate technique, but are so light that they float even in the customary zinc-sulfate-iodine mixture, and will only be seen if the area directly beneath the coverslip is examined carefully, with reduced illumination. Unless iodine stained, the oöcysts and contained material are quite transparent, and very difficult to recognize.

In summary, the following characteristics are of value in identification of *Isospora belli:*

In fresh stool or concentrate	oocysts; either immature, or mature containing two sporocysts; average size 30 by 12 microns.

Prior to the Second World War, infections with *Isospora* were considered to be of exceedingly rare occurrence. However, during and since that conflict large numbers of infections have been described from all parts of the world. It is now realized that while *Isospora* is not easily recognized in the feces, and is consequently seldom reported, it is not so rare as it was thought to be. Wherever a systematic search has been made for these parasites, they have been encountered. The majority of cases seem to be symptomless, but a number of workers have reported symptoms ranging from severe dysentery or diarrhea to mild gastrointestinal distress in patients infected with these parasites (Miller et al., 1971). The infection may evoke transitory eosinophilia, even in asymptomatic patients.

The loose, pale yellow and offensive stools are suggestive of a malabsorptive process. Fecal fat may be increased, and jejunal biopsy

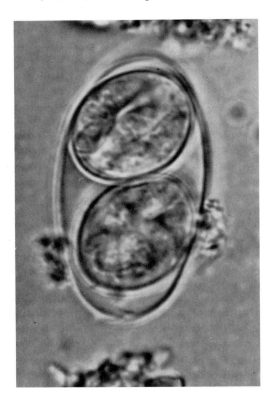

FIGURE 32.   Isospora belli. Oöcyst containing sporozoites. (Photomicrograph by Prof. John Gullberg.)

may reveal the villous atrophy commonly associated with the malabsorption syndrome (French et al., 1964). It will be remembered that this condition is also seen at times in giardiasis.

Although generally considered a mild and self-limited infection, oöcysts have been reported in the stools for as long as 120 days. No treatment is of proved value in human infections. Tetrachloroethylene and various antimalarial and antiamebic drugs have been found ineffective. The sulfonamides and nitrofurantoin (Furadantin) have been used to treat coccidian infections in various domestic animals.

Sarcocystis sp.

Unlike those of *Isospora belli,* the oöcysts of *Sarcocystis* are usually passed in the feces fully developed, and with the sporocysts ruptured out of the oöcyst. The sporocysts may occur singly, or may be seen in pairs in the feces, apparently held together by some sort of cement substance. Usually no vestige of an oöcyst wall is seen. The sporocysts average 15 by 10 microns, and each contains four sporozoites.

In summary, the following characteristics are of value in the identification of *Sarcocystis:*

In fresh stool or concentrate   sporocysts; 15 by 10 microns, each containing four sporozoites.

REFERENCES

Apley, J., Clarke, S. K. R., Roome, A. P. C. H., Sandry, S. A., Saygi, G., Silk, B., and Warhurst, D. C. 1970. Primary amoebic meningoencephalitis in Britain. Brit. Med. J., *1*:596–599.

Babb, R. R., Peck, O. C., and Vescia, F. G. 1971. Giardiasis: a cause of traveller's diarrhea. J.A.M.A., *217*:1359–1361.

Behrens, M. M. 1974. Optic atrophy in children after diiodohydroxyquin therapy. J.A.M.A. *228*:693.

Bhagwandeen, S. B., Carter, R. F., Naik, K. G., and Levitt, D. 1975. A case of hartmannellid amebic meningoencephalitis in Zambia. Am. J. Clin. Pathol., *63*:483–492.

Brandborg, L. L., Tankersley, C. B., Gottlieb, S., Barancik, M., and Sartor, V. E. 1967. Histological demonstration of mucosal invasion by *Giardia lamblia* in man. Gastroenterology, *52*:143–150.

Brandborg, L. L., Goldberg, S. B., and Breidenbach, W. C. 1970. Human coccidiosis—a possible cause of malabsorption. The life cycle in small bowel mucosal biopsies as a diagnostic feature. New Eng. J. Med., *283*:1306–1313.

Butt, C. G. 1966. Primary amebic meningoencephalitis. New Eng. J. Med., *274*:1473–1476.

Camp, R. R., Mattern, C. F. T., and Honigberg, B. M. 1974. Study of *Dientamoeba fragilis* Jepps & Dobell. I. Electronmicroscopic observations of the binucleate stages. J. Protozool., *21*:69–79.

Carter, R. F. 1969. Sensitivity to amphotericin B of a *Naegleria* sp. isolated from a case of primary amoebic meningoencephalitis. J. Clin. Path., *22*:470–474.

Carter, R. F. 1972. Primary amoebic meningoencephalitis. An appraisal of present knowledge. Trans. Roy. Soc. Trop. Med. & Hyg., *66*:193–208.

Center for Disease Control. 1975. Morbidity and Mortality. *24*:366;371. U.S. Department of Health, Education, and Welfare, Atlanta, Ga.

Chang, S., Holdebrandt, W., and Silvis, S. E. 1974. The accidental discovery that sodium diatrizoate (Hypaque) infusion will visualize amebic abscesses on hepatic tomograms. Am. J. Trop. Med. & Hyg., *23*:31–34.

Danziger, M., and Lopez, M. 1975. Numbers of *Giardia* in the feces of infected children. Am. J. Trop. Med. & Hyg., *24*:237–242.

Datta, D. V., Singh, S. A. K., and Chhuttani, P. N. 1974. Treatment of amebic liver abscess with emetine hydrochloride, niridazole and metronidazole. Am. J. Trop. Med. & Hyg., *23*:586–589.

DeCarneri, I. 1971. Perspectives in the treatment of protozoal diseases resistant to metronidazole. Trans. Roy. Soc. Trop. Med. & Hyg., *65*:268–269.

Duma, R. J., Ferrell, H. W., Nelson, E. C., and Jones, M. M. 1969. Primary amebic meningoencephalitis. New Eng. J. Med., *281*:1316–1323.

Elsdon-Dew, R. 1958. Factors influencing the pathogenicity of *Entamoeba histolytica*. Proc. World Congr. Gastroenterol., Vol. II, 770–773.

Elsdon-Dew, R. 1968. The epidemiology of amoebiasis. *In*: Dawes, B. (Ed.) *Advances in Parasitology*. Vol. 6. pp. 1–62. Academic Press, New York.

Elsdon-Dew, R., and Freedman, L. 1953. Coccidiosis in man: experiences in Natal. Trans. Roy. Soc. Trop. Med. & Hyg., *47*:209–214.

Fowler, M., and Carter, R. F. 1965. Acute pyogenic meningitis probably due to *Acanthamoeba* sp.: a preliminary report. Brit. Med. J., *2*:740–742.

French, J. M., Whitby, J. L., and Whitfield, A. G. W. 1964. Steatorrhea in a man infected with coccidiosis (*Isospora belli*). Gastroenterology, *47*:642–648.

Gelderman, A. H., Bartgis, I. L., Keister, D. B., and Diamond, L. S. 1971. A comparison of genome sizes and thermal denaturation-derived base composition of DNAs from several members of *Entamoeba* (histolytica group). J. Parasitol., *57*:912–916.

Gorbach, S. L., Kean, B. H., Evans, D. G., Evans, E. J., and Bessudo, D. 1975. Traveller's diarrhea and toxigenic *Escherichia coli.* New Eng. J. Med., *292*:933–936.

Honigberg, B. M. 1974. Study of *Dientamoeba fragilis* Jepps & Dobell. II. Taxonomic position and revision of the genus *Dientamoeba* Jepps & Dobell. J. Protozool., *21*:79–82.

Hoskins, L. C., Winawer, S. J., Broitman, S. A., Gottlieb, L. S., and Zamcheck, N. 1967. Clinical giardiasis and intestinal malabsorption. Gastroenterology, *53*:265–279.

Juniper, K., Worrell, C. L., Minshew, M. C., Roth, L. S., Cypert, H., and Lloyd, R. E. 1972. Serologic diagnosis of amebiasis. Amer. J. Trop. Med. & Hyg., *21*:157–168.

Kingston, D., and Warhurst, D. C. 1969. Isolation of amoebae from the air. J. Med. Microbiol., *2*:27–36.

MacLeod, I. N., Wilmot, A. J., and Powell, S. J., 1966. Amoebic pericarditis. Quart. J. Med., *35*:293–311.

Miller, F. H., Fizzuto, A. V., and McCauley, H. 1971. Human isosporosis: two cases. Amer. J. Trop. Med. & Hyg., *20*:23–25.

Moore, G. T., Cross, W. M., McGuire, D., Mollohan, C. S., Gleason, N. N., Healy, G. R., and Newton, L. H. 1969. Epidemic giardiasis at a ski resort. New Eng. J. Med., *281*:402–407.

Morecki, R., and Parker, J. G. 1967. Ultrastructural studies of the human *Giardia lamblia* and subjacent jejunal mucosa in a subject with steatorrhea. Gastroenterology, *52*:151–164.

Nagington, J., Watson, P. G., Playfair, T. J., McGill, J., Jones, B. R., and Steele, A. D. M. 1974. Amoebic infection of the eye. Lancet, *2*:1537–1540.

Neal, R. A. 1966. Experimental studies on *Entamoeba* with reference to speciation. *In*: Dawes, B. (Ed.) *Advances in Parasitology.* Vol. 4. pp. 1–51. Academic Press, New York.

Page, F. C. 1967a. Re-definition of the genus *Acanthamoeba* with description of three species. J. Protozool., *14*:709–724.

Page, F. C. 1967b. Taxonomic criteria for limax amoeba, with descriptions of 3 new species of *Hartmannella* and 3 of *Vahlkampfia.* J. Protozool., *14*:499–521.

Parmley, L. F., Sheehy, T. W., Johnston, G. S., and Boyce, H. W. 1968. Amebic abscess of the liver. The value of the isotope hepatoscan in diagnosis and management. Med. Ann. D.C., *37*:1–9.

Pittman, F. E., El-Hashimi, W. K., and Pittman, J. C. 1973. Studies of human amebiasis. I. Clinical and laboratory findings in eight cases of acute amebic colitis. Gastroenterology, *65*:581–587.

Powell, S. J., and Wilmot, A. J. 1966. Prognosis in peritonitis complicating severe amoebic dysentery. Trans. Roy. Soc. Trop. Med. & Hyg., *60*:544–548.

Powell, S. J., Wilmot, A. J., and Elsdon-Dew, R. 1967. Further trials of metronidazole in amoebic dysentery and amoebic liver abscess. Ann. Trop. Med. Parasit., *61*:511–514.

Powell, S. J., and Elsdon-Dew, R. 1971. Chloroquine in amoebic dysentery. Trans. Roy. Soc. Trop. Med. & Hyg., *65*:540.

Pritchard, J. H., Winston, M. A., Berger, H. G., and Blahd, W. H. 1974. Diagnosis of focal hepatic lesions. Combined radioisotope and ultrasound techniques. J.A.M.A., *229*:1463–1465.

Rustia, M., and Shubik, P. 1972. Induction of lung tumors and malignant lymphomas in mice by metronidazole. J. Natl. Cancer Inst., *48*:721–729.

Sargeaunt, P. G. 1971. The size range of *Balantidium coli.* Trans. Roy. Soc. Trop. Med. & Hyg., *65*:428.

Schultz, M. G. 1975. Giardiasis. J.A.M.A., *233*:1383–1384.

Sexton, D. J., Krogstad, D. J., Spencer, H. C., Jr., Healy, G. R., Sinclair, S., Sledge, C. E., and Schultz, M. G. 1974. Amebiasis in a mental institution: serologic and epidemiologic studies. Amer. J. Epidemiol., *100*:414–423.

Spencer, H. 1973. Amoebiasis. *In*: Spencer, H. et al. (Ed.) *Tropical Pathology*, p. 765. New York, Heidelberg & Berlin, Springer-Verlag.

Stillman, A. E., Alvarez, V., and Grube, D. 1974. Hepatic amebic abscess. Unresponsiveness to combination of metronidazole and surgical drainage. J.A.M.A., *229*:71–72.

Tsai, S. H. 1973. Experiences in the therapy of amebic liver abscess on Taiwan. Amer. J. Trop. Med. & Hyg., *22*:24–29.

Visvesvara, G. S., and Healy, G. R. 1975. Comparative antigenic analysis of pathogenic and free-living *Naegleria* species by the gel diffusion and immunoelectrophoresis techniques. Infection and Immunity, *11*:95–108.

Walter, P. D., Judson, F. N., Murphy, K. B., Healy, G. R., English, D. K., and Schultz, M. G. 1973. Balantidiasis outbreak in Truk. Amer. J. Trop. Med. Hyg., *22*:33–41.

Wang, S. S., and Feldman, H. A. 1967. Isolation of *Hartmannella* species from human throats. New Eng. J. Med., *277*:1174–1179.

Watson, R. B., Steel, R. K., and Spiegel, T. M. 1972. Amebic pericarditis consequent to amebic abscess of right lobe of liver. Amer. J. Trop. Med. & Hyg., *21*:889–894.

Weber, D. M. 1971. Amebic abscess of liver following metronidazole therapy. J.A.M.A., *216*:1339–1340.

Whittaker, L. R. 1973. Rupture of amebic liver abscess. Trans. Roy. Soc. Trop. Med. & Hyg., *67*:143.

Wolfe, M. S. 1975. Giardiasis. J.A.M.A., *233*:1362–1365.

World Health Organization. 1969. Amoebiasis. Report of a WHO expert committee. Technical Report Series, No. 421, 52 pp.

Zaman, V. 1968. Observations on human *Isospora*. Trans. Roy. Soc. Trop. Med. & Hyg., *62*:556–557.

6

Malaria

Several different clinical syndromes, now known to be caused by infection with malarial parasites, were first recognized centuries before the discovery of their etiological agents. Consequently, the diseases were referred to in terms of their outstanding clinical features, usually the type of febrile cycle. Thus, quotidian, tertian and quartan fevers denoted respectively twenty-four-, forty-eight- and seventy-two-hour cycles of fever. Other names designated various clinical features of the disease. The modern tendency is to refer to the various types of malaria by the names of their causative agents. Thus, benign tertian malaria is now usually called vivax malaria, as it is caused by infection with *Plasmodium vivax.* Similarly estivo-autumnal, malignant tertian or subtertian malaria is now known as falciparum malaria, from *P. falciparum.* Quartan malaria may be called malariae malaria after its etiological agent, *P. malariae*, but for the sake of euphony the old term is usually retained. Fortunately the fourth type, ovale malaria, was described so recently as to possess only the name derived from *P. ovale.* These four organisms and the diseases which they produce will be discussed separately. Many common features of general morphology and life cycle are shared by all plasmodia, and these will be considered first.

While human malarial parasites were first seen in 1880, and their development both in the anopheline mosquito and in the blood stream of man was thoroughly understood by 1900, the entire life cycle was more recently elucidated. In the intervening period many species of *Plasmodium* have been found in other animals, and from these non-human species much information of medical importance obtained. Of special interest from the standpoint of drug testing have been the organisms, such as *Plasmodium cathemerium*, causing bird malaria.

The life cycle of *Plasmodium*, in both man and mosquito, is shown in Figure 33. Various species of anopheline mosquitoes are definitive hosts of the malarial parasites. When the female mosquito bites an infected person, she draws into her stomach blood which may contain male and female gametocytes. In the mosquito, the male or micro-gametocyte undergoes a process of maturation, during which the microgametes appear. The extrusion of these delicate spindle-shaped gametes has been termed exflagellation. At the same time the female or macrogametocyte matures to become a macrogamete, after which it may be fertilized by the microgamete, forming a zygote. The zygote becomes elongated and active, and is called an oökinete. The oökinete penetrates through the stomach wall of the mosquito, and rounds up just beneath the outer covering of that organ to become an oöcyst. Growth and de-velopment of the oöcyst result in the production of a large number of slender, thread-like sporozoites, which break out and wander through-out the body of the mosquito. Those which enter the salivary glands of the mosquito may be inoculated into the next person bitten. Sporozoites, injected into the blood stream, leave the blood vascular system within a period of forty minutes and invade the parenchymal cells of the liver (Fig. 34). In the liver cells they undergo an asexual multiplication. After one or more generations of asexual development in the hepatic paren-chymal cells, parasites are liberated to invade the red cells and initiate the blood stream phase of the infection. The development in the liver prior to red cell invasion is referred to as the pre-erythrocytic cycle; if it con-tinues after red cell invasion has taken place it is called the exoerythro-cytic cycle. The two are not always distinguished, and both phases may be referred to as exo-erythrocytic.

Development of the parasites in the mosquito and in the hepatic parenchymal cells has been described as if it were exactly the same for all species of *Plasmodium*. There are differences in the asexual cycles in the liver, however, which are probably of more clinical significance. *Plasmodium falciparum* and *P. malariae* undergo only one asexual genera-tion before blood stream invasion, and it is probable that the hepatic cycle is not continued thereafter. In *P. vivax* infections, exo-erythrocytic development may continue for years, to provide a basis for the extended course and numerous relapses which can characterize infection with this species. The same may be true for *P. ovale*, but there is a high spontan-eous cure rate.

In the blood stream an asexual cycle takes place within the red cells. This process, known as schizogony, results in the formation, within a period of forty-eight to seventy-two hours, of from four to thirty-six new parasites in each infected cell. Details of this cycle differ for the various species, and will be given in more detail when each is described. At the end of the schizogonic cycle, the infected blood cells rupture, liberating

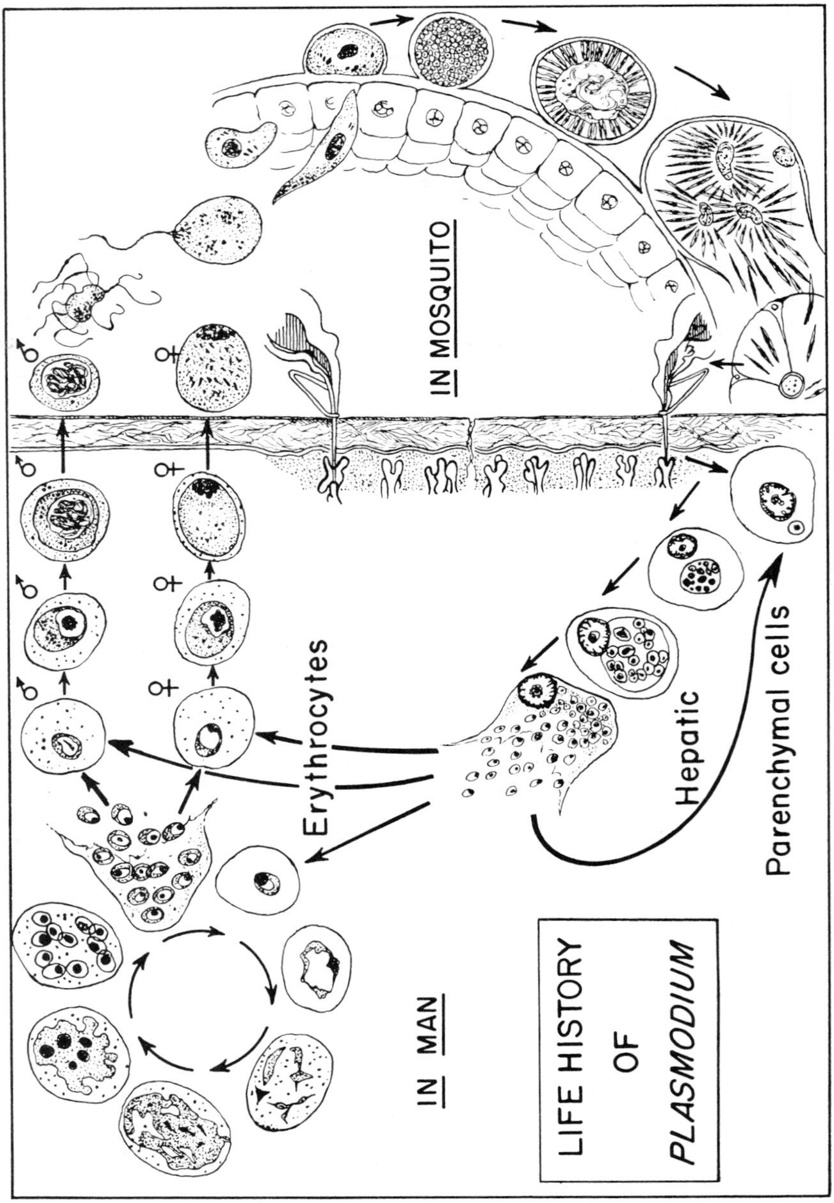

FIGURE 33. Life history of *Plasmodium.* (Adapted from Wilcox, Manual for the Microscopical Diagnosis of Malaria in Man. National Institutes of Health, U.S.P.H.S. Bulletin 180.)

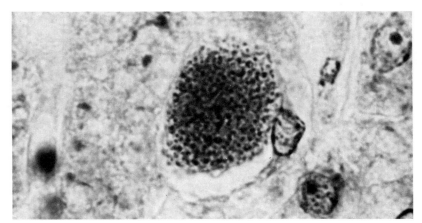

FIGURE 34. Exoerythrocytic stages of *Plasmodium vivax* in liver.

merozoites which in turn infect new red cells. Rupture of the red cells liberates products of metabolism of the parasites and of the red cells, and it is thought that if large numbers of infected cells rupture simultaneously, the volume of toxic materials thrown into the blood stream may be sufficient to bring about a malarial paroxysm. Generally, in the initial stages of infection, rupture of the infected cells is not synchronous, so that fever may be continuous or remittent, rather than intermittent in nature. It is theorized that the fever peaks may have a regulatory effect on the developmental cycle, speeding up those which are out of phase, so that after a number of days the febrile cycle becomes intermittent, with a forty-eight- or seventy-two-hour periodicity, depending upon the species of parasite. In mixed infections with two or more species, or in the early stages of infection with one species, there may be daily (quotidian) paroxysms, or even double paroxysms in one day.

Some time after the asexual parasites first appear in the blood stream, and usually not until after the patient has become clinically ill, gametocytes appear in the red blood cells. These forms are probably derived from merozoites quite similar in appearance to those which will continue the asexual cycle. However, instead of undergoing schizogony, they grow but do not divide, and finally form the male and female gametocytes. The gametocytes continue to circulate in the blood stream for some time, and, if ingested by a mosquito of the genus *Anopheles,* undergo the sexual cycle — gametogony — and subsequent development — sporogony — in the mosquito.

Plasmodium vivax

The predominant malarial parasite in most parts of the world is *Plasmodium vivax*. This species is found almost everywhere malaria is endemic, and is the only one which has a range extending into the temperate regions.

In blood smears from a patient infected with *Plasmodium vivax*, various stages in the asexual cycle of the parasite may be seen; gametocytes may also be present. The stages in the asexual cycle which are seen depend upon the time the blood is taken in relation to the febrile cycle. The paroxysm follows the somewhat synchronous rupture of the majority of infected cells, liberating merozoites which in turn infect new red cells. For the first few hours after the paroxysm, the majority of infected cells will contain very early forms of the parasite, referred to as trophozoites (Fig. 35). In a blood film correctly stained with Giemsa's, Field's, or Leishman's stain, the parasites appear first as minute blue disks with a red nucleus lying within the pink cytoplasm of the erythrocyte. Sometimes the parasites are first seen as crescentic masses at the periphery of the red cell—the so-called accolé forms. Shortly thereafter, an apparent vacuole forms in the blue cytoplasm of the parasite, pushing the nuclear chromatin to a peripheral position. The parasite now resembles a signet ring, and has grown to have a diameter about one-third that of the infected cell. Very active ameboid motility is exhibited during the growth period, and the parasite may assume bizarre and irregular forms within the red cell. It is this ameboid activity which suggested the specific name *vivax*. Between six and twenty-four hours after the beginning of the cycle the trophozoites have grown to approximately half the size of the infected cell, and granules of brownish pigment have begun to appear within

---

FIGURE 35. *Plasodium vivax; 1,* normal sized red cell with marginal ring form trophozoite; *2,* young signet ring form trophozoite in a macrocyte; *3,* slightly older ring form trophozoite in red cell showing basophilic stippling; *4,* polychromatophilic red cell containing young tertian parasite with pseudopodia; *5,* ring form trophozoite showing pigment in cytoplasm, in an enlarged cell containing Schüffner's stippling (Schüffner's stippling does not appear in all cells containing the growing and older forms of *P. vivax* as would be indicated by these pictures, but it can be found with any stage from the fairly young ring form onward); *6, 7,* very tenuous medium trophozoite forms; *8,* three ameboid trophozoites with fused cytoplasm; *9, 11, 12, 13,* older ameboid trophozoites in process of development; *10,* two ameboid trophozoites in one cell; *14,* mature trophozoite; *15,* mature trophozoite with chromatin apparently in process of division; *16, 17, 18, 19,* schizonts showing progressive steps in division ("presegmenting schizonts"); *20,* mature schizont; *21, 22,* developing gametocytes; *23,* mature microgametocyte; *24,* mature macrogametocyte. (Courtesy National Institutes of Health, U.S.P.H.S.)

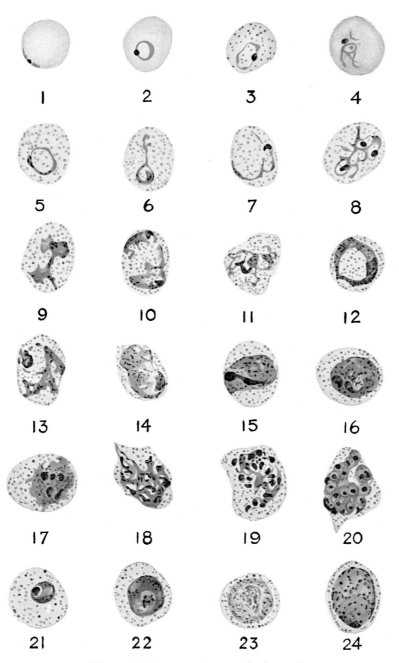

Figure 35. See opposite page for legend.

them. At the same time, the infected cell has become noticeably enlarged and pale, and may be seen to contain a number of fine red granules known as Schüffner's dots. Schüffner's dots will always be seen in a red cell infected fifteen to twenty hours or longer, if the slide has been properly stained. The nature of these dots is undetermined; if present, they are diagnostic of *P. vivax* or *P. ovale* infection. Increase in size continues during the second twenty-four hours, and the parasite comes very nearly to fill the infected cell, which may be enlarged to 10 to 12 microns. At about forty hours, the mature trophozoite largely ceases its ameboid activity and becomes compact, thus sometimes appearing smaller than the actively motile stages which preceded it. The single nucleus now divides repeatedly to give rise to a total of twelve to twenty-four nuclear masses, with average numbers which vary, according to the strain, from fourteen to twenty-two. During the stages of division, the parasite is known as a schizont. The cytoplasm finally segments to form separate small masses around each nucleus. The individual parasites thus produced are known as merozoites, and upon rupture of the infected cell at about forty-eight hours they are released to infect new red cells.

As the cycle is never entirely synchronous, parasites at more than one stage of development will usually be seen in the blood smear. In addition to the asexual forms mentioned above, gametocytes may be seen usually after the first few paroxysms. They mature more slowly than the asexual forms, do not exhibit as much ameboid activity, and develop more pigment. The infected cells enlarge, and Schüffner's granules may be seen. Fully mature gametocytes, in contrast to trophozoites about to undergo schizogony, fill the cell more completely and contain more pigment. One can differentiate the microgametocytes and macrogametocytes morphologically. The nucleus of the macrogametocyte is dense, while that of the microgametocyte forms a pale loose network.

All stages seen in thin films may be found also in thick-film preparations (Fig. 39), but the parasites appear somewhat distorted. Young trophozoites may be seen as typical rings, but more frequently are collapsed. A red dot of nuclear material may have a small wisp of blue cytoplasm at one side, or thin lines of cytoplasm may appear on either side of the nucleus. These distorted early trophozoites are known respectively as comma and swallow forms. However, if these forms alone are seen, they cannot be distinguished with certainty from similar stages of *Plasmodium ovale,* or from *P. falciparum* if the infection with this parasite is a light one. As the parasites become older their ameboid activity is reflected by the irregular shapes which they assume in thick film. The ghost-like shadows of lysed infected cells may be seen surrounding the parasites, and usually Schüffner's dots will be seen within them. Schizonts, if mature, can be recognized by the number of merozoites. Gametocytes of *P. vivax, P. ovale,* and *P. malariae* are very similar in appearance, except those of *P. malariae* are smaller and darker than the other two and do not contain Schüffner's dots. It is best to rely on asexual stages of the parasite for identification.

SYMPTOMATOLOGY. A primary clinical attack of vivax malaria usually has its onset ten to seventeen days after infection, although the average length of the incubation period may vary considerably from strain to strain of *P. vivax.* The last few days of the incubation period may be marked by prodromal symtpoms of a non-specific sort: headache, photophobia, muscular aches and pains, anorexia, nausea and sometimes vomiting. Frequently these symptoms are entirely absent. The onset of symptoms is determined by the sensitivity of the host, following the build-up of parasite concentration in the blood stream. Parasites may be found in blood films for one or two days prior to the onset of symptoms, or symptoms may occur before there are sufficient numbers of parasites to be readily detected in the blood. During the first few days of the primary attack, there are seldom typical paroxysms, and the patient will have a sustained or irregularly remittent fever. After a few days, usually not more than one week, the first typical paroxysm is experienced. A sudden, shaking chill, or rigor, ushers in the paroxysm. The chill lasts initially for ten to fifteen minutes, and may gradually become longer with succeeding paroxysms. During this stage the patient complains of extreme cold, although in actuality his temperature is elevated at the onset, and climbs during the period of the chill. The hot stage follows the cold without any respite, and the patient who a few moments before was huddled under a pile of blankets now throws them off. His skin, pale and cyanotic in the cold stage, becomes flushed. The patient frequently is excited; he may be restless and disoriented or even delirious. Severe frontal headache, and pains in the limbs and back are common. The hot stage lasts from two to six hours, and is followed by the sweating stage. Sweating is profuse and generalized, and with its onset the patient usually feels much better. This stage may last several hours; at its end the patient is usually weak and exhausted, and tends to fall asleep. When he awakes, his temperature is normal or slightly subnormal, and he usually feels quite well until the onset of the next paroxysm.

The periodicity of the paroxysms is often somewhat irregular at first and may then become quotidian, but after a variable time a regular forty-eight-hour cycle is established. Once the regular cycle is established it usually remains relatively fixed, but may occasionally change spontaneously. An untreated primary attack may last from three weeks to two months or longer before it subsides. As the attack wanes, paroxysms may become less severe, and often irregular in periodicity before they cease altogether. In perhaps one half of the cases, relapses occur following a period of weeks, months or even years without any symptoms. In vivax malaria, relapses may occur as long as five years after an initial attack, and there may be a long series of such relapses. Usually relapses follow somewhat the same pattern as the paroxysms, becoming shorter and less severe as time goes on, as a result of developing immunity.

Severe complications are fortunately rare in vivax malaria. Coma and sudden death or other manifestations of cerebral involvement such as hemiplegia, peripheral neuropathies, and gastrointestinal hemorrhage are reported (Hill et al., 1963), and probably depend upon the same mechanisms as in falciparum malaria.

PATHOGENESIS. The primary pathogenic effects of vivax infection are the result of hemolysis of infected and uninfected red cells, the liberation of the metabolites of the parasites, and the formation of malarial pigment. In *P. vivax* only reticulocytes are parasitized, so that a maximum of about 2 per cent of red blood cells may be infected at any one time. Rupture of the infected red cells, as previously mentioned, brings on the malarial paroxysm. Lysis of numerous uninfected cells during the paroxysm, plus enhanced phagocytosis of normal cells in addition to the cell remnants and other debris produced by schizogony, leads both to anemia and to enlargement of the spleen and liver. The spleen enlarges and becomes palpable during the first few weeks of infection, during which time it is soft and subject to rupture. If the infection is treated, the spleen returns to normal size, but in chronic infections it continues to enlarge and becomes hard. Malarial pigment (hemozoin) collects to give the organ a grayish to dark brown or black color. The liver becomes congested, and the Küpffer cells are packed with hemozoin, which indeed is seen throughout the viscera. Hemozoin is derived from the hemoglobin of the infected red cell, and, as it is insoluble in plasma, its formation depletes the iron stores of the body, thus adding to the anemia. Infected red cells have been reported to form thrombi in capillaries of the brain and other organs, though this process is much more characteristic of infections with *P. falciparum*.

A leukopenia is generally noted, though there may be leukocytosis during the febrile paroxysms. Total plasma proteins are unchanged or are slightly lower than normal during an attack of malaria; the albumin is generally lowered and the globulin increased. The globulin increase is in the gamma fraction and is associated with the appearance of antibodies measurable by the indirect immunofluorescence technique (Kuvin et al., 1963a). Serum potassium may increase with the lysis of red cells.

EPIDEMIOLOGY. In the subtropics and temperate zone, vivax malaria is more commonly seen than are the other types of infection; it is widespread in the tropics as well. Its transmission depends upon the presence both of suitable species of *Anopheles* mosquitoes and of infected (gametocyte-bearing) humans. In many temperate areas where suitable anopheline hosts still abound, endemic malaria has been eradicated and introduced malaria seldom results in transmission. Suitability of a mosquito as a vector of human disease depends not only upon physiologic adaptation to the infection, but also upon such factors as feeding preferences, hours of biting, and flight, resting and breeding habits. Thus, of over 200 known species of *Anopheles*, only approximately 60 are considered to be vectors of malaria.

Gametocytes appear in the circulating blood early in the course of a vivax infection and may appear with succeeding clinical relapses over a period of several months or years. In addition to gametocyte-induced, mosquito-transmitted malaria, transmission by means of transfusion is not unknown (Fisher and Schultz, 1969) and mechanical transmission through shared syringes is seen among drug users. Congenital transmission is rare.

Immunity in malaria is relative and generally strain-specific. Children exposed to repeated infections in hyperendemic areas develop a high degree of immunity, though this immunity does not imply an eradication of the infection but rather a balance between parasite and host. West African blacks and their descendants in the Americas and elsewhere possess a relative immunity to *P. vivax*, and also to experimental infection with *P. cynomolgi* (Coatney, 1963).

Miller et al. (1975) have found that Duffy blood group negative human erythrocytes are resistant to infection with *P. knowlesi*, whereas Duffy-positive erythrocytes are readily infected. They suggest that the high incidence of Duffy-negative erythrocytes in West Africans accounts for the resistance of these peoples, and of approximately 70 per cent of American blacks, to *P. vivax*. In East Africa, where there is a higher incidence of Duffy-positive red cells, *P. vivax* is seen.

A number of small epidemics of malaria have resulted from the shared use of hypodermic syringes by heroin addicts. One such epidemic, reported by Friedmann et al. (1973) from Bakersfield, California, involved a total of 47 cases, and probably originated with a returned soldier from Vietnam.

A strain of *P. cynomolgi,* usually parasitic in monkeys and morphologically identical to *P. vivax,* has been found to give rise to both natural and experimental human infections (Eyles et al., 1960; Kuvin et al., 1963), and it raises the possibility of subhuman reservoirs of malaria.

Treatment of malaria will be discussed at the end of the chapter.

Plasmodium ovale

Plasmodium ovale has been known only since 1922. It seems to be rather widely distributed in tropical Africa, and apparently supplants

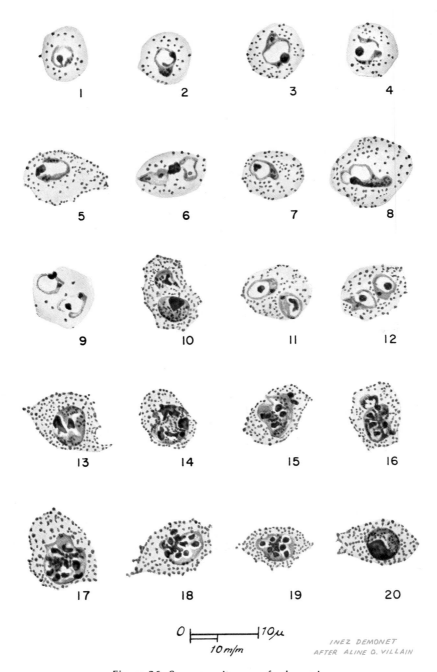

Figure 36. See opposite page for legend.

P. vivax almost entirely on the West African coast. It has also been reported from South America and Asia.

The morphological feature which originally led to the establishment of *P. ovale* as a separate species, an ovoid shape of many of the infected red cells, has been found to be variable (Fig. 36). Thin smears which because of excessive humidity have dried slowly may not show this characteristic at all. However, other criteria may be used to distinguish the two species. The parasite is not so ameboid as *P. vivax* and the nuclei in all stages are larger than in corresponding stages of that species. Pigment is scanty. In schizogony, typically four to twelve merozoites are produced, with an average of eight as in *Plasmodium malariae.* More rarely twelve to eighteen merozoites may be formed, with an average of fourteen to sixteen. The infected cells are enlarged, pale, and if properly stained exhibit Schüffner's dots. The margins of the infected cells are often ragged, and the cells distinctly elongated, ovoid or irregular in shape.

Thick films (Fig. 39) are very similar to those of *P. vivax.* If in such films schizonts larger than those of *P. malariae,* but with no more than twelve merozoites, are seen containing Schüffner's dots, a tentative diagnosis of ovale infection may be made.

SYMPTOMATOLOGY. Ovale and vivax malaria are clinically similar, but ovale is less severe, does not relapse frequently, and usually results in spontaneous recovery. The incubation period is similar to that of vivax malaria, and likewise may be prolonged for some months. Frequency and severity of prodromal symptoms are both much less than in vivax malaria, and likewise the initial periods of irregularly remittent fever and of quotidian paroxysms are less likely to occur. When the forty-eight-hour cycle is established, it is initiated by a chill which is not typically accompanied by the shaking rigor seen in *Plasmodium vivax* infections, and the fever does not often reach the height seen in the latter disease. Duration of the paroxysm is roughly the same as that in vivax malaria, but there is a high rate of sponta-

---

FIGURE 36. Plasmodium ovale: 1, young ring-shaped trophozoite; *2, 3, 4, 5,* older ring-shaped trophozoites; *6, 7, 8,* older ameboid trophozoites; *9, 11, 12,* doubly infected cells, trophozoites; *10,* doubly infected cell, young gametocytes; *13,* first stage of the schizont; *14, 15, 16, 17, 18, 19,* schizonts, progressive stages; *20,* mature gametocyte.

Free translation of legend accompanying original plate in "Guide pratique d'examen microscopique du sang appliqué au diagnostic du paludisme" by Georges Villain. Reproduced with permission from "Biologie Medicale" supplement, 1935.

(Plate courtesy of Aimee Wilcox. National Institutes of Health Bulletin no. 180.)

neous recovery, without medication, after no more than six to ten paroxysms. Ovale malaria has been used in the treatment of neurosyphilis, as the infection thus produced is a safer means of producing febrile attacks than is infection with any of the other human species. However, it frequently proved ineffective because of the low temperatures provoked, as well as high rates of spontaneous and early recovery. Malaria therapy for neurosyphilis has of course been superseded by the use of antibiotics.

Plasmodium malariae

Occurring primarily in those subtropical and temperate areas where other species of malaria are found, *Plasmodium malariae* generally has a much lower incidence than *P. vivax* or *P. falciparum*.

The asexual cycle of *P. malariae* occupies seventy-two hours, as compared to approximately forty-eight hours in the other species. Ring forms of *Plasmodium malariae* (Fig. 37) are not readily distinguished from those of *P. vivax*. As the parasite grows it exhibits little ameboid activity. It tends to assume an elongate form, stretching part way or entirely across the red cell. The infected cell is not enlarged. As the parasite grows, it may nearly completely fill the red cell prior to schizogony. The cytoplasm of the red cell may rarely contain dust-fine pale pink dots, called Ziemann's stippling. This stippling is seen only in heavily stained slides. Pigment is produced in some quantity, and is rather dark in color. Schizogony results in the formation of six to twelve merozoites. The average number of merozoites is eight, and they may be arranged in a rosette, symmetrically around a central mass of pigment, but more typically are irregularly dispersed within the mature schizont.

Gametocytes of *P. malariae* are difficult to distinguish from the growing trophozoites, but when mature may be slightly larger than the

FIGURE 37. *Plasmodium malariae: 1,* young ring form trophozoite of quartan malaria; *2, 3, 4,* young trophozoite forms of the parasite showing gradual increase of chromatin and cytoplasm; *5,* developing ring form trophozoite showing pigment granule; *6,* early band form trophozoite—elongated chromatin, some pigment apparent; *7, 8, 9, 10, 11, 12,* some forms which the developing trophozoite of quartan may take; *13, 14,* mature trophozoites—one a band form; *15, 16, 17, 18, 19,* phases in the development of the schizont ("presegmenting schizonts"); *20,* mature schizont; *21,* immature microgametocyte; *22,* immature macrogametocyte; *23,* mature microgametocyte; *24,* mature macrogametocyte. (Courtesy National Institutes of Health, U.S.P.H.S.)

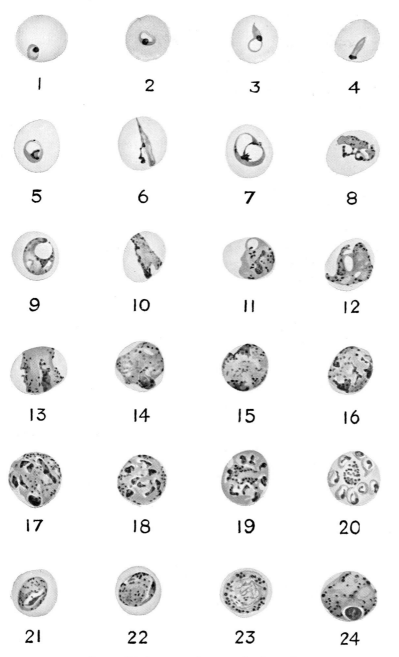

Figure 37. See opposite page for legend.

mature trophozoites, and tend to be ovoid. They contain proportionately more pigment than the trophozoites at all stages.

In the thick film (Fig. 39) trophozoites of *P. malariae* do not assume the ameboid, comma or swallow forms seen in the other species, but because of their compact nature usually appear as small dots of nuclear material with rounded or slightly elongate masses of cytoplasm. The older trophozoites of *P. malariae* are also compact, and the predominant color seen may be that of the abundant pigment. The fully developed schizont, containing an average of eight merozoites, is readily recognized.

SYMPTOMATOLOGY. *Plasmodium malariae* seems preferentially to invade aging red cells, and this puts a natural limit on the degree of infection. The lower reproductive potential inherent in the prolonged cycle and small number of merozoites produced is probably basic to the long incubation period in this infection. The time elapsing between infection and the onset of symptoms ranges from about twenty-seven to forty days, and during the last few days there may be prodromal symptoms similar to those seen in *vivax* infections. Parasites may nearly always be found in the blood for several days prior to the initial attack, which commences with a paroxysm. A regular periodicity is the rule from the onset. The paroxysm is similar to that in vivax malaria, but in general tends to be more severe. The cold stage may be of longer duration, and is more frequently accompanied by headache, nausea and vomiting than in vivax malaria. A true rigor may or may not be seen. The hot stage is again similar to that seen with *P. vivax* infections, but usually more severe and lasting for six hours or more. Nausea, vomiting, diarrhea and delirium are frequently seen during this stage. Collapse during the sweating stage is not uncommon. Proteinuria during the period of clinical attack is common in this type of malaria, and in children may be associated with massive edema and other clinical signs of the nephrotic syndrome. It is suggested (Kubukamusoke et al., 1967) that the renal lesions may be secondary to deposition within the glomeruli of circulating antigen-antibody complexes in the antigen-excess situation which may occur in a chronic low-grade quartan infection. Unlike most forms of the nephrotic syndrome, that associated with quartan malaria is essentially unaffected by the administration of steroids.

Spontaneous termination of attacks in quartan malaria induced for the treatment of neurosyphilis has been reported to occur in 19 to 169 days in white patients; the average time in blacks is somewhat shorter. A primary attack may result in elimination of the parasites, or there may be a recrudescence or succession of recrudescences over a period of years. In some cases the subsidence of clinical infection leaves the patient with a latent infection and persisting low-grade parasitemia. This may never bring about a clinical recrudescence, or do so only when the patient has become greatly debilitated from other causes. However, if blood from such a patient is used for transfusion, the recipient will probably experience a typical attack.

Plasmodium brasilianum, a quartan type of parasite, is another species of monkey malaria which has been transmitted to man by the bite of infected mosquitoes (Contacos et al., 1963). Infection in man is mild or asymptomatic. Both Caucasians and blacks can be infected with this parasite, in contrast to the *vivax*-like *P. cynomolgi* which has been transmitted only to Caucasians. Coatney (1971) discusses the several monkey malarias which from time to time cause human infections, as well as those probably of human origin which have become established in simian hosts.

Plasmodium falciparum

Falciparum malaria is almost entirely confined to the tropics and subtropics. Clinically, falciparum malaria is quite sharply differentiated from the other malarias in a number of ways. Morphologically, there are certain differences as well. The gametocytes of *Plasmodium falciparum* are elongate or sausage shaped in contrast to the spherical or ovoid gametocytes of the other species. On the basis of the shape of the gametocytes, *Plasmodium falciparum* was placed by some workers in a separate genus, *Laverania*.

Schizogony does not usually take place in the peripheral blood in falciparum malaria. Therefore, the only stages of the parasite seen ordinarily are young trophozoites and gametocytes. Double and even triple infections of red cells are not uncommon, and as *P. falciparum* will attack all stages of red cells the number of cells parasitized may be very great. The young trophozoites are minute rings (Fig. 38). Much more frequently than in other species, the ring may have two small chromatin dots. Occasionally the earliest stages do not assume a ring form but lie spread out along the periphery of the red cell. Such parasites are referred to as accolé forms. The parasites may grow somewhat in size and become irregular in outline, although still retaining the ring form, while in the circulating blood. Pigment is rarely seen in the forms normally found in the circulating blood. The infected red cells, which retain their original size, may develop a few irregular dark-red rod- or wedge-shaped markings, known as Maurer's dots. Gametocytes are quite characteristic, being crescentic in outline. The ends of the gametocyte may be pointed, or bluntly rounded, and the remains of the red cell may be seen in the concavity formed by the arched body of the parasite. In very heavy infections, generally occurring only in moribund

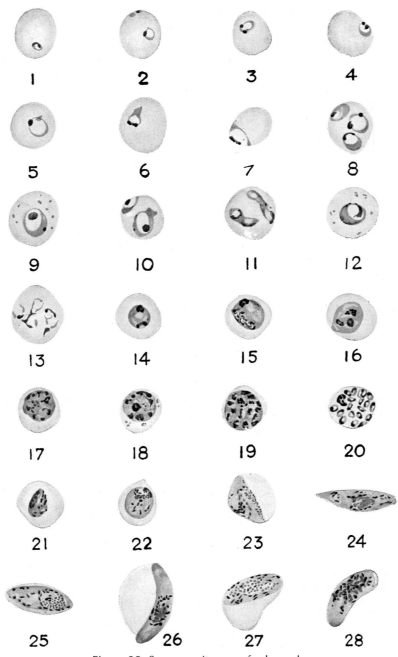

Figure 38. See opposite page for legend.

patients, schizonts may be seen in the peripheral blood. The mature schizont forms from eight to thirty-six merozoites, with an average of about twenty-four, although varying from twelve to twenty-eight with different strains.

In the thick film (Fig. 39) one is usually impressed with the large number of early trophozoites. As these are delicate, they frequently collapse to assume the comma or swallow shape. Gametocytes are easily recognizable by their shape, which is much the same as in the thin film.

SYMPTOMATOLOGY. *P. falciparum* seems to invade all ages of red cells indifferently, instead of being limited to the reticulocytes as is *P. vivax*, or the aging cells as *P. malariae*. Thus there is no limit on its invasive powers, and infection can proceed until a considerable percentage of red cells has been parasitized. Schizogony occurs in the internal organs rather than the circulating blood, and vessels of these organs may become plugged by masses of parasitized red cells. Ischemia consequent upon plugging of the vessels will produce symptoms which will vary depending upon the organs involved. Miller et al. (1972) suggest that decreased deformability of the infected red cells may lead to their inability to pass through capillaries or the splenic filter.

An uncomplicated attack of falciparum malaria will have its onset eight to twelve days after infection. It is usually preceded by a prodromal period of three or four days, during which the patient experiences vague aches and pains, often has some headache, is tired and depressed and may have anorexia and nausea. The onset of the attack is marked by fever and exaggeration of the prodromal symptoms, especially of the headache. There may be a paroxysm, with initial rigor and chills, but these are usually not severe. Frequently there will be only a sensation of chilliness at the onset of fever. Nausea and vomiting are frequently seen, and there may be severe epigastric pain. Early in the attack, fever

---

FIGURE 38. Plasmodium falciparum: 1, very young ring form trophozoite; *2,* double infection of single cell with young trophozoites, one a "marginal form," the other "signet ring" form; *3, 4,* young trophozoites showing double chromatin dots; *5, 6, 7,* developing trophozoite forms; *8,* three medium trophozoites in one cell; *9,* trophozoite showing pigment, in a cell containing Maurer's dots; *10, 11,* two trophozoites in each of two cells, showing variation of forms which parasites may assume; *12,* almost mature trophozoite showing haze of pigment throughout cytoplasm; Maurer's dots in the cell; *13,* estivo-autumnal "slender forms"; *14,* mature trophozoite, showing clumped pigment; *15,* parasite in the process of initial chromatin division; *16, 17, 18, 19,* various phases of the development of the schizont ("presegmenting schizonts"); *20,* mature schizont; *21, 22, 23, 24,* successive forms in the development of the gametocyte—usually not found in the peripheral circulation; *25,* immature macrogametocyte; *26,* mature macrogametocyte; *27,* immature microgametocyte; *28,* mature microgametocyte. (Courtesy National Institutes of Health, U.S.P.H.S.)

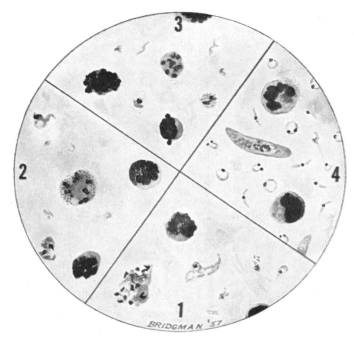

FIGURE 39. The human plasmodia as seen in thick film: *1, Plasmodium vivax:* young and older trophozoites and schizont; *2, P. ovale:* developing trophozoite and schizonts, one within a "ghost cell"; *3, P. malariae:* trophozoites and schizont; *4, P. falciparum:* young trophozoites and gametocyte.

may be continuous, remittent or intermittent. If intermittent there may be a tertian cycle resembling vivax malaria, or a quotidian fever. In some cases, there will be double rises in fever daily, resembling somewhat the fever pattern of kala-azar. Rarely, there is no appreciable fever until late in the attack, when parasitemia has developed to a high level. If the fever develops a definite synchronous cycle, it will usually be noted that febrile peaks are somewhat less than forty-eight hours apart.

An untreated primary attack of *P. falciparum* malaria tends to run its course quickly, and seldom exceeds two or three weeks in duration. True relapses probably do not occur; clinical recrudescences are infrequent after a year and are usually confined to a six-month period after infection. In recrudescences, the fever may exhibit an initial quotidian periodicity.

Severe or even fatal complications of a *P. falciparum* infection may occur at any time during the course of the disease. As mentioned above, these complications are largely the result of occlusion of blood vessels by masses of infected red cells. The symptoms may be expected to vary according to the portion of the body involved.

PATHOGENESIS. Disseminated intravascular coagulation is a feature of many diseases marked by intravascular hemolysis, especially those in which bacterial endotoxins play an etiologic role. McKay (1965) suggests that the same process occurs in malaria. Thrombocytopenia and decreased prothrombin levels are characteristic of these conditions, including falciparum malaria. Whether or not the "sludging" of parasitized red cells is a separate phenomenon is unclear, but focal ischemia produced by one of, or a combination of, the above factors is fundamental to the pathologic processes in most complications of falciparum malaria.

Cerebral malaria is most commonly seen as a complication of *P. falciparum* infection, but may occur and even prove fatal in other types of the disease. It will be remembered that headache, disorientation and other signs of cerebral involvement were mentioned in connection with the paroxysm of vivax and of quartan malaria. Coma may develop suddenly in the course of a malaria attack, or even in patients exhibiting no clinical symptoms. If the onset is more gradual, the patient may become confused and violent, or may develop severe headache and quietly pass into coma. Physical signs of central nervous system involvement may be quite variable, and any degree of parasitemia may be found in the blood. Unless prompt treatment is instituted, this condition is usually fatal.

Malarial hyperpyrexia may be seen during the course of an uncomplicated attack, or may develop as a further complication of the cerebral form of the disease. Injury to the heat-controlling mechanism in the hypothalamus, either by toxic products of the parasites or more probably because of a vascular lesion, brings about this condition. The temperature rises to 107° F. or higher, and the patient quickly becomes comatose and expires unless energetic treatment is instituted.

Bilious remittent fever is a form of the disease in which the chief organ affected is the liver. The patient usually complains of abdominal pain from the onset, with nausea and severe and persistent vomiting. The vomitus contains bile and sometimes altered or fresh blood. There is usually copious diarrhea and sometimes dysentery; the patient quickly becomes dehydrated. The liver becomes enlarged and tender, the skin becomes icteric and the urine contains bile. The fever usually assumes a remittent form. This is one of the most serious complications of malaria.

Dysenteric malaria has gastrointestinal manifestations similar to those of bilious remittent fever, but the liver is not involved and there is no jaundice. A malabsorptive state has been described (Karney and Tongi, 1972) characterized by decreased absorption of D-xylose and vitamin B_{12}, and low serum carotene. Jejunal biopsy showed edema, round cell infiltration of the lamina propria, and blunting of villi.

The syndrome of algid malaria may develop during the course of an apparently uncomplicated falciparum attack. The temperature falls rapidly, and the patient may become delirious. Symptoms of generalized vascular collapse and shock develop quickly. There may be severe abdominal pain, vomiting and diarrhea, and muscular cramps. Death may ensue very rapidly in spite of supportive therapy, or the disease may pursue a more subacute course. In the subacute stage, and after recovery from an acute attack of algid malaria, a percentage of patients develops signs resembling Addison's disease. It is generally considered that adrenal failure is basic to the development of the algid form of the disease.

Blackwater fever is most frequently seen in falciparum malaria, although it sometimes develops in patients suffering from vivax or quartan malaria as well. Usually there is a history of previous malaria attacks, and occasionally of prior bouts with blackwater fever. The onset is generally during a paroxysm of falciparum malaria, but it may take place without accompanying symptoms. A sudden intravascular hemolysis results in the passage of hemoglobin in the urine; however, the onset of the condition may be missed, as hemoglobinuria *per se* does not give rise to symptoms. There may be but one hemolytic crisis, or there may be several in the course of an attack. Destruction of red cells can be quite rapid, leading in a short time to profound degrees of anemia, or it may be relatively minor in nature. Quinine sensitivity has been considered by some as a factor inducing hemolysis; it has also been suggested that invaded red cells may function as antigens, giving rise to antibodies which act as hemolysins.

Acute renal failure may result from an attack of blackwater fever, but it may also occur unassociated with hemolytic anemia in other cases of falciparum malaria (Sitprija, 1970). It is thought to follow acute tubular necrosis, which is brought on by renal anoxia. Without aggressive treatment, this complication may rapidly prove fatal. The nephrotic syndrome, due to acute glomerulonephritis, with typical renal biopsy findings by light microscopy, has been reported in cases of falciparum malaria (Berger et al., 1967).

Fluid retention, secondary to parenteral fluid administration in oliguric or anuric patients, may lead to acute pulmonary edema, but this condition can occur (Brooks et al., 1968; Punyagupta et al., 1974) without evidence of fluid retention or cardiac decompensation, possibly secondary to intravascular coagulation affecting the pulmonary microcirculation. Pulmonary edema may be rapid in onset and refractory to treatment. Deaton (1970) recommends the use of dexamethasone.

EPIDEMIOLOGY. Falciparum malaria is primarily a disease of the tropics, as is ovale, while vivax and malariae may occur extensively in the subtropics and temperate zone as well. In cooler parts of the endemic areas, development of *P. falciparum* cannot take place in the spring, and attacks of malaria caused by this species occur primarily in the hot weather of summer and early autumn. From this characteristic seasonal appearance comes the old name of estivo-autumnal malaria.

Gametocytes of *P. falciparum* appear in the circulating blood approximately ten days after the onset of parasitemia, and they are not infectious for mosquitoes for another four days. Thus, the patient with falciparum malaria is infectious later than is the case with vivax malaria, and he is less likely already to have infected mosquitoes at the time the infection is discovered and treated. A single pre-erythrocytic cycle, without subsequent liver involvement, theoretically makes treatment of this type of malaria less difficult. The development of resistance to the synthetic antimalarials, which also characterizes falciparum malaria, considerably complicates the therapeutic picture.

Luzzatto et al. (1969) found glucose-6-phosphate dehydrogenase (G-6-PD)–deficient cells to be from two to eighty times as resistant to invasion by *P. falciparum* as normal erythrocytes. Various hemoglobinopathies, and especially the presence of hemoglobin S, have been found to be related to increased resistance to *P. falciparum* infection. Motulsky (1964) indicated that malaria mortality in patients with the sickle-cell trait was less than one-twentieth of that expected. These hemoglobinopathies (as well as thalassemia and hemoglobin C or E, also considered by some to be associated with increased resistance to *P. falciparum* infection) have a geographic distribution such that their presence could be readily explained if they confer a selective advantage to their possessors in a hyperendemic malaria zone. The mechanism by which they may afford protection against infection with *P. falciparum* is uncertain.

TREATMENT. A brief synopsis of recommended treatment is given at the end of this section. Quinine and its related alkaloids were the only specific antimalarials available prior to World War I. Subsequently a large number of synthetic drugs were produced, some of which have become mainstays of therapy. Resistance was noted early to certain of these drugs (chlorguanide, pyrimethamine), but this was of little clinical significance until, in South America and Southeast Asia, chloroquine was found ineffective in the treatment of certain strains of *P. falciparum*. Frequently, resistance to chloroquine means resistance to other synthetic antimalarials as well, and successful treatment may require the use of quinine. Unfortunately, some strains now have developed a partial resistance to quinine as well (Clyde et al., 1970) and require the use of combination therapy.

Rational use of the antimalarial drugs is based on a knowledge of their effects upon the various stages of the life cycle. Suppressive therapy involves repeated use of small doses of drugs effective against the erythrocytic stages in order to destroy the parasites as they invade the blood stream. A clinical cure employs larger doses of the same types of drugs to eliminate the greater number of erythrocytic parasites present in a clinical attack. Radical cure, on the other hand, requires the use of agents which will eliminate the tissue stages in the liver as well. Drugs effective against the asexual erythrocytic stages are not necessarily gametocytocidal, nor are they effective against the exo-erythrocytic stages; the patient may be cured of his schizogonic parasites but still be infectious because gametocytes remain in his circulating blood, or relapse because of reinfection of the blood stream from the tissues.

Quinine, the 4-aminoquinoline drugs chloroquine (Aralen), hydroxychloroquine (Plaquenil) and amodiaquine (Camoquin), and the acridine dye quinacrine (Atabrine) are all effective against the asexual erythrocytic stages of the human malarias, but are ineffective against their exo-erythrocytic stages or the gametocytes of *P. falciparum*. The mechanism of action of this group of drugs is thought to involve inhibition of the enzymatic synthesis of DNA and RNA.

The 8-aminoquinoline drugs, of which primaquine is the least toxic, are most effective against the pre- and exo-erythrocytic stages and gametocytes of the various species of human malaria. They are relatively ineffective against the asexual erythrocytic parasites. Their mechanisms of action are unknown but are thought to be related to that by which they produce hemolysis of glucose-6-phosphate dehydrogenase-deficient red cells. Certain strains of *P. vivax* from Central America (Miller et al., 1974), as well as the Vietnam strain, have a significant relapse rate (3.5 to 7.5 per cent) following primaquine treatment.

Chlorguanide (Paludrine), a biguanide, and the structurally related diaminopyrimidine, pyrimethamine (Daraprim), are relatively slow-acting drugs of limited value in the treatment of the sexual erythrocytic stages of malaria; they are most effective against the tissue stages of susceptible strains of *P. falciparum*, but they have a less certain effect upon these stages in *P. vivax*. Both of these drugs inhibit the metabolism of folic acid and affect nuclear division of the parasites.

The sulfonamides and sulfones have been known for many years to have antimalarial properties, but they were not extensively tested until the emergence of resistant strains of *P. falciparum* created an acute need for new and effective antimalarials. Both the longer-acting sulfonamides, such as sulphormethoxine (Fanzil) and sulfalene, and the sulfone Dapsone (diaminodiphenylsulfone, DDS) have been clinically tested and found to have some schizonticidal activity, especially against *P. falciparum*. The sulfonamides and sulfones are PABA antagonists; their effect on the malarial parasite apparently derives from their ability to block the synthesis of folic acid from para-aminobenzoic acid. Dapsone and other sulfones inhibit intraerythrocytic-parasite glycolysis and the utilization of adenosine, apparently by blockage at the red-cell membrane.

Colchicine was first used as an antimalarial during World War II; at that time it was discarded because of the availability of more effective drugs. With the development of resistance on the part of *P. falciparum,* it has been employed again and, in combination with quinine, seems to lessen the tendency to recrudescence of this parasite. Colchicine interferes with the metabolism of folic acid as well as with the mitotic process.

It will be seen that the three separate stages of the plasmodial life cycle which occur in man cannot be treated successfully with any single drug. The pre- and exo-erythrocytic cycles are sensitive to primaquine and also to chlorguanide and pyrimethamine. The asexual erythrocytic stages respond to treatment with a variety of agents: quinine, chloroquine, hydroxychloroquine, amodiaquine and quinacrine, chlorguanide and pyrimethamine, sulfonamides and sulfones, and colchicine. Primaquine, again, is the most effective gametocidal agent. A combination therapy should be devised bearing in mind the spectrum of activity of the various drugs and, in some cases, their modes of action. Thus, if a combination of drugs effective against a single stage is desired, one should combine agents with different modes of action, as indicated in Table 6.

A note of warning regarding combinations of drugs with the same mode of action is issued by Hall (1973), who noted substantially less radical cures in falciparum malaria from Southeast Asia when a combination of chloroquine and quinine was used, as compared with treatment with quinine alone.

Various drugs can be used for malaria suppression. A generally effective regimen is chloroquine diphosphate, 0.5 gm., with pyrimetha-

Table 6. Antimalarial Drug Combinations

Stage Affected	Action by Interference With			
	FOLIC ACID SYNTHESIS	FOLIC ACID METABOLISM	NUCLEIC ACID METABOLISM	UNKNOWN*
Erythrocytic cycle (Schizonts)	Sulfonamides Sulfones	Chlorguanide Pyrimethamine Colchicine	Quinine Chloroquine Amodiaquine	
Erythrocytic cycle (Gametocytes)				Primaquine
Exo-erythrocytic cycle		Chloroquine Pyrimethamine		Primaquine

*Nucleic acid precursor synthesis?

mine, 25 mg. once weekly, starting on arrival in a malarious area. Chloroquine should be continued for six weeks after leaving the area and may be combined with primaquine (80 mg. weekly) for the same period in order to achieve a radical cure during suppression. Hydroxychloroquine (Plaquenil) is equally effective for suppression and treatment; 200 mg. of hydroxychloroquine is the equivalent of 250 mg. of chloroquine.

In areas where resistance to chloroquine has been noted, other suppressive regimens have been advocated. In Vietnam, the U.S. military forces added a daily dose of 25 mg. of Dapsone to the weekly 0.5 gm. of chloroquine with 75 mg. of pyrimethamine. This improved its effectiveness, but Dapsone was found to produce agranulocytosis in a very small percentage of cases. Dapsone may produce hemolytic anemia when administered in large doses to normal individuals and in smaller doses to glucose-6-phosphate dehydrogenase-deficient individuals. In healthy G-6-PD-deficient individuals, doses of 25 mg. daily are usually well tolerated.

Clinical cure, except in the presence of resistant strains (unfortunately no longer rare for *Plasmodium falciparum* in some areas of Southeast Asia and South America and reported also from Central America) may be achieved in all types of malaria with chloroquine diphosphate. The initial dose is 1.0 gm. (600 mg. of chloroquine base) followed six hours later with 0.5 gm. and an additional 0.5 gm. on each of the two succeeding days. If there is not a prompt response to therapy, resistance to chloroquine should be suspected, and quinine added at the rate of 0.65 gm. three times daily for seven to fourteen days. In the presence of resistant strains of *P. falciparum*, Dapsone may be administered for an additional 30 days at the rate of 25 mg. daily.

Other regimens advocated for the treatment of resistant falciparum malaria utilize conventional doses of quinine or of chloroquine, to which are added pyrimethamine and a long- or short-acting sulfonamide, or colchicine (Bartonelli et al., 1967; Berman, 1969; Reba and Sheehy, 1967). A promising combination is that of the long-acting sulfonamide, sulfalene, and trimethoprim, a dihydrofolic acid reductase inhibitor, which is effective against some resistant strains of *P. falciparum* (Clyde et al., 1971). The potential for production of erythema multiforme (Stevens-Johnson syndrome) by the long-acting sulfonamides must be borne in mind if their use is contemplated. Tetracycline and its derivatives (Doxycycline, alpha-6-deoxytetracycline, and Minocycline, 7-dimethylamino-6-deoxy-6-dimethyl-tetracycline) have some antimalarial activity (Rieckmann et al., 1971) and when combined with quinine give excellent results in acute falciparum malaria (Colwell et al., 1972).

Local experience may well dictate the therapeutic regimen of choice, but if resistant falciparum malaria is a possibility, quinine sulfate may be employed initially in full dosage as given above. If there is not an adequate response within 24 hours, or if there is a recrudescence of parasitemia after an adequate course of quinine, pyrimethamine (25 mg. every 12 hours for three days) may be added along with Dapsone (25 mg. daily for 30 days), or an alternative form of therapy may be undertaken.

It has been conclusively demonstrated that, rather than presenting a danger to pregnancy, the administration of antimalarials constitutes "the single most important antenatal medical procedure in a country where malaria is endemic" (Gilles et al., 1969).

If questions arise concerning drug resistance or the response of a specific strain of malarial parasite to various treatment regimens, estimates of parasite levels may be of value (see Chapter 15). If the level determined before administration of a certain drug or combination does not drop within 24 hours thereafter, the regimen in question is probably ineffective for the strain of parasite being treated.

Parenteral therapy is seldom necessary but may be lifesaving in cerebral malaria. Chloroquine hydrochloride (not available commercially, but obtainable from the Winthrop Laboratories as Aralen hydrochloride, in ampoules containing 120 mg. of chloroquine base) may be administered intramuscularly at the rate of 200 to 400 mg. every 6 hours. The total intramuscular dose for the first 24 hours should not exceed 900 mg. of the base, and oral administration should be begun as soon as possible. In infants and children, dosage of chloroquine by any route must not exceed 5 mg. per Kg. at any one time. Quinine dihydrochloride is also available for intravenous use; it is given by slow intravenous drip, 0.65 gm. in 250 ml. or more of physiological saline every 6 to 8 hours. Chloroquine is less toxic and is preferred to quinine unless a resistant strain is being treated.

Radical cure may be achieved in falciparum and quartan malaria by any drug or combination of drugs which will sterilize the blood stream, as there is no continuation of the tissue pre-erythrocytic cycle. Relapse cannot occur, but there may be a recrudescence after inadequate treatment of the erythrocytic phase or when inadequate or no treatment combines with a waning host immunity. In vivax and ovale malaria, administration of a course of the 8-amino-quinoline, primaquine phosphate, 26.3 mg. (1 tablet or 15 mg. of primaquine base) daily for 14 days, started during or immediately following chloroquine therapy as previously outlined will produce a radical cure in most cases. An alternative method of administration is to give 80 mg. (3 tablets) with the second dose of chloroquine, and 80 mg. as a single dose once weekly thereafter for seven additional weeks. The latter method of administration is said to give better results with the Southwest Pacific strains of vivax malaria. Primaquine may cause intravascular hemolysis in persons with glucose-6-phosphate dehydrogenase deficiency, and should be used with caution in blacks and other groups in which this deficiency occurs. A test for this deficiency can be performed, and whenever possible this should be done before starting treatment with primaquine. Severe toxicity is rare at any rate if a daily dose of 15 mg. primaquine base is given for not more than two weeks, or if the weekly dosage is limited to 30 mg. of the base. It should not be administered at the same time as quinacrine, nor within three weeks of terminating a course of that drug, as quinacrine increases toxicity.

In addition to therapy directed at the malarial infection itself, attention must be given to treatment of the complications of that infection, especially if caused by *P. falciparum.* The two most vulnerable target organs are the brain and kidneys.

Dexamethasone has proved effective in the management of edema of the brain occurring in cerebral malaria (Blount, 1967). It is administered as in other forms of cerebral edema. The use of this drug or other steroids in massive hemolysis with hemoglobinuria has been advocated. Heparin in sufficient dosage to produce a satisfactory prolongation of the prothrombin time is also effective in patients with hemolysis as well as in other situations suggestive of disseminated intravascular coagulation (McKay, 1965; Blount, 1967). When acute renal failure supervenes in a case of falciparum malaria, peritoneal (Canfield et al., 1968) or other methods of dialysis may prove lifesaving.

The following regimens are recommended for chemoprophylaxis and initial treatment of malaria:

Drugs: Chloroquine phosphate (Aralen), 500 mg. tabs. (300 mg. base)

Dapsone (Avlosulfon) 25 mg. tabs.

Hydroxychloroquine sulfate (Plaquenil), 200 mg. tabs. (155 mg. base)

Primaquine phosphate, 26.3 mg. tabs. (15 mg. base)

Pyrimethamine (Daraprim), 25 mg. tabs.

Quinine sulfate, 195 mg. and 325 mg. caps. and 325 mg. tabs.

Ampules: Chloroquine hydrochloride (120 mg. base) and quinine dihydrochloride

I. In areas from which chloroquine resistance has not yet been reported.
   A. *Chemoprophylaxis*
      1. Adults: chloroquine base 300 mg. or hydroxychloroquine base 400 mg., once weekly starting on or shortly before arrival in malarious area, and continuing for 6 weeks after leaving endemic area.

2. Children: chloroquine or hydroxychloroquine (the former is generally enteric coated, the latter more easily divided for pediatric dosage), 5 mg. per kg. of body weight weekly, as above.
3. To the above may be added pyrimethamine:
    a) 25 mg. weekly for adults and children over 10 years of age.
    b) children 4–10 years old, 12.5 mg. weekly
        children under 4 years of age, 6.25 mg. weekly.

B. *Clinical cure*

Mild cases:

1. Adults: chloroquine base 600 mg. initially, followed by 300 mg. 6 hours later, and a single dose of 300 mg. on each of two consecutive days thereafter.
2. Children: chloroquine or hydroxychloroquine base, 10 mg. per kg. of body weight initially, followed by 5 mg. per kg. 6 hours later, and 5 mg. per kg. daily on each of two consecutive days thereafter.

Severe Cases:

1. Adults: chloroquine hydrochloride 250 mg. (200 mg. base) IM every 6 hours until oral therapy possible.
2. Children: chloroquine hydrochloride, 5 mg. base per kg. body wieght, IM every 6 hours until oral therapy possible.

C. *Radical cure* (for vivax or ovale malaria only)

1. Adults: 15 mg. primaquine base daily — may be given near the end of the chemoprophylactic regimen, or concurrently with treatment for a clinical attack.
2. Children: 1 to 3 years old: 1/6 tab. daily
              4 to 6 years old: 1/3 tab. daily
              7 to 10 years old: 1/2 tab. daily
              11 to 15 years old: 3/4 to 1 tab. daily

II. In areas from which chloroquine resistance has been reported.

A. *Chemoprophylaxis*

1. Chloroquine, in dosage recommended for patient's age, plus primaquine three times daily dose for patient's age, once weekly, *and* dapsone 25 mg. daily for persons over 9 years of age.
2. Weekly chloroquine in dosage recommended for patient's age, plus dapsone:
   Patients 9 years of age and older: 25 mg. per day
   Patients under 9 years of age: 1/4 to 1/2 tab. daily

B. *Clinical cure*

Mild cases: treatment as in *IB* above; if not improved within 24 hours:

1. Adults: quinine sulfate 650 mg. three times daily for 14 days
2. Children:
   under 1 year: 80 mg. every 6 hours for 14 days
   1–3 years: 80 mg. every 4 hours for 14 days
   3–6 years: 160 mg. every 6 hours for 14 days
   6–12 years: 325 mg. every 8 hours for 14 days

Severe cases:

1. Adults: quinine dihydrochloride 600 mg. in 300 ml. normal saline IV over 30 minutes. Monitor pulse and BP, preferably with electrocardiography. Repeat every 6 to 9 hours until able to take *per os,* then as above.

2. Children: quinine dihydrochloride 10 mg. per kg., in normal saline diluted to 1 mg. per ml., administered at 1 mg. per minute. Repeat every 12 hours until able to take *per os,* then as above.

REFERENCES

Bartelloni, P. J., Sheehy, T. W., and Tigertt, W. D. 1967. Combined therapy for chloroquine-resistant *Plasmodium falciparum* infection. J.A.M.A., *199*:173–177.

Berger, M., Birch, L. M., and Conte, N. F. 1967. The nephrotic syndrome secondary to acute glomerulonephritis during falciparum malaria. Ann. Intern. Med., *67*:116–117.

Berman, S. J. 1969. Chloroquin-pyrimethamine-sulfisoxazole therapy of *Plasmodium falciparum* malaria. J.A.M.A., *207*:128–130.

Blount, R. E. 1967. Management of chloroquine-resistant falciparum malaria. Arch. Intern. Med., *119*:557–560.

Brooks, M. H., Kiel, F. W., Sheehy, T. W., and Barry, K. G. 1968. Acute pulmonary edema in falciparum malaria. A clinicopathologic correlation. New Eng. J. Med., *279*:732–737.

Canfield, C. J., Miller, L. H., Bartelloni, P. J., Eichler, P., and Barry, K. G. 1968. Acute renal failure in *Plasmodium falciparum* malaria. Treatment by peritoneal dialysis. Arch. Intern. Med., *122*:199–203.

Clyde, D. F., Miller, R. M., DuPont, H. L., and Hornick, R. B. 1970. Treatment of falciparum malaria caused by strain resistance to quinine. J.A.M.A., *123*:2041–2045.

Clyde, D. F., Miller, R. M., Schwartz, A. R., and Levine, M. M. 1971. Treatment of falciparum malaria with sulfalene and trimethoprim. Amer. J. Trop. Med. & Hyg., *20*:804–810.

Coatney, G. R. 1963. Simian malaria, its importance to world-wide eradication of malaria. J.A.M.A., *184*:876–877.

Coatney, G. R. 1971. The simian malarias: zoonoses, anthroponoses, or both? Amer. J. Trop. Med. & Hyg., *20*:795–803.

Colwell, E. J., Hickman, R. L., Intraprasert, R., and Tirabutana, C. 1972. Minocycline and tetracycline treatment in acute falciparum malaria. Amer. J. Trop. Med. & Hyg., *21*:144–149.

Contacos, P. G., Lunn, J. S., Coatney, G. R., Kilpatrick, J. W., and Jones, F. E. 1963. Quartan-type malaria parasite of New World monkeys transmissible to man. Science, *142*:676.

Deaton, J. G. 1970. Fatal pulmonary edema as a complication of acute falciparum malaria. Amer. J. Trop. Med. & Hyg., *19*:196–201.

Eyles, D. E., Coatney, G. R., and Getz, M. E. 1960. Vivax-type malaria parasite of macaques transmissible to man. Science, *131*:1812–1813.

Fisher, G. U., and Schultz, M. G. 1969. Unusual host-parasite relationship in blood donors responsible for transfusion-induced falciparum malaria. Lancet, *2*:716–718.

Friedmann, C. T., Dover, A. S., Roberto, R. R., and Kearns, O. A. 1973. A malaria epidemic among heroin users. Amer. J. Trop. Med. & Hyg., *22*:302–306.

Gilles, H. M., Lawson, J. B., Sibelas, M., Voller, A., and Allen, N, 1969. Malaria, anaemia and pregnancy. Ann. Trop. Med. & Parasit., *63*:245–263.

Garnham, P. C. C. C. 1966. *Malaria Parasites and Other Haemosporidia.* 1114 pp. Blackwell Scientific Publication, Oxford, England.

Hall, A. P. 1973. Quinine and chloroquine antagonism in falciparum malaria. Trans. Roy. Soc. Trop. Med. & Hyg., *67*:425.

Hill, G. J., II, Knight, V., Coatney, G. R., and Lawless, D. K. 1963. Vivax malaria complicated by aphasia and hemiparesis. Arch. Intern. Med., *112*:863–868.

Karney, W. W., and Tongi, M. J. 1972. Malabsorption in *Plasmodium falciparum* malaria. Amer. J. Trop. Med. & Hyg., *21*:1–5.

Kibukamusoke, J. W., Hutt, M. S. R., and Wilks, N. E. 1967. The nephrotic syndrome in Uganda and its association with quartan malaria. Quart. J. Med., *36*:393–408.

Kuvin, S. F., Beye, H. K., Stohlman, F., Jr., Contacos, P. G., and Coatney, G. R. 1963. Malaria in man, infection by *Plasmodium vivax* and the B strain of *Plasmodium cynomolgi*. J.A.M.A., *184*:1018–1020.

Kuvin, S. F., Tobie, J. E., Evans, C. B., Coatney, G. R., and Contacos, P. G. 1963. Production of malarial antibody. Determination by the fluorescent-antibody technique. J.A.M.A., *184*:943–945.

Luzzatto, L., Usanga, E. A., and Reddy, S. 1969. Glucose-6-phosphate dehydrogenase-deficient red cells: resistance to infection by malarial parasites. Science, *164*:839–841.

McKay, D. G. 1965. *Disseminated Intravascular Coagulation*. 493 pp. Paul B. Hoeber, Inc., New York.

Miller, L. H., Chien, S., and Usami, S. 1972. Decreased deformability of *Plasmodium coatneyi*-infected red cells and its possible relation to cerebral malaria. Amer. J. Trop. Med. & Hyg., *21*:133–137.

Miller, L. H., Wyler, D. J., Glew, R. H., Collins, W. E., and Contacos, P. G. 1974. Sensitivity of four Central American strains of *Plasmodium vivax* to primaquine. Amer. J. Trop. Med. & Hyg., *28*:309–310.

Miller, L. H., Mason, S. J., Dvorak, J. A., McGinniss, M. H., and Rothman, I. K. 1975. Erythrocyte receptors for (*Plasmodium knowlesi*) malaria: Duffy blood group determinants. Science, *189*:561–562.

Motulsky, A. G. 1964. Hereditary red cell traits and malaria. Amer. J. Trop. Med. & Hyg., *13*:147–158.

Punyagupta, S., Srichaikul, T., Nitiyanant, P., and Petchelai, B. 1974. Acute pulmonary insufficiency in falciparum malaria: summary of 12 cases with evidence of disseminated intravascular coagulation. Amer. J. Trop. Med. & Hyg., *23*:551–559.

Reba, R. C., and Sheehy, T. W. 1967. Colchicine-quinine therapy for acute falciparum malaria acquired in Vietnam. J.A.M.A., *201*:553–556.

Rieckmann, K. H., Powell, R. D., McNamara, J. V., Willerson, D., Jr., Kass, L., Frischer, H., and Carson, P. E. 1971. Effects of tetracycline against chloroquine-resistant and chloroquine-sensitive *Plasmodium falciparum*. Amer. J. Trop. Med. & Hyg., *20*:811–815.

Sitprija, V. 1970. Renal involvement in malaria. Trans. Roy. Soc. Trop. Med. & Hyg., *64*:695–699.

7

Other Blood- and Tissue-Dwelling Protozoa

While a strictly taxonomic approach seems unwarranted in a book emphasizing the medical aspects of parasitology, it must be understood that any other is equally arbitrary. We have already considered, as lumen-dwellers, both the tissue-invasive *Entamoeba histolytica* and (for convenience) those free-living amebae whose only medical importance comes from their ability on occasion to invade the central nervous system. We now take up a number of flagellates, lumen-dwellers in their insect hosts, which invade the tissues or blood stream of man. Additionally, we will consider the sporozoa *Toxoplasma, Pneumocystis, Sarcocystis,* and *Babesia.*

THE HEMOFLAGELLATES

The family Trypanosomidae, which includes the hemoflagellates, contains a number of genera, only two of which parasitize man. The primitive structure in this group is probably represented by the genus *Leptomonas,* parasitic in insects. These organisms (Fig. 40) have a fusiform body, with the nucleus central in position and a single anterior flagellum arising from a kinetoplast near the anterior end. In the genus *Trypanosoma* those forms which are seen in the blood of man have been rather profoundly modified from the leptomonad type (also known as a promastigote). The kinetoplast has assumed a position near the posterior

124

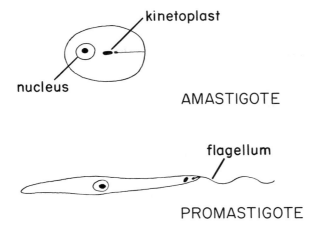

AMASTIGOTE

PROMASTIGOTE

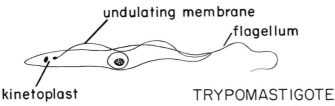

TRYPOMASTIGOTE

FIGURE 40. Morphological types seen in various hemoflagellates of man.

end of the body, and the flagellum passes anteriorly, forming the outer edge of the undulating membrane, a thin protoplasmic sheet running along one side of the organism. Anterior to the body of the trypanosome, the flagellum may project free of the undulating membrane. One species of trypanosome parasitizing man may be found both in the circulating blood and intracellularly in cardiac muscle. It has the typical trypanosome form (trypomastigote) as a blood parasite, while the stages found in cardiac muscle are more nearly rounded, have lost both undulating membrane and all trace of an external flagellum, and are known as leishmania forms, or amastigotes. In these minute parasites the only structures which can be distinguished are the nucleus and the kinetoplast, with sometimes a remaining short intracytoplasmic portion of the flagellum. This type of organization is also seen in members of the genus *Leishmania,* which are always intracellular parasites, primarily in cells of the reticuloendothelial system. They may at times be present in the blood stream in large mononuclear cells.

The hemoflagellates were in all probability originally parasites of insects. As evidence for this we see that these organisms are transmitted by insects, in which they undergo a developmental cycle. Some genera are still exclusively insect parasites. The forms of the parasites which occur in the insect host are often quite different from those found in the vertebrate. In culture, leishmanias assume a promastigote form, while trypanosomes also exhibit forms similar to those which occur naturally in the insect host. The Old World forms of leishmaniasis are transmitted by the bite of various species of sandflies of the genus *Phlebotomus;* the South American leishmaniases are likewise carried by sandflies. African sleeping sickness is transmitted by bites of several species of *Glossina,* or tsetse flies; the American forms of trypanosomiasis are carried by reduviid bugs, and transmission occurs when infective feces of the bug contaminate the wound made by the insect's bite or an abrasion of the skin.

Trypanosoma

Two distinctly different forms of this genus occur in man, represented on the one hand by the species associated with African sleeping sickness, and on the other by Chagas' disease or American trypanosomiasis. In both the Gambian and Rhodesian forms of African trypanosomiasis, the parasites occur in the blood stream in the trypomastigote form, and as amastigotes in the choroid plexus and possibly in other organs, whereas in Chagas' disease trypomastigotes are found in the blood stream and amastigotes occur intracellularly in cardiac muscle and other tissues.

Several species of trypanosomes are important parasites of cattle, horses and other domestic animals in Africa; the effects of these diseases on the economy of Central Africa can hardly be overestimated.

Trypanosoma brucei gambiense

African sleeping sickness occurs in what must have been originally two distinctly separate geographical areas, and in two clinically distinguishable forms. The causative agents of the two types of disease are not readily differentiated, and there has been considerable controversy over their status. *Trypanosoma brucei gambiense* (Fig. 41) causes the Gambian or West African form of the disease. It is a highly pleomorphic organism, frequently showing in a single blood smear a variety of forms ranging from slender-bodied organisms with a long free flagellum, reaching a length of 30 microns or more, to fatter, stumpier forms without a free flagellum which average about 15 microns in length. The same pleomorphism characterizes *T. brucei rhodesiense,* the cause of Rhodesian or East African sleeping sickness, and *T. brucei brucei,* which produces a rela-

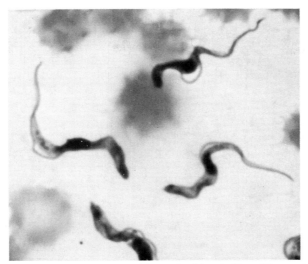

FIGURE 41. Trypanosoma gambiense in blood film. (Photomicrograph by Zane Price.)

tively mild disease in native game animals, a severe infection in many domestic animals, and apparently does not infect man. These three organisms, morphologically indistinguishable except under special and somewhat debatable circumstances, cannot be differentiated by serological means with any certainty. As their pathogenicity for man and laboratory animals is the only criterion for separating these organisms, some authorities prefer to consider all three as varieties of *Trypanosoma brucei*. Others grant specific status to *T. gambiense* and *T. rhodesiense*.

SYMPTOMATOLOGY. Following the bite of an infected tsetse fly, most frequently *Glossina palpalis*, there is an asymptomatic incubation period of a few days to several weeks. Occasionally there will be ulceration in the area of the bite, with formation of an indurated, painful "trypanosomal chancre," which slowly disappears. Trypanosomes may be demonstrated in fluid aspirated from the ulcer. At the end of the incubation period the patient is still in apparent excellent health, but examination of a blood film will reveal trypanosomes. Often they are rather scanty, and may even be difficult to find on thick-film examination. The essentially symptom-free period of low-grade parasitemia may continue for several weeks or perhaps a number of months. The infection may be abortive, and terminate during this period without the development of symptoms, or the parasites may invade the lymphatic tissues. Invasion of the lymph nodes is usually accompanied by the onset of febrile attacks. The fever is usually rather irregular, and may be initiated by a rigor. Malaise and headache usually accompany the fever, and there is often anorexia and generalized weakness, and sometimes nausea and vomiting. Night sweats are frequent. A febrile attack will last a few days to a week, and is followed by an asymptomatic interval, usually of some weeks' duration. During the fever, trypanosomes may be found in large numbers in the circulating blood, but in the afebrile periods they are few in number. With the commencement of febrile attacks there is usually some glandular enlargement. Any lymph node may be affected, but those of the posterior cervical region are most frequently involved. Enlargement of these nodes is known as Winterbottom's sign (Fig. 42). Trypanosomes may be found on aspiration of the enlarged nodes. An irregular erythematous rash, suggestive of erythema multiforme, sometimes with underlying edema and frequently accompanied by pruritus, may appear and disappear during attacks of fever. The rash usually lasts only a few hours.

The infection may terminate without overt nervous involvement, or this may occur at any time after the patient first develops symptoms of infection. The increasing lassitude and apathy common in the later stages of the glandular phase of the disease probably point to beginning nervous involvement. Usually these symptoms are not sufficiently far advanced to be recognized as a separate phase of the disease for six months to a year after the first symptoms are seen. There is steady progression in

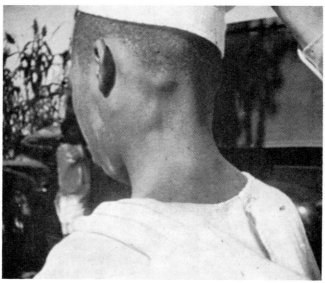

FIGURE 42. Enlargement of posterior cervical lymph nodes — Winterbottom's sign. (Courtesy of Dr. James R. Busvine, London School of Hygiene and Tropical Medicine.)

development of a meningoencephalitis, with a general deterioration of the patient, increase of apathy and fatigability, confusion and somnolence. Extreme emaciation is seen in patients who do not have strict nursing supervision. The face, in contrast to the rest of the body, is usually edematous. Neurological signs develop late. Motor changes may include fibrillation of the muscles of the face, lips and fingers, and incoordination leading to a slurred speech and ataxic gait. Sensory changes are frequently less marked; paresthesias and loss of kinesthetic sense sometimes are observed. Pressure on the palms of the hands or over the ulnar nerve may be followed by severe pain a short time after the pressure is removed. This is known as Kerandel's sign.

In the final stages of the disease there may be profound character changes and mental deterioration. Motor involvement may lead to convulsions, hemiplegia or paraplegia, and incontinence of urine and feces; severe paresthesias often occur. The patient is gradually more and more difficult to arouse, and finally becomes comatose. The progression of the central nervous symptoms is usually continuous, but there may be remissions and exacerbations with a course extending over several years.

Diagnosis depends upon demonstration of the trypanosomes in blood, fluid aspirated from lymph nodes, or in spinal fluid. Clinical history and physical findings may be of considerable value; cell counts and protein determinations of spinal fluid are of prognostic interest in evaluation of the response to therapy. If the parasites cannot be demonstrated in thick or thin films of blood, a concentration method, described in Chapter 15, may be of value.

Trypanosoma brucei gambiense can seldom be isolated by inoculation into the usual laboratory animals (rats, mice, hamsters), although *T. brucei rhodesiense* infects these animals readily. Serologic tests include indirect immunofluorescence and complement fixation techniques; serum and spinal fluid IgM measurements are of diagnostic value.

PATHOGENESIS. Until recently, it was believed that trypomastigotes were the only developmental stages of the *T. brucei* complex found in the mammalian host. It is now known that, at least in experimental animals, amastigotes of *T. brucei* are found early in infection in the choroid plexus. There they may block capillaries, causing localized edema and obstruction to the flow of cerebrospinal fluid, and possibly by this means producing the headache seen early in human infections. During the first flush of trypomastigotes in the blood, amastigotes disappear from the choroid plexus, to become reestablished there later in the course of infection. They may also occur in the lung. (Ormerod and Venkatesan, 1971a,b,c.) Overt infection involves particularly the lymphoid tissues early in the disease and the central nervous system in its later stages. There is generalized lymphoid hyperplasia as the result of proliferation of the parasites within the lymph nodes; aspiration of an enlarged node will often reveal trypanosomes when they are too few in numbers to be found in blood films. An anemia is usually noted; the white blood count is essentially normal with a relative lymphocytosis. Thrombocytopenia is often seen, a consequence of hypertrophy of the reticuloendothelial system, and of the presence of disseminated intravascular coagulation (Robins-Browne et al., 1975). Hypergammaglobulinemia is characteristic; immunoelectrophoresis or ultracentrifugation of the serum of infected persons will usually demonstrate an IgM level greater than four times that found in pooled normal serum. Such an increase, otherwise associated with Waldenström's macroglobulinemia or other dysproteinemias, may, however, be found occasionally in Africans without evidence of these diseases or of trypanosomiasis. *Absence* of an elevated serum IgM level effectively rules out trypanosomiasis, whereas the presence of detectable levels in the cerebrospinal fluid is diagnostic for CNS trypanosomiasis. Invasion of the central nervous system is marked by a progressive leptomeningitis, with perivascular round-cell infiltration of the Virchow-Robin spaces, an increased spinal fluid protein, and a cell count of 15 to 500 white blood cells per cu.mm. Growth of the parasites in this location is reported (Goodwin, 1970) to lead to localized antigen-antibody reactions with the release of kinin, disruption of collagen fibers and destruction of fibroblasts. Trypanosomes may occur outside the blood stream and spinal fluid, in the gray and white matter of the brain, and have been reported to invade other organs and tissues as well. The exact mechanism by which these parasites cause death of the host has long been debated and is still uncertain. Both cellular and humoral immunity are depressed in patients with Gambian trypanosomiasis, and Greenwood et al. (1973) note that such immunosuppression may contribute to the increased susceptibility to secondary infection characteristic of the disease. Exacerbation of a clinically inapparent and unsuspected infection (with the production of ascites and presence of trypomastigotes in the ascitic fluid) was noted (Francis, 1972) in a patient treated with steroids for an unrelated condition.

EPIDEMIOLOGY. *Trypanosoma brucei gambiense* is most frequently transmitted to man by the bite of the tsetse flies *Glossina palpalis* and *G. tachinoides.* These species dwell on the banks of shaded streams, generally in proximity to human habitation. Consequently Gambian sleeping sickness is likely to assume an endemic form, affecting those persons whose daily activities bring them in contact with such streams. No animal reservoirs are known or suspected for *T. brucei gambiense.* Control of the spread of infection is brought about by control of the vector, either by elimination of its breeding grounds through clearing away of streamside underbrush or by means of insecticides.

Throughout the endemic areas, available figures indicate a low prevalence rate, generally well under one per cent of the population at present. However, there remain foci with high rates of transmission and areas in which the disease has shown some resurgence in the past few years (WHO Report, 1969).

TREATMENT. While some authorities recommend the use of melarsoprol*, Mel B or melarsen oxide complexed with dimercaprol (BAL) for treatment of all stages of Gambian sleeping sickness, less toxic drugs may be substituted in the early stages during which there is no evidence of neurologic involvement. Pentamidine* (Lomidine or 4–4'-diaminodiphenoxypentane di-β-hydroxyethane sulfonate) is effective in the hemolymphatic stages of the infection, and is also used as a chemoprophylactic. This drug does not penetrate the blood brain barrier, and therefore it is ineffective during the later stages of the disease. It is administered by intramuscular injection at the rate of 4 mg. per Kg. of body weight daily for ten days. Rather marked toxic reactions have been noted with intravenous administration of the drug; its intramuscular injection may be marked by mild and transient cardiovascular (hypotension, tachycardia) and gastrointestinal (nausea, vomiting) symptoms. Reactions of the Herxheimer type have been reported and, as in treatment with melarsoprol, might be prevented or modified by pretreatment with corticosteroids. A single injection of pentamidine, 4 mg. per Kg. of body weight (maximum 300 mg. per person), is reported to give protection against infection for about six months. The drug is not available for this purpose in the United States, but it may be obtained in the endemic areas.

Melarsoprol has the trypanosomicidal activity of melarsen oxide and also has that drug's ability to penetrate the blood brain barrier, but because of its combination with BAL it is considerably less toxic. It is the drug of choice for treatment of Gambian sleeping sickness with neurologic involvement. In early cases with minimal CNS symptoms, the drug is given in two three-day courses of 3.6 mg. per Kg. of body weight daily, separated by an interval of two weeks. It is administered by the intravenous route. Herxheimer reactions are not uncommon, and to prevent them pre-treatment with corticosteroids is suggested. Nausea and vomiting, also common, may be suppressed by administration of prochlorperazine or other antiemetic drugs. Further neurologic complications are seen in about one-fifth of patients following melarsoprol therapy. BAL is recommended in such cases.

In patients with moderately advanced to severe neurologic involvement, the treatment schedule is modified, and pre-treatment with sur-

---

*Available at present in the United States only from the Parasitic Disease Service, Center for Disease Control, U.S. Public Health Service, Atlanta, Ga. 30333.

amin* (Bayer 205, antrypol), a complex organic urea compound, may be necessary. Detailed instructions for treatment of the various stages of the disease are supplied by the Parasitic Disease Service.

Trypanosoma brucei rhodesiense

In Eastern and Central Africa a more virulent form of trypanosomiasis is seen; it is sporadic in occurrence and generally has a discontinuous distribution. The etiologic agent of this type of infection is *Trypanosoma brucei rhodesiense;* it is carried by *Glossina morsitans* and occasionally other species of game-attacking tsetse flies.

SYMPTOMATOLOGY. The disease picture is similar to that in Gambian trypanosomiasis, but is much more rapidly progressive; patients frequently die before the full development of the meningoencephalitic signs and symptoms seen in the former disease. The incubation period is commonly short, and clinical symptoms may be ushered in with a rigor and severe fever. Trypanosomes appear in the blood early in the infection, and are often present in some numbers. There is usually little obvious glandular involvement, and Winterbottom's sign may not be present. Weight loss is rapid, and the central nervous system is involved early. Untreated persons usually die within nine months to a year after the onset of the disease.

Diagnosis is made as in Gambian trypanosomiasis. The parasites are more readily found in the peripheral blood in the Rhodesian form of the disease. A differential diagnosis can frequently be made on geographical grounds, but there are some areas, such as Uganda, where the two infections are coexistent.

PATHOGENESIS. Development of the infection is similar in Rhodesian to that in Gambian sleeping sickness, save that in the former the infection is more acute, trypanosomes are numerous in the peripheral blood, and there is little lymphadenopathy. CNS invasion takes place relatively early in the course of the Rhodesian infection.

EPIDEMIOLOGY. The vectors of Rhodesian sleeping sickness are game-feeding tsetses. They breed in the lightly covered "bush" rather than along river banks. Control is more difficult than that of *G. palpalis* and its relatives, depending primarily upon the elimination of the wild game, which is their chief source of food, or the widespread use of insecticides.

Unlike *T. brucei gambiense,* the Rhodesian species has a number of animal reservoirs. It has been isolated from the bushbuck, hartebeest, and domestic ox, carried by cyclic transmission through sheep and tsetse

---

*Available at present in the United States only from the Parasitic Disease Service, Center for Disease Control, U.S. Public Health Service, Atlanta, Ga. 30333.

flies for many years (with repeated infections of human volunteers), and there is strong circumstantial evidence of natural human infections from game animals in the bush.

T. brucei rhodesiense infection is sporadic, usually affecting only individuals or small numbers of persons, although localized epidemics may occur. Because the infection tends to be acute rather than chronic, asymptomatic carriers do not play the role in transmission of the disease that they do in Gambian trypanosomiasis.

TREATMENT. Suramin is the drug of choice for treatment of early Rhodesian sleeping sickness. It is a toxic drug, to which a very small percentage of patients will exhibit a marked idiosyncrasy consisting of nausea, vomiting, loss of consciousness and seizures. If a test dose of not more than 200 mg., administered intravenously, is well tolerated, it is given by the same route in a dosage of 10 to 15 mg. per Kg. of body weight to children, or 1 gm. for adults, on treatment days 1, 3, 7, 14 and 21. It should not be given to patients with pre-existing renal disease; if proteinuria appears, the course of treatment should be discontinued. Less severe side effects of suramin treatment include fever, hepatitis, rash, pruritus and edema, pains in the palms and soles of the feet, blepharitis, conjunctivitis, photophobia and tearing. If an early response to suramin is not apparent, consideration should be given to the administration of pentamidine or melarsoprol as used in Gambian sleeping sickness.

In the later stages of the disease, during which there is evidence of CNS involvement, melarsoprol should be used as in the corresponding stages of Gambian sleeping sickness, following the recommendations of the Parasitic Disease Service as to dosage and administration.

Trypanosoma rangeli

Human cases of an apparently asymptomatic trypanosomal infection have been reported from Brazil, Venezuela, Colombia, Panama, El Salvador and Guatemala. The organism has been known as *Trypanosoma ariari* and *T. guatemalensis,* but seems to be correctly named *T. rangeli.* In Panama, *T. rangeli* is found six times more frequently than *T. cruzi,* in a population in which the average combined infection rate is 3.4 per cent *T. rangeli* infections are most common in persons less than 16 years old, being encountered in some 75 per cent of that age group (Sousa and Johnson, 1971). It is transmitted by the bite of the reduviid bug *Rhodnius prolixus* and a few related species. No evidence of pathogenicity has been noted in any of the natural infections, or in human volunteers. The parasites may be isolated from the blood stream for some months after infection. They are about 30 microns in length, with a nucleus anterior to the middle of the body, and a small kinetoplast. Natural infections have been found in dogs, and *T. rangeli* will multiply in a number of laboratory, domestic and wild animals, in none of which it seems to cause disease.

Trypanosoma cruzi

From the southern parts of the United States through Mexico and Central America, and in South America as far south as Argentina, various wild rodents, opossums and armadillos may be found infected with a trypanosome which is also capable of producing disease in man. The organism was first found in the reduviid bug *Panstrongylus megistus* and later in human cases, by the Brazilian worker Chagas, in whose honor the disease has been named. Chagas' disease is caused by *Trypanosoma cruzi*, an organism which differs from other trypanosomes infecting man in that it has an intracellular amastigote stage in cardiac muscle, and other tissues, as well as trypanosome forms in the circulating blood.

The trypomastigotes average 20 microns in length, ranging in their proportions from rather short and stubby to long, slender forms. The nucleus is usually positioned centrally and the large oval kinetoplast is located posteriorly. In stained blood films they characteristically assume a C or U shape (Fig. 43).

T. cruzi develops successfully in a large number of insects, but it is considered that reduviid bugs are the only vectors of importance, and that only those species which invade houses, and which habitually defecate during the process of feeding or immediately thereafter, are major vectors of the human disease. The importance of time of defecation lies in the fact that the trypanosomes develop in the hindgut of the

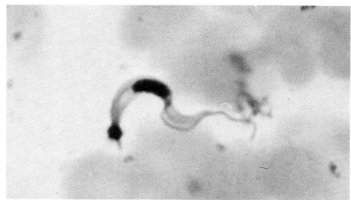

FIGURE 43. Trypanosoma cruzi in blood film. (Photomicrograph by Zane Price.)

insect and are carried in the feces. Unless the insect deposits infective feces near the bite, it is unlikely that parasites will be introduced into the skin through scratching the intensely pruritic lesions.

SYMPTOMATOLOGY. The disease is seen most commonly, and in its most severe form in children under five years of age, in whom symptoms of central nervous system involvement may predominate. In older children and adults the disease usually occurs in a milder, subacute or chronic form, which generally follows an acute attack.

At the site of infection the organisms proliferate, producing an erythematous indurated area, known as a chagoma. This lesion occurs most frequently on the face, but may appear elsewhere on the body. On the trunk, the chagoma may reach a diameter of several centimeters, and become very painful. The lesions reach their full size in a few days, and then gradually subside over a period of two or three months. Trypomastigotes or amastigotes may be aspirated from the chagoma in the early stages of the infection. They spread rapidly to the regional lymph nodes, which become enlarged and palpable within three days. The nodes are hard, and moderately tender, and usually contain amastigote forms. Similar lesions may appear in the first few weeks of infection, apparently by hematogenous spread, and localized areas of hard non-pitting edema may develop in various parts of the body. These appear suddenly, and may subside within a few days or persist for months. While such edematous patches may develop anywhere on the body, they most frequently involve one side of the face. Unilateral edema, affecting both upper and lower eyelid, usually with conjunctivitis, is known as Romaña's sign. The edema usually spreads to involve the cheek and sometimes the neck of the same side; occasionally the eyelids of the other side may be involved, and rarely there is bilateral facial edema. Unilateral ocular and facial edema, involving the submaxillary lymph nodes, is also known as the oculoglandular syndrome (ophthalmoganglionary complex).

Symptoms of generalized infection may appear from four days to two weeks or more after the bite. Organisms appear in the blood at about ten days, and persist during the acute stage; however, they are usually sparse in patients over one year of age. When the infection occurs in infants, parasites will be found in the blood in considerable numbers. Generalized malaise, chills, high fever which may be continuous, intermittent or remittent, muscular aches and pains and increasing exhaustion characterize the acute stage. Epistaxis is common in young children. There is usually a moderate degree of generalized glandular enlargement early in the infection; amastigotes may be found in any enlarged lymph node, but are frequently scanty in all but the regional nodes which drain the chagoma. The spleen becomes palpable, but is generally not greatly enlarged; the liver may be felt several fingerbreadths below the costal margin. A rash may make its appearance approximately two weeks after infection. Pinhead-sized, well-defined red spots, appearing on chest and abdomen, are neither painful nor pruritic and fade in seven to ten days.

The most severe infections are usually seen in infants and are characterized by high fever (sometimes with the "dromedary" curve, or double daily peak, seen in kala-azar) and the development of generalized lymphadenitis, hepatosplenomegaly, and anasarca. These young children may develop signs and symptoms of meningoencephalitis and die of central nervous involvement within a few days or weeks. Older children and adults may show no signs of nervous involvement. Electrocardiographic changes are seen in over 40 per cent of acute cases (Laranja et al., 1956) and consist of prolongation of the P-R and Q-T intervals, low voltage of QRS complexes, S-T depression, and T-wave inversion. Tachycardia, various arrhythmias and cardiac failure may be evident. There is usually a lymphocytosis, though the total white blood cell count may be normal, low, or high. The serum globulin is increased, and albumin is decreased.

An acute attack of Chagas' disease may terminate in a few weeks in death or recovery, or the patient may enter the chronic stage of the infection. Variable periods of remission, and exacerbations marked by fever and the appearance of trypanosomes in the circulating blood, may serve to separate the two stages of the disease, or the chronic phase may be initially asymptomatic. Although trypanosomes are seldom seen in the circulating blood, transmission of the disease by means of blood transfusions has been a problem in certain endemic areas. Chronic infections may be seen in patients who have no history of the acute stage; and if patients are asymptomatic at times, the infection may be diagnosed by electrocardiographic changes. Characteristic alterations in the ECG are seen in a large percentage of patients in the chronic stage of the disease. A majority of such patients will show partial or complete A-V block, complete right bundle branch block or premature ventricular contractions, along with abnormalities of the QRS complexes and of the P- and T-waves (Fig. 44). Symptomatic infections exhibit the signs and symptoms of progressive congestive cardiac failure, primarily right-sided failure, and may occur at any age but are rare in patients under 25 years old. Syncope is common, probably due to complete heart block, and sudden death is not infrequent.

Less common than the cardiac involvement is dilatation of the digestive tract caused by chronic Chagas' disease. Mega-esophagus, usually characterized by dysphagia, and megacolon with symptoms of prolonged constipation, fecal impaction, or volvulus are most frequent, though other parts of the digestive tract may be involved. In endemic

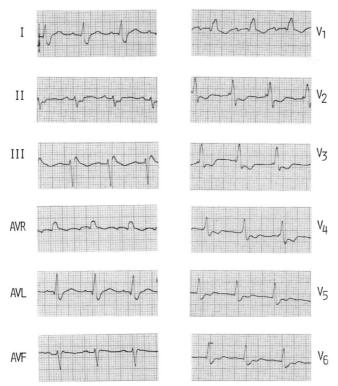

FIGURE 44. Electrocardiographic changes in chronic Chagas' disease. Patient is a 21-year-old Brazilian male. See text for discussion of abnormalities. (Tracings courtesy of Dr. A. Prata, University of Bahia Medical School, Bahia, Brazil.)

areas, it is probable (Atías et al., 1963) that most cases of acquired dilatation of the digestive tract are related to infection with *T. cruzi*. In addition, some authorities recognize forms of the disease which affect the central nervous system, thyroid, and so forth (Köberle, 1968). Most of the symptoms ascribed to these forms of the disease are typical of endemic goiter, which is prevalent in many of the areas where Chagas' disease occurs.

Administration of immunosuppressive drugs to a patient with Chagas' disease may be expected to result in exacerbation of the infection. Kumar et al. (1970) noted that the administration of cyclophosphamide to mice in the early, the subacute and the late subacute stages of experimental infections uniformly increased mortality, parasitemia and severity of the myocarditis.

Definitive diagnosis of *T. cruzi* infection must be based upon demonstration of the parasites. In young children they may be detected in the blood with ease, particularly at the height of the acute stage. In older children and adults, the parasites are frequently very difficult to find. They may be demonstrated by special concentration techniques, by culture or by the method of xenodiagnosis. Various serological methods, which are mainly group-specific for hemoflagellates, are also available. The Machado-Guerreiro test, a complement fixation test using *T. cruzi* antigen, is more specific. These specialized diagnostic techniques are described in Chapter 16. Biopsy of enlarged lymph nodes may reveal parasites in the amastigote stage.

PATHOGENESIS. Upon its entry into the vertebrate host, *T. cruzi* produces an acute local inflammatory reaction. Lymphatic spread then carries the organisms to regional lymph nodes, where upon ingestion by histiocytes or other cells they transform into amastigotes. After local multiplication, the organisms may assume the trypomastigote form to invade the blood stream, carrying the infection to all parts of the body. In the amastigote form, parasites can multiply within the cells of virtually every organ and tissue. Cells of the reticuloendothelial system, the cardiac, skeletal and smooth muscle, and neuroglia cells are preferentially invaded.

The chagoma consists of an intense inflammatory reaction, with invasion of histiocytes, adipose cells of the subcutaneous tissue, and the adjacent muscle cells by the proliferating amastigotes, and of the area by neutrophilic leukocytes and round cells. Eventually a lipogranuloma forms, but not before there has been lymphatic spread of the parasites to the regional nodes.

As infection spreads beyond the regional lymph nodes, trypanosomes appear in the circulating blood, infecting other organs and tissues as they are carried throughout the body. Küpffer cells of the liver, the macrophages of the spleen, and cardiac muscle are especially prone to infection. Within the cardiac muscle, the amastigotes proliferate to form pseudocysts; there is loss of muscle substance, a diffuse inflammatory exudate, and proliferation of interstitial connective tissue. Invasion of the central nervous system is marked by inflammation of the cortex and meninges, with perivascular round cell infiltrates, and small granulomas formed around trypomastigotes or amastigotes in the brain substance around the small vessels.

Early in the chronic stage of infection the heart may be normal in size or only slightly enlarged, although later massive cardiomegaly may develop. There is diffuse inflammation of the myocardium as well as fibrosis and infiltration of lymphocytes, macrophages and plasma cells. The heart weight increases and all chambers, especially the right ventricle, become dilated. Damage to the autonomic nervous system of the heart parallels that to Auerbach's plexus in the walls of the digestive tract. Hypertrophy of the muscle layers and diminution in numbers of the ganglion cells are seen in affected portions of the digestive tract, most frequently in the esophagus and colon.

Levels of both IgG and IgM rise during an acute infection, but decline with treatment (Hanson et al., 1974). Experimental *T. cruzi* infections are not characterized by the sustained elevations of IgM seen in African trypanosomiasis. In the latter, sustained high IgM levels are thought to be due to antigenic variation, presumably less common in *T. cruzi* (Seah et al., 1974).

Circulating antibodies reacting against endocardium, blood vessels, and the interstitium of striated muscle (EVI antibody) have been found by Szarfman et al. (1974) in 95 per cent of patients with chagasic cardiomyopathy, in 45 per cent of asymptomatic patients infected with *T. cruzi,* and to be absent in uninfected persons and those suffering from other types of cardiomyopathy. The antibody is known to cross-react with *T. brucei rhodesiense.*

EPIDEMIOLOGY. The reduviids (also known as cone-nose bugs or triatomids) which carry *Trypanosoma cruzi* are widespread throughout the Americas, and the infection has been reported in a variety of mammalian hosts from the United States southward to Argentina and Chile (WHO Report, 1960). Human infection occurs in the same areas, but the highest prevalence is in Brazil; the disease is nearly unknown north of the Tropic of Cancer. *T. cruzi* has been reported (Kagan et al., 1966) from 14 different species of mammalian hosts in the United States in localities extending from California, Arizona and Utah through the southernmost tier of states to Florida and Georgia and also in Maryland. Only two autochthonous cases have been reported from north of the Rio Grande; both were from Texas. There is serologic evidence for human infection in Georgia as well (Farrar et al., 1972). Sporadic infections are of course encountered in persons coming from endemic areas (Massumi and Gooch, 1965).

In the endemic areas of South America, the prevalence rate is estimated at about 20 per cent of the population at risk, resulting in approximately seven million persons infected. In Mexico the prevalence rate is unknown, but autopsy figures place it under 0.2 per cent of the general population (Tay et al., 1961), and in the United States it is vanishingly small. In South America 20 to 30 per cent of reduviids are infected, and in North America infection rates are similar. However, the loose methods of construction used in human habitations in the endemic areas of South America are much more favorable for domiciliation of the vector than those methods generally employed in house construction in the United States. Certain species of reduviids do not ordinarily defecate at the time of feeding, as do the important vectors of Chagas' disease. The lack of domestic species of reduviids, with proper defecation habits, may explain the fact that this disease seldom infects man in North America. In California, woodrat burrows are frequently very heavily infested with the local reduviid, *Triatoma protracta*, an animal which does not ordinarily defecate while feeding, and it is known that the animals can become infected by eating the insects or licking infected feces from their fur.

The severity of Chagas' disease also lessens with its northward spread. In South America approximately 10 per cent of infected persons die during the acute stage or develop serious myocardiopathy in the chronic stage of the disease. Some workers consider that the demonstrable strain differences in *T. cruzi* from various areas and hosts are reflected in the apparent difference in incidence of cardiopathy, mega-esophagus and megacolon in different areas. More extensive surveillance is needed before this theory can be confirmed or denied.

TREATMENT. The only medication of any value in treatment of Chagas' disease is the nitrofurfurylidine derivative Bayer 2502*, which has shown promise in the treatment of acute or early chronic cases.

Bayer 2502, 3-methyl-4(5'-nitrofurfurylidenamino)-tetrahydro-(1,4)-thiazine-1,1-dioxide, inhibits the intracellular development of *T. cruzi* in tissue culture. It is given orally over an extended period of time, and it is better tolerated in young than in older patients. Informational material furnished by the Parasitic Disease Service should be consulted for dosages.

Leishmania

Among the trypanosomes we recognize complexes of closely related forms, morphologically almost or quite indistinguishable, which produce strikingly different diseases, or which may have entirely different hosts. It is debatable whether those which produce different clinical diseases in man, yet are morphologically indistinguishable, should be considered as the same or as different species. The problem is even more vexatious when it comes to the leishmanias. No morphological differences can be observed between one *Leishmania* and another, and serologic separation of the various types has not yielded clear-cut results. We can, however, distinguish between viscerotropic and dermatotropic species or species-complexes. The various species of *Leishmania* are transmitted by the bite of sandflies belonging to the genus *Phlebotomus*. Amastigotes, liberated from host cells in the insect's gut, transform into promastigotes which multiply and finally pass forward into the

---

*Available at present in the United States only from the Parasitic Disease Service, Center for Disease Control, U.S. Public Health Service, Atlanta, Georgia, 30333.

pharynx and buccal cavity from which they are introduced into a new host when the sandfly again feeds. Host specificity is marked; if more than one species of leishmania occurs in an area, they will be transmitted by different species of sandflies.

Leishmania tropica

The prototype of the dermatotropic forms is *Leishmania tropica*, and all forms which do not invade the viscera may be considered as belonging to the *L. tropica* species-complex. The various entities which may be distinguished on geographic and clinical grounds are considered by some as subspecies and by other authorities as separate species. Lacking a basis on which to make a firm zoological classification of this group, we may consider the various clinical entities as caused by closely related leishmanias, without committing ourselves as to the degree of relationship.

The classical form of cutaneous leishmaniasis is oriental sore, which occurs in almost all countries bordering on the Mediterranean, in Asia Minor, in the Sudan, Ethiopia, the Congo basin and on the West Coast of Africa, in Central and Northern India and in Turkestan. Oriental sore is transmitted by various species of sandflies, belonging to the genus *Phlebotomus*. In man, the amastigotes are ovoid or spherical intracellular bodies, parasitizing monocytes, polymorphonuclear leucocytes and endothelial cells of the capillaries of the skin. The organisms are 1.5 to 4 microns in diameter and contain a rounded nucleus and elongate parabasal body.

SYMPTOMATOLOGY. After an incubation period which is extremely variable in length (as short as two weeks or possibly less, as long as three years; average two to six months), a small red papule appears at the site of inoculation. It may itch intensely, and slowly grows in size to an average diameter of 2 cm. or more (Fig. 45). A serous exudate forms a dry scab which varies in color from whitish to red-brown, and is usually scaly. The surface epithelium, at first covered by dried exudate, finally breaks down completely to form an ulcer. The ulcer enlarges centrifugally, so that it remains more or less circular. It remains shallow, with a bed of granulation tissue and sharply defined, raised edges surrounded by a zone of erythema. The discharge is serous, or sero-purulent if secondary bacterial infection has taken place. Under ordinary circumstances the ulcers are always secondarily infected. The regional lymph nodes may become enlarged and tender; sometimes leishmanias will be found in the nodes but more frequently their enlargement is a response to bacterial infection. If the infection is left untreated, it will gradually heal, usually within a year, leaving a depressed and depigmented scar.

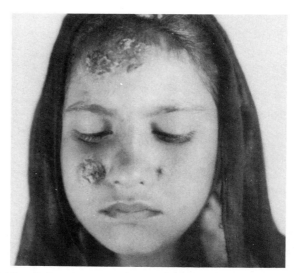

FIGURE 45. Oriental sores on face and forehead. (Courtesy of Ash and Spitz. Pathology of Tropical Diseases, Armed Forces Institute of Pathology, #80,717.)

Usually, a single sore appears. Occasionally there may be more than one, either because of multiple infective bites or through contamination of other areas from the primary sore before any immunity has been developed. Rarely, hundreds of sores may be seen, covering large areas of the body. Since one sore usually confers immunity to reinfection, vaccination of children, on parts of the body where the scar will not be disfiguring, is often practiced in endemic localities (Naggan et al., 1972).

Two forms of oriental sore are recognized. *L. tropica major* causes the rural form, chiefly found as a zoonotic infection among desert rodents, with human disease consequent upon encroachment into their territory, which extends from the Sahara through Syria, Iran, Afghanistan and the Southeastern Soviet Republics. In man, ulcers are of the "wet" type described above. *L. tropica minor* causes the urban form of the disease, chiefly spread from man to man, with dogs as a reservoir. It is seen commonly in Southern Russia, the Middle East and North Africa, and also in Italy. The "dry" lesions characteristic of this type of infection ulcerate late if at all, and heal slowly, while the "wet" lesions are of more rapid onset, and ulcerate early. Infection with *L. tropica major* prevents subsequent infection with *L. tropica minor,* though the reverse does not seem to confer such an immunity.

In South and Central America, several distinct types of cutaneous and mucocutaneous leishmaniasis occur. One type which is primarily cutaneous, and is representative of infections of this nature, is the Chiclero ulcer of Guatemala, British Honduras and Southern Mexico. The lesions are similar to those of oriental sore, but tend to be smaller. They develop slowly, are shallow, and do not cause much tissue damage except when they occur on the ear, for which the parasites seem to have a predilection. Lesions on the ear are slow to heal, and may result in destruction of most of the pinna. The parasite which causes this type of infection is distinguished by some as *L. tropica mexicana* or *L. mexicana.*

Mucocutaneous leishmaniasis is considered sufficiently distinct to justify creation of a separate species, *Leishmania braziliensis*, for its etiological agent. The outstanding feature of this disease, known in Brazil as espundia, is the development, in a variable percentage of patients, of ulcers on the oral or nasal mucosa. In some parts of Brazil, such lesions are said to occur in about one fifth of cases of the disease. The rate of mucous membrane involvement for the endemic area as a whole is considerably lower. The cutaneous lesions develop exactly as does oriental sore, but they are more frequently multiple and may become very large. Secondary infection plays a prominent role in the persistence of these ulcers, and the size which they may attain. Sometimes ulcerations of adjacent areas extend to involve mucosal surfaces, but more frequently these lesions seem to develop by metastasis. The cutaneous lesions may be completely healed at the time mucosal lesions are first seen, or the two types may coexist. In fact, mucosal lesions sometimes develop many years after the patient has left an endemic area, in persons with no history of cutaneous lesions (Walton et al., 1973). If mucosal ulcerations develop, progress of the infection, while slow, is steady. Unless effective treatment is given, the entire nasal mucosa, and that of the hard and soft palates, will eventually be affected (Fig. 46). The nasal septum is destroyed, but unlike similar syphilitic lesions, the bones are not involved. Ulceration may result in loss of all soft parts of the nose, the lips, the soft palate, and so forth. Death usually occurs from secondary infection.

In the mountainous regions of Ecuador, Bolivia and Peru a form of cutaneous leishmaniasis known as uta, which is characterized by dry, generally non-ulcerating cutaneous plaques, has been described. The etiologic agent is considered to be a variety of *L. braziliensis*, but it is sometimes referred to as *L. peruviana.*

In Venezuela, as well as elsewhere in South and Central America, and in Ethiopia (Bryceson, 1969, 1970), another clinical variety of cutaneous leishmaniasis has been recognized. Referred to as diffuse cutaneous leishmaniasis, it is caused by an organism known variously as *L. braziliensis pifanoi*, *L. tropica pifanoi*, and *L. pifanoi*. The initial lesion is a single one, and often a period of months or years (during which the initial lesion may ulcerate or even disappear) passes before it spreads both locally and to distant parts of the body. The irregularly shaped

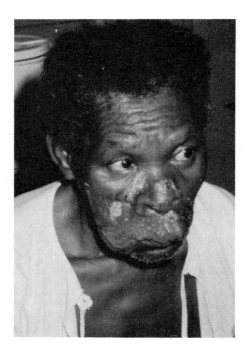

FIGURE 46. Patient with mucocutaneous leishmaniasis. (Courtesy of Dr. Q. H. Geiman, Stanford University Medical School, Palo Alto, California.)

papules, which bear a resemblance to the lepromatous lesions of leprosy, spread slowly and do not ulcerate or heal. The organisms do not invade the viscera, and the patient remains in general good health. The characteristic lesions of diffuse cutaneous leishmaniasis have been considered (Convit et al., 1972) as an expression of an immunologic defect in the host. Patients with this disease react normally to tuberculin, but do not react to the leishmanin skin test, and have normal levels of IgM.

It is very difficult to assess the significance of the different clinical pictures of leishmaniasis seen in various areas. Mucocutaneous lesions have been reported occasionally in true oriental sore. As noted above, they occur in only a small percentage of espundia cases, and the more typical picture varies but little from that seen in Old World oriental sore. Espundia occurs almost exclusively in the hot, moist, rain-forest areas of Brazil, and it may be that climatic factors are of paramount importance in determining the extent and progression of the ulcers, and in predisposing toward mucous membrane involvement. On the other hand, true strain differences cannot be ruled out.

Diagnosis of oriental sore is usually made in endemic areas on clinical grounds, but this requires much familiarity with the disease. It is usually possible to demonstrate the organisms, rounded or oval in shape, 1.5 to 4 microns in diameter, and having a typical amastigote structure, within large monocytic cells obtained by aspiration of fluid from beneath the ulcer bed. Scrapings taken from the ulcer surface will not reveal the organisms, destroyed in areas secondarily infected with bacteria. Culture of N.N.N. medium of material obtained by aspiration or biopsy (Chapter 15) may demonstrate promastigote forms. The Montenegro test, involving the intradermal injection of a killed suspension of promastigotes, is positive in a high percentage of *L. tropica* infections, and in over 95 per cent of *L. braziliensis.* Indirect fluorescent antibody and other serologic tests are also available.

PATHOGENESIS. Upon the bite of an infected sandfly, liberating promastigotes into the skin, the parasites proliferate as amastigotes in the macrophages and the endothelium of the capillaries and other small blood vessels of the immediate area. A granulomatous reaction results in formation of a localized nodule, which ulcerates when the blood supply to the area is compromised by parasite-induced damage to the local blood supply. A pyogenic infection, generally of a trivial nature, develops in the open ulcer bed, and as host immunity increases, the ulcer heals. Whereas in man infection with *L. tropica* is confined to the skin and heals spontaneously, the hamster is unable to develop any tissue resistance and is ultimately killed by the infection which spreads to the viscera. Resistance following a primary infection is nearly absolute, although as mentioned previously infection with *L. tropica minor* may not protect against the *major* variety.

In *L. braziliensis* infections, and very rarely in *L. tropica* as well, the local lesion may undergo typical evolutionary changes and finally disappear, only to have the infection, possibly after a prolonged period of dormancy, appear in adjacent or distant areas. In espundia, organisms may be obtained from scrapings of the nasal mucosa before any tissue damage results from the metastatic infection, suggesting a situation analogous to that in tuberculosis, in which the tissue damage is an effect of hypersensitivity rather than a direct consequence of cellular invasion. On the other hand the extensive indolent lesions of the diffuse cutaneous type suggest a lack of host response to the parasite.

EPIDEMIOLOGY. Although sandflies are the natural vectors of all types of leishmaniasis, contact infection is possible, and vaccination is practiced in certain areas by inoculating serum from naturally acquired lesions into an inconspicuous location on the body of a non-immune person. Mechanical transmission through the bites of flies such as *Stomoxys* has also been documented.

In parts of Central Asia, gerbils are reservoirs of *L. tropica.* The dog and cat are naturally infected in many areas, and in India transmission from dog to man has been demonstrated. In the chicle forests of Mexico and Central America, a number of rodents serve as reservoirs of infection; the role of reservoirs in *L. braziliensis* infection is less clear, although natural rodent infections have been noted.

TREATMENT. Antimony sodium gluconate (Pentostam),* less toxic than the earlier pentavalent antimonials, is the most effective compound presently available for treatment of all the cutaneous infections except the Ethiopian form of diffuse cutaneous leishmaniasis, which is reported (Bryceson, 1970) to respond best to Pentamidine.* Pentostam is administered either intravenously or intramuscularly; the dosage is 10 mg. (0.1 ml.) per Kg. of body weight (maximum 600 mg.) daily for six to ten days. The course may be repeated at ten-day intervals in resistant cases; a maximum of three courses is advised. Pentamidine is administered as outlined below for the treatment of kala-azar. Cycloguanyl pamoate (CI-501; Camolar) is reported to be effective in the treatment of *L. braziliensis* infections when administered intramuscularly at the rate of 300 mg. for adults, 280 mg. for children one to five years of age, and 140 mg. for infants (Peña Chavarria et al., 1965). Amphotericin B (Fungizone) is also reported to yield good results when administered intravenously at the rate of 0.25 to 1.0 mg. per Kg. of body weight, daily or every other day, for periods up to eight weeks.

Coughing, headache and vomiting may be noted with either antimonials or amphotericin; renal damage and bone marrow depression are frequently seen when amphotericin is given for extended periods.

Leishmania donovani

Visceral leishmaniasis, widely known by its Indian name of kala-azar, is prevalent in various parts of that country, especially in Assam and Bengal, in China north of the Yangtze River, in the USSR in Transcaucasia and areas around the Caspian Sea, in countries bordering the Mediterranean, Ethiopia, the Sudan, Kenya and various parts of West Africa, and in widely scattered parts of South America. As in cutaneous and mucocutaneous leishmaniasis, the causative organisms are parasites of the reticuloendothelial system. Unlike those which have been discussed previously, the parasites which cause kala-azar are not confined to reticuloendothelial cells of the subcutaneous tissues and mucous membranes, but may be found throughout the body (Fig. 47). Because of this difference in tissue affinities, a separate species seems justified for the viscerotropic leishmanias. Several different clinical varieties of visceral leishmaniasis may be distinguished, but it seems best to consider that all are caused by *Leishmania donovani*, which may,

---

*Available from the Parasitic Disease Service, Center for Disease Control, U.S. Public Health Service, Atlanta, Georgia 30333.

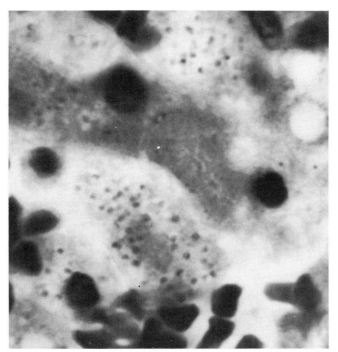

FIGURE 47. Leishmania donovani parasites in Küpffer cells. (Photomicrograph by Zane Price.)

like *L. tropica*, be either a single species or a complex of closely related forms.

SYMPTOMATOLOGY. As in the cutaneous and mucocutaneous leishmaniases, the parasites causing kala-azar are transmitted by various species of sandflies. Promastigote forms of the parasite multiply in the gut of the *Phlebotomus* and migrate anteriorly to escape from the proboscis when the fly feeds. The onset of the disease is gradual, after an incubation period which may vary between two weeks and eighteen months. Frequently the patient may present with a complaint of abdominal swelling, which has taken place without any definite illness. On examination, he will be found to have enlargement of the liver and spleen. Sometimes there is an acute onset, which may closely mimic an attack of malaria, even to the exhibition of a tertian or quartan periodicity. There is sometimes diarrhea, and an onset resembling typhoid fever. If the onset is insidious, there may be only an indefinite feeling of ill health during the earlier stages of the disease. Fever may be continuous, intermittent, or remittent, and recur at irregular intervals. A double or "dromedary" or even triple fever peak daily is characteristic, but is not always seen, as the temperature must be taken every three hours day and night to detect the sometimes transitory peaks. There is progressive loss of weight as the disease pursues its course. The body becomes emaciated, with the abdomen hugely swollen by the enlarged liver and spleen. Both organs are frequently soft, and generally non-tender. Ascites may occur in advanced stages of the disease. Kala-azar means literally black fever, having reference to a characteristic darkening of the skin, which has been most often noted in light-colored Indians and is difficult to distinguish in persons with either very dark or very light skins. It is most marked on the forehead, over the temples and around the mouth.

Leishmania donovani does not under ordinary circumstances cause skin lesions, but a condition known as dermal leishmanoid (Fig. 48) is sometimes seen in patients who have been treated for visceral leishmaniasis, and may occur in persons who deny any history of disease. In the light of the insidious course which kala-azar may exhibit, it is difficult to rule out the possibility of earlier, abortive visceral disease in such cases. The dermal lesions may be erythematous or depigmented macules, distributed over the entire body or in patches. A butterfly

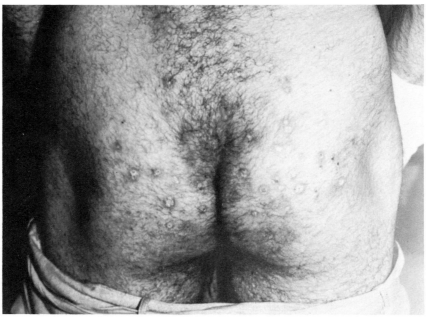

FIGURE 48. Dermal leishmanoid lesions on buttocks. (Courtesy of Ash and Spitz, Pathology of Tropical Diseases, Armed Forces Institute of Pathology, #84,447.)

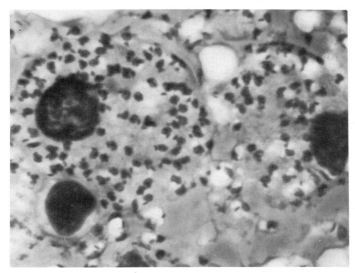

FIGURE 49. *Leishmania donovani,* organisms in spleen impression preparation from infected hamster. (Photomicrograph by Zane Price.)

distribution over the nose is not uncommon. Later the lesions tend to become nodular, and at this stage may be mistaken for leprosy nodules. Organisms may be found in the dermal lesions, and it has been suggested that patients with such lesions represent an important source of infection for the sandfly.

The clinical picture may be suggestive, but a definitive diagnosis rests upon demonstration of the parasites. Splenic puncture is undoubtedly an effective method for securing reticuloendothelial cells for study, but is a risky procedure. Liver puncture is safer, but possibly not so productive. Sternal marrow aspiration may likewise reveal the parasites and is considered by some the diagnostic procedure of choice. Buffy coat films, prepared from venous blood, are sometimes of value. Culture of venous blood, or of specimens of sternal marrow, liver or spleen may reveal the parasites when they are scanty in the original material. Hamsters are very susceptible to the disease, and can be infected by intraperitoneal inoculation (Fig. 49). The Napier formol-gel reaction, performed on serum, is a good presumptive screening test, depending upon the presence of increased amounts of globulin in the serum. In kala-azar and trypanosomiasis, gamma globulins may constitute 60 to 70 per cent of the serum proteins. Interestingly, the Montenegro (leishmanin) test is negative in active kala-azar, but it becomes positive within two months following successful treatment. Presumably it likewise is positive after spontaneous cure; in surveys a leishmanin-positive rate of over 5 per cent is considered evidence of endemic kala-azar. Fluorescent antibody tests have also been developed. Details of the more important diagnostic procedures are given in Chapter 16.

PATHOGENESIS. Although members of the *L. tropica* species-complex have poor invasive powers in man, the same is not true of *L. donovani*, which may parasitize cells of the reticuloendothelial (RE) system throughout the body. The disease is progressive, and the mortality rate in untreated cases ranges from 75 to 95 per cent; death usually occurs within two years. In a relatively mild form, the disease may persist for many years; spontaneous cures undoubtedly occur.

Proliferation of the RE cells, particularly of the spleen and liver, leads to massive hypertrophy of these organs, which may return essentially to normal size after successful treatment. The bone marrow may be involved, resulting in anemia and leukopenia. The white blood cell count is generally below 4000 per cu. mm., often ranging from 2000 to 3000 per cu. mm., accompanied by a progressive monocytosis. Splenomegaly with stasis of blood in the sinusoids may result in increased destruction of both red and white blood cells. Glomerular involvement, with deposition of immune complexes resembling those found in the kidney in human cases of hepatosplenic schistosomiasis, is described by DeBrito et al. (1975). IgG, IgM, and C_3 have been identified from these glomerular complexes. Death usually is the result of intercurrent infection.

EPIDEMIOLOGY. Various clinical forms of visceral leishmaniasis are characteristic of different localities. In general, two different forms of transmission are observed. In the urban form, transmission is primarily from man to man. In this situation younger age groups are primarily affected, the disease is endemic, and dogs may be a reservoir of infection. During an outbreak of kala-azar in Northern Italy in 1971–72, Pampiglione et al. (1975) found that 64 per cent of asymptomatic household contacts, and 40 per cent of neighbors of these patients had positive leishmanin skin tests. They suggest that clinical cases represent that minority of infected persons who do not develop an immune response, allow the parasites to multiply unchecked, and will die without treatment. A rural form of transmission, seen in other areas, is primarily a zoonosis. The infection is epizootic in rodents or other wild animals; man is a sporadic and somewhat accidental victim.

In the region around the Mediterranean, the disease is primarily found in small children, and there is a high incidence of canine infection. This was the first area in which a reservoir host was noted; a separate specific name was suggested for the agent of this infection, *Leishmania infantum*, but it has not generally been accepted. This type of transmission is also seen in China and South America. In India, the infection is primarily one of the adult population, and reservoirs do not play an important role. In the semi-arid Transcaucasian areas, wild jackals serve as a reservoir of infection, which in rural areas occurs primarily in adults. In cities the disease conforms to the urban pattern; the younger age groups are affected and dogs are reservoirs of infection. In Africa a rural form of transmission is generally seen; rats in the Sudan (Hoogstraal and Heyneman, 1969) and gerbils and ground squirrels in East Africa carry the infection which sporadically infects man. Epidemics have occurred in these areas, however. The African forms of kala-azar differ in several ways from those seen elsewhere. Primary skin lesions (leishmaniomas) are characteristic; they generally occur on the legs and represent healed ulcerations at the site of infection. The Montenegro test is often positive in the early stages of the disease, a consequence presumably of the dermatotrophic nature of *L. donovani* strains in this area. Response to therapy with the pentavalent antimonials is generally not as favorable as that seen in other areas.

The ground squirrel strain of *L. donovani* isolated in Kenya is apparently non-viscerotropic in man. Introduced into the skin, it will give rise to a leishmanioma, but it will not extend to produce a visceral infection. At least a temporary immunity is produced against viscerotropic strains of *L. donovani* by this means.

TREATMENT. Antimony sodium gluconate (Pentostam),* administered as described for *L. tropica* infections, is the drug of choice for initial therapy in all but Sudanese infections. Strains acquired in the Sudan are generally resistant to antimonials, and treatment should be initiated with Pentamidine* at the rate of 2 to 4 mg. per Kg. of body weight, given in daily intramuscular doses for 10 to 15 days. Also effective in this disease is ethylstibamine, diethylamine-p-amino-phenylstibamate (obtainable in Switzerland from Bayer under the name Neostibosan), given in daily intravenous dosage, 0.1 gm. the first day, 0.2 gm. the second, and 0.3 gm. daily thereafter until clinical response is noted. A total of 12 to 24 doses may be necessary.

THE TISSUE COCCIDIA

Isospora, discussed in Chapter 5, with species which are intestinal parasites of man and various other animals, is a rather typical coccidian. Two other genera, *Toxoplasma* and *Sarcocystis*, were not until recently recognized as coccidia, because the stages seen in man did not suggest coccidian affinities.

---

*Available from the Parasitic Disease Service, Center for Disease Control, U.S. Public Health Service, Atlanta, Ga. 30333.

While in all three genera oöcysts essentially identical in appearance are produced, details of life cycles of the three genera, and appearance of the tissue stages may vary considerably (Frenkel, 1974). In *Isospora,* the enteric stage is of greatest importance, and oöcysts readily infect members of the species in which they developed. *Toxoplasma* oöcysts, on the other hand, more readily infect a variety of other species (including man); they may also infect the definitive hosts (cats), but with a long pre-patent period. *Sarcocystis* is obligatorily heteroxenous, its oöcysts not being infectious for the host of origin.

Toxoplasma gondii

Toxoplasma is a parasite of cosmopolitan distribution, able to develop in a wide variety of vertebrate hosts, but its definitive host is the house cat and certain other Felidae (Frenkel et al., 1970). It was originally described from a North African rodent called the gundi, from which it derives its specific name. Serologic evidence indicates that human infections are common in many parts of the world, but most are of a benign nature or completely asymptomatic.

Within the mucosal cells of the small intestine of the cat, the organisms develop first to produce schizonts and gametocytes (Fig. 50, *A*) and finally oöcysts which are passed in the feces. These oöcysts, 9 to 11 microns in width by 11 to 14 microns in length, similar in appearance to those of *Isospora belli* but smaller, contain two sporocysts, each of which encloses four sporozoites (Fig. 50, *B*).

Toxoplasma trophozoites may be found in the mesenteric lymph

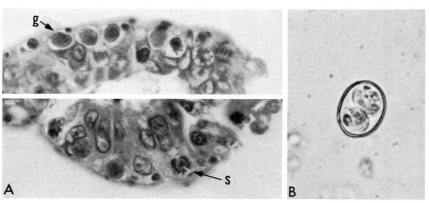

FIGURE 50. *Toxoplasma gondii* in intestine of cat. A, Gametocytes (g) and schizonts (s); 1000×. B, Oocyst containing two sporocysts with sporozoites; 1600×. (Courtesy of Dr. J. K. Frenkel, University of Kansas School of Medicine, Kansas City.)

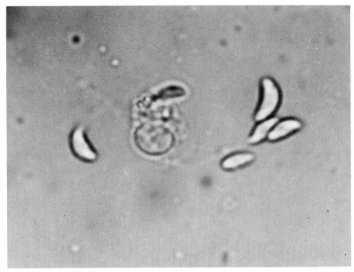

FIGURE 51. *Toxoplasma gondii* from peritoneal exudate of mouse. (Photomicrograph courtesy of Dr. Leon Jacobs, National Institutes of Health.)

nodes and in other organs of the cat, while in other vertebrates these non-intestinal forms are the only stages seen. They are crescentic in shape, and as seen apparently free in the peritoneal exudate of experimentally infected mice (Fig. 51) vary in length from 4 to 6 microns, and in breadth from 2 to 3 microns. Intracellular forms are somewhat smaller, and tend to be less pointed at the ends. Many different tissues may be parasitized by these organisms, especially lung, heart, lymphoid organs, and the cells of the central nervous system. Multiplication of the parasites within an infected cell usually leads to death and rupture of the cell, freeing the parasites to spread the infection to new cells, or may lead to formation of a cyst. Two terms are used for the trophozoites of *Toxoplasma*. The quickly multiplying forms responsible for initial spread of infection and tissue destruction are known as tachyzoites, while the more slowly developing bradyzoites form cysts. Although cysts (Fig. 52) are more characteristic of older infections, perhaps forming as a consequence of increased host immunity, they are present at least in small numbers early in the course of experimental infections.

In zoites stained by any routine method, a spherical nucleus is seen, situated closer to the rounded than to the pointed end. A smaller, dark-staining mass may be visible at the end opposite the nucleus, in organisms stained with certain silver stains, giving a superficial resemblance to the amastigote form of hemoflagellates. The small mass is a structure of unknown function termed a conoid.

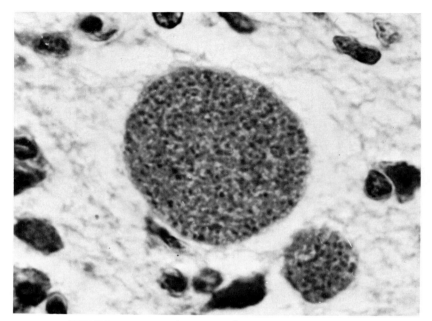

FIGURE 52.   Toxoplasma gondii cyst in brain of mouse.

SYMPTOMATOLOGY. It has been mentioned that the majority of human infections with *Toxoplasma* are benign. In adults, and in children past the neonatal period, the disease is usually asymptomatic. Nevertheless, a generalized infection probably occurs. In a small percentage of cases, symptoms, ranging from mild to severe, will result. Most frequently when symptoms are seen, they are mild in nature. The disease picture may simulate infectious mononucleosis, with chills, fever, headache, myalgia, lymphadenitis and extreme fatigue. Rarely the infection may be severe, with a maculopapular rash in addition to the above symptoms, and sometimes evidence of encephalomyelitis or myocarditis. In a very few cases chorioretinitis will occur, and may progress to produce blindness. In intra-uterine and neonatal infections, however, the picture is the reverse of that seen in older patients. Instead of a majority of asymptomatic infections, most infections contracted during this period are quite severe, and in only a small percentage is there complete recovery. Retinochoroiditis, encephalomyelitis and hydrocephalus or microcephaly are such common sequelae of infection at this stage as to be highly suggestive of toxoplasmosis when seen in very young children. *Toxoplasma* encephalomyelitis may result in cerebral calcifications, demonstrable in x-rays (Fig. 53). Infection in the newborn is marked by fever, pneumonitis and often the development of hepatosplenomegaly. Convulsions are common. There is seldom complete recovery, most infections resulting in blindness or severe visual impairment and mental retardation. In a small percentage of cases there would appear to be a milder systemic infection, with complete recovery. A more extended discussion of clinical aspects of the disease is given by Kean (1972). Recent reports of Kagan et al. (1974) and Samuels and Reitschel (1976) suggest a causal relationship between polymyositis and toxoplasmosis, with improvement of the polymyositis after treatment of the infection and coincident with serologic improvement.

Diagnosis is seldom made by recovery of the organisms, although inoculation of tissues into suitable laboratory animals, such as mice, may demonstrate the infection. The only laboratory tests of value are the various serologic procedures which have been employed for diagnostic purposes. The first of these techniques to be employed was the Sabin-Feldman dye test, a reaction based on the fact that serum from a patient who has had toxoplasmosis will affect toxoplasmas in such manner that they become refractory to staining with a solution of methylene blue. This test requires the use of living *Toxoplasma*, obtained from the peritoneal fluid of infected mice, and is not adapted for use in the average laboratory. The dye test, like the toxoplasmin skin test which is prepared from a saline extract of mouse peritoneal exudate, does not necessarily indicate present infection. As in the tuberculin skin

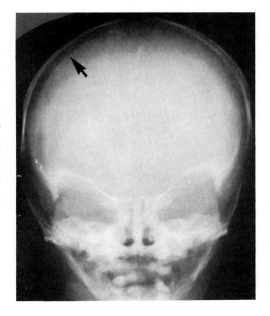

FIGURE 53. X-ray of skull with congenital toxoplasmosis showing calcifications and hydrocephalus. Curvilinear calcific plaque is seen in the right parietal area (arrow). (Courtesy A. Tucker, 1961. Amer. J. Roentg. Rad. Ther., 86:458.)

test, positive reactions may denote either previous exposure or active disease. Indirect fluorescent antibody, complement fixation and hemagglutination tests are also available; the IFA test is now most widely used.

Indirect fluorescent and dye test antibodies are first demonstrable within the first two weeks after infection and may rise to levels of 1:4096 or greater early in infection, falling slightly thereafter but persisting at an elevated level for many months before declining to low levels after many years. The indirect fluorescent and hemagglutination antibodies appear slightly later than the dye test, but parallel it in titer and duration. The complement fixation (CF) test usually appears late in the course of the active infection, generally at a time when the dye test titer is high and stable. A rising CF titer under these circumstances is valuable in demonstrating active infection. The CF titer usually becomes negative within a few years after infection. The skin test usually becomes positive some months after the acute infection; for this reason a positive result excludes a diagnosis of acute toxoplasmosis.

PATHOGENESIS. These obligate intracellular parasites disseminate via the blood stream to many organs and tissues, throughout which they invade the cells, multiply and finally disrupt them. Focal areas of necrosis, surrounded by lymphocytes, monocytes and plasma cells, result from death of the infected cells. Cysts form in many organs, but particularly the muscles and brain, probably as a response to developing host immunity. In the central nervous system, including the eye, an active infection may persist much longer than elsewhere.

In the brain, minute scattered necrotic areas may later calcify, producing a characteristic x-ray picture. Retinochoroiditis may be either a hypersensitivity response to cyst rupture (the more sporadic and evanescent attacks) or a chronic progressive effect of the proliferation of tachyzoites in the retina, an immunologically deficient tissue.

EPIDEMIOLOGY. Toxoplasmosis occurs in a wide variety of both carnivorous and herbivorous mammals and in birds. In man, evidence of infection has been found in all population groups investigated. Prevalence rates vary from place to place for reasons which remain largely obscure. The highest recorded rate (93 per cent) occurs in Parisian women who prefer undercooked or raw meat; at least 50 per cent of their children (in infancy often fed the juices expressed from raw meat) are likewise infected. At a yearly seroconversion rate of from 3 to 5 per cent, such as is seen in central France, fetal risk is highest (Frenkel, 1973), because more mothers in the childbearing range of 20 to 30 years become infected. In areas having such rates, more than 40 fetuses are at risk per 10,000 pregnancies. Lower seroconversion rates, such as are seen in the United States, or considerably higher ones, are both associated with less fetal risk. A small epidemic among medical students in New York apparently resulted from the consumption of undercooked meat, presumably beef (Kean et al., 1969). Contamination of the beef with pork or mutton, from which *Toxoplasma* has more commonly been isolated, could not be excluded. While ingestion of cyst-containing meat may be a common means of infection among carnivores, herbivorous animals must acquire the infection by ingestion of oöcysts. Oöcysts shed in the feces are immature, becoming infective in from 1 to 5 days. They are resistant to acids, alkalis and common laboratory detergents, but are killed by drying or exposure to 55°C for 30 minutes (Dubey et al., 1970). Sporulated oöcysts will survive a temperature of −21°C for 28 days, though the muscle cysts are killed by freezing at −6°C for one day, or immediately at −21°C (Frenkel and Dubey, 1973). Of perhaps great epidemiologic significance is the observation by Frenkel and others (1975) that oöcysts in cat feces survive for a year in the soil in Costa Rica, and up to 18 months (including two winters) in Kansas.

Transplacental transmission usually takes place in the course of an acute but inapparent or undiagnosed maternal infection. In some domestic animals chronic toxoplasmosis may lead to habitual abortion, and it has been suggested that this may take place in man. If so, it is probably quite rare.

Although the complete life cycle of *Toxoplasma* is believed to occur only in felines (Fig. 54), the role of domestic and other cats in dissemination of the infection has not been fully assessed. Wallace (1973) has noted that on Pacific atolls, serologic evidence of infection in the rat population depends upon the presence of cats. On those islands devoid of cats, there is no evidence for infection among the rats. A similar correlation between toxoplasma antibodies in man and the presence of cats was noted in New Guinea by Wallace et al. (1974), who consider that Neotropical Felidae are involved in the spread of infection among Columbian Indians. It is interesting that in the cat, the period which must elapse between ingestion of toxoplasmas and their appearance as oöcysts in the feces varies considerably with the stage ingested. This period is short (3 to 10 days) when the cat ingests cysts from a chronic infection and longer (21 to 24 days) when the infection is initiated with oöcysts. Oöcysts are effective in producing a generalized infection as cysts in a variety of animals.

PREVENTION. Human infection with *Toxoplasma* may come either from consumption or handling of infected meat, or contact with cat feces, in litterpans or soil. Frenkel and Dubey (1972) suggest that meat should be heated throughout to 150°F (66°C) before consumption, and that hands should be washed with soap and water after handling uncooked meat. Indoor cats, fed on dry, canned or boiled food, are unlikely to be infected, whereas those which can hunt, or are fed uncooked food are liable to infection. Such cats' litterpans should be cleaned daily, with feces flushed down the toilet and the pans disinfected with boiling

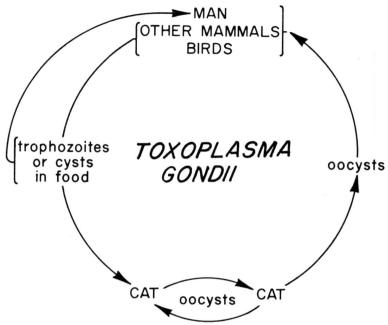

FIGURE 54. Diagram of life cycle of *Toxoplasma gondii.*

water. Pregnant women, unless they have evidence of *old* toxoplasma infection, should avoid contact with cats whose source of food is not controlled, and should not empty litterpans. Disposable gloves should be worn when cleaning litterboxes, and working in soil which may have been contaminated with cat feces. Children's sandboxes should be cat-proofed.

TREATMENT. The only accepted treatment for toxoplasmosis is a combination of pyrimethamine at the rate of 25 to 50 mg. daily for one month, with trisulfapyrimidines, 2 to 6 gm. daily for the same period. Folinic acid may be administered to counteract the bone marrow depression caused by pyrimethamine. In acute retinochoroiditis, a loading dose of 75 mg. of pyrimethamine daily may be used for 3 to 5 days. Corticosteroids may be of value for their anti-inflammatory action.

Sarcocystis lindemanni

Parasites belonging to the genus *Sarcocystis* were first described from mice over 100 years ago, and since that time have been reported from numerous other mammals, especially sheep, cattle and pigs and rarely horses. They occur as elongated cylindrical bodies, sometimes large enough to be visible to the naked eye, in striated and sometimes in unstriated muscle.

Human sarcosporidia were named for Lindemann, credited with the first description of the parasite in man. It is interesting that the organisms described by Lindemann are not now believed to be *Sarcocystis* (Jeffrey, 1974), and indeed of the 28 cases which have been reported, only 16 can be accepted as valid. The scarcity of reported cases is not thought to reflect the true prevalence of this parasite, as many cases are believed to be asymptomatic, and pathologic examination of "normal" muscle tissue is not frequently performed.

Details of cyst morphology and size make it possible to differentiate *Sarcocystis* from *Toxoplasma* cysts in many, though not in all cases. Some sarcocysts may measure less than the 100 microns considered to be the upper limit of size for *Toxoplasma*, but they may attain a length of 5 cm. The limiting membrane may show radial striations (Fig. 55) not seen in *Toxoplasma*, and septa may divide the cyst into compartments. Neither of these characteristics is uniformly seen in *Sarcocystis*, however. The contained trophozoites are considerably larger than those of *Toxoplasma*, measuring 4 to 9 microns in breadth and 12 to 16 microns in length.

It is thought that most human cases are completely asymptomatic, and in 7 of the 16 recognized cases the finding was an incidental one. In 5 cases local symptoms were described, and in at least two of these a myositis seemed associated with presence of the parasite. Frenkel (1971)

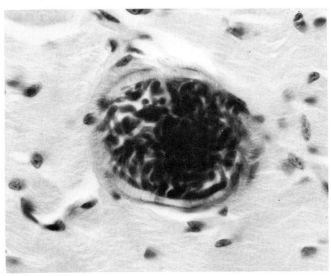

FIGURE 55. Sarcocystis in section of muscle. Note radial striations of limiting membrane. (Photomicrograph by Zane Price.)

describes such a myositis in laboratory animals, accompanying cyst degeneration, and characterized by infiltration of lymphocytes, plasma cells and eosinophils. More generalized symptoms have been described in three of the human cases, including pain and swelling of an isolated muscle, dyspnea and wheezing, associated with eosinophilia.

It will be recalled that the organism previously known as *Isospora hominis* (see Chapter 5) has been found to be the sporocyst stages of two species of *Sarcocystis* from cattle and swine. There are at least three *Sarcocystis* species in cattle, one of which develops in the intestine of dogs and coyotes (Fayer, 1974), and another in cats. Another species of *Sarcocystis* which develops in the cat intestine produces sarcocysts in the muscles of mice (Ruiz and Frenkel, 1976). Much remains to be learned concerning the interrelationships of the *Isospora-Toxoplasma-Sarcocystis* group, the complexities of which have only been touched upon here.

OTHER SPOROZOA

Pneumocystis carinii

Pneumocystis, a small organism of uncertain affinities, generally classed with the sporozoa, causes pulmonary infections in a variety of domestic and wild animals. The first human isolations were from European infants suffering from interstitial plasma cell pneumonia; subsequently it has been reported from all parts of the world. It has come into prominence in recent years as an important cause of pneumonia in patients with congenital and acquired immunologic disorders as well as in the increasing group subjected to immunosuppressive therapy for indications ranging from neoplasia or collagen diseases to organ transplantation (Western et al., 1970).

The organism may be demonstrated in impression smears of lung tissue obtained by open or brush biopsy, or in smears made from tracheobronchial aspirates, stained by the silver methenamine technique of Gomori, but is not ordinarily seen in the sputum, except at times following chemotherapy. They occur in the form of cysts, 5 to 12 microns in diameter, each containing eight nuclei scattered irregularly or arranged in a rosette formation. More frequently seen are single ovoid organisms, 2 to 4 microns in diameter, with a doubly contoured outer membrane (Fig. 56).

SYMPTOMATOLOGY AND PATHOGENESIS. The causative agents of interstitial plasma-cell pneumonia in infants include not only *Pneumocystis* but *Treponema pallidum* and *Toxoplasma gondii*. Descriptions of the clinical and pathological picture in pneumocystis infections are based on fatal cases; what relationship fatal, or even symptomatic, cases may bear

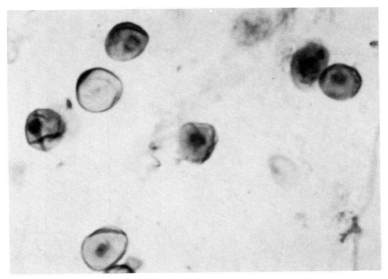

FIGURE 56. *Pneumocystis carinii* from tracheobronchial aspirate; stained with methenamine silver.

to the total infections is not known. As formerly seen in its epidemic form in European hospitals, and now reported from Korea and Iran, the disease primarily affects children between six weeks and six months of age; it seems to have an incubation period of from two to six weeks, and a mortality of from 30 to 40 per cent. It chiefly strikes malnourished premature babies, though full-term infants may be infected. Weakness, followed by progressive dyspnea, tachypnea and cyanosis, is seen, with radiographic evidence of a patchy infiltration of the lungs, classically spreading out from the hilar areas but tending to spare the peripheral parts of the lower lobes (Fig. 57). However, the x-ray picture may be quite variable. A more sporadic form of the disease is seen in immuno-suppressed children and adults, superimposed upon some other chronic debilitating illness. Frenkel (1974) gives a detailed classification of the types of *Pneumocystis* infection.

Physical signs and laboratory findings are not particularly helpful, although blood gas determinations may be of value, indicating hypoxia without acidosis or hypercapnea, along with x-ray evidence of a diffuse pulmonary infiltrate. Both complement-fixation and fluorescent anti-body tests have been described, but are not generally available.

Post-mortem examination reveals an almost homogenous, gray-white consolidation of the lungs characterized histologically by a foamy ground substance containing the parasites either singly or in masses.

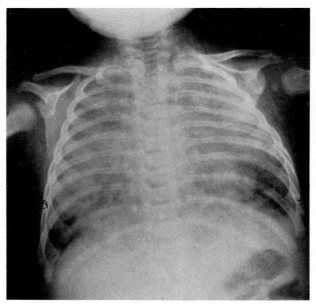

FIGURE 57. Chest x-ray of 10-week-old child with *Pneumocystis* pneumonia. Note sparing of peripheral areas of lower lobes. (From Sternberg, S. D., and Rosenthal, J. H. 1955. Interstitial plasma cell pneumonia. J. Pediat., 46:380–393.)

Intracellular parasites may be found in phagocytic cells in the septa, primarily following chemotherapy. Diffuse interstitial fibrosis may develop in the lungs of patients recovering from *Pneumocystis* pneumonia (Whitcomb et al., 1970).

EPIDEMIOLOGY. *Pneumocystis* pneumonia occurs in two distinct settings. That first recognized was the overcrowded orphanage or hospital situation in which premature and malnourished children were the victims. Epidemics of this sort have now been reported from many areas. A second setting for this type of infection is that of the chronic disease ward, especially those in which malignancies are being treated, or those in which patients are immunologically compromised, either naturally or in the course of treatment of chronic illness. The sporadic way in which such infections occur suggests that an occasional host may have been a long-time carrier of the parasite, which remained inactive until a lowered resistance enabled its unchecked multiplication to begin, and that patient-to-patient infection may then take place.

While air-borne infection seems most common, transplacental passage of the organisms has been reported, resulting in infection of the fetus and stillbirth.

TREATMENT. Pentamidine* is generally considered as the drug of choice for treatment of *Pneumocystis* pneumonia. It is administered by intramuscular injection at the rate of 4 mg. per Kg. of body weight daily for 12 to 14 days. Intravenous administration is apparently accompanied by an increased incidence of severe side effects.

Side effects are common, and must be considered in the light of the severely ill and debilitated patients in which this disease generally develops. Immediate reactions include hypotension, nausea, vomiting, flushing, urticaria, an unpleasant metallic taste, and transitory hallucinations. Pain at the injection site, sterile abscesses, skin rashes, azotemia, hypoglycemia and abnormal liver function tests have also been reported.

An alternate method of treatment involves the oral administration of sulfadiazine, 1 gm. four times daily, and of pyrimethamine 25 mg. once or twice a day, for 14 to 28 days, with 6 mg. of leucovorin daily. The combination of trimethoprim 20 mg. per Kg. body weight with sulfamethoxazole 100 mg. per Kg. of body weight daily, given in four equal doses at 6-hour intervals for 14 days, is reported to be very effective (Hughes et al., 1975).

Babesia

Sporozoan parasites belonging to the genus *Babesia* have long been known as parasites of domestic and wild animals, causing at times inapparent infections, but also causing such economically important diseases as Texas cattle fever and malignant jaundice in dogs. The organisms infect the red cells, in which they appear as somewhat pleomorphic ringlike structures (Fig. 58). Infection is transmitted by various species of ticks, in which a sexual multiplicative cycle occurs.

Few human cases are known, the four reported prior to 1969 having all been in splenectomized persons, three of whom died as a result of the infection (Garnham et al., 1969). Since 1969, seven cases have been found on Nantucket Island, Massachusetts. All of these patients had intact spleens (Western et al., 1970; Morbid. & Mortal. Weekly Report, Sept. 19, 1975).

Clinical illness in the Nantucket cases began 10 to 20 days after a tick bite, and continued for several weeks. It was characterized by the gradual onset of malaise followed by fever, shaking chills, drenching sweats, arthralgias, myalgias, fatigue and weakness. There was hepatosplenomegaly, and five patients had a hemolytic anemia with mild elevations of serum bilirubin or transaminase levels.

---

*Available from the Parasitic Disease Service, Center for Disease Control, U.S. Public Health Service, Atlanta, Georgia 30333.

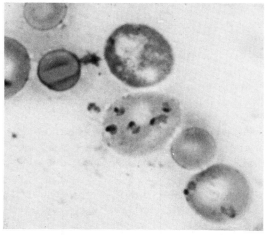

FIGURE 58. *Babesia* in red blood cells. (Photomicrograph by Zane Price.)

All of these patients recovered after being treated with an initial oral dose of 1.5 gm. of chloroquine phosphate, followed by 0.5 gm. daily for two to four weeks.

REFERENCES

Atías, A., Neghme, A., Aguirre MacKay, L., and Jarpa, S. 1963. Mega-esophagus, mega-colon and Chagas' disease in Chile. Gastroenterology, *44*:433–437.

Biagi, F. F. 1953. Algunos comentarios sobre las leishmaniasis y sus agentes etiologicos. Leishmania tropica mexicana, nueva subspecie. Medicina (Mexico), *33*:401–406.

Bryceson, A. D. M. 1969. Diffuse cutaneous leishmaniasis in Ethiopia: I. The clinical and histological features of the disease. Trans. Roy. Soc. Trop. Med. & Hyg., *63*:708–737.

Bryceson, A. D. M. 1970. Diffuse cutaneous leishmaniasis in Ethiopia: II. Treatment. Trans. Roy. Soc. Trop Med. & Hyg., *64*:369–393.

Convit, J., Pinardi, M. E., and Rondón, A. J. 1972. Diffuse cutaneous leishmaniasis: a disease due to an immunologic defect of the host. Trans. Roy. Soc. Trop. Med. & Hyg., *66*:603–610.

DeBrito, T., Hoshino-Shimizu, S., Amato Neto, V., Duarte, I. S., and Penna, D. O. 1975. Glomerular involvement in human kala-azar. Amer. J. Trop. Med. & Hyg., *24*:9–18.

Dubey, J. P., Miller, N. L., and Frenkel, J. K. 1970. Characterization of the new fecal form of *Toxoplasma gondii.* J. Parasitol., *56*:447–456.

Farrar, W. E., Gibbins, S. D., and Whitfield, S. T. 1972. Low prevalence of antibody to *Trypanosoma cruzi* in Georgia. Amer. J. Trop. Med. & Hyg., *21*:404–406.

Fayer, R. 1974. Development of *Sarcocystis fusiformis* in the small intestine of the dog. J. Parasit., *60*:660–665.

Francis, T. I. 1972. Visceral complications of Gambian trypanosomiasis in a Nigerian. Trans. Roy. Soc. Trop. Med. & Hyg., *66*:140–144.

Frenkel, J. K. 1971. Protozoal diseases of laboratory animals. *In*: Marcial-Rojas, R. A., (Ed.) *Pathology of Protozoal and Helminthic Diseases.* 1010 pp. Williams and Wilkins Co., Baltimore.

Frenkel, J. K. 1973. Toxoplasma in and around us. BioSci., 23:343–352.

Frenkel, J. K. 1974. Toxoplasmosis and pneumocystosis: clinical and laboratory aspects in immunocompetent and compromised hosts. In: Prier, J. E., and Friedman, H. (Eds.) Opportunistic Pathogens. pp. 203–259. University Park Press, Baltimore, Maryland.

Frenkel, J. K. 1974. Advances in the biology of sporozoa. Z. Parasitenkd., 45:125–162.

Frenkel, J. K., and Dubey, J. P. 1972. Toxoplasmosis and its prevention in cats and man. J. Inf. Dis., 126:664–673.

Frenkel, J. K., and Dubey, J. P. 1973. Effects of freezing on the viability of toxoplasma oöcysts. J. Parasitol., 59:587–588.

Frenkel, J. K., Dubey, J. P., and Miller, N. L. 1970. Toxoplasma gondii in cats: fecal stages identified as coccidian oöcysts. Science, 167:893–896.

Frenkel, J. K., Good, J. T., and Schultz, J. A. 1966. Latent pneumocystis infection of rats, relapse and chemotherapy. Lab. Invest., 15:1559–1577.

Frenkel, J. K., Ruiz, A., and Chinchilla, M. 1975. Soil survival of toxoplasma oöcysts in Kansas and Costa Rica. Amer. J. Trop. Med. & Hyg., 24:439–443.

Garnham, P. C. C., Donnelly, J., Hoogstraal, H., Kennedy, C. C., and Walton, G. A. 1969. Human babesiosis in Ireland: further observations and the medical significance of this infection. Brit. Med. J., 4:768–770.

Goodwin, L. G. 1970. The pathology of African trypanosomiasis. Trans. Roy. Soc. Trop. Med. & Hyg., 64:797–812.

Greenwood, B. M., Whittle, H. C., and Molyneux, D. H. 1973. Immunosuppression in Gambian trypanosomiasis. Trans. Roy. Soc. Trop. Med. & Hyg., 67:846–850.

Hanson, W. L., Devlin, R. F., and Roberson, E. L. 1974. Immunoglobulin levels in a laboratory-acquired case of human Chagas' disease. J. Parasit., 60:532–533.

Hoogstraal, H., and Heyneman, D. 1969. Leishmaniasis in the Sudan Republic. 30. Final Epidemiologic Report. Amer. J. Trop. Med. & Hyg., 18:1091–1210.

Hughes, W. T., Feldman, S., and Sanyal, S. K. 1975. Treatment of Pneumocystis carinii pneumonitis with trimethoprim-sulfamethoxazole. J. Canad. Med. Assoc., 112:475–505.

Jeffrey, H. C. 1974. Sarcosporidiosis in man. Trans. Roy. Soc. Trop. Med. & Hyg., 68:17–29.

Kagan, L. J., Kimball, A. C., and Christian, C. L. 1974. Serologic evidence of toxoplasmosis among patients with polymyositis. Amer. J. Med., 58:186–191.

Kagan, I. G., Norman, L., and Allain, D. 1966. Studies on Trypanosoma cruzi isolated in the United States: a review. Rev. Biol. Trop., 14:55–73.

Kean, B. H. 1972. Clinical toxoplasmosis—50 years. Trans. Roy. Soc. Trop. Med. & Hyg., 66:549–567.

Kean, B. H., Kimball, A. C., and Christenson, W. N. 1969. An epidemic of acute toxoplasmosis. J.A.M.A., 208:1002–1004.

Köberle, F. 1968. Chagas' disease and Chagas' syndromes: The pathology of American trypanosomiasis. In: Dawes, B. (Ed.) Advances in Parasitology. Vol. 6. pp. 63–116. Academic Press, New York.

Kumar, R., Kline, I. K., and Abelman, W. H. 1970. Immunosuppression in experimental acute and subacute chagasic myocarditis. Amer. J. Trop. Med. & Hyg., 19:932–939.

Laranja, F. S., Dias, E., Nobrega, G., and Miranda, A. 1956. Chagas' disease. A clinical, epidemiologic, and pathologic study. Circulation, 14:1035–1060.

Massumi, R. A., and Gooch, A. 1965. Chagas' myocarditis. Arch. Intern. Med., 116:531–536.

Naggan, L., Gunders, A. E., and Michaeli, D. 1972. Follow-up study of a vaccination programme against cutaneous leishmaniasis. II. Vaccination with a recently-isolated strain of L. tropica from Jericho. Trans. Roy. Soc. Trop. Med. & Hyg., 66:239–243.

Ormerod, W. E., and Venkatesan, S. 1971a. The significance of the choroid plexus in African trypanosomiasis. Trans. Roy. Soc. Trop. Med. & Hyg., 65:231–232.

Ormerod, W. E., and Venkatesan, S. 1971b. The occult visceral phase of mammalian trypanosomes with special reference to the life cycle of Trypanosoma (Trypanozoon) brucei. Trans. Roy. Soc. Trop. Med. & Hyg., 65:722–735.

Ormerod, W. E., and Venkatesan, S. 1971c. An amastigote phase of the sleeping sickness trypanosome. Trans. Roy. Soc. Trop. Med. & Hyg., 65:736–741.

Pampiglione, S., Manson-Bahr, P. E. C., LaPlaca, M., Borgatti, M. A., and Musumeci, S.

1975. Studies in Mediterranean leishmaniasis. 3. The leishmanin test in kala-azar. Trans. Roy. Soc. Trop. Med. & Hyg., *69*:60–68.

Peña Chavarria, A., Kotcher, E., and Lizano, C. 1965. Preliminary evaluation of cycloguanil pamoate in dermal leishmaniasis. J.A.M.A., *194*:1142–1144.

Robins-Browne, R. M., Schneider, J., and Metz, J. 1975. Thrombocytopenia in trypanosomiasis. Amer. J. Trop. Med. & Hyg., *24*:226–231.

Ruiz, A., and Frenkel, J. 1976. Recognition of cyclic transmission of *Sarcocystis muris* by cats. J. Inf. Dis. *133*:409–418.

Samuels, B. S., and Rietschel, R. L. 1976. Polymositis and toxoplasmosis. J.A.M.A., *235*: 60–61.

Seah, S. K. K., Marsden, P. D., Voller, A., and Pettitt, L. E. 1974. Experimental *Trypanosoma cruzi* infection in rhesus monkeys—the acute phase. Trans. Roy. Soc. Trop. Med. & Hyg., *68*:63–69.

Sousa, O. E., and Johnson, C. M. 1971. Frequency and distribution of *Trypanosoma cruzi* and *Trypanosoma rangeli* in the Republic of Panama. Amer. J. Trop. Med. & Hyg., *20*:405–410.

Szarfman, A., Cassio, P. M., Diez, C., Arana, R. M., and Sadun, E. 1974. Antibodies against endocardium, vascular structures and interstitium of striated muscle that cross-react with *T. cruzi* and *T. rhodesiense*. J. Parasit., *60*:1024.

Tay, J., Goycoolea, O., and Biagi, F. 1961. Observaciones sobre enfermedad de Chagas en la Mixteca Baja, nuevo caso humano en la Republica Mexicana. Biol. Ofic. Sanit. Panamer., *51*:322–327.

Wallace, G. D. 1973. The role of the cat in the natural history of *Toxoplasma gondii*. Amer. J. Trop. Med. & Hyg., *22*:313–322.

Wallace, G. D., Zigas, V., and Gajdusek, D. C. 1974. Toxoplasma and cats in New Guinea. Amer. J. Trop. Med. & Hyg., *23*:8–14.

Walton, B. C., Valverde Chinel, L., and Equia y Equia, O. 1973. Onset of espundia after many years of occult infection with *Leishmania braziliensis*. Amer. J. Trop. Med. & Hyg., *22*:696–698.

Western, K. A., Benson, G. D., Gleason, N. N., Healy, G. R., and Schultz, M. G. 1970. Babesiosis in a Massachusetts resident. New Eng. J. Med., *283*:854–856.

Western, K. A., Perera, D. A., and Schultz, M. G. 1970. Pentamidine isethionate in the treatment of *Pneumocystis carinii* pneumonia. Ann. Intern. Med., *73*:695–702.

Whitcomb, M. E., Schwarz, M. I., Charles, M. A., and Larson, P. H. 1970. Interstitial fibrosis after *Pneumocystis carinii* pneumonia. Ann. Intern. Med., *73*:761–765.

World Health Organization. 1960. *Chagas' Disease. Report of a Study Group.* 21 pp. W.H.O. Technical Report Series No. 202. Geneva.

World Health Organization. 1969. *Comparative Studies of American and African Trypanosomiasis.* 39 pp. W.H.O. Technical Report Series No. 411. Geneva.

8

The Trematodes

The Trematoda, or flukes, comprise one class of the phylum Platyhelminthes. Adult trematodes are parasites of vertebrates. Most are hermaphroditic, and many are capable of self-fertilization. Most adult trematodes are dorsoventrally flattened. All flukes have complex life cycles, involving one or more required intermediate hosts. Eggs laid by the adult within the vertebrate host pass outside, and a larva develops within them. This larva, called a miracidium, may eventually hatch and swim away or, depending upon the species, its emergence may have to wait upon ingestion by the next host. In either case, development cannot proceed unless the proper first intermediate host is available—a mollusc (snail or clam). Each of the thousands of species of trematodes requires certain species of intermediate hosts for development, lacking which it will die. A complex series of generations follows within the mollusc, resulting in the liberation of large numbers of larvae of a different type, known as cercariae. Again, depending upon the species of trematode, the cercaria must proceed in a certain way for completion of the life cycle. In some species, it must penetrate directly through the skin of the vertebrate host; in others it enters an insect, fish, or other second intermediate host; in still others it must attach to vegetation and secrete a resistant cyst, waiting to be eaten by the final host. Life cycles of trematodes are among the most varied of all parasites, and they illustrate an extraordinary range of evolutionary adaptations. A "typical" life cycle is shown in Figure 59.

Most trematodes are described as leaf-shaped, but, like leaves, they may vary considerably in form (see Figs. 64, 67, 70, and 71). The largest human parasite belonging to this group is *Fasciolopsis buski*, which may attain a length of 75 mm. and breadth of 20 mm. while not over 3 mm. in thickness. *Heterophyes heterophyes*, the smallest, is under 2

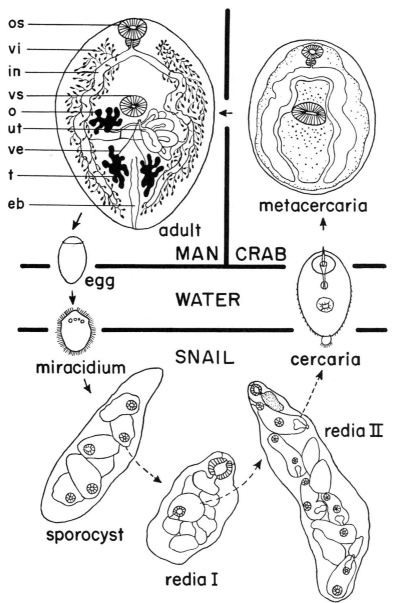

FIGURE 59. *Paragonimus,* an example of a trematode life cycle: *eb,* excretory bladder; *in,* intestine; *o,* ovary; *os,* oral sucker; *t,* testis; *ut,* uterus; *ve,* vas efferens; *vi,* vitellaria; *vs,* ventral sucker. (Adapted from Porter in Burrows, Textbook of Microbiology.)

mm. in length and 0.5 mm. in breadth. The body of a trematode is covered with a resistant cuticle, which may be smooth or spiny. There are two suckers or attachment organs: an anterior one surrounding the mouth, called the oral sucker, and a more posterior one on the ventral surface, called the acetabulum or ventral sucker. The oral cavity leads to a muscular esophagus, from which the thin-walled intestine branches to form two intestinal ceca, which run parallel to each other ending blindly near the posterior end of the worm. Most of the rest of the body is taken up with reproductive organs and associated structures. There are usually two testes leading, by means of long thin ducts, to the genital pore, which usually lies in the region of the ventral sucker. There is a single ovary, from which arises a tubule differentiated near its origin to form a seminal receptacle. A series of glandular structures called vitellaria, usually in two masses lying lateral to the intestinal ceca, produce the shell material. Vitelline ducts lead inward from the vitellaria to the region of the ovary; the ducts from the ovary, the seminal receptacle and the vitellaria come together at Mehlis' gland, and here the shell is formed over the ovum. The uterus arises from Mehlis' gland, and winds forward to the genital pore. In most trematodes, the uterus is the largest organ in the body, filled with many thousands of eggs.

Trematode eggs have a smooth hard shell, which is transparent and generally of a yellow-brown or brown color. They range in length from under 30 microns to as much as 175 microns, depending upon the species. The majority are close to what would be considered a conventional egg shape. Most have an operculum or cap at one end, an "escape hatch" through which the miracidium emerges. This operculum may be difficult to detect, but it can usually be seen by careful focusing with reduced illumination. The miracidium is covered with cilia, and in some species can be seen to be fully developed when the eggs are passed in the feces. The shell may be smoothly continuous in outline, or there may be a slight flare, marking the line of cleavage between shell and operculum. The flared portion of the shell, into which the operculum fits, is known as the opercular shoulders. Possession of these shoulders is characteristic of the eggs of certain species. Spines may be present, either very small and inconspicuous as in *Opisthorchis*, or large and striking as in certain species of *Schistosoma*. Eggs of the schistosomes are non-operculate, and the egg is irregularly ruptured in hatching. Trematode eggs cannot successfully be concentrated by the zinc-sulfate technique, as both operculate and non-operculate forms rupture and fail to float. Formalin-ether concentrates are quite satisfactory, or the sediment of the zinc-sulfate concentrate may be examined for the eggs which are still recognizable even when ruptured.

We shall describe only the most common infections of man. A listing of rarer ones is given by Healy (1970).

INTESTINAL FLUKES

Fasciolopsis buski

The giant intestinal fluke, *Fasciolopsis buski* (Fig. 60), is found in China (including Taiwan), Vietnam, Thailand and in parts of Indonesia and the Indian subcontinent. Adult worms live attached to the bowel wall, primarily in the duodenum and jejunum; in heavy infections they may be found throughout the intestinal tract.

Infection is acquired by ingestion of the metacercariae, encysted on fresh-water vegetation (Fig. 61) such as bamboo shoots or water chestnuts, which may be consumed raw or peeled with the teeth. Reservoir hosts include pigs, dogs, and rabbits.

Adult worms will be seen only following purgation after specific anthelmintic treatment. They are fleshy worms, 2 to 7.5 cm. in length by 0.8 to 2 cm. in width. The ellipsoid eggs (Fig. 62) are yellowish-brown in color. The shell is transparent, with a small operculum at the more pointed end. Eggs are unembryonated when first passed, containing early cleavage stages; they measure 130 to 140 microns in length by 80 to 85 microns in breadth.

SYMPTOMATOLOGY AND PATHOGENESIS. Attachment of these large worms to the mucosa of the bowel causes local inflammation and ulceration, sometimes accompanied by hemorrhage. A few worms will not give rise to any recognizable symptoms, but with heavier infections there may be abdominal pain, at times suggestive of duodenal

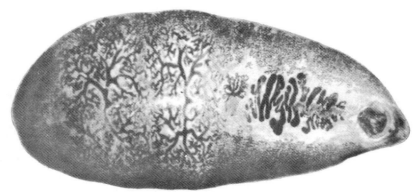

FIGURE 60. *Fasciolopsis buski*. (Photomicrograph by Zane Price.)

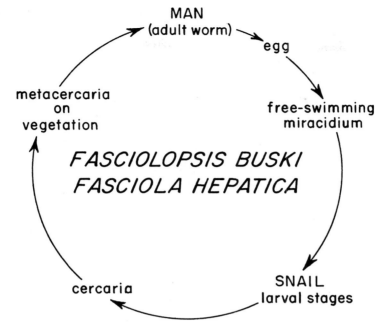

FIGURE 61. Schematic representation of life cycle of those trematodes acquired by man through ingestion of raw aquatic vegetation.

ulcer disease, and diarrhea. In heavy infections (with hundreds or perhaps thousands of worms in the bowel) the stools are profuse and light yellow in color, and contain much undigested food; they are suggestive of a malabsorptive process, such as seen in giardiasis. Intestinal obstruction may occur. Edema and ascites, which may develop in severe infections, have traditionally been considered as secondary to the absorption of worm toxins, but these symptoms can perhaps more rationally be ascribed to a hypoalbuminemia resulting from long-continued malabsorption, or from a protein-wasting enteropathy. A marked eosinophilia is usually seen.

TREATMENT. Hexylresorcinol crystoids, available in the form of hard gelatine capsules containing 0.1 and 0.2 gm. of the drug, and tetrachloroethylene, which comes in soft gelatine capsules containing 0.5 and 1.0 ml. of the drug, are both effective in treatment of fasciolopsiasis, but repeated courses may be necessary. Unfortunately tetrachloroethylene, while approved for human use, is generally available only as a veterinary product (which, however, meets all USP standards).

Hexylresorcinol is administered in the morning before the patient has anything to eat, in doses ranging from 0.4 gm. for children 1 to 7 years of age to 1.0 gm. for children over 13 and adults. A saline purge

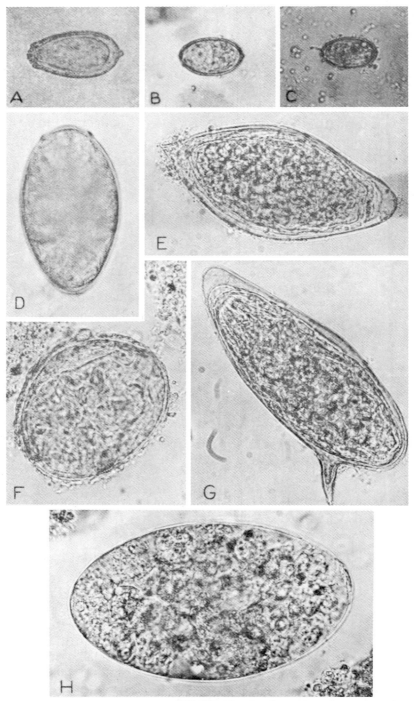

FIGURE 62. See legend on the opposite page.

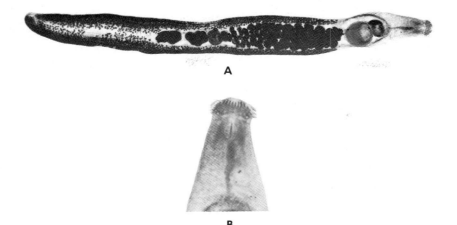

FIGURE 63. *A, Echinostoma* sp; *B,* anterior end of *Echinostoma,* showing circumoral spines. (Photomicrographs by Zane Price.)

may be given two hours after administration of the drug. Tetrachloroethylene is given on an empty stomach, in a dose of 0.10 to 0.12 ml. per Kg. of body weight. Purgation is neither necessary nor desirable, as it increases toxicity of the drug. No alcoholic beverages should be taken before or for 24 hours after treatment.

The Echinostomes

A number of medium-sized intestinal flukes, belonging to the genus *Echinostoma* and to several related genera, have been reported from the Philippines, Malaya, the Celebes and a few other localities in Asia. They live attached to the wall of the small intestine, where they may produce an inflammatory reaction and ulceration, leading to diarrhea. They average under 1 cm. in length and 0.2 cm. in width, and are distinguished by possession of a collarette of spines on a disk surrounding the oral sucker (Fig. 63). The most important species is *Echinostoma ilocanum*, which occurs in the Philippines. Human infections are accidental; the worms are found in a variety of mammals whose food habits promote infection.

FIGURE 62. Some trematode eggs: *A, Opisthorchis sinensis; B, Heterophyes heterophyes; C, Metagonimus yokogawai; D, Paragonimus westermanii; E, Schistosoma haematobium; F, S. japonicum; G, S. mansoni; H, Fasciolopsis buski.* All figures 500× except *A,* which is 830×. (Courtesy of Hunter, G. W., Swartzwelder, J. C., and Clyde, D. F. 1976. Tropical Medicine. 5th Ed. W. B. Saunders Company, Philadelphia.)

The worms are acquired through ingestion of the second intermediate host, which may be any of a number of large, edible fresh-water snails or other molluscs in which the metacercariae encyst.

The adult worms are seen only after treatment, but can be recognized by the circumoral spines. The unembryonated eggs are similar in shape to those of *Fasciolopsis,* and vary in size in the different species. Some species overlap the size range of *Fasciolopsis,* and therefore an exact identification cannot be made from examination of the eggs. Frequently a diagnosis can be established on the basis of the patient's past history or the clinical findings.

Tetrachloroethylene, as used in the treatment of fasciolopsiasis, is effective in echinostome infections.

The Heterophyids

Two minute flukes, *Heterophyes heterophyes* and *Metagonimus yokogawai* (Fig. 64), occur in Japan, Korea, China (including Taiwan), and the

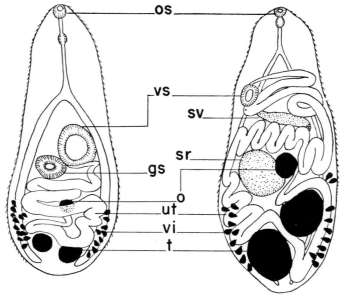

Heterophyes   **Metagonimus**

FIGURE 64.   Heterophyes heterophyes and *Metagonimus yokogawai:* gs, genital sucker; o, ovary; os, oral sucker; sr, seminal receptacle; sv, seminal vesicle; t, testis; ut, uterus; vi, vitellaria; vs, ventral sucker. Drawings made with the aid of a camera lucida, magnification approximately 40×.

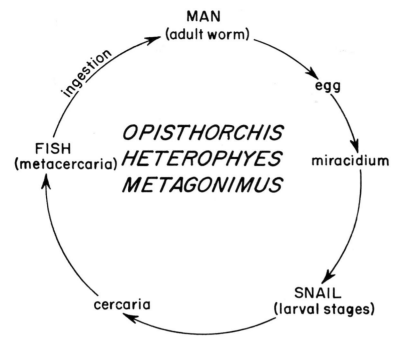

FIGURE 65. Schematic representation of life cycles of trematodes acquired by man through ingestion of raw fish.

Philippines. *Heterophyes* has also been reported from Egypt and Israel, and *Metagonimus* from the Balkans, Spain, Israel, the U.S.S.R. and Indonesia. The parasites live attached to the wall of the small intestine, where they produce no apparent symptoms unless present in very large numbers. Chronic intermittent diarrhea, nausea, and vague abdominal complaints have been reported. *Metagonimus* is somewhat larger than *Heterophyes*, but does not exceed 2.5 mm. in length by 0.75 mm. in width. *Heterophyes* has a third sucker, surrounding the genital pore; this structure is not present in *Metagonimus.*

Heterophyids are acquired through ingestion of raw or pickled fresh-water fish of a large number of kinds (Fig. 65). Metacercariae of the heterophyid flukes encyst under the scales or in the flesh of fish, and are not killed by the various pickling processes to which fish is sometimes subjected. Thorough cooking will, of course, kill them. A variety of fish-eating mammals serve as reservoir hosts for both of the heterophyids which infect man.

The adult worms will be seen in the feces only following anthelmintic treatment. The eggs which contain fully developed miracidia and possess prominent opercular shoulders, are brownish-yellow in color. Those of *Heterophyes* average very slightly larger than those of *Metagonimus*, but differences are too slight to be of value. The size range for the two species is 26.5 to 30 microns in length, by 15 to 17 microns in breadth. The eggs closely resemble in size and shape those of worms belonging to the genus *Opisthorchis*.* Some morphological differences have been described, but these are slight and not constant.

Tetrachloroethylene, as used in the treatment of fasciolopsiasis, is effective in heterophyid infections, as is bephenium hydroxynaphthoate in a single oral dose of 5 gm.

THE LIVER FLUKES

Three genera of quite dissimilar trematodes are parasites of the biliary passages of man. Two of them, *Opisthorchis* and *Dicrocoelium*, are relatively elongate and narrow-bodied worms, which tend to localize in the smaller, more distal parts of the biliary tree. Only in heavy infections are these worms found in the common duct or gallbladder. *Fasciola*, a much larger worm, is confined by its size to the larger passages.

These worms all produce hyperplastic changes in the epithelium of the bile ducts and fibrosis around them. Massive infection by any of these worms may lead to portal cirrhosis, with all its associated manifestations.

The eggs of the opisthorchid flukes are very similar in appearance to those of the heterophyids, while those of *Fasciola* closely resemble both *Fasciolopsis* and the echinostomes. If eggs of one of these forms are found in the stool, and a differential diagnosis between hepatic and intestinal infection cannot be made on clinical grounds, examination of bile obtained by duodenal drainage will provide the correct answer. If one is successful in obtaining uncontaminated bile, and eggs are found in this material, they must have been produced by worms in the liver or gallbladder.

Opisthorchis sinensis

The Chinese liver fluke, *Opisthorchis sinensis* (Figs. 66 and 67), occurs in large areas of China, including Taiwan, Japan and Korea, and Vietnam. It is of moderate size, from 1 to 2.5 cm. in length by 0.3 to 0.5 cm. in width. It is broadest in the mid-portion of the body,

---

*Most modern authorities (Dawes, 1946) consider *Clonorchis* to be a synonym of *Opisthorchis*. We will therefore refer to the Chinese liver fluke as *Opisthorchis sinensis*.

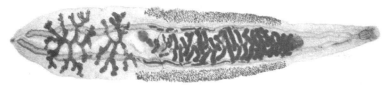

FIGURE 66. *Opisthorchis sinensis.* (Photomicrograph by Zane Price.)

tapering toward both ends. Adult worms live in the bile ducts, and apparently localize first in the more distal portions, just under the capsule of the liver. In more massive infections they will occupy most of the bile passages, and may even be found in the gallbladder and pancreatic duct.

Human infection results from the consumption of fresh-water fish containing the encysted metacercariae (Fig. 65). Fish may be eaten raw,

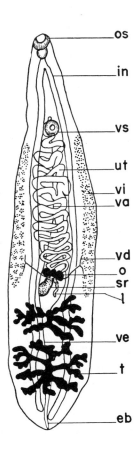

FIGURE 67. *Opisthorchis sinensis: eb,* excretory bladder; *in,* intestine; *l,* Laurers' canal; *o,* ovary; *os,* oral sucker; *sr,* seminal receptacle; *t,* testis; *ut,* uterus; *va,* vas deferens; *vd,* vitelline duct; *ve,* vas efferens; *vi,* vitellaria; *vs,* ventral sucker. Drawing made with the aid of a camera lucida.

pickled, smoked or dried. The disease has been reported in native Hawaiians as a result of consumption of infected fish imported from the Orient. Dogs and cats are the most important reservoir hosts.

The adult worms are seen only at autopsy, or rarely upon surgical removal. Eggs are found in the feces, and as the average daily output per worm is probably over 2400 eggs, they may be very numerous. Eggs of *Opisthorchis sinensis* (Fig. 62, *A*) resemble very closely those of *Heterophyes* and *Metagonimus*, but may have a small comma-shaped process at the abopercular end. This process, if present, is diagnostic of *Opisthorchis*. The average length is 29 microns, and breadth 16 microns, which falls within the *Heterophyes-Metagonimus* range. The extreme measurements are significantly higher than those of the heterophyid worms, being about 35 microns in length and 19.5 microns in breadth for eggs of *O. sinensis*.

Diagnosis is by recovery of the eggs from the feces or in duodenal aspirates. Complement fixation and intradermal tests have been described, but they are not generally available.

SYMPTOMATOLOGY. Light infections, which are the rule, are generally asymptomatic. Heavier infections, if acquired over an extended period of time, seldom cause early symptoms. The ingestion of large numbers of metacercariae over a short period of time may produce symptomatic early infections (Koenigstein, 1949). The acute period lasts less than a month and may be characterized by fever, diarrhea, epigastric pain, anorexia, enlargement and tenderness of the liver, and sometimes jaundice. There may be a leukocytosis, and eosinophilia is generally present. Eggs appear in the feces in about a month, and the acute symptoms subside. Strauss (1962) has emphasized that patients acutely infected and not subject to repeated reinfection do not generally have any recognizable symptoms from their chronic low-grade infections.

Heavy worm burdens—the result of repeated infection over a period of years—may result in a degree of functional impairment of the liver; this impairment is secondary to localized biliary obstruction and is at times aggravated by intrahepatic stone formation, cholangitis, and the formation of multiple liver abscesses (Hou, 1955). Cholecystitis and cholelithiasis may be the result of invasion of the gallbladder by these worms, which have also been considered to cause acute pancreatitis (MacFadzean and Yeung, 1966). Cirrhosis is probably a rare complication, related more to chronic malnourishment than to the parasitic infection.

PATHOGENESIS. Thickening and localized dilatation of the bile ducts is seen in heavy infections, accompanied by a moderate to quite marked hyperplasia of the small mucinous glands of the duct mucosa. The degree to which both of these changes may take place bears a direct relationship to the degree of infection. However, these adenomatous changes may persist for many years in patients whose infections have become very light. Hou (1956) described adenocarcinomas arising from the hyperplastic bile duct mucosa in persons infected with *O. sinensis* and concluded that they had been induced by the infection.

TREATMENT. At present there is no satisfactory treatment for this infection. Chloroquine has been widely used for this purpose; it is probably not curative, but it produces a temporary inhibition of egg production. Hetol, or 1,4-bis (trichloromethyl) benzene, has been used in China and Japan (Yokogawa et al., 1967) but is unavailable in the United States. Bithionol* is a drug which, on the basis of preliminary trials as well as its usefulness in related infections, may deserve further clinical trials. See discussion under treatment of paragonimiasis.

A comprehensive account of clonorchiasis was published by Komiya (1966).

Opisthorchis felineus

As the name suggests, *Opisthorchis felineus* parasitizes cats. In central and eastern Europe and in Siberia it is prevalent in both cats and dogs; in various sectors where the human population eats raw or pickled fish, man is also infected. It is particularly prevalent as a human parasite in East Prussia, Poland and parts of Siberia. Human infections have also been reported from the Philippines, Korea, Japan, North Vietnam and India, although there is some question as to whether or not the parasite is indigenous to all of these areas. Like *O. sinensis*, *O. felineus* inhabits the bile ducts, and much the same disease picture is produced by both parasites. The life cycle of the two parasites is likewise similar.

The adult *Opisthorchis felineus* differs from *O. sinensis* only in some relatively minor details of structure. Eggs of *O. felineus* are narrower than those of *O. sinensis*, averaging 30 microns in length by only 11 to 12 microns in width. They are otherwise indistinguishable.

Opisthorchis viverrini

A third species of *Opisthorchis* has been extensively investigated by Sadun (1955) and others. *Opisthorchis viverrini* has been reported only from northern Thailand, where it is a major public health problem. It is quite possible, however, that *O. felineus* infections reported from neighboring areas, such as North Vietnam, may in reality be caused by *O. viverrini*. Details of life cycle and host-parasite relationships are similar to those of the other two species.

*Available from the Parasitic Disease Service, Center for Disease Control, U. S. Public Health Service, Atlanta, Ga. 30333.

The adult *O. viverrini* differs only slightly in structure from the other two species. The eggs are relatively short and broad, with an average length of 26.7 microns and breadth of 15 microns.

Dicrocoelium dendriticum

A common parasite of the biliary tree of herbivores in many parts of the world is *Dicrocoelium dendriticum* (Fig. 68), a fluke of about the same size and shape as *Opisthorchis*. Many human infections with this parasite have in fact been spurious, the result of consumption of infected liver with subsequent appearances of the ingested eggs in the feces. Other reports, from many parts of the world, have been true *Dicrocoelium* infections. As will be seen from a consideration of the life cycle, such human infections must be uncommon. *Dicrocoelium* is similar to *Opisthorchis* both as regards localization and the pathological lesions produced. After ingestion, the metacercariae excyst in the duodenum and pass through the common bile duct to invade the biliary system (Krull, 1958). Human infections are usually light, and symptoms are not generally severe.

The life cycle of this parasite (Krull and Mapes, 1952) is most unusual. Eggs of this parasite, fully embryonated when passed in the feces, are ingested by land snails, in which they undergo a developmental cycle. Cercariae are liberated from the snails during rainy periods, and become massed in "slime balls," shed on vegetation as the snail crawls. These slime balls, each of which contains large numbers of cercariae, are eaten by ants. In this host, the cercariae become encysted to form metacercariae. For man to acquire this disease, he must ingest an infected ant.

The adult worm is easily distinguishable from *Opisthorchis* in that its testes are situated in the anterior third of the body, while in *Opisthorchis* they are in the posterior third. The eggs, passed in the feces, are dark

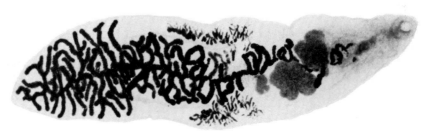

FIGURE 68. Dicrocoelium dendriticum. (Photomicrograph by Zane Price.)

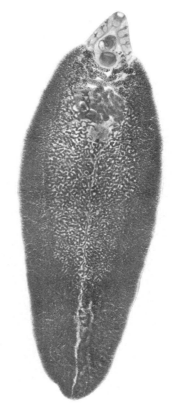

FIGURE 69. *Fasciola hepatica.* (Photomicrograph by Zane Price.)

brown in color, thick shelled, and with a large operculum. They measure 38 to 45 microns in length by 22 to 30 microns in breadth.

Bithionol* and thiabendazole are reported to be effective against dicrocoeliasis in sheep; no effective treatment is known for this condition in man.

Fasciola hepatica

The sheep liver fluke *Fasciola hepatica* (Figs. 69, 70) is a common parasite of herbivores, and one which is cosmopolitan in its distribution. Human infections (Hadden and Pascarelli, 1967) have been reported from many parts of the world. In Southern France and Algeria, as well as Cuba and some other Latin American countries, this parasite

---

*Available from the Parasitic Disease Service, Center for Disease Control, U.S. Public Health Service, Atlanta, Ga. 30333, but only for treatment of paragonimiasis.

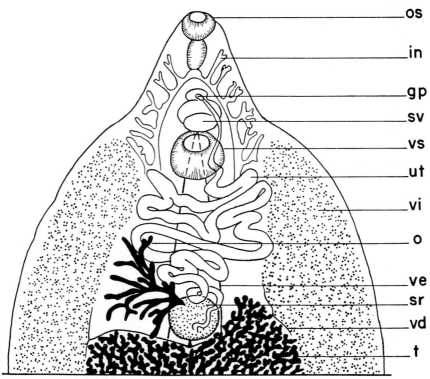

FIGURE 70. *Fasciola hepatica,* anterior end of worm: *gp,* genital pore; *in,* intestine; *o,* ovary; *os,* oral sucker; *sr,* seminal receptacle; *sv,* seminal vesicle; *t,* testis; *ut,* uterus; *vd,* vitelline duct; *ve,* vas efferens; *vi,* vitellaria; *vs,* ventral sucker. Drawing made with the aid of a camera lucida but somewhat diagrammatic.

has become of considerable public health importance. *Fasciola* is a large fluke, measuring as much as 3 cm. in length and nearly 1.5 cm. in width. Its shape is characteristic, by virtue of a "cephalic cone" at the anterior end. The adult worms reside in the larger biliary passages and gallbladder.

Unlike the opisthorchids, which enter the biliary tree in a conventional manner by passage through the ampulla of Vater and ascent of the common bile duct, *Fasciola* metacercariae burrow into and through the duodenal wall, migrate actively across the peritoneal cavity, and enter the bile ducts via Glisson's capsule and the liver parenchyma. It is not surprising that some are lost on the way, and occasionally may develop in the peritoneal cavity or other ectopic foci. In human infections, symptoms are occasionally seen which suggest that there may be considerable local irritation during the migration of the young worms to the liver. In sheep, migration through the liver parenchyma gives rise to such massive tissue destruction that the disease at this stage is known as liver rot. Once established in the bile ducts, the worms may produce both mechanical and toxic effects, which differ from those seen with infection by the opisthorchids or *Dicrocoelium* only inasmuch as *Fasciola* is a larger and more powerful worm. Mechanical irritation, the effects of toxic metabolites of the worms on host tissue and mechanical obstruction may bring about hyperplasia of the biliary epithelium, proliferation of connective tissue around the ducts, and partial or total biliary obstruction. The adult worms may erode through the walls of the bile ducts to invade once again the liver parenchyma. Secondary bacterial infection may occur; portal cirrhosis is usually the final outcome in severe infections. Light infections may, however, be almost asymptomatic.

Infection occurs following the consumption of aquatic vegetation upon which metacercariae of *Fasciola* have become encysted (Fig. 61). Human cases can usually be traced to infected water cress, which should never be grown for human use in water to which herbivores have access.

Eggs of *Fasciola* will be found in the feces, but cannot readily be differentiated from those of *Fasciolopsis* (Fig. 62) and the echinostomes. They are operculated and measure 130 to 150 microns in length and 63 to 90 microns in breadth.

Emetine hydrochloride has been used for many years in the treatment of this infection, at dosages ranging from 30 mg. daily for 18 days, to 1 mg. per Kg. (maximum 65 mg.) daily for 10 to 12 days. Dehydroemetine* is reportedly likewise effective, and less toxic. On the basis of preliminary studies, bithionol* may be effective in treatment of this condition. It is administered orally at the rate of 50 mg. per Kg. of body weight every other day for 20 days.

Fasciola gigantica

The giant liver fluke, *Fasciola gigantica*, may attain a length of 7.4 cm. It has a more attenuated shape than *F. hepatica*, from which it also differs in some details of structure. *Fasciola gigantica* is a parasite of herbivores, particularly camels, cattle and water buffalo in Africa and the Orient. It has been introduced into other areas, and human cases have been reported from several regions, including Hawaii.

The life cycle of the parasite is very similar to that of *F. hepatica*,

---

*Available from the Parasitic Disease Service, Center for Disease Control, U.S. Public Health Service, Atlanta Ga. 30333, but only for treatment of paragonimiasis.

and the clinical picture in the two infections is also much alike. The eggs of *F. gigantica* are large, measuring 150 to 190 microns in length by 70 to 90 microns in breadth.

THE BLOOD FLUKES

Three species of schistosomes which parasitize man are of major importance. They are *Schistosoma mansoni, S. japonicum,* and *S. haematobium.* Of lesser significance are *S. intercalatum* and perhaps the *S. japonicum*-like infection in the Mekong Basin. Although the adult worms live in the blood vascular system, the eggs of *S. mansoni, S. japonicum* and *S. intercalatum* are generally found in the feces. Eggs of *S. haematobium* are occasionally seen in the stool but usually occur in the urine.

The schistosomes differ in a number of ways from other trematodes. They are diecious, and the two sexes are dissimilar in appearance. Female worms are long and slender, 1.2 to 2.6 cm. in length, with a body almost circular in cross section and 0.3 mm. or less in diameter. Male worms (Fig. 71) are from 0.6 to 2.2 cm. long, and while the body is flattened behind the ventral sucker, it looks cylindrical, as it is characteristically incurved ventrally to form a gynecophoral canal in which the female reposes (Figs. 72 and 73).

Body structure of the schistosomes, and particularly that of the long thin females, seems clearly an adaptation to an intravascular existence. The females leave the male worms to deposit their eggs in

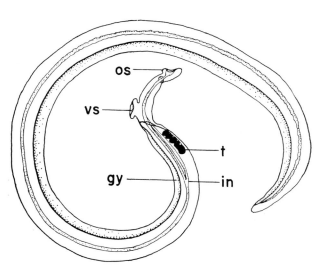

FIGURE 71. *Schistosoma mansoni,* male: *gy,* gynecophoral canal; *in,* intestine; *os,* oral sucker; *t,* testes; *vs,* ventral sucker.

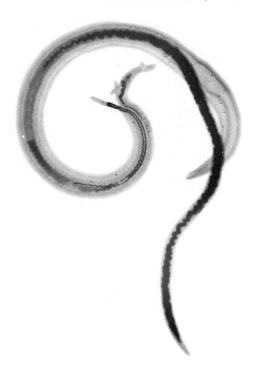

FIGURE 72. *Schistosoma mansoni*, male and female *in copula*. (Photomicrograph by Zane Price.)

small venules, close to the lumen of the intestine or bladder. The worms dilate the vessel when they penetrate into them for oviposition, and withdraw as the eggs are laid, so that the eggs are wedged firmly into the small vessels. Retention in the vessels is facilitated in the case of *Schistosoma mansoni* and *S. haematobium* by the fact that the eggs bear long sharp spines. An enzyme is elaborated by the miracidium, and this diffuses through the egg shell and helps to digest the overlying tissue. The action of this enzyme, plus necrosis of the tissue caused by pressure and the effect of the spine, work together to liberate the egg from the tissues into the lumen of the intestine or bladder. Schistosome eggs are not operculated, and hatch by rupture if liberated into fresh water. The miracidium that escapes swims in search of an appropriate snail host (Fig. 74). If successful, it penetrates an appropriate snail where it undergoes a cycle of development, giving rise to a large number of cercariae infective for man.

All other trematode parasites of man are acquired through ingestion of metacercariae, but infection with schistosomes follows exposure to water in which infected snails have liberated their cercariae. Human infection takes place by direct penetration of the cercariae through the skin to invade the circulatory system. After penetration and invasion of

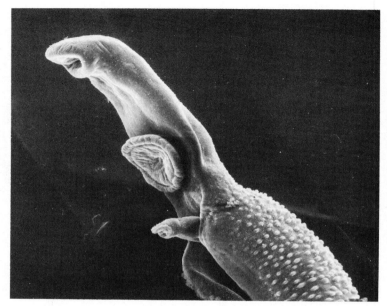

FIGURE 73. Scanning electron micrograph of the anterior end of a male and female *Schistosoma mansoni*. (Courtesy of Dr. Wilmar Jansma.)

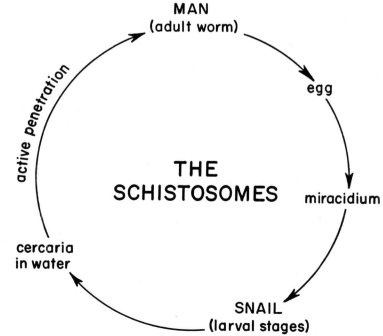

FIGURE 74. Schematic representation of schistosome life cycle.

a blood vessel, the young flukes are carried to the liver sinusoids, where they begin their growth. Two weeks or longer after infection the maturing worms commence a migration against the flow of the blood in the portal system to their final location in mesenteric or vesicular veins. Their final location in the host differs in the different species, and will be discussed separately for each.

Cercariae of the schistosome parasites (Fig. 75), both of man and of lower animals, have a forked tail, and glands at the anterior end which assist penetration through the skin.

SYMPTOMATOLOGY. Following penetration of the skin by cercariae of a human schistosome, a transient reaction may be seen. Petechial hemorrhages occur at the site of penetration, with some localized edema and pruritus, which reach a maximum in twenty-four to thirty-six hours and disappear in four days or less. During the succeeding three weeks there may be transient toxic and allergic manifestations. These may be very mild, and pass unnoticed, or there may be generalized malaise, fever, giant urticaria, vague intestinal complaints, and so forth. Migration of the worms through the lungs may cause cough or hemoptysis. Soon after the developing schistosomes reach the liver, acute hepatitis may develop.

When the flukes reach their final location in the mesenteric or vesical venules and egg laying commences, the acute stage of the disease

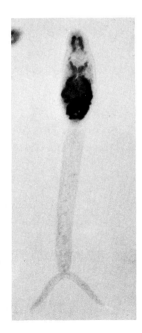

FIGURE 75. Cercaria of *Schistosoma mansoni* showing penetration glands. (Courtesy Dr. David Bruckner.)

is seen. The onset of this stage may be from one to three months after infection. Symptoms of the acute stage may range from very mild to rather severe, and the degree of reaction seems to depend as much upon constitutional factors in the host as upon numbers of parasites involved. With the extrusion of eggs through the wall of the intestine or bladder, there may once again be generalized malaise, fever, urticaria, abdominal pain and liver tenderness. In *Schistosoma mansoni* or *S. japonicum* infections there may be diarrhea or dysentery at this stage, while in *S. haematobium* infections there is often hematuria at the end of micturition, and sometimes dysuria.

The third stage, in which the disease becomes chronic, comes on gradually. It is consequent upon fibrosis and hyperplasia in the tissues in which the eggs are deposited. Egg deposition takes place in the smaller vessels, close to the lumen of the intestine or bladder. Many eggs remain where deposited; secretions of the contained miracidia evoke the formation of minute abscesses around them, and the eggs are liberated into the lumen of the affected organ. Other eggs are dislodged and swept into the circulation; the characteristic pathologic effects produced by these embolic eggs will be discussed separately for each species.

A leukocytosis in the early stages of infection is generally accompanied by eosinophilia, which persists after the total white blood cell count returns to normal. Liver function tests are often abnormal in acute and sometimes in chronic cases of *S. mansoni* and *S. japonicum* infections. Gamma globulin levels may be increased, and albumin may be slightly decreased.

Schistosoma mansoni

A by-product of the African slave trade was the establishment of *Schistosoma mansoni* in the Western Hemisphere. This fluke, which occurs over extensive areas of Africa, and in the Arabian peninsula and Malagasy, has also become well established in Brazil, Surinam and Venezuela, as well as in parts of the West Indies. Of special interest is the heavy rate of infection in Puerto Rico. The influx of people from this island into New York and other large cities in the past few years has resulted in schistosomiasis mansoni being seen with some frequency in this country. It does not seem to present a public health problem, however, and there is little reason to expect that the infection could become successfully established in North American snail hosts.

Adults of *S. mansoni* usually live in the smaller branches of the inferior mesenteric vein in the region of the lower colon. They may be found elsewhere in the portal system, in the vesical venous plexus or in other ectopic foci on occasion. They subsist on ingested blood. Lawrence (1973) showed that a female *S. mansoni* in the laboratory mouse ingested as many as 330,000 red cells per hour, while the male ingested only 39,000 hourly. *S. mansoni* is the smallest of the human schistosomes, males reaching a length of only 1 cm., and females an extreme length of 1.6 cm. While they have been found on rare occasions infecting both African and West Indian monkeys, and rodents of both Africa and South America, it is not thought that any of these animals is of importance as a reservoir host.

Diagnosis during the acute period of the disease is based upon the recovery of the characteristic eggs in the stool. The light yellow brown eggs (Fig. 62, G) measure 114 to 180 microns in length by 45 to 73 microns in breadth. They are elongate, regularly ovoid, and possess a large lateral spine, shaped rather like a rose thorn, which projects from the side of the egg near one pole. In the chronic stage of the disease, eggs may not be found in the stools. Rectal biopsy (Fig. 76) may be of value in such cases, as eggs can be demonstrated in the tissue by flattening it between two glass slides and examination under the microscope. The zinc-sulfate technique is not recommended for isolation of schistosome eggs, as they rupture and do not float. They may be found upon examination of the sediment, but the formalin-ether technique is preferable. A stool specimen may be diluted with water to allow the eggs to hatch, following which an examination is made for miracidia. This procedure is helpful when few eggs are present, but will obviously reveal only those containing living miracidia. Intradermal tests and a variety

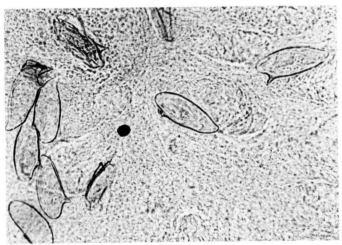

FIGURE 76. Schistosoma mansoni eggs, as seen in rectal biopsy. (Photomicrograph by Zane Price.)

of serologic procedures have been recommended for diagnosis of this infection. The more useful of these procedures are discussed in Chapter 16.

PATHOGENESIS. Early in the infection, local damage caused by egg deposition and abscess formation may give rise to schistosomal dysentery, accompanied by abdominal pain, cramping, and frequent bloody or blood-flecked stools. There may be considerable hypertrophy of the affected sections of bowel (Fig. 77), and papilloma formation. Fibrosis of the submucosa in areas of egg deposition has long been advanced to explain the decrease in egg passage which is noted as the infection progresses. This concept is questioned by Cheever and Andrade (1967), who found such fibrosis to be rare and explain decreased egg production as secondary to worm death or decreased fecundity.

Eggs swept back to the liver with the portal blood flow lodge in the finer branches of the portal system. Around them develop granulomas and, if the infection is heavy enough, a periportal fibrosis develops also. This fibrous tissue may finally come to surround the branches of the portal vein in a thick white layer, visible grossly as the "clay-pipe-

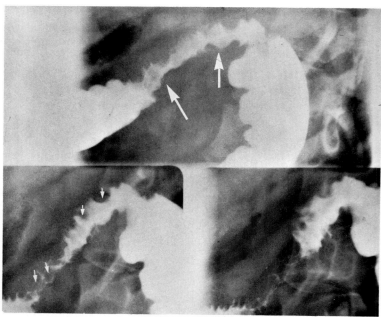

FIGURE 77. Schistosomiasis of the colon. There is segmental narrowing of the distal transverse colon (large arrows), which was irritable and contained many thickened folds (small arrows). (Courtesy of W. Seaman: Radiology *85*:682, 1965.)

stem" fibrosis of Symmers. Such periportal fibrosis was reported in about 20 per cent of patients dying of schistosomiasis or its complications in Cheever and Andrade's series (loc. cit.). The majority of their patients exhibited granuloma formation around eggs in the liver and fibrosis of small portal tracts, but there was no generalized liver involvement. Cirrhosis was no more common than in uninfected controls. On the other hand, cirrhosis is very commonly seen in Egyptian patients with this disease, possibly because of nutritional factors. Even if cirrhosis does not develop, evidence of marked portal hypertension (splenomegaly, esophageal varices) is seen in nearly all patients with Symmers' fibrosis. Cor pulmonale (Fig. 78) has been noted in over 15 per cent of patients with periportal fibrosis, with evidence of arteriolitis secondary to schistosomal pulmonary fibrosis. Intestinal involvement was minor, and largely asymptomatic. Light infections, even of many years' duration, seem to be of little consequence (Cheever, 1968). A correlation between the occurrence of hepatosplenic schistosomiasis and follicular lymphoma of the spleen was reported by Andrade and Abreu (1971) from patients in Brazil.

Transverse myelitis has been reported in patients in whom granuloma-producing *S. mansoni* eggs were found in the spinal cord. This type of lesion is more frequently seen in schistosomiasis japonica. Schistosomiasis as a cause of glomerulonephritis was studied by Queiroz et al. (1973), who observed schistosomiasis patients with hepatomegaly or splenomegaly, and the nephrotic syndrome. Lehman et al. (1975) observed proteinuria associated with *S. mansoni* infection but apparently not related to hepatic or splenic enlargement. Patients with schistosomiasis had a higher mean urinary protein than those without. Falcão and Gould (1975) described immune complex nephropathy in a patient with hepatosplenic schistosomiasis and kidney disease, and demonstrated the presence of schistosomal antigen, immunoglobulin, and complement in the glomeruli of this patient.

An association between *S. mansoni* and chronic *Salmonella paratyphi* infection is discussed by Young et al. (1973), who also cultured the bacteria from the tegument of adult schistosomes removed from a patient with chronic salmonellosis.

EPIDEMIOLOGY. Even though *Schistosoma mansoni* is widely distributed throughout the world, man is apparently the only important host in most areas of high endemicity. In Africa, non-human primates, insectivores, and wild rodents are found to harbor the schistosomes, while in Brazil several species of marsupials and rodents carry the infection. The importance of these reservoir hosts in maintaining and spreading the disease to humans probably varies from one area to the next and depends on the precise ecological interactions between man and his environment.

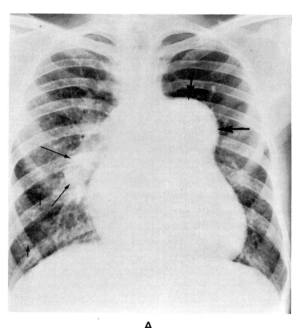

A

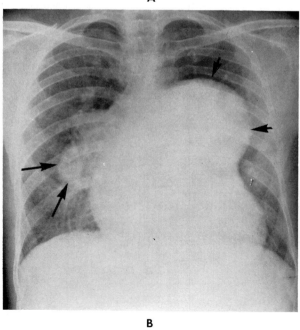

B

Figure 78. See legend on the opposite page.

Extension of the disease into new areas still occurs upon migration of infected people and the agricultural development of virgin land where the snail vector is present. Irrigation and the establishment of artificial bodies of water, combined with unsanitary practices, may quickly result in new foci of high endemicity. Since the snail intermediate host is entirely aquatic, the aqueous environment (water flow, vegetation, water temperature and pH) will determine snail density and distribution. Extensive discussion of the ecology of schistosomiasis mansoni is given by Maldonado (1967).

TREATMENT. Potassium antimony tartrate, or tartar emetic, a trivalent antimony compound, has been the mainstay of treatment in the schistosomal infections. It is given by slow intravenous injection as a 0.5 per cent solution in distilled water. The usual dosage schedule is to start with 8 ml. of the drug, administering it on alternate days and increasing each dose by 4 ml. until a daily dose of 28 ml. is reached, then continuing at 28 ml. for a total of 10 doses at this level. The entire course consists of 15 doses. The drug usually produces coughing; vomiting, prostration and bradycardia are seen occasionally, and require a reduction in dosage or discontinuation of therapy.

Stibophen (Fuadin), sodium antimony bis-catechol-2,4-disulfonate heptahydrate, is somewhat less toxic than tartar emetic. It is also less effective. It is supplied in a solution containing 8.5 mg. of antimony per ml.; the adult dosage is 4 ml. intramuscularly daily, five days per week, for a total dose of 80 to 100 ml.

Sodium antimony dimercaptosuccinate (Astiban)* is less toxic than potassium antimony tartrate or stibophen and may be administered in a shorter course of injections. A series of five injections given at weekly or twice-weekly intervals comprises the standard course. The amount given is 8 mg. per Kg. of body weight in adults, 10 mg. per Kg. in children, per injection.

---

*Available from the Parasitic Disease Service, Center for Disease Control, U.S. Public Health Service, Atlanta, Ga. 30333.

FIGURE 78. Pulmonary schistosomiasis: Progressive pulmonary hypertension and cor pulmonale. A, There are numerous linear and nodular densities in the pulmonary parenchyma (short arrows). The heart is enlarged, and the right pulmonary arteries are greatly enlarged (arrows). The main pulmonary artery (large arrows) is almost aneurysmal. B, Three years later the main pulmonary artery (short arrows) has increased further in size; the heart and right pulmonary artery (arrows) are also much larger. The pulmonary markings are considerably decreased, owing to obliteration of the peripheral pulmonary vasculature. The extreme dilatation of the pulmonary artery caused by pulmonary schistosomiasis is unequalled by almost any other disease. (Courtesy of Z. Farid, Cairo, Egypt.)

Side effects of antimony administration include nausea and vomiting in a high percentage of patients, coughing during administration, abdominal pain, anorexia, weakness, diarrhea headache, lassitude and myalgia, which seldom necessitate termination of treatment. Increasing proteinuria, persistent joint pain, rash, or intercurrent infection calls for its cessation.

Antimonials are contraindicated in the presence of severe cardiac or renal disease, also if there is hepatic disease unrelated to the schistosomal infection. The organic compound lucanthone hydrochloride, 1-diethylaminoethylamino-4-methylthiaxanthone hydrochloride, also known as Nilodin or Miracil D, is not as effective as tartar emetic or stibophen, except possibly in the treatment of the Puerto Rican strain of S. mansoni. Hycanthone, the hydroxymethyl derivative of lucanthone, was thought to be more effective and less toxic than lucanthone, but was shown to be a potent mutagen (Hartman and Hulbert, 1975), as well as a carcinogen (Haese and Bueding, 1976). It is not approved for use in this country.

Recently, a new drug, oxamniquine, a hydroxyquinoline derivative, has proved to be curative in a large number of cases. It is administered orally as a single dose of 12.5 mg./Kg. body weight on an empty stomach (Dominguez and Coutinho, 1975). The drug is well tolerated and, except for occasional nausea and dizziness, no serious side effects were noted. The drug is not yet available in the United States.

Goldsmith et al. (1967) have successfully removed numbers of adult schistosomes by cannulization, and extracorporeal filtration of the portal blood. The worms were "mobilized" from their sites in the intestinal venules by administration of a single dose of potassium antimony tartrate. Kessler et al. (1970) have further refined this technique.

Schistosoma japonicum

The Oriental blood fluke, *Schistosoma japonicum*, is confined to the Far East, where it occurs in parts of China (including Taiwan), Japan, the Philippines and Celebes, and probably Laos and Cambodia. Unlike *S. mansoni*, which rarely infects other animals, *S. japonicum* is found in virtually all mammals exposed to infected water. During World War II, large numbers of American and Australian troops serving on the island of Leyte in the Philippines acquired the infection.

S. japonicum adults inhabit the branches of the superior mesenteric vein adjacent to the small intestine; the inferior mesenterics and caval system may also be invaded, as the worms tend in time to migrate farther and farther from the liver. The males may reach a length of 2.2 cm., and the females 2.6 cm. Egg production is higher in this species than in the other two schistosomes, and the eggs are smaller and more nearly spherical. For a combination of these reasons, more eggs become free in the general circulation, to be filtered out in the liver, lungs or other organs. Infection even with a few worms of this species may be very serious. Hepatic and pulmonary cirrhosis are commonly seen in the chronic stage of this infection, and central nervous system symptoms may occur following lodgment of eggs in nervous tissue.

Diagnosis may be made by identification of the eggs in the stool. The eggs are spherical to oval in shape (Fig. 62, *F*). They may have a minute lateral spine (Fig. 79) but this structure may be absent in some strains. The size range is from 74 to 106 microns in length by 55 to 80 microns in breadth. Examination for eggs should be carried out as indicated for *S. mansoni*. Rectal biopsy is sometimes helpful in making the diagnosis in chronic cases.

SYMPTOMATOLOGY. Schistosomiasis japonica differs clinically from the generalized type described previously in that it has a rather severe early course and also neurologic involvement. The early stages of infection, known locally as Katayama disease and Yangtze River fever, are characterized by the development of fever, malaise, cough, and giant urticaria. The same signs and symptoms may accompany the early migration and establishment of the other species but tend to be more pronounced in *S. japonicum* infection. A tender and enlarged liver is seen early, but portal cirrhosis with splenomegaly and ascites come on gradually.

Cerebral involvement of two general types is seen. Early in the course of the disease more generalized neurologic symptoms, such as lethargy, confusion and coma, may occur and have been thought to be on a toxic basis. Later, focal neurologic symptoms, including jacksonian seizures and transverse myelitis, are probably secondary to egg deposition in the brain and spinal cord.

PATHOGENESIS. The adult worms, generally concentrated in the

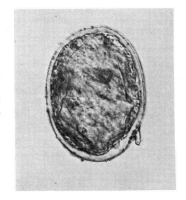

FIGURE 79. Egg of *Schistosoma japonicum*. Material for this figure courtesy the Shanghai Institute for Parasitic Diseases, The People's Republic of China. (Photomicrograph by Zane Price.)

superior mesenteric veins, produce eggs readily embolized to the liver, which early develops periportal fibrosis. Portal hypertension, spleno-megaly, and hypersplenism may result, accompanied by esophageal varices, a caput medusae, and ascites. Lung involvement may occur, but it is relatively rare and light. Anastomoses between the mesenteric and spinal veins allow both worms and their eggs to reach the central nervous system, where granulomas forming around them may produce focal lesions.

EPIDEMIOLOGY. The complexity of the epidemiologic problems of schistosomiasis are further enhanced in *S. japonicum* because so many domestic animals are efficient reservoirs of the infection. Cats, dogs, cattle, horses, and pigs, as well as some wild mammals, are susceptible and may show a high infection rate in certain areas. Prevention of the disease is further complicated by the semiaquatic habits of the snail intermediate host which visits water only for the purpose of egg laying so that molluscicides applied to the water are virtually useless. Rice, the staple crop in almost all areas where *S. japonicum* is endemic, grows in water so that infection of the agricultural population is a constant occupational hazard. It is estimated that about 70 million people are infected with *S. japonicum.*

A somewhat modified form of the disease is encountered in the Mekong river basin. The Mekong schistosome is carried by a different snail intermediate host, the disease produced in man is usually milder, and the adult worms differ slightly from the *S. japonicum* seen in other parts of Asia.

TREATMENT. Potassium antimony tartrate is the drug of choice in *S. japonicum* infections. Astiban is also effective. Both are administered as outlined for treatment of *S. mansoni.* Stibophen is relatively ineffective in well-tolerated doses.

Schistosoma haematobium

Urinary schistosomiasis is generally caused by *Schistosoma haematobium,* although as mentioned above the other two species may sometimes inhabit the vesical plexus. The original focus of this disease was apparently the Nile Valley, where it is highly endemic. From there it has spread widely throughout Africa, and occurs also in the islands off the east coast of that continent, in Asia Minor, on the island of Cyprus and in Southern Portugal. There is also an isolated focus in India.

After the worms mature in the sinusoids of the liver, they migrate from that organ, and in the case of *S. haematobium* the majority of them reach the vesical, prostatic and uterine plexuses, by way of the haemorrhoidal veins. Adult male worms may reach a length of 1.5 cm., and the females a length of 2 cm. Their eggs are deposited in the walls of the bladder, or to a lesser extent the uterus, prostate or other organs. Those deposited in the wall of the bladder may break through into the lumen, and escape with the urine.

Diagnosis is most readily made by recovery of the characteristic eggs (Fig. 62), either by sedimentation or centrifugation of the urine. Containers used for collection of urine specimens must not contain preservatives, if the hatching test is to be done. The eggs contain a fully developed miracidium when deposited, and are from 112 to 170 microns in length, and 40 to 70 microns in breadth. They have a conspicuous terminal spine, and are a light yellowish-brown in color. Terminal hematuria in a patient from the endemic areas should make one highly suspicious of this infection. It may be possible to find the eggs in biopsy material from the bladder wall. Intradermal tests and certain serological procedures are of value, and are given in Chapter 16.

SYMPTOMATOLOGY. The clinical picture associated with penetration of the cercariae into the body, and development of the young worms in the liver, differs in no essentials in S. *haematobium* infection from that observed in infection by other species of schistosomes. Urinary symptoms usually are not seen for three to six months after infection, and may not develop for a year or more. The bladder wall becomes increasingly infiltrated with eggs, some of which pass out into the lumen while others are trapped and become encapsulated in the tissues. There is some bleeding from the bladder wall as it contracts, so that the patient may begin to have intermittent terminal hematuria. As the bladder wall becomes more and more involved, papillomas appear and there may be areas of ulceration. The hematuria becomes more severe, and clots may be passed in the urine. Eventually there can be partial calcification of the wall of the bladder. Obstruction of the ureters or the neck of the bladder leads to back-pressure, and predisposes to ascending bacterial infection. The subsequent involvement of ureters and kidneys is similar to that seen when there is urinary tract obstruction from any cause.

Eggs may fail to lodge in the venules when they are deposited, or become dislodged from them, and be carried into the general circulation. Venous blood from the vesical, prostatic and uterine plexuses enters the hypogastric vein, from which it goes via the common iliac to the vena cava. Thus it does not enter the portal circulation, and eggs carried as emboli will be filtered out in the lungs, rather than the liver. Hepatic involvement is rare in urinary schistosomiasis, but fibrosis of the lungs is not uncommon, and may lead to cor pulmonale.

PATHOGENESIS. Eggs which escape into the lumen of the bladder cause little damage. If they do not escape, they die within a few weeks and around them form granulomas. Fibrosis of the surrounding tissue leads to the appearance of yellowish schistosomal tubercles or papillomas of the bladder wall; these are especially common in the area of the trigone and are readily seen by cystoscopy. Caseation or calcification of these fibrotic egg masses may take place. The ureteral openings into the bladder may become partly or completely occluded, with the development of hydronephrosis and hydroureter. In the male, heavy infections may involve the urethra, prostate, seminal vesicles and even the spermatic cord and penis. Elephantiasis of the penis may follow blockage of scrotal lymphatics by egg deposition. In the female, the urethra as well as the entire reproductive tract may be affected. Cystitis, pyelitis and pyelonephritis (Smith et al., 1974; von Lichtenberg et al., 1971) may be consequences of the impeded urinary drainage. Pyogenic infections of the surrounding tissues and sinus and fistula formation may occur in advanced and neglected cases. Death from intercurrent infection is not uncommon in such cases.

Worms invading the inferior mesenteric veins may deposit their eggs in the large bowel from the appendix to the rectum; these eggs may be passed in the feces.

Small numbers of eggs are at times carried by the portal circulation to the liver, in which they produce a periportal fibrosis. Larger numbers of eggs, and even adult worms, pass through the hypogastric and iliac veins to the inferior vena cava, the heart and the lungs. In the lungs granuloma formation and fibrosis lead to blockage of the finer pulmonary circulation, arteriolitis with increasing pulmonary blood pressure, hypertrophy of the right ventricle, and right heart failure—cor pulmonale. An extensive discussion of the pathogenesis and pathology of schistosomiasis may be found in Mostofi (1967) and Warren (1973).

EPIDEMIOLOGY. As far as is known, man is the only important host for *S. haematobium*. The snail intermediate host apparently has less stringent requirements for water temperature than the snail host of *S. mansoni*. This may partly explain the relatively wide distribution of *S. haematobium* on the African continent. In some areas of high endemicity in East Africa, the snail lives in relatively small bodies of water which may dry up during part of the year. The snails then estivate while buried in the mud but retain the infection and resume shedding of cercariae when the rainy season begins. Thus, special adaptations of the snail host may be of prime importance in maintaining and perpetuating the disease in foci where water is not plentiful at all times.

TREATMENT. Metrifonate in three oral doses of 7.5 mg. per Kg. body weight, administered at intervals of two weeks, is effective but is unavailable in the United States. Stibophen and astiban are administered as outlined for the treatment of schistosomiasis mansoni.

Niridazole (Ambilhar), a nitrothiazole derivative, used for treatment in some parts of the world, is a potent mutagen (Legator et al., 1975) and a potent suppressor of delayed hypersensitivity (Mahmoud et al., 1975). It is not available for use in the United States.

Schistosoma intercalatum

This species occurs in man in Western and Central Africa. Adult worms are found in the mesenteric vessels and eggs are voided in the feces. The eggs of *S. intercalatum* closely resemble those of *S. haematobium* but can be differentiated by a slight bend in the terminal spine, with the egg shell being Ziehl-Neelsen positive while those of the other schistosomes are not. An extensive description of this species is given by Wright et al. (1972).

The disease produced by this infection is relatively benign and hepatomegaly is usually not marked. There may be severe digestive disturbances accompanied by pain and bloody stools. The most effective treatment remains to be determined.

Schistosomal dermatitis

Many schistosome cercariae which ordinarily infect birds and semi-aquatic mammals are capable of penetration into the skin of man, although not of producing a permanent infection. A dermatitis may be produced by penetration of the cercariae of the human species of schistosomes, and is frequently very severe when caused by non-human species (Chu, 1958). Fresh-water lakes as well as some marine beaches are plagued by the presence of cercariae of the blood flukes of aquatic birds, which cause a severe dermatitis known as "swimmer's itch" (Fig. 80).

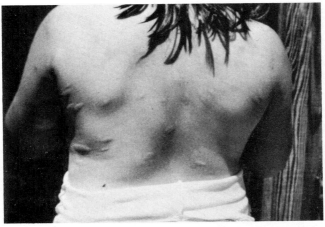

FIGURE 80. Swimmer's itch. Papular eruption caused by penetration of skin by cercariae of various schistosome parasites of lower animals.

There is suggestive evidence that exposure to these non-human schistosome cercariae, many of which are present in the endemic areas of human schistosomiasis, may increase man's resistance to infection with the human species.

THE LUNG FLUKE

Paragonimus westermani (Fig. 81) is the best known of the lung flukes parasitizing man, but it is clearly not the only lung fluke of medical importance (Yokogawa, 1969). In Thailand and in China *P. heterotremus* occurs in man in addition to *P. westermani,* and in Central and South America lung flukes of different species have been found in humans (Miyazaki, 1974a; Sogandares-Bernal and Seed, 1973). Other species of *Paragonimus* have been reported from wild and domestic mammals in different parts of the world, including the United States (Miyazaki, 1974b).

Human infection with *P. westermani* occurs throughout the Far East and in Indonesia. In Africa, it has been reported from the Congo, Cameroon, and Nigeria. It has also been reported from United States troops

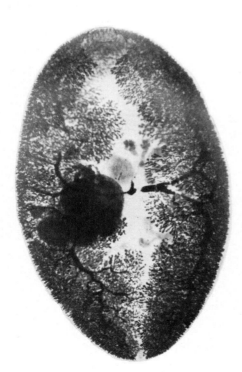

FIGURE 81.   *Paragonimus westermani.* (Photomicrograph by Zane Price.)

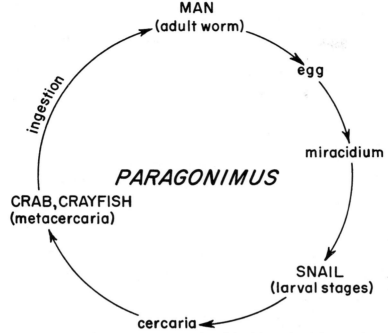

FIGURE 82. Schematic representation of the life cycle of *Paragonimus westermani.*

who were stationed in the South Pacific during World War II. Animal infection is extensive; human cases are less common, as the dietary habits of most parts of the world preclude the acquisition of this parasite. The adult worms are reddish brown in color, and very thick-bodied. They are from 0.8 to 1.6 cm. in length, 0.4 to 0.8 cm. in width, and from 0.3 to 0.5 cm. in thickness. They are found typically encapsulated in cystic structures adjacent to the bronchi. The eggs are discharged into the bronchi or bronchioles; they may be expectorated, or if swallowed will appear in the feces.

Infection results from the ingestion of raw or improperly cooked crayfish or fresh-water crabs (Fig. 82) in which the encysted metacercarial stage occurs. Animal reservoirs include a wide variety of crustacean-eating mammals. In many endemic areas, these crustaceans are pickled for human consumption with various agents which do not kill the encysted parasites. It has been suggested that fresh water may become contaminated with metacercarial cysts following death and disintegration of the crustacean second intermediate host, and that infection can be acquired through drinking such water. Metacercariae excyst in the small intestine, penetrate through its wall into the peritoneal cavity, and make their way through the diaphragm and pleura into the lungs. A cyst-like capsule surrounds the developing parasite, which grows to maturity in a period of about six weeks. Rupture of the cyst capsule into a bronchiole leads to a discharge of eggs, but not the parasite, which continues to produce eggs for a long time. Chronic infections may persist for many years after the patient has left an endemic area.

SYMPTOMATOLOGY. No recognizable symptoms attend the migration of the parasites. As they grow in the lungs, there is an inflammatory reaction, which may be sufficient to produce fever. When the cysts rupture, a cough develops, and there may be increased production of sputum. The sputum is frequently blood tinged, and may contain numerous dark brown eggs. The appearance of the eggs in sputum has suggested iron filings to some observers. Hemoptysis may occur after paroxysms of coughing. There may be severe chest pain. Severity and progression of symptoms will depend upon the numbers of parasites present and upon whether or not the infection is treated successfully, but as time goes on there is increasing dyspnea, and chronic bronchitis develops. Bronchiectasis may result, and pleural effusion sometimes is seen. Increasing fibrosis of the lungs occurs with long-standing infections.

If, in their migration from the small intestine to the lungs, the parasites become sidetracked, they may encyst elsewhere in the body. They have been found in the liver, throughout the abdomen and in the wall of the intestine, in the muscles or subcutaneous tissues, and in the brain and spinal cord. Symptoms will of course vary depending upon the location of the parasites.

Diagnosis depends upon identification of the characteristic dark golden-brown eggs (Fig. 62, *D*) in sputum or feces, although the clinical picture may be suggestive. The ovoid eggs have a flattened operculum, distinctly set off from the rest of the shell by raised opercular shoulders. They measure 80 to 120 microns in length by 48 to 60 microns in breadth, and are immature when found in the sputum or feces. Various serologic tests have been developed but are not generally available. An intradermal test has also been described.

The chest film (Fig. 83) may show a patchy infiltrate with nodular cystic shadows or calcification; pleural effusion may be seen. Cerebral calcifications may also occur.

PATHOGENESIS. Migration of larval *Paragonimus* through the intestinal wall and into the pleural cavity is generally accomplished in experimental animals within five to ten days. Some young flukes wander about in the peritoneal cavity for 20 days or more, growing considerably in size and penetrating into various organs en route. Those reaching

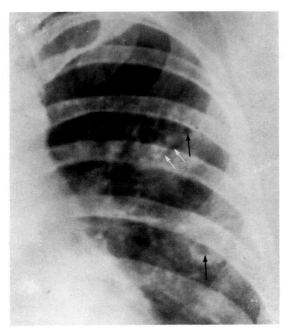

FIGURE 83. Pulmonary paragonimiasis with ring shadows (black arrows) and linear lucency (white arrows) representing burrow tract. (Courtesy R. Suwanik, Dhonburi, Thailand.)

sexual maturity in ectopic sites apparently remain there. Worms reaching the brain do so via the soft tissues of the neck and the cranial foramina. Passage of worms through the tissues produces local hemorrhage and leukocytic infiltration of a transitory nature and without clinical significance except for rare cases in which they wander subcutaneously.

When the worms settle down, either in the lungs or in ectopic foci, more pronounced tissue reactions occur. In the lungs a leukocytic infiltrate forms around the parasite and fibrous tissue surrounds the infiltrate to form a cyst wall. Communication of the cyst with the respiratory tree may result from inclusion of a bronchiolar branch within the cyst or erosion of the cyst into adjacent bronchioles. Eggs may infiltrate the surrounding pulmonary tissues or may be carried by the circulation to other parts of the body, in which they evoke a granulomatous reaction similar to that seen surrounding schistosome eggs in tissues. Such lesions have been reported from many organs and tissues, including both pericardium and myocardium, but they are apparently rare in the central nervous system.

Worm cysts in the peritoneal cavity or other sites outside the lungs are similar to pulmonic cysts. Peritonitis and abdominal adhesions resulting from infection have been reported, although there is usually little or no inflammatory reaction, and suppurative and ulcerative lesions are uncommon.

In the brain, lesions may occur in both gray and white matter, and sometimes they are connected by passageways. Lesions in the gray matter may cause a thickening of the pia and adhesive arachnoiditis. In older lesions a more or less definite cyst wall develops. For a discussion of cerebral paragonimiasis see Miyazaki and Nishimura (1975).

Since the majority of worms migrate to the lungs, and since most human infections are light, extrapulmonary paragonimiasis is rarely seen in man. Cysts, in whatever location, may contain living or dead worms, a yellow to brownish-colored thick fluid, sometimes hemorrhagic, eggs and Charcot-Leyden crystals. If the worms die or escape, the cysts gradually shrink as their contents are absorbed, eventually leaving a nodule of fibrous tissue and eggs, which may partly calcify.

EPIDEMIOLOGY. The importance of non-human vertebrate reservoir hosts in the maintenance of human paragonimiasis in different parts of the world is still largely unknown, since the specific identity of some *Paragonimus* found in man remains to be established. Transmission of the infection to humans is based on the consumption of pickled or raw fresh-water crabs. In different parts of the world, different species of crabs are vectors of human and of animal paragonimiasis. Thus, endemicity of the disease rests on dietary habits, the distribution of eggs by unsanitary practices and lack of sanitation, the presence of appropriate snail hosts, of fresh-water crustaceans, and possibly on the presence of reservoir hosts.

TREATMENT. Bithionol* (2,2'-thiobis-[4,6-dichlorophenol]), formerly widely used in the formulation of medicated soaps, shampoos and cosmetics, is no longer used for this purpose because of its association with contact dermatitis. It has been found effective in the treatment of paragonimiasis, and it is administered orally at the rate of 15 to 25 mg. per Kg. of body weight, twice daily, on alternate days for a total of 10 to 15 days.

Skin rashes and urticaria are not infrequently seen in the course of bithionol treatment. Abdominal cramps, nausea and vomiting, and diarrhea are rather frequent side effects, as are dizziness and headache. Hepatic and renal involvement, hypertension, extrasystoles and first degree heart block have all been reported to occur during the course of treatment but are apparently transient. Bithionol is contrain-

---

*Available from the Parasitic Disease Service, Center for Disease Control, U.S. Public Health Service, Atlanta, Ga. 30333.

dicated in patients with a clear history of sensitization to preparations containing this drug. A list of such preparations is given in the informational leaflet supplied by the Parasitic Disease Service.

REFERENCES

Andrade, Z. A., and Abreu, W. N. 1971. Follicular lymphoma of the spleen in patients with hepatosplenic schistosomiasis mansoni. Amer. J. Trop. Med. & Hyg., 20:237–243.

Cheever, A. W., and Andrade, Z. A. 1967. Pathological lesions associated with Schistosoma mansoni infection in man. Trans. Roy. Soc. Trop. Med. & Hyg., 61:626–639.

Cheever, A. W. 1968. A quantitative postmortem study of schistosomiasis mansoni in man. Amer. J. Trop. Med. & Hyg., 17:38–64.

Chu, G. W. T. C. 1958. Pacific area distribution of fresh-water and marine cercarial dermatitis. Pacific Science, 12:229–312.

Dawes, B. 1946. The Trematoda. 644 pp. Cambridge University Press, London.

Domingues, A. L. C., and Coutinho, A. 1975. Tratamento da esquistossomose mansonica com oxamniquine oral. Rev. Inst. Med. Trop. (São Paulo), 17:164–180.

Falcão, H. A., and Gould, D. B. 1975. Immune complex nephropathy in schistosomiasis. Ann. Int. Med., 83:148–154.

Goldsmith, E. I., Carvalho Luz, F. F., Prata, A., and Kean, B. H. 1967. Surgical recovery of schistosomes from the portal blood. J.A.M.A., 199:235–240.

Hadden, J. W., and Pascarelli, E. F. 1967. Diagnosis and treatment of human fascioliasis. J.A.M.A., 202:149–151.

Haese, W., and Bueding, E. 1976. Longterm hepatotoxicity effects of hycanthone and of two other antischistosomal drugs in mice infected with Schistosoma mansoni. J. Pharmacol. Exper. Ther., 197:703–713.

Hartman, P. E., and Hulbert, P. B. 1975. Genetic activity spectra of some antischistosomal compounds, with particular emphasis on thioxanthenones and benzothiopyrano-indazoles. J. Toxicol. Environ. Health, 1:243–270.

Healy, G. R. 1970. Trematodes transmitted to man by fish, frogs, and crustacea. J. Wildlife Dis., 6:255–261.

Hou, P. C. 1955. The pathology of Clonorchis sinensis infestation of the liver. J. Path. & Bact., 70:53–64.

Hou, P. C. 1965. The relationship between primary carcinoma of the liver and infestation with Clonorchis sinensis. J. Path. & Bact., 72:239–246.

Kessler, R. E., Amadea, J. H., Tice, D. A., and Zimmon, D. S. 1970. Filtration of schistosomes in unanesthetized man. J.A.M.A., 214:519–524.

Koenigstein, R. P. 1949. Observations on the epidemiology of infections with Clonorchis sinensis. Trans. Roy. Soc. Trop. Med. & Hyg., 42:503–506.

Komiya, Y. 1966. Clonorchis and Clonorchiasis. In: Dawes, B. (Ed.) Advances in Parasitology. pp. 53–106. Academic Press, New York.

Krull, W. H., and Mapes, C. R. 1952. Studies on the biology of Dicrocoelium dendriticum (Rudolphi, 1819) Looss, 1899 (Trematoda: Dicrocoeliidae), including its relationship to the intermediate host Cionella lubrica (Muller). VII. The second intermediate host of Dicrocoelium dendriticum. Cornell Vet., 42:603–604.

Krull, W. H. 1958. The migratory route of the metacercaria of Dicrocoelium dendriticum (Rudolphi, 1819) Looss, 1899 in the definitive host: Dicrocoeliidae. Cornell Vet., 48:17–24.

Lawrence, J. D. 1973. The ingestion of red blood cells by Schistosoma mansoni. J. Parasit., 59:60–63.

Legator, M. S., Connor, T. H., and Stoeckel, M. 1975. Detection of mutagenic activity of metronidazole and niridazole in body fluids of humans and mice. Science, 188:1118–1119.

Lehman, J. S., Jr., Mott, E. K., DeSouza, C. A. M., Leboreiro, O., and Muniz, T. M. 1975. The association of schistosomiasis mansoni and proteinuria in an endemic area. A preliminary report. Amer. J. Trop. Med. & Hyg., 24:616–618.

Mahmoud, A. A. F., Mandel, M. A., Warren, K. S., and Webster, L. T., Jr. 1975. Niridazole. II. A potent long-acting suppressant of cellular hypersensitivity. J. Immunol., *114*: 279–283.

Maldonado, J. F. 1967. *Schistosomiasis in America.* 119 pp. Editorial Científico Medica, Barcelona, Spain.

McFadzean, A. J. S., and Yeung, R. T. T. 1966. Hypoglycemia in suppurative pericholangitis due to *Clonorchis sinensis.* Trans. Roy. Soc. Trop. Med. & Hyg., *59*:179–185.

Miyazaki, I. 1974a. Occurrence of the lung fluke, *Paragonimus peruvianus* in Costa Rica. Jap. J. Parasit., *23*:280–284.

Miyazaki, I. 1974b. V. Lung flukes in the world. Morphology and life history. A symposium on epidemiology of parasitic diseases. pp. 101–135. International Medical Foundation of Japan, Tokyo.

Miyazaki, I., and Nishimura, K. 1975. Cerebral paragonimiasis. *In*: Hornabrook, R. W. (Ed.) *Topics in Tropical Neurology* (Contemporary Neurology Series, No. 12). pp. 109–132. F. A. Davis Company, Philadelphia.

Mostofi, K. F. (Ed.) 1967. *Bilharziasis.* 357 pp. Springer-Verlag, Inc., New York.

Neves, J., Marinho, R. P., DeAranjo, P. K., and Raso, P. 1973. Spinal cord complications of acute schistosomiasis mansoni. Trans. Roy. Soc. Trop. Med. & Hyg., *67*:782–792.

Queiroz, F. P., Brito, E., Marinelli R., and Rocha, H. 1973. Nephrotic syndrome in patients with *Schistosoma mansoni* infection. Amer. J. Trop. Med. & Hyg., *22*:622–628.

Sadun, E. H. 1955. Studies on *Opisthorchis viverrini* in Thailand. Amer. J. Hyg., *62*:81–115.

Smith, J. H., Kamel, I. A., Elwi, A., and von Lichtenberg, F. 1974. A quantitative post mortem analysis of urinary schistosomiasis in Egypt. I. Pathology and pathogenesis. Amer. J. Trop. Med. & Hyg., *23*:1054–1071.

Sogandares-Bernal, F., and Seed, J. R. 1973. American paragonimiasis. *In*: Cheng, T. (Ed.) *Current Topics in Comparative Pathobiology,* Vol. 2. pp. 1–56. Academic Press, Inc., New York.

Strauss, W. G. 1962. Clinical manifestations of clonorchiasis. A controlled study of 105 cases. Amer. J. Trop. Med. & Hyg., *11*:625–630.

von Lichtenberg, F., Edington, G. M., Mwabuebo, I., Taylor, J. R., and Smith, J. H. 1971. Pathologic effects of schistosomiasis in Ibadan, Western State of Nigeria. II. Pathogenesis of lesions of the bladder and ureters. Amer. J. Trop. Med. & Hyg., *20*:244–254.

Warren, K. S. 1973. The pathology of schistosome infections. Helm. Abst. Ser. A., *42*: 591–633.

Wright, C. A., Southgate, V. R., and Knowles, R. J. 1972. What is *Schistosoma intercalatum* Fisher, 1934? Trans. Roy. Soc. Trop. Med. & Hyg., *66*:28–56.

Yokogawa, M. 1969. *Paragonimus* and Paragonimiasis. *In*: Dawes, B. (Ed.) *Advances in Parasitology.* Vol. 7. pp. 375–387. Academic Press, New York.

Yokogawa, M., Tsuji, M., Koyama, H., Wakejima, T., Ozu, S., and Ogino, Y. 1967. Chemotherapy of *Clonorchis sinensis* infections. III. Treatment of clonorchiasis sinensis with 1,4-bis-trichloromethylbenzol. Z. Tropenmed. Parasit., *18*:82–88.

Young, S. W., Higashi, G., Kamel, R., El Abdin, A. Z., and Mikhail, I. A. 1973. Interaction of salmonellae and schistosomes in host-parasite relations. Trans. Roy. Soc. Trop. Med. & Hyg., *67*:797–802.

9

The Cestodes

The cestodes or tapeworms comprise a class of the phylum Platy-helminthes. Those commonly found in man include a variety of forms, all of which have as adults a body that may be characterized as flat and ribbon-like. Living worms are white or yellowish in color. The cestode body consists of an anterior attachment organ or scolex followed by a chain of segments or proglottids (Fig. 84). This chain of proglottids is called the strobila. The strobila grows throughout the life of the tape-worm by continuous proliferation of new segments or proglottids in the region immediately posterior to the scolex. The new segments are referred to as immature because they do not yet contain fully devel-oped internal structures. The mature segments are larger than imma-ture ones and are found near the middle of the chain. Each mature segment may contain either one or two sets of both male and female reproductive organs. The terminal portion of the strobila contains the ripe or gravid segments usually filled with eggs. The eggs are enclosed in the uterus, a structure which varies in shape and size in different cestode species. The form of the uterus is quite characteristic, and serves as an important diagnostic feature. Terminal proglottids of some species may become detached in the intestine and pass out with the stool; some types may be too small to be seen in gross examination.

Adult tapeworms inhabit the small intestine, where they live attached to the mucosa. Tapeworms do not have a digestive system; their food is absorbed from the host's intestine. Attachment is accom-plished by means of the scolex, an organ which varies in morphology from species to species. However, with the exception of *Diphyllobothrium latum*, the broad fish tapeworm, all cestodes of man have four muscu-lar, cup-shaped suckers on the scolex. In addition to suckers, the scolex

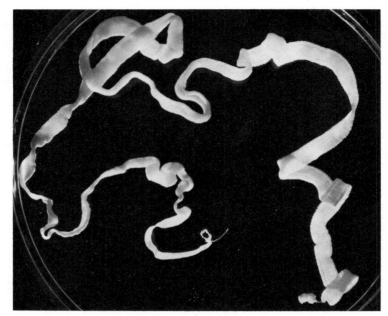

FIGURE 84. Entire tapeworm—*Hymenolepis diminuta*. (Photograph by Zane Price.)

may have an elongate and protrusible structure, the rostellum, situated in the center of the scolex. In some species the rostellum bears hooks and is referred to as armed. While precise identification of the tapeworms of man is usually made on the basis of eggs or proglottids, the scolex of each species is quite characteristic and is sufficient for specific diagnosis. Of greater practical importance is the recognition of the scolex in a stool specimen from a patient who has received anthelmintic treatment. Therapy has been successful only when the *whole* worm has been expelled. Recovery of the scolex from treated patients is essential because the strobila regrows if the scolex remains in the intestine. If, for any reason, expulsion of the whole worm is uncertain, the patient should have another stool examination three or four weeks after treatment.

The cestodes parasitizing man have complex life cycles that generally require a second or intermediate host. Infective larvae, when ingested accidentally or with food, will hatch in the small intestine and begin to grow. Infection with adult tapeworms is always accomplished via the oral route. Transport from one host to the next is generally passive. While man usually harbors the adult stage of the parasite in the intestine, extra-intestinal infection with certain larval forms does occur.

Unlike the trematodes, in which the egg is usually operculated, the tapeworms, with one exception, do not have operculate eggs. Cestode eggs vary considerably in the appearance of the external shell as well as in the number and thickness of the embryonic membranes. These membranes serve as protective coverings of the embryo, which is called an oncosphere and bears six elongate hooks.

Diphyllobothrium latum

The broad or fish tapeworm of man is world-wide in distribution, occurring in north temperate areas of the world where pickled or improperly cooked fresh-water fish is prominent in the diet. A high incidence of *Diphyllobothrium latum* in man is seen in Scandinavia and Finland, as well as in Alaska and Canada. In the United States, *D. latum* occurs in the lakes region of Minnesota and Michigan. While infection with *D. latum* is, in many instances, relatively harmless, it may produce in some persons a condition closely resembling pernicious anemia. One of the reasons for this may be found in the relatively high vitamin B_{12} content of the adult worm. This vitamin is selectively absorbed from the host's intestinal tract by *Diphyllobothrium latum*. An extensive review of this subject is given by von Bonsdorff (1956).

The life cycle of this tapeworm requires not one but two intermediate hosts (Fig. 85). Eggs are passed in the feces and hatch into small ciliated coracidium larvae which swim about until ingested by copepods, in which growth and development of the first larval stage are completed. When these infected fresh-water crustaceans are ingested by fish, the larvae continue development in the flesh of the fish, eventually developing to a stage called the sparganum. The sparganum, when ingested by man or some other fish-eating mammal, will grow to adulthood in the small intestine.

The adult worm may be some meters in length. The scolex of *Diphyllobothrium latum* (Fig. 86) is elongate, spoon-shaped, and characterized by the possession of two longitudinally situated grooves. Mature and gravid segments (Fig. 87) are wider than long. In freshly passed or formalin-preserved segments, one frequently observes a pronounced central elevation which marks the site of the egg-filled uterus. The uterus of *D. latum* is a coiled tube confined to a relatively small area in the center of the segment. This arrangement of the uterus is unlike that of the other tapeworms of man; it has been frequently likened to a rosette. Ripe eggs escape through a uterine pore and are discharged into the intestine. Both eggs and proglottids may be found in the stool. Eggs of *D. latum* (Fig. 93, *B* and *C*) are ovoid in shape and possess an operculum for the escape of the larva. Eggs are about 70 microns long

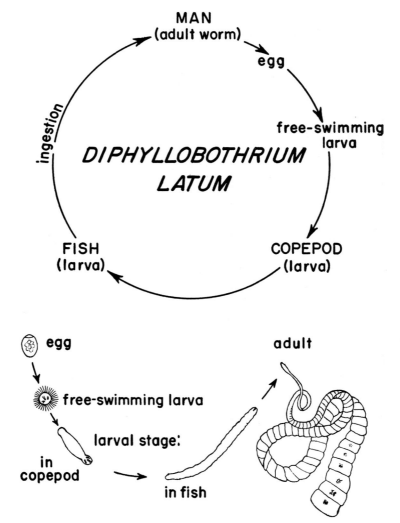

FIGURE 85. Schematic representation of life cycle of *Diphyllobothrium latum*.

and 50 microns wide. The shell is smooth, of moderate thickness and yellowish-brown in color.

SYMPTOMATOLOGY. Presence of adult worms in the intestinal tract causes no symptoms in most infected persons. Some rather non-specific abdominal symptoms have been ascribed to this infection, but the only significant consequence is seen as the result of chance localization of the parasite in the proximal portion of the jejunum. If the worm attaches in this area, clinical B_{12} deficiency develops in a small percentage of those parasitized. Such tapeworm anemia is most frequently

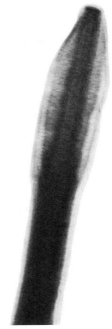

FIGURE 86. *Diphyllobothrium latum, scolex.* (Photomicrograph by Zane Price.)

seen in areas such as Finland, where many persons have a genetic predisposition to pernicious anemia, suggesting that B_{12} deprivation through *D. latum* infection is seldom sufficient to produce clinical symptoms in an otherwise normal patient.

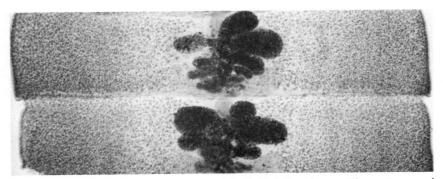

FIGURE 87. Gravid proglottid of *Diphyllobothrium latum.* (Photomicrograph by Zane Price, from material furnished by Dr. Justus F. Mueller.)

Another species of *Diphyllobothrium*, *D. pacificum*, is endemic in the coastal areas of Peru. The infection is apparently acquired from eating raw marine fish steeped in lime juice, "cebiche," which is considered a great delicacy (Baer, 1969). Another diphyllobothriid, *Diplogonoporus*, is encountered fairly frequently in Japan (Kamo, et al., 1971), probably acquired by the consumption of raw anchovies or sardines.

TREATMENT. Niclosamide (Yomesan*) is very effective in treatment of diphyllobothriasis. It acts by inhibition of oxidative phosphorylation in the mitochondria of the worm. The scolex and proximal segments, killed on contact with the drug, are dislodged and may be digested by the host. Thus, the scolex may not be identifiable in the feces after successful treatment. The drug is administered by mouth after a light breakfast. It must be chewed thoroughly. The adult dose is 2.0 gm. in a single dose; children weighing more than 35 Kg. are given 1.5 gm., and those between 10 and 35 Kg. receive 1.0 gm. No special dietary restrictions are necessary before or after treatment, but a mild laxative may be administered to facilitate evacuation and identification of the worm. Side effects of administration of the drug have been minimal, almost entirely limited to queasiness, abdominal cramps, and nausea and vomiting in a small proportion of patients. Clinical trials with this drug are described by Perera et al. (1970).

Quinacrine hydrochloride is also effective. Its main disadvantage lies in the fact that in the dose used it produces nausea in a high percentage of patients; this can usually be controlled by premedication with barbiturates or antinauseant drugs such as prochlorperazine. Prochlorperazine should be used with caution in children because like other phenothiazine derivatives it may produce extrapyramidal effects.

The day before treatment, the patient should have a liquid diet, with nothing but coffee, tea or bouillon for the evening meal. A cleansing enema should be taken in the evening. The treatment is given on an empty stomach; phenobarbital 50 mg. or prochlorperazine 10 mg. may be given by mouth one-half hour earlier. The adult dose of quinacrine is 1.0 gm.; it is administered in divided doses, 0.2 gm. with 0.5 gm. sodium bicarbonate and a little water every 10 minutes for five doses. Children weighing 18 Kg. or more receive 0.4 gm. total dose; those 35 Kg. or over; 0.6 gm.; and the adult dose is given to those weighing over 45 Kg. Frequently, this amount of quinacrine will stimulate a bowel movement, but if there has been none two hours after taking the last dose, a saline purge should be administered. After the bowels have moved, the patient may eat. If the entire worm, including scolex, is not found in the stool, treatment may still have been success-

---

*Available from the Parasitic Disease Service, Center For Disease Control, U.S. Public Health Service, Atlanta, Ga., 30333.

ful, and should not be repeated until the presence of eggs or proglottids in the stool makes failure obvious.

If, in spite of premedication, the patient is unable to retain the quinacrine, the drug may be pulverized and suspended in 100 ml. of water, and administered through a duodenal tube.

Sparganosis

The genus *Diphyllobothrium* is a large one, and man is an acceptable second intermediate host for certain species that normally develop to the adult stage in other mammals. Sparganosis in man is cosmopolitan, though rarely seen in most parts of the world. The infection may be acquired by drinking water containing copepods infected with the larval stage of the parasite, in which case the larva penetrates the gut wall and works its way into the muscles or subcutaneous tissues, where it grows into the sparganum larva. Certain spargana, which cannot become adult worms in man, are capable of infecting a person who may eat them; they remain in the sparganum stage. In various areas snakes or tadpoles are consumed raw for medicinal reasons. If they happen to be infected with spargana, these parasites may be capable of penetration through the intestinal wall to infect man. A third manner in which human infections have been known to take place is through the practice of placing poultices of frog or snake flesh on open wounds or other lesions, especially of the eyes. If the flesh is infected with sparganum larvae, these may actively penetrate into the poulticed lesion. Ocular sparganosis, acquired in this manner, is said to be not uncommon in parts of the Orient, especially in China and Vietnam.

The sparganum is a wrinkled, whitish, ribbon-shaped object, a few millimeters in width and up to several centimeters in length. The anterior end is capable of invagination, and bears suggestions of the sucking grooves of the mature scolex. In a few instances in Japan and Florida, human infections with a peculiar budding type of larva, known as *Sparganum proliferum*, have been reported. These larvae may occur almost anywhere in the body, and the branched proliferating larvae may break up into segments capable of further independent development. Infection with this form of parasite is extremely serious.

The early migratory stages in development of the sparganum are asymptomatic, but when the sparganum has reached its final site and begins to grow, its presence elicits a painful inflammatory reaction of the surrounding tissues. The larvae apparently do not become encysted. Ocular sparganosis produces an especially intense reaction, with periorbital edema. If the larvae are retrobulbar in position, the orbit may be forced out so that the lids are unable to close, and corneal ulcers will develop.

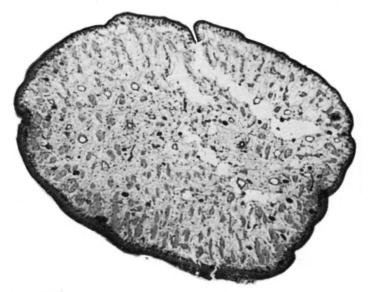

FIGURE 88.   Cross section of sparganum removed at surgery.

Diagnosis is made following surgical removal of the worms, which on section will be seen to possess a rather homogeneous parenchyma, in which are scattered the laminated, intensely basophilic calcareous corpuscles, characteristic of cestode tissue (Fig. 88). A presumptive preoperative diagnosis might be made on demonstration of a painful migratory subcutaneous nodule.

Taenia solium

The pork tapeworm of man occurs wherever people eat cured or insufficiently cooked pork. Infection with *Taenia solium* is rarely encountered in the United States, but is prevalent in certain parts of Mexico and in Central Europe. The life cycle of this tapeworm (Fig. 89) requires one intermediate host, the pig. Embryonated eggs, when ingested by a pig, develop into the infective larval stages or cysticerci in the muscles. A cysticercus is essentially a thin-walled bladder which contains a scolex. These larvae are one-half centimeter or more in diameter. Man becomes infected by eating pork containing these larvae which develop into adults in the small intestine.

While the adult tapeworm develops in man after ingestion of infected meat, infection with the larval stage or cysticercus occurs upon ingestion of eggs, either from exogenous sources or from his own stools. Although not proved, it is thought that reverse peristalsis may

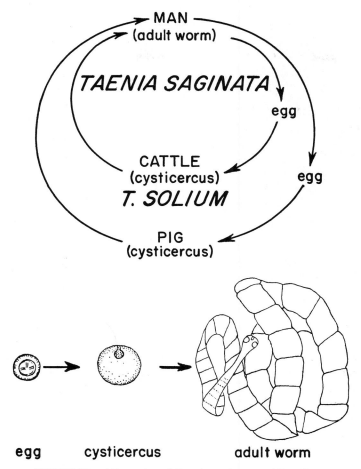

FIGURE 89.   Life cycles of Taenia saginata and T. solium.

carry intestinal contents with eggs to the upper portions of the duodenum, where after hatching the oncospheres penetrate directly into the
intestinal wall. For these reasons, infection with adults of *Taenia solium*
is dangerous both to the patient and to those with whom he comes in
contact. Prompt and efficient treatment, so administered as to minimize the chance of reverse peristalsis, is essential.

Adult *T. solium* may attain a length of several meters. The scolex
(Fig. 90) is muscular and bears in addition to the four suckers a double
crown of prominent hooks which function in attachment to the intestinal mucosa. Mature segments (Fig. 91) are wider than long, and contain one set of male and female reproductive organs. Gravid segments
(Fig. 92) are usually longer than wide, and contain a branched uterus

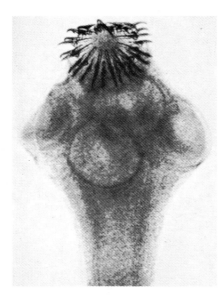

FIGURE 90. *Taenia solium* scolex.
(Photomicrograph by Zane Price.)

filled with eggs. A central uterine stem extends throughout the length of the gravid segment. From this stem arise side branches which project laterally and extend toward the lateral margin of the proglottid. These main side branches may have a variable number of smaller secondary branches. In *T. solium*, the number of main branches on one side of the central stem varies from seven to thirteen. Specific diagnosis of *Taenia solium* is made by counting the number of uterine side branches, which may be done in living or in stained preparations.

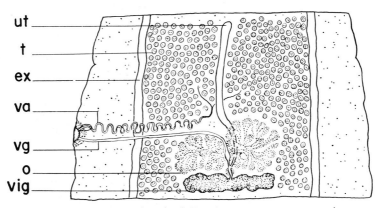

FIGURE 91. Mature proglottid of *Taenia:* ex, excretory canal; o, ovary; t, testis; ut, uterus; va, vas deferens; vg, vagina; vig, vitelline gland.

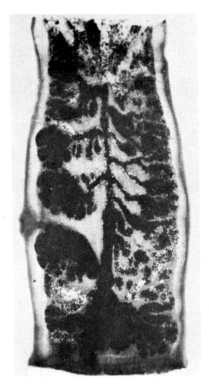

FIGURE 92. Taenia solium, gravid proglottid. (Photomicrograph by Zane Price.)

While gravid segments and eggs may be found in stool specimens, specific identification cannot be made on eggs alone, but only on examination of gravid proglottids. Eggs and mature proglottids of *T. solium* and of *T. saginata* described below are very much alike and do not provide a means of specific differentiation. *Taenia* eggs (Fig. 93,*A*) may be found free in the feces. They may also be recovered by means of a Scotch Tape swab (refer to *Enterobius*). The oncosphere is enclosed in a thick radially striated coat called the embryophore, usually dark brown in color. The six-hooked larva can be easily seen in living eggs but frequently becomes shriveled and opaque in preserved material. The radially striated coat is, however, sufficiently characteristic so that *Taenia* eggs cannot be confused with any of the other eggs of human helminths.

The whole stool specimen, or specimens, passed after treatment, should be examined carefully for the presence of the scolex, which is relatively small when compared to the strobila or individual proglottids. The scolex of *T. solium* has hooks, which serves to differentiate this species from *T. saginata.*

SYMPTOMATOLOGY. The adult worm probably causes no symptoms in the majority of patients. Vague abdominal discomfort, hunger pains, and chronic indigestion have been reported but are undoubtedly seen more often in patients who are aware of their parasitic infection than in those who are not. A moderate eosinophilia frequently occurs.

TREATMENT. The accepted standard of treatment is quinacrine, administered as outlined for diphyllobothriasis, with all precautions to prevent nausea and vomiting. Niclosamide is probably as effective and safe in this as in other tapeworm infections.

Taenia saginata

The beef tapeworm or *Taenia saginata* has a world-wide distribution. In contrast to *T. solium*, infection with *T. saginata* is frequently encountered in the United States. The life cycle is very similar to that

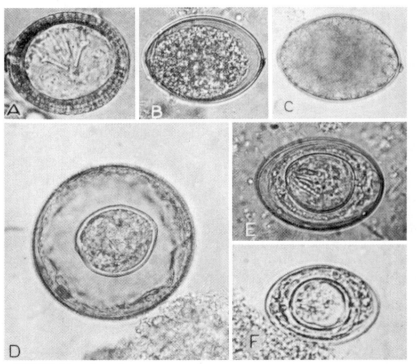

FIGURE 93. Cestode eggs: *A, Taenia* sp. *B, C, Diphyllobothrium latum; D, Hymenolepis diminuta; E, F, H. nana. A, E* and *F,* 750×; *D,* 650×; *C,* 500×. (Courtesy of Hunter, G. W., Swartzwelder, J. C., and Clyde, D. F. 1976. Tropical Medicine. 5th Ed. W. B. Saunders Company, Philadelphia.)

of *T. solium* (Fig. 89). Embyronated eggs are passed with the feces and must be ingested by cattle. The larva grows in the flesh of cattle and eventually develops into an infective cysticercus. It is acquired by man through the ingestion of raw or insufficiently cooked beef. The prevalent (and from a parasitologist's, if not a gourmet's, point of view, deplorable) liking for rare steak is one means of successful survival of this species in the United States. An important difference between *T. solium* and *T. saginata* is that cysticercosis of man due to *T. saginata* apparently occurs quite rarely.

Adults of *T. saginata* may attain a length of 25 meters but they are usually about one-half this size. The scolex (Fig. 94) bears four muscular suckers and a small rostellum without hooks. Presence or absence of hooks may thus serve to differentiate the two species of *Taenia*. Mature proglottids are either wider than long or nearly square, while gravid proglottids, which are eventually passed out in the stool, are considerably longer than they are wide. Usually, the gravid proglottids of *T. saginata* (Fig. 95) are longer than are those of *T. solium*. The structure of the uterus is very much like that in *T. solium* but the number of main side branches on each side of the central stem is fifteen to twenty. Eggs are similar to those of *T. solium*; specific identification may be made by examination of the gravid segments, as outlined for *T. solium*.

The radiographic demonstration of taeniasis has been reported by Fetterman (1965).

Symptomatology is as outlined for taeniasis solium, and treatment is identical to that given for diphyllobothriasis.

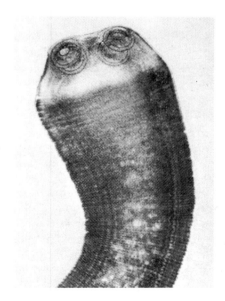

FIGURE 94. *Taenia saginata*, scolex. (Photomicrograph by Zane Price.)

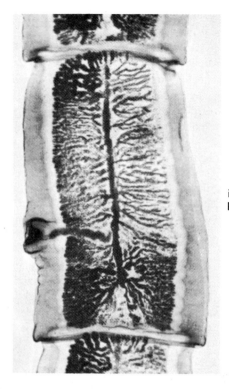

FIGURE 95. Taenia saginata, gravid proglottid. (Photomicrograph by Zane Price.)

Cysticercosis

The common larval stage of tapeworms of the genus *Taenia* is known as a cysticercus, or bladder worm. When these stages were first discovered, their relationship to the adult worm was not known, and so they were given generic and specific names of their own. Thus, the bladder worm of *Taenia solium* was known as *Cysticercus cellulosae*; it is still sometimes referred to by this old name, which no longer has any taxonomic validity.

The life cycle of *T. solium* (Fig. 89) commonly involves swine as the intermediate host. The eggs may remain viable for many weeks in the soil, after they are passed in the feces. Upon ingestion by hogs or by man, the outer shell disintegrates in the small intestine, and the contained larva, or oncosphere, penetrates into the intestinal wall. The oncosphere is able to invade the intestinal wall and enter a blood vessel by means of the six hooklets which it bears. It may be carried in the blood stream to all parts of the body and it may lodge in any tissue, but it most frequently develops in voluntary muscle. The larva completes development in about two months. It is semi-transparent, an opalescent white in color, elongate-oval in shape, and may reach a length of 0.6 to 1.8 cm. (Fig. 96). The bladder is fluid filled, and on one side is seen a denser area containing the scolex. If improperly cooked cysticercus-infected meat is eaten by man, all but the scolex portion will be digested, and that organ will attach itself to the intestinal wall, to grow a chain of proglottids.

SYMPTOMATOLOGY. Light infections with the bladder worm may cause no symptoms in man, unless the cysts become lodged in some vital area. In heavier infections, the chances of larvae developing in the brain (Fig. 97) or eye, where they are most likely to provoke symptoms, are greater. They rarely cause trouble, unless lodged in the orbit, while still alive, but they will begin to die and degenerate within three to five years. In muscle, the cysts frequently calcify without giving trouble. In the brain or spinal cord they rarely calcify, but often evoke tissue reactions leading to focal epileptic attacks, or other motor or sensory involvement. Internal hydrocephalus may develop if cerebrospinal fluid drainage is blocked.

Diagnosis may be made by surgical removal of subcutaneous nodules, radiographic demonstration of calcified cysts in the muscle (Fig. 98) or by visualization of the cysticercus within the orbit. Signs and symptoms of a space-occupying lesion of the central nervous system may be highly suggestive of cysticercosis in the presence of demonstrable cysticerci elsewhere in the body, or of a positive serologic test for cysticercosis (the more important of these tests are mentioned in Chapter 16). The diagnosis will ultimately depend upon demonstration of the organism after surgical removal of the cysts. Electroencephalography and pneumoencephalography may be of value in locating the

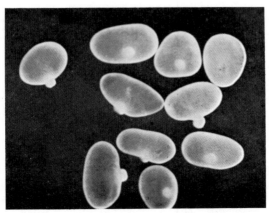

FIGURE 96.   Cysticercus larvae of *Taenia solium*. (Photograph courtesy of U.S. Department of Agriculture.)

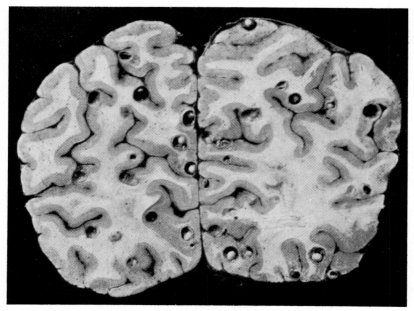

FIGURE 97. Cerebral cysticercosis. (Courtesy of Prof. C. H. Hu.)

parasites. It should be noted that cysticerci developing within the central nervous system are frequently abnormal, showing excessive and irregular proliferation of the bladder wall (Fig. 99). These cysts are called "racemose" and they frequently lack the characteristic scolex and hooks.

The larva of *Taenia saginata,* sometimes known as *Cysticercus bovis,* may exceptionally develop in the tissues of man. Symptoms should parallel those seen in *T. solium* cysticercosis, but heavy infections would not be expected to occur. For a detailed discussion of cysticercosis in man and animals, see Šlais (1970).

FIGURE 98. Extensive calcified cysticercosis of muscle. Numerous elliptical calcifications having variable sizes are evident in the muscle planes of the pelvis and lower extremities and are aligned along the long axis parallel to the muscle planes (large arrows). Nearly all the calcifications have a small lucent center (small arrows). When viewed from the side, they resemble a ring calcification. (Courtesy of T. Keats, Missouri Med. *58*:457, 1961.)

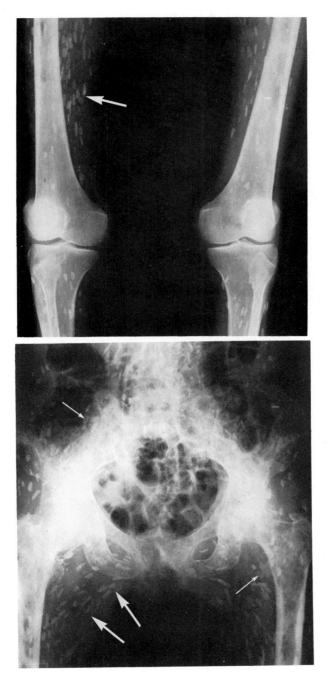

Figure 98. See legend on the opposite page.

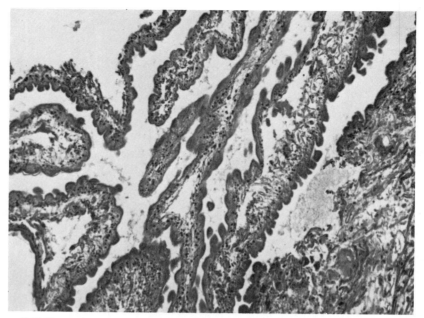

FIGURE 99. Section of "racemose" cysticercus removed from ventricle of human brain. Note scalloped surface of bladder wall. (Photomicrograph by Zane Price.)

Echinococcus granulosus and E. multilocularis (Hydatid Disease)

The minute tapeworm *Echinococcus granulosus* lives as an adult in the intestine of dogs and other Canidae. Its larval stage (Fig. 100), the hydatid cyst, may be found in many mammals, chiefly herbivores. Hydatid infection follows closely in distribution the occurrence of its most important intermediate host, the sheep. In some areas the hydatid is also a common parasite of hogs and cattle. Human infection is seen in the sheep-raising areas of South America, Algeria, Tanzania and South Africa, Asia Minor, Central Asia and North China, and in New Zealand and southern Australia. A few cases are reported each year from southern Canada and the United States, while more are seen in northern Canada and Alaska.

The adult worm (Fig. 101) is seen only in dogs and closely related animals, and cannot develop in man. The entire worm is 0.6 cm. or less in length, and possesses a scolex, neck and usually three proglottids. One proglottid is immature, one mature, and one is gravid. The eggs cannot be distinguished from those of *Taenia*. When ingested, they hatch in the small intestine and penetrate its wall in the same manner as do

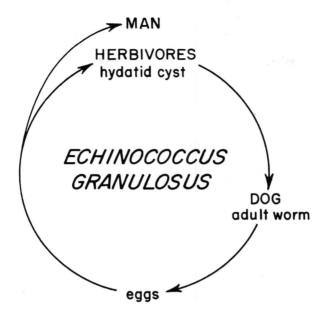

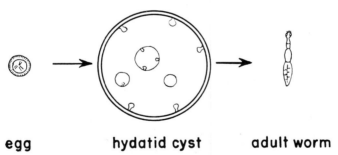

egg   **hydatid cyst**   **adult worm**

FIGURE 100. Schematic representation of life cycle of *Echinococcus granulosus*.

those of *Taenia*. *Echinococcus* embryos may lodge in any organ or tissue, but most frequently are found in the liver and lungs. In man, 80 to 95 per cent of hydatids develop in these two organs, the majority of them in the liver. The embryo develops slowly into the hydatid cyst, reaching a diameter of 1 cm. in five months or so, and thereafter enlarging steadily so that at the end of ten or more years' growth they may contain some liters of fluid. Ultimate growth will depend upon location, as in some areas they will be unable to expand freely, while in others even a modest

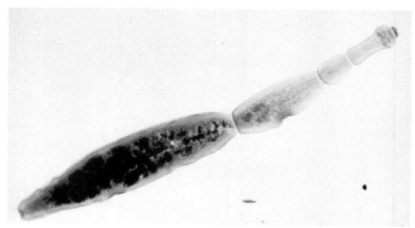

FIGURE 101. Echinococcus granulosus, adult worm.

growth will result in serious impairment to the function of vital structures, or even death. By the time the cyst has reached the diameter of 1 cm., its wall is differentiated into a thick outer laminated, non-cellular layer, which covers the thin germinal epithelium. From the germinal epithelium, masses of cells grow into the cavity of the cyst. They become vacuolated, and are known as the brood capsules. Scolices are budded from the inner wall of the brood capsule. Occasionally, daughter cysts

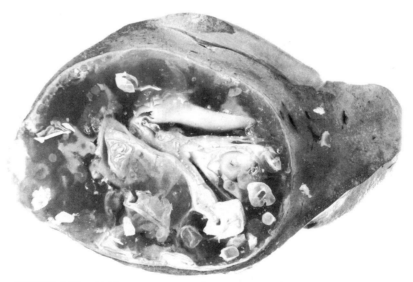

FIGURE 102. Echinococcus granulosus, section through unilocular hydatid cyst containing daughter cysts. (Courtesy of Ash and Spitz, Pathology of Tropical Diseases, Armed Forces Institute of Pathology, #31,977.)

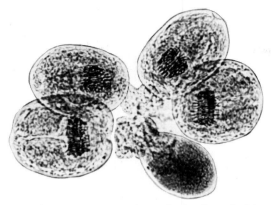

FIGURE 103. *Echinococcus granulosus,* hydatid sand. (Photomicrograph by Zane Price.)

appear within the hydatid (Fig. 102); these in turn produce brood capsules which may contain scolices. The daughter cysts are replicas in miniature of the complete hydatid, possessing even the laminated outer layer; their mode of development is obscure. Gradually the brood capsules and daughter cysts break down, liberating the developed scolices. A granular material, consisting of free scolices, daughter cysts, and amorphous material, is found in older cysts. It is the "hydatid sand" (Fig. 103) which is sometimes aspirated for diagnostic purposes. Some cysts may never produce brood capsules, or the brood capsules may fail to produce scolices. In other cases hydatids may become sterile because of secondary bacterial infection, or they may die and become calcified.

A second type of hydatid formation is the so-called alveolar or multilocular cyst, in which there is either a breakdown or a failure in formation of the closed limiting membrane, so that the cyst may proliferate in any direction, and even metastasize. It has long been thought that this type of development was the result of some untoward escape of germinal tissue through the ruptured limiting membrane, with budding thereafter in the manner of a malignant growth. Work by Rausch (1954) and others in Alaska and northern Canada has demonstrated that in that area as in certain of the northern states, the U.S.S.R., much of Europe, and elsewhere, alveolar cysts in man and animals may be produced by an entirely distinct species, *Echinococcus multilocularis.* A typical case report is that of LaFond et al. (1963). This species exhibits slight morphological differences from *E. granulosus* in the adult stage. The common intermediate hosts of *E. multilocularis* are rodents.

A third type of hydatid is the osseous type (Hutchison et al., 1962), so called because it develops in bone. Here, as might be expected, development is markedly abnormal, and the limiting membrane is not formed. The hydatid develops in the bony canal, and frequently erodes large areas of bone. It is probable that this type could be formed by either species.

SYMPTOMATOLOGY. Symptoms of hydatid disease will vary according to the location of the cyst. If, as is most commonly the case, the cyst is in the liver, it may cause no symptoms, and will only be noted when its increasing size calls attention to its presence. Hepatic cysts may cause early symptoms if the location within the liver is such that their expansion produces pressure on a major bile duct or blood vessel. Cysts in the lungs ordinarily are asymptomatic until they become large enough to give rise to cough, shortness of breath or pain in the chest. Cysts within the central nervous system will produce serious damage; symptoms will vary depending upon location. Leakage of the hydatid fluid produces sensitization, and provokes eosinophilia. If extensive sudden leakage occurs, spontaneously or as a result of trauma or operative procedure, an anaphylactic reaction of severe or fatal nature may result.

Many asymptomatic hydatid cysts are first discovered on radiologic examination (Fig. 104). The cyst shows a sharp outline, and fluid levels

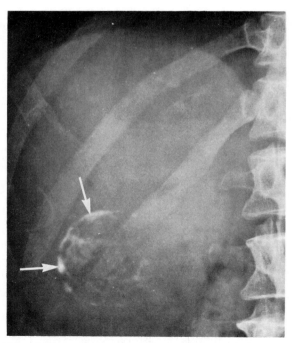

FIGURE 104. Echinococcus cyst of liver. There is a single, round, partially calcified, echinococcus cyst in the inferior portion of the right lobe (white arrows). (Courtesy of J. G. Teplick, et al., Roentgenologic Diagnosis, Vol. 1, 3rd Ed. Philadelphia, W. B. Saunders Co., 1976, Figure 7–29A.)

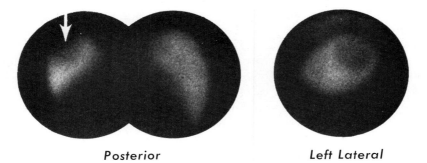

Posterior   *Left Lateral*

FIGURE 105. Radioisotope scan, echinococcus cyst of spleen. Spleen and liver images separated photographically for clarity. (Courtesy of Nuclear Medicine Division, Kaiser Permanente Medical Center, Oakland, California.)

can sometimes be detected within it. Photoscans may indicate the presence of space-occupying lesions of the liver (Sodeman and Haynie, 1964), or spleen (Fig. 105). If abdominal and large, a characteristic thrill can sometimes be elicited. The intracutaneous Casoni test is a valuable diagnostic aid, and is described in Chapter 16. After surgical exposure of a presumed hydatid cyst, aspiration of a portion of its contents can be performed, and examination of fluid removed in this manner may reveal hydatid sand. It should be remembered that a proportion of hydatid cysts are sterile, and will contain no sand. Cryosurgical stabilization of the fragile cyst wall prior to evacuation of its contents is recommended by Saidi and Nazarian (1971). These authors also recommend instillation of a 0.5 per cent solution of silver nitrate into the exocyst space after removal of the hydatid, for sterilization of any residual larval tissue.

EPIDEMIOLOGY. While hydatid disease caused by *Echinococcus granulosus* is most prevalent in sheep-raising areas, such as Australia and New Zealand, other domestic and wild animals serve as reservoir hosts of the parasite elsewhere. In North Africa, Iraq and Iran, hydatid cysts occur with high frequency in the lungs of camels. They may also be found in goats, in cattle and in wild herbivores. The adult worms are acquired by sheep dogs, or stray dogs feeding on infected entrails which lie about abattoirs or which are discarded by families after slaughtering animals at home. Feral dogs and other canids acquire the infection by scavenging or by preying on sheep or wild herbivores. Transmission to man may occur whenever infected dogs live in close proximity to humans.

Hydatid disease is widely distributed throughout the South American continent. In North America, *E. granulosus* occurs in Alaska, Canada, and the United States. Animal reservoirs are dogs, coyotes and wolves; the hydatid cysts occur in sheep, pigs, deer, and other wild herbivores. Reports by Brunetti and Rosen (1970) and by Liu et al.

(1970) contain data on incidence of *E. granulosus* in wild mammals in California. Endemicity of the disease in California is discussed by Schwabe et al. (1972), and in Utah by Spruance et al. (1974).

Echinococcus multilocularis is somewhat more restricted in distribution than is *E. granulosus.* Leiby et al. (1970) summarize host occurrence and endemic foci of this species in the Northern United States. Reservoir hosts of *E. multilocularis* in nature are dogs, wolves, foxes, and cats; the larval stages occur in wild rodents, particularly voles, which are an important food item of wild carnivores as well as of dogs and cats in rural areas. Leiby and Kritsky (1972) note a domestic life cycle involving adult worms in house cats, hydatids in mice. Thus, transmission to man can occur via the accidental ingestion of eggs passed by dogs or cats. In addition, hunters and trappers could become infected while handling foxes or wolves. It should be noted that both *E. granulosus* and *E. multilocularis* may occur simultaneously in dogs and other canids (Rausch, 1967). A summary of the different species of *Echinococcus* and their hosts may be found in Smyth (1964). A review of the different species and their prevalence in the Americas was given by Williams et al. (1971).

TREATMENT. There is no effective medical treatment for hydatid disease. Surgical removal is usually preceded, after adequate exposure of the cyst, by aspiration of a portion of its contents, injection of a quantity of 10 per cent formalin solution to sterilize the germinal epithelium and remaining contents of the cyst, and its withdrawal after five minutes. Intraventricular cysts frequently are unattached and may be removed with relative ease. Blind needling of what may be a hydatid cyst should never be attempted, as fluid leakage may lead to serious anaphylactic reactions, and if scolices or germinal tissue become implanted outside the cyst they may continue to grow, forming new hydatid cysts (Schiller, 1966).

Multiceps multiceps (Coenurus Disease)

The adult of *Multiceps multiceps,* a taeniid worm of moderate size, is found in dogs and other Canidae; the larvae occur in a variety of herbivorous mammals, and have been reported occasionally from man in various parts of the world, including the United States. It is possible that more than one species of *Multiceps* can produce human disease, but it is very difficult to distinguish species in this genus.

Following ingestion of the ovum of *Multiceps,* the oncosphere hatches in the small intestine, and makes its way into a blood vessel in the intestinal wall, in the same manner as larvae of *Taenia* or *Echinococcus.* The embryo is carried in the blood stream to various parts of the body, but most frequently develops in the central nervous system. The larval form is intermediate between the cysticercus and hydatid: multiple scolices bud from the inner surface of its wall, instead of the single one which characterizes the bladder worm: neither brood capsules nor daughter cysts are formed. The coenurus larva is larger than a cysticercus; it is semi-transparent, a glistening white in color, and is filled with fluid. Numerous denser white spots on the wall indicate the position of the attached scolices. The coenurus may form a single vesicle, or be branched to a greater or lesser degree.

In sheep, the most common intermediate host, the parasite produces a disease known as gid, from the unstable gait, or giddiness, which marks the infected animals. In man, most reported cases have had coenuri in the brain or spinal cord, with symptoms suggestive of space-occupying lesions of the central nervous system. In a few cases coenurus larvae, which may have been those of species other than *Multiceps multiceps*, have been found in the muscles or subcutaneous tissues. A preoperative diagnosis of coenurus infection is unlikely. It is probable that the Casoni test would be positive in this disease.

Dipylidium caninum

Dipylidium caninum is common in cats and dogs all over the world. Occasionally it is found in man, particularly in small children. *D. caninum* may cause mild intestinal disturbances in some individuals. Man usually acquires the infection through association with infected pets. The larvae of this species are known as cysticercoids. The cysticercoid develops when the ovum is ingested by a larval cat or dog flea and is retained within the adult flea. Infection takes place through the accidental ingestion of these fleas. The cysticercoids grow into adult worms in the small intestine. The gravid proglottids possess a remarkable degree of motility and may migrate actively from the anus. They contract and expand vigorously upon reaching the exterior of the host and may remain attached to the fur surrounding the anal area for some time. It is probable that these contractions function in the release of the eggs which are then ingested by the flea larvae. Children may become infected while hugging or kissing their pets.

Adults of *D. caninum* are relatively small in size, averaging about 15 cm. in length. They may reach a length of 80 cm. Many specimens may be present in one individual host. The scolex bears four suckers and a conical, retractile rostellum with several circles of small hooks. Mature proglottids (Fig. 106) are longer than they are wide, and contain two sets each of male and female reproductive organs. The developing uterus appears in the form of a network which, as the segment becomes gravid, eventually breaks up into discrete units called egg packets. Each of these egg packets may contain from five to thirty eggs. Gravid segments

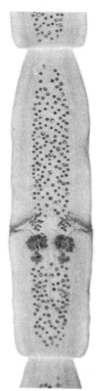

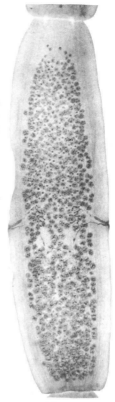

Fig. 106   Fig. 107

FIGURE 106. Dipylidium caninum, mature proglottid. (Photomicrograph by Zane Price.)

FIGURE 107. Dipylidium caninum, gravid proglottid. (Photomicrograph by Zane Price.)

(Fig. 107) are considerably longer than wide and are barrel-like in outline.

Diagnosis of this species is made upon finding the characteristic proglottids, or, more rarely, egg packets in the stool.

TREATMENT. Quinacrine is curative, and niclosamide would be expected to be equally effective. Both are administered as outlined for *Diphyllobothrium latum* infections.

Hymenolepis nana

Hymenolepis nana, the dwarf tapeworm of man, is a common parasite of the house mouse and is found in man all over the world. Infec-

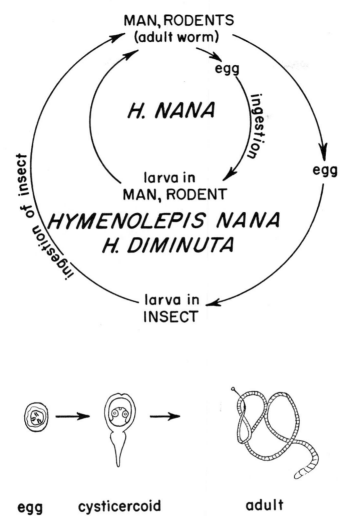

FIGURE 108. Schematic representation of life cycles of *Hymenolepis nana* and *H. diminuta*.

tion with *H. nana* is seen frequently in children but occurs in adults as well. A relatively high prevalence of this tapeworm in man has been reported in surveys conducted in central Europe and in Latin America.

Apparently, *H. nana* is unique in that the adult worm develops following ingestion of the egg by man (Fig. 108). Eggs when swallowed hatch in the small intestine. The six-hooked oncosphere burrows into the villi of the intestinal mucosa where, within a few days, it develops into a cysticercoid larva. When fully grown, the larvae break out of the villi into the lumen of the small intestine, where they grow into adult worms. Experimental evidence obtained from studies on mice (Heyneman, 1962) suggests that in these animals a certain degree of immunity to reinfection results from the occurrence in them of the tissue phase.

Eggs of *H. nana* may also develop into infective cysticercoids in various intermediate hosts, particularly grain beetles. When ingested accidentally with contaminated grain products, the larvae will grow into adult worms in mice and probably in man also. Since such an infection through ingestion of larval stages is not preceded by a tissue phase, no immunity is built up in the mammalian host. Eggs from adult worms acquired in this fashion may hatch in the small intestine of the same host individual, and the oncospheres invade the villi. In this manner, a second generation of adult worms may be produced from the initial infection within the same person. This phenomenon is called hyperinfection and may in some persons be responsible for the presence of very large numbers of adult worms. It is believed that infection in man is commonly the result of ingestion of eggs. Successful treatment therefore must involve, in addition to appropriate anthelmintic therapy, preventive measures against the possibility of reinfection. Apparently successful treatment should always be followed by a stool examination approximately three weeks following the administration of the anthelmintic. Adults of *Hymenolepis nana* are relatively small worms, only a few centimeters in length. The scolex has four suckers and a rostellum armed with one circle of hooks. All segments are wider than they are long. Mature proglottids contain one set of male and female reproductive organs. Gravid segments contain a sac-like uterus filled with eggs. Eggs are usually liberated from the gravid segments before they become detached. The eggs of *H. nana* (Fig. 93, *E* and *F*) are broadly ovoid, have a thin and smooth outer shell and measure 30 to 47 microns. They contain the six-hooked oncosphere within a rigid membrane. This membrane has two polar thickenings or knobs from which project four to eight long and thin filaments called polar filaments. The presence of these polar filaments is diagnostic and serves to differentiate *Hymenolepis nana* from *H. diminuta* described below.

SYMPTOMATOLOGY. Light infections are asymptomatic. When large numbers of worms are present, they may give rise to abdominal pain, diarrhea, headache, dizziness, anorexia and various non-specific symptoms.

TREATMENT. Niclosamide (Yomesan*) is the treatment of choice.

---

*Available from the Parasitic Disease Service, Center for Disease Control, U.S. Public Health Service, Atlanta, Ga. 30333.

It is administered at the rate of 40 to 80 mg. per Kg. daily for five days (Most et al., 1971). Paromomycin sulfate (Humatin) has been used successfully by Wittner and Tanowitz (1971), who recommend 45 mg. per Kg. body weight daily for five days, after a light breakfast.

Hymenolepis diminuta

Hymenolepis diminuta, despite its specific name, is much larger than *H. nana*. While *H. diminuta* commonly parasitizes rats, it may occasionally be encountered in human beings, cases having been reported from many parts of the world including several areas of the United States. Completion of the life cycle requires an arthropod intermediate host. More than twenty different species of insects have been shown to serve as suitable hosts for the development of the cysticercoid larvae. The most important are flour moths and flour beetles. Upon ingestion of infected insects from flour contaminated by the droppings of infected rats, larvae will grow into adults in the small intestine of man or rat.

H. diminuta seems to produce few or no definite symptoms. The size of adult worms varies considerably and, as in other tapeworm species, depends in part on the number of worms present in the intestine. The greatest length reported for an adult specimen of *H. diminuta* from man is 1 meter. Usually, adults are from 20 to 50 cm. long and as much as 4 mm. wide. The scolex bears four suckers and a small rostellum without hooks. Diagnosis of this species is made on finding the characteristic eggs (Fig. 93, *D*) in the stool. Eggs are slightly ovoid in shape and brown in color. The egg shell is relatively thick. In some specimens fine concentric striations may be observed in the outer shell. The oncosphere is enclosed in a membrane which has two polar thickenings but no polar filaments. The absence of polar filaments readily differentiates this species from *Hymenolepis nana*.

TREATMENT. Quinacrine or niclosamide is the treatment of choice, administered as outlined for treatment of *Diphyllobothrium latum*.

Key to the Gravid Proglottids of the Major Human Tapeworms

a. Uterus forms rosette in center of proglottid .... *Diphyllobothrium latum*
   Uterus otherwise disposed... b
b. Uterus with central stem running length of proglottid.......................... c
   Uterus without central stem... d
c. Central stem with seven to thirteen main lateral branches ...... *Taenia solium*
   Central stem with fifteen to twenty main lateral branches .... *T. saginata*
d. Proglottid wider than long .... *Hymenolepis* spp.
   Proglottid longer than wide .... *Dipylidium caninum*

REFERENCES

Baer, Jean G. 1969. *Diphyllobothrium pacificum,* a tapeworm from sea lions endemic in man along the coastal area of Peru. J. Fish Res. Bd. (Canada), *26*:717–723.

Brunetti, O. A., and Rosen, M. N. 1970. Prevalence of *Echinococcus granulosus* hydatid in California deer. J. Parasit., *56*:1138–1140.

Fetterman, L. E. 1965. Radiographic demonstration of *Taenia saginata*—an unsuspected cause of abdominal pain. New Eng. J. Med., *272*:364–365.

Heyneman, D. 1962. Studies on helminth immunity. IV. Rapid onset of resistance by the white mouse against a challenging infection with eggs of *Hymenolepis nana* (Cestoda: Hymenolepididae). J. Immun., *88*:217–220.

Hutchison, W. F., Thompson, W. B., and Derian, P. S. 1962. Osseous hydatid (echinococcus) disease. Report of an indigenous case. J.A.M.A. *182*:81–83.

Kamo, H., Hatsushika, R., and Yamane, Y. 1971. Diplogonoporiasis and diplogonadic cestodes in Japan. Yonago Acta Med., *15*:234–246.

LaFond, D. J., Thatcher, D. S., and Handeyside, R. G. 1963. Alveolar hydatid disease. J.A.M.A., *186*:35–37.

Leiby, P. D., Carney, W. P., and Woods, C. E. 1970. Studies on sylvatic echinococcosis. III. Host occurrence and geographic distribution of *Echinococcus multilocularis* in the North Central United States. J. Parasit., *56*:1141–1150.

Leiby, P. D., and Kritsky, D. C. 1972. *Echinococcus multilocularis:* A possible domestic life cycle in Central North America and its public health importance. J. Parasit., *58*:1213–1215.

Liu, I. K. M., Schwabe, C. W., Schantz, P. M., and Allison, M. N. 1970. The occurrence of *Echinococcus granulosus* in coyotes (*Canis latrans*) in the Central Valley of California. J. Parasit., *56*:1135–1137.

Most, H., Yoeli, M., Hammond, J., and Scheinesson, G. P. 1971. Yomesan (Niclosamide) therapy of *Hymenolepis nana* infections. Am. J. Trop. Med. & Hyg., *20*:206–208.

Perera, D. R., Western, K. A., and Schultz, M. G. 1970. Niclosamide treatment of cestodiasis. Clinical trials in the United States. Am. J. Trop. Med. & Hyg., *19*:610–612.

Rausch, R. 1954. Studies on the helminth fauna of Alaska. XX. The histogenesis of the alveolar larva of *Echinococcus* species. J. Infect. Dis., *94*:178–186.

Rausch, R. L. 1967. On the occurrence and distribution of *Echinococcus* spp. (Cestoda: Taeniidae), and characteristics of their development in the intermediate host. Ann. Parasit., *42*:19–63.

Saidi, F., and Nazarian, I. 1971. Surgical treatment of hydatid cysts by freezing of cyst wall and instillation of 0.5 per cent silver nitrate solution. New Eng. J. Med., *284*:1346–1350.

Schiller, C. F. 1966. Complications of *Echinococcus* cyst rupture. J.A.M.A., *195*:220–222.

Schwabe, C. W., Ruppanner, R., Miller, C. W., Fontaine, R. E., and Kagan, I. G. 1972. Hydatid disease is endemic in California. Cal. Med., *117*:13–17.

Šlais, J. 1970. The Morphology and Pathogenicity of the Bladder Worms *Cysticercus cellulosae* and *Cysticercus bovis.* 144 pp. Dr. W. Junk, N. V. Publishers, The Hague.

Smyth, J. D. 1964. The biology of the hydatid organism. *In*: Dawes, B. (ed.) *Advances in Parasitology.* Vol. 2. pp. 169–219. Academic Press, New York.

Sodeman, W. A., Jr., and Haynie, T. P. 1964. Hepatic photoscanning in hydatid liver cysts. J.A.M.A., *188*:318–320.

Spruance S. L., Klock, L. E., Chang, F., Fukushima, T., Andersen, F. L., and Kagan, I. G. 1974. Endemic hydatid disease in Utah. Rocky Mtn. Med. J., *71*:17–23.

von Bonsdorff, B. 1956. *Diphyllobothrium latum* as a cause of pernicious anemia. Exp. Parasit., *5*:207–230.

Williams, J. F., Lopez-Adaros, H., and Trejos, A. 1971. Current prevalence and distribution of hydatidosis with special reference to the Americas. Am. J. Trop. Med. & Hyg., *20*:224–236.

Wittner, M., and Tanowitz, H. 1971. Paromomycin therapy of human cestodiasis with special reference to hymenolepiasis. Am. J. Trop. Med. & Hyg., *20*:433–435.

10

The Intestinal Nematodes

The nematodes have been said to be the most worm-like of the various groups of parasitic animals lumped under the loose title of worms. This is perhaps a reflection of the fact that they are shaped like the common earthworm, which seems the prototype for all worms. Actually, the earthworm is not a nematode, being a representative of the segmented worms, or annelids. Nematodes are non-segmented, generally cylindrical in shape, tapering at both ends, and covered by a tough protective covering or cuticle. They have a complete digestive tract, with both oral and anal openings. The sexes are separate; generally males are much smaller than female worms. Reproductive organs are tubular, and lie coiled within the body cavity. In the male there is a single tubule, which at its smaller end consists of testicular cells; it extends into a vas deferens and seminal vesicle, and terminates in an ejaculatory duct opening into the cloaca. The female worm has two cylindrical ovaries, which expand into uteri. The uteri may open to the exterior through a single vulva, or there may be a common vagina between the vulva and uteri. The vulva is frequently located near the middle of the body, but varies in position in different species. In contrast to the trematodes and cestodes, all of which are parasitic, the majority of nematodes are free living. There are an estimated 500,000 species of nematodes. Many are of considerable economic importance as plant parasites, others as causes of disease in animals, and approximately one dozen are commonly encountered in man.

The parasitic nematodes are generally a light creamy-white color, but the females of the smaller forms may appear darker when filled

237

with dark-colored eggs. Certain structural modifications are of importance in identification of various species. The mouth in primitive forms is surrounded by three lips, but in hookworms has become modified into a buccal capsule furnished with cutting plates or teeth. The anterior portion of the digestive tract, or the esophagus, is muscular in most forms. In one group, of which *Trichuris* and *Trichinella* are examples, the esophagus is much reduced and has the appearance of a fine tubule running lengthwise through a column of large cuboidal cells. The muscular esophagus of certain nematodes is of uniform caliber throughout; this type is called filariform. If the esophagus is expanded posteriorly into a bulb, which contains a valve mechanism, it is referred to as rhabditiform. Male nematodes usually have a pair of copulatory spicules, which lie in pouches near the ejaculatory duct and may be inserted into the vagina of the female. In some forms, the posterior end of the male is expanded into a thin-walled copulatory bursa, supported by thickened rays. The arrangement of these rays may be of importance in identification of the worms.

Stages in the life cycle of nematodes include the egg, larvae which undergo several molts, and adults. The filariform type of esophagus generally characterizes infective stage larvae, which in their free-living stages (or those passed in intermediate hosts) may have been rhabditiform.

As has been mentioned, the majority of nematodes are free living. The parasitic forms include representatives of several different groups of nematodes, which may be assumed to have independently evolved a parasitic mode of existence. The nematodes exemplify, as does no other group, many of the stages which may be considered to lead from a wholly free-living to an obligate parasitic existence. If one desires to set up such a series, at one end might be placed the vinegar eel, *Turbatrix aceti*. *Turbatrix* is a free-living nematode, which frequently was found multiplying to enormous numbers in vinegar, in the era when that commodity was dispensed from wooden casks and not sterilized when bottled at the factory. The vinegar eel has been found on occasion in the vagina, where it apparently is able to survive for some time if introduced in a douche. This organism exhibits some potentialities of becoming a parasite but cannot establish itself permanently in the vagina. *Strongyloides stercoralis* is a small nematode which, if conditions are suitable, may pass several free-living generations in the soil, but sooner or later produces larvae of a type which must complete their development as parasites of man. The hookworms are invariably parasitic in the adult stage, but their larvae must undergo a free-living developmental period in the soil. *Ascaris* eggs must develop for a period outside the body before they mature and become infective, but then are ingested and no stages of the life cycle are free living. Finally the

filarial worms, such as *Wuchereria*, might be considered perfect examples of obligate parasitism, having larval stages which develop in
an insect and adults in man or other mammals. At no time can the
worm exist outside the body of one or the other host.

The nematode parasites of man are moderately long-lived worms.
Ascaris will usually die out in about a year in the absence of reinfection,
while *Trichuris* lives several times that long, and hookworm infections
may persist for as long as 8 to 16 years. Autoinfection is seen in *Strongyloides* (and perhaps *Enterobius*), enabling these parasites to persist for
indefinite periods in the absence of reinfection.

Diagnosis of intestinal nematode infection is generally made by
demonstration of the characteristic eggs in the feces. Occasionally adult
worms are found in the stools, but except for *Ascaris* they are so small
that they are frequently overlooked unless a special search is made.

Ascaris lumbricoides

The specific name of the large intestinal roundworm, *Ascaris lumbricoides* (Fig. 109), is a tribute to its superficial resemblance to the
common earthworm, *Lumbricus*. Female worms range from 20 to 35 cm.
in length, while males are seldom over 30 cm. long. The female worms
may be as thick as a lead pencil; the males are definitely more slender
and may be distinguished by an incurved tail. Both sexes are creamy-

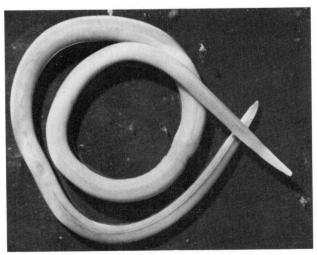

FIGURE 109. *Ascaris lumbricoides,* female worm passed spontaneously (natural size). (Photograph by Zane Price.)

white in color, sometimes with a pinkish cast, and the cuticle has fine circular striations.

Ascaris infections are found throughout the temperate and tropical areas of the globe, and under conditions of poor sanitation virtually one hundred per cent of the population may be found to harbor the parasite. The per capita worm burden may reach staggering levels, with hundreds or even a thousand or more worms in a single individual. A graphic illustration of *Ascaris* density is given by Stoll (1947), who calculated a total of 18,000 tons of ascaris eggs produced annually by those worms affecting the people of China alone. The total is perhaps higher today.

When fully embryonated eggs are swallowed, they hatch in the duodenum and then undergo an extraordinary migration through the body before returning to settle down in the intestine and grow to adulthood. The larvae first penetrate the wall of the duodenum and enter blood or lymphatic vessels to be carried to the liver, heart, and thence into the pulmonary circulation. They are filtered out by the capillaries of the lungs, and break from them into the alveoli. There they grow and molt, and after about ten days migrate through the respiratory passages to reach the esophagus and eventually once again the small intestine. Two or three months after ingestion of the ova, the mature worms commence egg-laying in the intestine. There is suggestive evidence that while infection may take place constantly, and the larvae undergo a migratory cycle, they will not be able to grow to adulthood in the intestine as long as any considerable number of worms remain from a previous infection. Batches of adult worms may succeed each other in hyperendemic areas at periods dependent upon the longevity of the adult worms in the intestine. *Ascaris* eggs are unsegmented when passed; under favorable conditions they require a period of about two or three weeks outside of the host to develop to the infective stage. Excessive heat and dryness will soon kill them, but they will remain viable in moist soil for long periods.

Mature female worms have been estimated to produce an average of 200,000 eggs daily. In all but the rare infections in which only male worms are present, diagnosis can usually be made with ease on examination of even the unconcentrated stool. The fertilized ovum of *Ascaris* (Fig. 110, 3) is readily recognized. It is broadly oval, measuring 45 to 75 microns in length by 35 to 50 microns in breadth. The outer covering is an albuminoid coat, usually stained a golden brown by bile as seen in the fresh stool. The outer coat is coarsely mammillated, and lies directly on top of a thick smooth shell, which is usually not easily distinguished. Some eggs will be seen to have lost the outer albuminoid coat (Fig. 110, 5) and in these the thick yellowish inner shell is obvious. It is thicker than the shell of a hookworm egg, which these decorticated

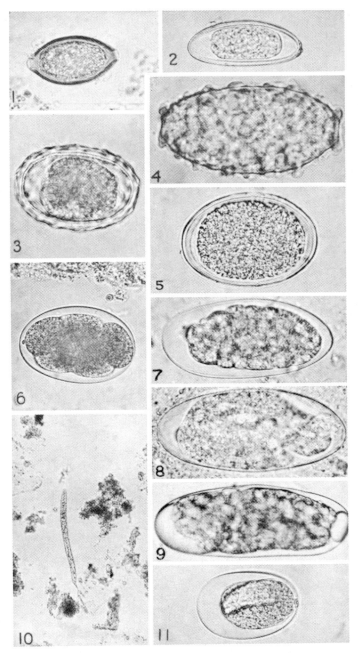

FIGURE 110. Nematode eggs: *1, Trichuris trichiura; 2, Enterobius vermicularis; 3, Ascaris lumbricoides,* fertilized egg; *4, Ascaris,* unfertilized egg; *5, Ascaris,* decorticated egg; 6, hookworm; *7, Trichostrongylus orientalis;* immature egg; *8, Trichostrongylus,* embryonated egg; *9, Heterodera marioni; 10, Strongyloides stercoralis,* rhabditiform larva; *11,* Strongyloides egg (rarely seen in stool). All figures 500 × except *10* (75 ×). Courtesy of Hunter, G. W., Swartzwelder, J. C., and Clyde, D. F., 1976. Tropical Medicine. 5th Ed. W. B. Saunders Company, Philadelphia.

Ascaris eggs otherwise resemble. Infertile eggs (Fig. 110, *4*) are longer and narrower than the fertile ones. They may measure about 90 by 40 microns. Both the inner shell and outer albuminous coat may be thin, and if the latter is absent and the inner shell very thin they may resemble *Trichostrongylus* eggs (Fig. 110, *7, 8*).

Ascaris infections are sometimes diagnosed roentgenologically, either as worm-shaped radiolucent areas in a barium-filled intestine (Fig. 111), or more spectacularly with their own intestinal tracts outlined as well by barium which they have ingested.

SYMPTOMATOLOGY. Small numbers of adult worms in the intestine often cause no symptoms, but may give rise to vague abdominal pains, or to intermittent colic, especially in children. The worms, irritated by medication into excesses of activity, can penetrate through the wall of the intestine, or into the appendix, and travel up the common bile duct which they may block or traverse to enter the gallbladder or liver. They may enter the stomach and be vomited, or even crawl up the esophagus to enter the nasopharynx or trachea. The symptoms caused by migratory worms will depend upon the organs involved. Large numbers of worms may give rise to more or less severe allergic symptoms. Eosinophilia is generally present but seldom impressive. Serum IgE has

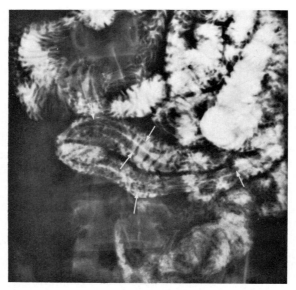

FIGURE 111. Ascariasis of the small intestine. Multiple worms are clearly outlined (arrows) in the middle segment and contrast clearly with the barium. No abnormalities of the mucosal pattern are apparent. (Courtesy of Teplick, J. G., et al. 1976. Roentgenologic Diagnosis, Vol. 1, 3rd Ed. W. B. Saunders Company, Philadelphia, Figure 7–41.)

been reported to reach very high levels in children infected with *Ascaris* (Johansson et al., 1968).

PATHOGENESIS. Small numbers of infecting larvae will produce no obvious symptoms. Larger numbers may give rise to a transient hepatitis; with rupture into the alveoli, a pneumonitis may develop (Gelpi and Mustafa, 1967). X-ray changes are non-specific, with infiltrates and patchy areas of pneumonitis, increased bronchovascular markings, and widening of the hilar shadows. These pulmonary findings, when accompanied as is usual by an eosinophilia, fulfill the rather ill-defined criteria for tropical eosinophilia. Later in the course of infection, the presence of large numbers of worms may lead to intestinal obstruction; this complication is most common in smaller children.

TREATMENT. Pyrantel pamoate (Antiminth) is the most effective drug presently available for the treatment of ascariasis. Its administration requires no special diet or pre- or post-treatment purgation. It may be given with milk or fruit juice. Gastrointestinal reactions, including nausea, vomiting, abdominal cramps and diarrhea, are sometimes seen, and transient elevation of the SGOT has been reported. Pyrantel is administered at the rate of 11 mg. per Kg. of body weight in a single oral dose (to a maximum dose of 1.0 gm.). A cure rate of over 95 per cent is reported (Villarejos et al., 1971). Piperazine citrate (Antepar) is also effective, and requires no special diet, and no purgation. Side effects are few: dizziness and urticarial reactions are occasionally seen, visual disturbances are rare; epilepsy may be exacerbated by the drug. For uncomplicated intestinal ascariasis, piperazine may be given orally at the rate of 75 mg. per Kg. of body weight daily for two days (the maximum daily dose is 3.5 gm.). Intestinal obstruction due to ascarids is treated by nasogastric suction until vomiting is controlled. One or two hours after the suction is discontinued an initial dose of piperazine is administered through the nasogastric tube, which is allowed to remain in place. This dose may be 150 mg. per Kg. of body weight; again, the maximum dosage is 3.5 gm. If vomiting recurs and suction must be resumed, additional doses may be given at the rate of 65 mg. per Kg. (maximum 1.0 gm.) every 12 hours for six doses. If there is no vomiting, the second dose is given by mouth, 24 hours after the first, and is repeated at 12-hour intervals for six doses. The amount given is again 65 mg. per Kg. If this treatment is not successful or if the obstruction is complete, surgical intervention will probably be necessary.

An alternate form of therapy for uncomplicated intestinal ascariasis is the administration of thiabendazole (Mintezol) by mouth. It is given at the rate of 25 mg. per Kg. of body weight, twice daily for two days. Nausea, vomiting and vertigo are fairly frequent side effects of treatment with this drug. Levamisole, administered at the rate of 2.5 mg.

per Kg. of body weight in a single oral dose, is still more effective than any of those listed above, but is as yet unavailable in the United States.

In mixed infections of *Ascaris* and other intestinal worms, it is good practice to treat initially with a drug effective against *Ascaris*. Some of the medications specific for other worms, while ineffective ascaricides, are thought to stimulate *Ascaris* to unusual bursts of activity during which they may cause considerable damage to their host. Perforation of the bowel wall or invasion of the bile duct are examples of such untoward migratory activity.

Enterobius vermicularis

The pinworm *Enterobius vermicularis* (Fig. 112) is by all odds the most common helminth parasite of those temperate regions where sanitation is at a high level. Spread of pinworm infection is no doubt facilitated by crowded indoor living in temperate climates, but it is also common in the tropics. Less attention is paid to pinworm in tropical areas, probably because of the relative prevalence of more important parasites. Conversely, the importance of *Enterobius* is frequently over-rated in the United States.

The male pinworm is inconspicuous, about 2 to 5 mm. in length, and at most 0.2 mm. in width. The female reaches a length of 8 to 13

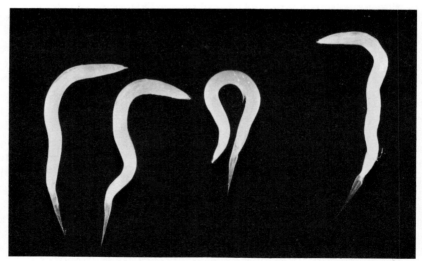

FIGURE 112. Enterobius vermicularis adult female worms. Note shapes and the clear, attenuated and pointed posterior end. (Courtesy of The Louisiana State University School of Medicine.)

mm., and a width up to 0.5 mm. They are a light yellowish-white in color; the female is distinguished by a long thin and sharply pointed tail, which characteristic gave rise to the common name. The adult worms inhabit the cecum and adjacent portions of large and small intestine. The female worms, when fully gravid, migrate down the intestinal tract to pass out the anus and deposit their eggs. The worms may migrate several inches out of the anus, depositing eggs as they crawl, or liberating masses of them as the worms dry and literally explode. The eggs are fully embryonated, and infective within a few hours of the time they are deposited; if climatic conditions are suitable they will survive for some weeks outside of the body. The eggs live longest under conditions of fairly high humidity and moderate temperature. Reinfection of the patient by contamination of the hands is common, and makes control of the parasite very difficult. Development of the adult worms is stated to require about six weeks; shorter periods have, however, been reported. Infection of others through contaminated clothing, bedding, and so forth, is frequently the cause of familial outbreaks. The eggs may survive for some days in dry dust, and airborne eggs may serve to infect persons at some distance. A type of autoinfection described by Schüffner and Swellengrebel (1949) as "retrofection" involves hatching of the embryonated eggs after their deposition in the perianal region, and their subsequent migration back into the rectum and large intestine.

Diagnosis of pinworm infection is made on recovery of the characteristic eggs, although it may be suspected in children who have pruritus ani. Occasionally, the adult female worms will be seen crawling in the perianal region, or in the feces. Eggs may be found in the stools, but this is exceptional, as the females ordinarily do not oviposit until they leave the intestinal tract. Various methods of recovery of eggs from the perianal region provide the most efficient means of diagnosis. The best known of these is the Scotch tape swab or Graham technique, described in Chapter 15. The eggs (Fig. 110, 2) are 50 to 60 microns in length, and 20 to 32 microns in breadth, and have a translucent shell of moderate thickness. They are usually conspicuously flattened on one side, and this flattening and consequent reduction in diameter, plus the thicker shell, serves to differentiate the eggs from hookworm ova.

SYMPTOMATOLOGY. The multiplicity of symptoms charged against *Enterobius* are legion, and in some cases fantastic. Migration of the female worms from the anus will in some persons produce pruritus, which may at times be severe. In small children, the worms may invade the vagina after leaving the rectum, thereby producing a local irritation. The local itching undoubtedly may interfere with the sleep of children or adults who are infected, as the worms migrate from the anus during the resting hours. It is probable that *Enterobius* causes no symptoms in the majority of infected adults and children.

PATHOGENESIS. *Enterobius* may for all practical purposes be considered a commensal in all save those persons whose hypersensitivity to the secretions and excretions of the worms leads to rectal pruritus. Attachment of the adult worms to the intestinal wall may produce some inflammation. Invasion of the appendix might be expected to be the common occurrence which it is, but any relationship between this invasion and appendicitis remains unproven. Invasion of the peritoneal cavity via the female reproductive system has been reported (Brooks et al., 1962), and it may result in the formation of granulomas around eggs or worms; these are rarely of clinical significance. Granuloma formation around pinworm eggs in the liver was reported by Little et al. (1973) in a patient whose worms presumably gained access to the peritoneal cavity via a necrotic area in an adenocarcinoma of the bowel. An adult female pinworm found on thoracotomy for a non-calcified pulmonary nodule (Beaver et al., 1973) is thought to have gained access to the lung via the respiratory tract.

TREATMENT. The worms may be eliminated by a variety of drugs, and by means as simple as warm tap water enemas, yet their eggs are so resistant and widespread that their reintroduction into a household containing small children is generally only a matter of time. In a family situation in which reintroduction of the parasite seems probable, only those persons who are symptomatic need generally be treated. Tap water enemas, repeated as necessary, will control symptoms. For those patients who, for a variety of reasons, need more dramatic treatment, pyrvinium pamoate (Povan) is recommended, as it not only is effective but colors the stools a bright red. Pyrvinium pamoate is administered in a single dose, at the rate of 5 mg. per Kg. of body weight. Administration of this drug is occasionally accompanied by vomiting or diarrhea; rarely it is associated with photosensitization. Pyrvinium is available in both tablet and liquid form. The tablets are less likely to cause emesis, but have a coating which contains acetylsalicylic acid.

THE HOOKWORMS

Ancylostoma duodenale

The Old World hookworm, *Ancylostoma duodenale*, is the only hookworm of Europe and the areas bordering the Mediterranean, of the west coast of South America, and of parts of India and China. It is found together with *Necator americanus* in certain areas in Brazil, a part of India, most of China, and throughout southeast Asia, Indonesia and the islands of the South and the Southwest Pacific. Within these areas, it is generally confined to those parts of the Northern hemisphere south of the thirty-sixth parallel, and of the Southern hemisphere north of the thirtieth parallel, except where local conditions may be especially favorable, as in mines.

Ancylostoma adults are of a grayish-white or pinkish color. The head has a slight bend in relation to the rest of the body. The male worm measures nearly 1 cm. in length by 0.5 mm. in greatest width; the female is somewhat longer and stouter. The mouth is well developed (Fig. 113) with a pair of teeth on either side of the median line, and a smaller pair in the depths of the buccal capsule. The male worm is provided with a prominent copulatory bursa posteriorly.

Hookworm eggs when passed in the feces are unsegmented or in the early cleavage stages. Under optimal conditions, when deposited on moist sandy soil, the larva develops and hatches within twenty-four to forty-eight hours. Growth and development take place in the soil, as the larva feeds on bacteria and organic material and undergoes a first molt. After about seven days the worm stops feeding and molts a second time, transforming from a rhabditiform to a filariform or infective larva. The infective larvae do not eat, and probably can live for only about two weeks if they do not find a host. They usually live in the upper layers of the soil, and when the soil is cool and moist climb to the highest point covered by a film of moisture. They extend their bodies into the air and remain waving about in this position until driven down by drying of their surroundings or by heat, or until they come in contact with the skin of a suitable host. It is probable that man is the only normal host of *Ancylostoma duodenale;* although larval penetration

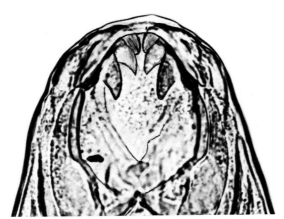

FIGURE 113. Ancylostoma caninum, mouth parts showing teeth. (Photomicrograph by Zane Price.)

can take place in other mammals, development to the adult stage does not occur.

Diagnosis of hookworm infection depends upon recovery of the eggs from the stools. The hookworm egg is unsegmented or in an early segmentation stage when passed. In specimens which have been allowed to stand at room temperature for a period of hours, especially if the weather is warm, a larva may be seen within the egg shell. Rarely, eggs may hatch and liberate larvae, which are then found free in the stool and must be differentiated from those of *Strongyloides*. If a stained smear is made of the stool, it is easy to differentiate between hookworm and *Strongyloides* larvae (Fig. 114), as the former have a distinct, long buccal capsule between the oral opening and the esophagus, while in *Strongyloides* this structure is very short. The eggs (Fig. 110, 6) are regularly oval, and 56 to 60 microns in length by 36 to 40 microns in breadth. The shell is thin and colorless. Although *Ancylostoma* eggs average somewhat smaller than those of *Necator*, no attempt at differentiation of the two genera is ordinarily made on stool examination. Rough estimates of the numbers of worms present may be made on the basis of egg counts, as described in Chapter 15.

In man, larval penetration usually takes place through the feet, though the larvae can penetrate through any skin areas with which they

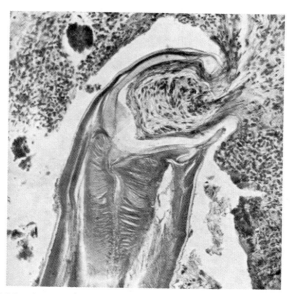

FIGURE 114. Longitudinal section through hookworm attached to intestinal mucosa. (Courtesy of Hunter, G. W., Swartzwelder, J. C., and Clyde, D. F. 1976. Tropical Medicine. 5th Ed. W. B. Saunders Company, Philadelphia.)

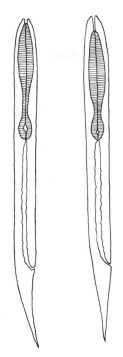

FIGURE 115. Diagram of hookworm and *Strongyloides* larvae from stool, showing differentiation on basis of buccal cavities.

STRONGYLOIDES   HOOKWORM

come in contact. The larvae make their way into cutaneous venules and are carried passively to the lungs, where they break out into alveoli. From the lungs, the larvae migrate up the trachea to be swallowed and reach the small intestine, where they mature. They attach by means of their stout mouth parts to the intestinal mucosa (Fig. 115), and suck blood and tissue juices of the host. The average prepatent period is seven or eight weeks. However, Nawalinski and Schad (1974) report a strain from India having a prepatent period of approximately 30 weeks.

SYMPTOMATOLOGY. In penetrating the skin, the larvae may cause an allergic reaction known as ground itch. This is less common with *Ancylostoma* than with the New World hookworm, *Necator americanus.* Hookworm larvae are smaller than those of *Ascaris,* and do not usually cause as severe pulmonary symptoms. If the infecting dose was large, pneumonitis may be produced by numbers of larvae breaking into the alveoli in a short space of time. Maturation of the worms may be marked by diarrhea, particularly when a previously uninfected person first acquires a heavy infection. This may be seen in persons from non-hookworm areas if they acquire an infection in the tropics. Other symptoms of early infection may be vague abdominal pains, colic or nausea. In chronic infections, if the number of worms is considerable, blood loss will be serious. If the diet is adequate in protein, and sufficient iron is taken to replace that lost through the activity of the hookworms, there may still be no evident symptoms. If iron intake is insufficient, symptoms of iron deficiency anemia will gradually develop. Eosinophilia is variable, ranging up to 70 per cent.

PATHOGENESIS. Roche and Layrisse (1966) point out that in any carefully analyzed representative series of patients infected with hookworm, a significant negative correlation between worm burden and hemoglobin can be demonstrated. When anemia is present, it is of the microcytic hypochromic type. The bone marrow is generally markedly hyperplastic, and there may be erythroid and myeloid hyperplasia of the spleen. Radioisotopic measurements indicate a host blood loss in the order of 0.15 ml. per day (0.26 ml. daily according to the measurements of Farid et al., 1965) per *Ancylostoma duodenale;* this is considerably greater than the 0.03 ml. per day calculated for *Necator americanus.* Histologic changes in the mucosa of the affected intestine appear to be minimal. Flattening or atrophy of the intestinal villi has been noted on occasion, but more frequently capsule biopsies demonstrate a completely normal mucosal pattern. Malabsorption is apparently uncommon, and malnutrition does not seem to be characteristic of pure hookworm disease in areas where a good diet is available. Emaciation, and mental and physical retardation frequently associated with this disease are more properly ascribed to a combination of other nutritional and disease factors which are associated with hookworm anemia and are common in many endemic areas.

TREATMENT. Bephenium (Alcopara) is the most effective drug presently available for treatment of *Ancylostoma duodenale.* Its administration is simple, as pre-treatment preparation is unnecessary, and post-treatment purging is contraindicated. It is administered in the morning on an empty stomach. The dose for both adults and children is a single 5 gm. packet of granules, shaken into one-half glass of water. A light meal is allowed three hours later, and a second dose may be administered in mid-afternoon. Alternatively, a single daily dose may be given for four to seven days. Vomiting and diarrhea are occasional side effects of treatment.

Thiabendazole (Mintezol) is effective in the treatment of both *Ancylostoma* and *Necator.* It is administered orally at the rate of 25 mg. per Kg. of body weight, as in ascariasis. Pyrantel pamoate is likewise effective in the treatment of *Ancylostoma* infections. The dose employed is that used for treatment of ascariasis. Either thiabendazole or pyrantel can be used in mixed ascaris-hookworm infections.

Cutaneous Larva Migrans

If man comes in contact with larvae of the dog hookworms *Ancylostoma braziliense* or *A. caninum*, penetration of the skin may take place, but the larvae are then unable to complete their migratory cycle. Trapped larvae may survive for some weeks or even months, migrating through the subcutaneous tissues. They may evoke a fairly severe reaction (Fig. 116), forming serpiginous tunnels through the tissues, erythematous and sometimes vesicular at the advancing end, fading out and becoming dry and encrusted in the older portions. There is often intense pruritus, and scratching may lead to secondary bacterial invasion. This syndrome is referred to as creeping eruption, or as cutaneous larva migrans, to distinguish it from the visceral type of larva migrans, discussed in Chapter 11.

TREATMENT. The oral administration of thiabendazole, at the

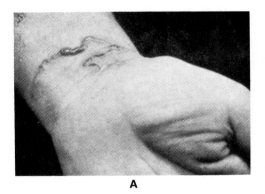

A

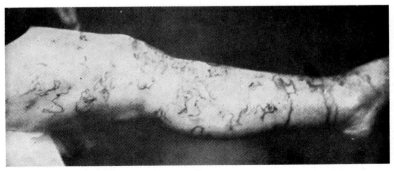

B

FIGURE 116. Creeping eruption: *A,* lesions on wrist (Courtesy of Drs. J. B. and Bedford Shelmire); *B,* extensive lesions on leg of three weeks' duration. (Courtesy of Dr. J. Lee Kirby-Smith.)

rate of 25 mg. per Kg. of body weight, twice daily for two days, is recommended for treatment of creeping eruption.

Necator americanus

The New World hookworm, *Necator americanus*, while prevalent over large portions of the Western hemisphere, was probably introduced from Africa with the slave trade. In addition to being the only hookworm found in North America and large areas of South America, it is the native hookworm of Africa south of the Sahara, and the only one found in parts of India. *Ancylostoma* and *Necator* occur together elsewhere in India, in much of China, in southeast Asia, in Indonesia, in the islands of the South and Southwest Pacific and in parts of Australia. With increasing rapidity of communications, and exposure of large numbers of persons to the hazards of infection in various parts of the world, it is probable that the geographic boundaries between the two genera of human hookworms will disappear.

Hookworm infection is still prevalent in some parts of the United States. Gloor et al. (1970) report a 14.8 per cent infection rate in upper elementary grade school students in rural Kentucky, and Martin (1972) found that on the coastal plain of Georgia 12 per cent of rural school children were infected. He did not find these infections to be associated with anemia.

Adults of *N. americanus* resemble those of *Ancylostoma*, but are slightly smaller. The males range from 5 to 9 mm. in length while females are usually about 1 cm. long. The head is sharply bent in relation to the rest of the body, forming a definite "hook" at the anterior end, from which the worms derive their common name. The buccal capsule of *Necator* (Fig. 117) is armed with a pair of cutting plates, while *Ancylostoma* has teeth. There are also decided differences in the structure of the rays supporting the copulatory bursa in the two genera. However, with a little practice one may be able to distinguish with the eye between adults of *Necator* and *Ancylostoma*, as the anterior hook is very much more pronounced in the former genus.

The life cycles of the two genera of hookworms are very similar. *Necator* larvae are more likely to produce irritation when they penetrate the skin, and ground itch more frequently accompanies infection by this parasite. The adult *Ancylostoma* is larger than *Necator*, and worm for worm is more likely to bring about iron deficiency. Eggs of *Necator* closely resemble those of *Ancylostoma*, but are slightly larger, averaging 64 to 76 microns in length by 36 to 40 microns in breadth.

SYMPTOMATOLOGY AND PATHOGENESIS are essentially as outlined for *Ancylostoma duodenale*, the chief difference between the two

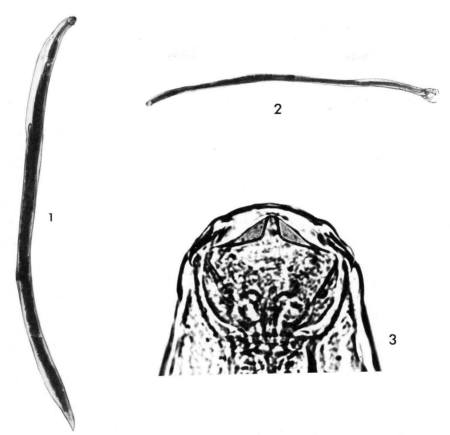

FIGURE 117. *Necator americanus* adults: *1,* female worm; *2,* male worm showing copulatory bursa; *3,* frontal view of head showing cutting plates. Male and female worms photographed at same magnification. (Photomicrographs by Zane Price.)

types of infection arising from the considerably smaller blood loss per worm produced by *Necator americanus.*

TREATMENT. According to Botero and Castaño (1973), pyrantel pamoate, administered at the rate of 10 mg. per Kg. of body weight daily for three days, is more effective than either tetrachloroethylene or bephenium in *Necator* infections. Tetrachloroethylene, an inexpensive medication which comes in gelatine capsules containing 0.5 and 1.0 ml. of the drug, is relatively difficult to obtain in a form manufactured for human use in this country. However, the veterinary product (which meets all USP standards) is readily available. Tetrachloroethylene is administered on an empty stomach, in a dose of 0.12 mg. per Kg. of body weight. Post-treatment purgation is contraindicated, as it increases toxicity of the drug. No alcoholic beverages should be taken during the day of treatment, or for 24 hours thereafter. Nausea, dizziness and headache are common side effects of treatment with tetrachloroethylene; diarrhea is sometimes seen, and liver damage may result, as with the ingestion of any chlorinated hydrocarbon. A combination of tetrachloroethylene, with bephenium administered as for treatment of *A. duodenale* infection, is said to give excellent results. Bephenium may be given alone, but it is less effective than in *Ancylostoma* infections.

Thiabendazole is effective in *Necator* infections, and is given in the dosage used for *Ancylostoma* or *Ascaris* infection. Mixed hookworm-ascaris infections may also be treated with pyrantel pamoate.

Philippine Capillariasis

This infection, which seems to be restricted to a small area in the Philippines, is caused by the roundworm *Capillaria philippinensis*. The illness is frequently protracted, and the fatality rate is high.

The adult worms are slender, approximately 4 to 5 mm. in length. They live in the intestinal mucosa, primarily in the jejunum (Fig. 118), where they may occur in enormous numbers. The finding of larval stages, and oviparous as well as larviparous females in the bowel, suggests that the parasite multiplies in the intestine and that overwhelming infections are the result of auto-infection. Eggs voided by infected individuals develop outside the host and are ingested by freshwater and brackish-water fish in which larval stages have been found. The complete life cycle is unknown. Laboratory diagnosis is made by finding the characteristic eggs (Fig. 119) in the stool.

SYMPTOMATOLOGY. Although asymptomatic or mildly symptomatic cases occur, many infected persons exhibit a rather characteristic

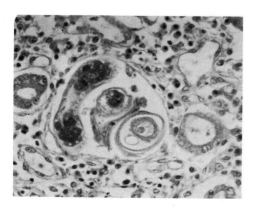

FIGURE 118. Section through intestinal mucosa containing *Capillaria philippinensis.*

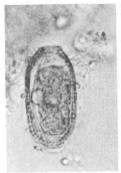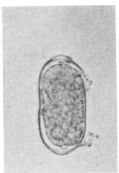

FIGURE 119. Eggs of *Capillaria philippinensis;* fully formed shell (left) and incomplete shell development (right).

clinical picture. Abdominal pain, borborygmus (gurgling) and diarrhea appear early. The diarrhea may be protracted and may be accompanied by anorexia, nausea and vomiting, and hypotension. The patient may become cachectic, with generalized anasarca. Visible peristaltic waves may be seen over the distended abdomen.

PATHOGENESIS. A pronounced eosinophilia, surprisingly, does not seem to be a consistent feature of this disease. Hypoproteinemia, low blood calcium, potassium and cholesterol levels, and other features of a protein-wasting enteropathy are encountered and are reflected in the pathologic picture (Dauz et al., 1967; Fresh et al., 1972; Watten et al., 1972). The villi are blunted, flattened or completely obliterated, with deepening of the crypts of Lieberkühn and an inflammatory submucosal infiltrate. Total thickness of the mucosa is generally reduced. These non-specific changes are seen in various malabsorption stages, and have been mentioned in relation to giardiasis and coccidiosis.

TREATMENT. Prolonged treatment with thiabendazole (25 mg. per Kg. of body weight twice daily for 30 days, followed by 1 gm. every other day for six months) has proved effective (Whalen et al., 1971). Protracted anthelmintic therapy is essential to prevent recurrence of the disease, as developmental forms in the mucosa may not be eliminated, and relapses are frequent. In management of the acute illness, fluid and electrolyte replacement and a high protein diet are important. A comprehensive review of Philippine capillariasis was published by Cross et al., 1970.

Strongyloides stercoralis

The temperature and moisture requirements of *Strongyloides stercoralis* during the free-living phase of its life cycle are similar to those of hookworm, and their geographical distribution is likewise similar. However, the incidence of strongyloidiasis is generally lower than that of hookworm disease. A number of species of *Strongyloides* are known, and generally they are quite host-specific. Cats and dogs may both be infected with *S. stercoralis,* and human infection from a canine source has been reported (Georgi and Sprinkle, 1974).

When environmental conditions are optimal, *Strongyloides* may exist for some time as a free-living nematode, completing two or more generations in this manner. The adults of the free-living generations, like other soil nematodes, are very small, being only about 1 mm. in length (Fig. 120). More frequently, perhaps, there is but a single free-living generation, producing rhabditiform larvae which transform into infective filariform larvae. The filariform larvae are incapable of further development in the soil, and must penetrate the skin of their host to continue the life cycle. Rhabditiform larvae which pass out of the host in the stools may also transform into filariform larvae directly, without developing into free-living adults. Penetration through the skin and the subsequent migration through the lungs and eventually to the small intestine is similar to that seen in hookworms. The parasitic males are eliminated from the body early in the infection, if indeed they exist. It seems likely that the larvae, produced over a period of months, develop parthenogenetically. The females (Fig. 121), which may attain a length of slightly over 2 mm., burrow into the mucosa of the intestinal tract, where they lay their eggs (Fig. 110, *11*). The eggs, similar in appearance to those of hookworms, hatch in the mucosa and liberate rhabditiform larvae, which make their way to the lumen of the intestine. The larvae may feed and molt once before being passed in the feces. When they molt within the intestinal tract they usually retain their rhabditiform characteristics, but may transform into infective filariform larvae.

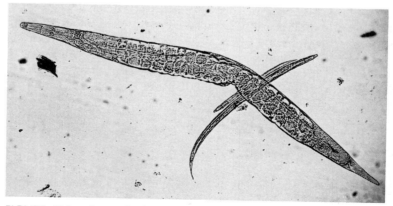

FIGURE 120. *Strongyloides stercoralis,* free-living female and larvae. (Photomicrograph by Zane Price.)

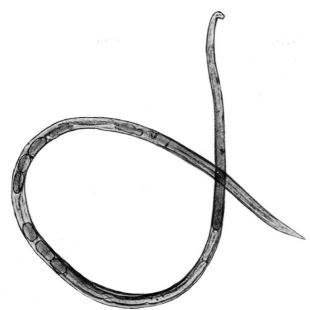

FIGURE 121. *Strongyloides stercoralis,* parasitic female. (Photomicrograph by Zane Price.)

If filariform larvae are formed, they may penetrate immediately into the wall of the gut and enter the blood stream, where they begin the same type of migratory cycle as the larvae which penetrate the skin from the soil.

Diagnosis is by demonstration of the characteristic larvae in the stools (Fig. 122). Larvae resemble those of hookworms, but can be differentiated from them through possession of a very short buccal

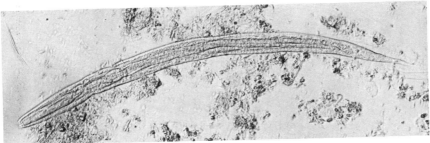

FIGURE 122. *Strongyloides stercoralis.* Larva in stool specimen preserved in formalin. (Photomicrograph by Zane Price, from material furnished by Dr. Lawrence Ash.)

cavity (Fig. 114). In severe diarrhea, the embryonated eggs may be present in the stools, and can be differentiated from hookworm eggs by the fact that they always contain well-developed larvae. If larvae are scarce, it may be necessary to concentrate the stool. The larvae may be concentrated with zinc sulfate, but a more efficient means of recovery is the Baermann technique, described in Chapter 15. Duodenal aspiration will occasionally reveal larvae when the stools remain consistently negative.

A characteristic x-ray picture is reported in severe strongyloidiasis, with loss of mucosal pattern, rigidity, and tubular narrowing (Fig. 123).

SYMPTOMATOLOGY. Lesions resembling the ground itch of hookworm infection are sometimes seen following penetration of the skin by *Strongyloides* larvae. Pneumonitis may be produced by the larvae, but as in hookworm infection is generally less severe than in ascariasis. The adult worms in the intestine may give rise to no demonstrable symptoms, or to moderate or severe diarrhea. A malabsorption syndrome with steatorrhea is described by O'Brien (1975). Ulceration of

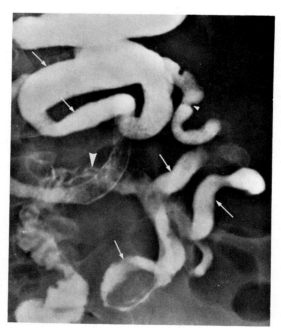

FIGURE 123. Strongyloidiasis of duodenum and jejunum. The upper small bowel appears smooth and tubular without a mucosal pattern (white arrows). The narrowing is almost uniform but areas of local constriction can be seen (small arrowhead). Note the abrupt transition to a more nearly normal mucosal pattern (large arrowhead). (Courtesy G. Arantis Pereira, Rio de Janeiro, Brazil.)

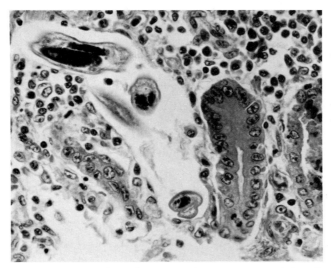

FIGURE 124. Section through intestinal mucosa containing *Strongyloides stercoralis*.

the intestinal mucosa may give rise to symptoms resembling those of duodenal ulcer, sometimes with melena and anemia, or ulcerative colitis (Stemmerman, 1967). Hyperinfection may lead to severe debilitation or death. It is probable that such heavy internal auto-infections occur primarily in patients whose resistance is lowered by intercurrent disease (Rogers and Nelson, 1966) or immunosuppressive therapy (Cruz et al., 1966). Some reported fatalities have occurred in persons who, because of their long residence in areas where exogenous infection was extremely unlikely, must have been infected for many years.

PATHOGENESIS. While local lesions occur on penetration of the larvae into the skin, these are generally minor. More severe skin lesions, including giant hives, are rare. The pulmonary response to larval migration is generally not severe; in heavy infections there may be a patchy pneumonitis. The adult female worms may be found in all parts of the intestinal tract, although they are most common in the jejunum. The young female worms lodge in the intestinal crypts and as they mature they penetrate the mucosa (Fig. 124). They remain embedded in the mucosa, laying eggs from which hatch rhabditiform larvae that migrate to the intestinal lumen. An inflammatory infiltration of the mucosa may lead to the x-ray picture seen in Fig. 123). Heavy infections can produce extensive ulceration and sloughing of the mucosa, and fibrosis and inflammatory infiltration of the submucosal layers. In the more severe infections, transformation of rhabditiform to filariform larvae seems to proceed very rapidly (Grové and Elsdon-Dew, 1958), and filariform larvae may be found in many organs and tissues.

Eosinophilia from 10 to 40 per cent is common; in occasional patients it will be higher. Lack of eosinophilic response is occasionally seen; this generally occurs in overwhelming infections. Early in the infection there may be a polymorphonuclear leukocytosis.

TREATMENT. Thiabendazole is the drug of choice in treatment of strongyloidiasis (Cahill, 1967). The recommended dose is 25 mg. per Kg. of body weight, twice daily for two days. Nausea, vomiting and vertigo are frequent side effects of this drug. In patients who are taking immunosuppressive medications, treatment for strongyloidiasis must be prolonged, and may be unsuccessful (Seabury et al., 1971).

Trichuris trichiura

The whipworm, *Trichuris trichiura,* has a world-wide distribution, but is more common in tropical areas and regions where sanitation is poor. The common name of whipworm is most descriptive, the thick posterior part of the body forming the stock, and the long thin anterior portion the lash (Fig. 125). The generic name (*Trichuris* = thread tail) is less fortunate, having been applied under the impression that the attenuated portion of the worm was its posterior end. Subsequently the name *Trichocephalus* was given to the genus, and has been adopted by

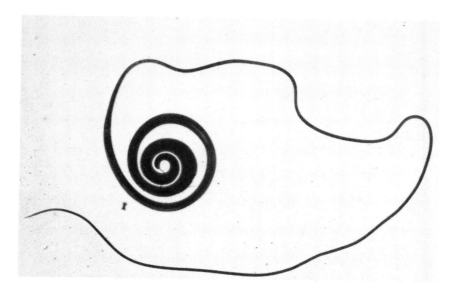

FIGURE 125. *Trichuris trichiura,* adult male. (Photomicrograph by Zane Price.)

some workers. It is much more apt, but unfortunately should not be used, as the name *Trichuris* has priority.

The adult worms are from 3 to 5 cm. in length. As is usual among the nematodes, the females are larger than the males. The thin almost colorless anterior three-fifths of the body consists of the much reduced esophagus. The expanded posterior part of the worm is pinkish-gray in color, and contains the intestine and reproductive organs.

Infection is acquired by ingestion of the fully embryonated eggs. These are passed in the unsegmented condition and require a period of ten days or more outside the body to reach the infective stage. The shell is digested in the small intestine, where the larvae lodge temporarily. After a period of growth, larvae pass to the cecal area, where they attach permanently with their attenuated anterior ends embedded in the mucosa. In heavy infections, worms may be found as far down as the rectum.

Diagnosis is by demonstration of the characteristic barrel-shaped eggs in the feces (Fig. 110, *1*). Each female worm produces from 3000 to 7000 eggs daily. The eggs measure 50 to 54 microns in length, with refractile prominences (usually referred to as polar plugs) at either end. The zinc-sulfate flotation method is extremely efficient in demonstrating them.

SYMPTOMATOLOGY. Light whipworm infections are usually asymptomatic. Heavier infections may be characterized by abdominal pain and distention, a bloody or mucoid diarrhea, tenesmus, weight loss and weakness. Prolapse of the rectum is occasionally seen, usually in children with heavy infections. Worms may be visible on the prolapsed, edematous rectum. Anemia and a moderate eosinophilia may be seen in heavy infections.

PATHOGENESIS. The anterior ends of the worms, interlaced in the colonic mucosa, apparently produce little damage to the host unless present in large numbers. Some authorities consider that bacterial invasion of the mucosa is facilitated by the penetration of the worms. Appendicitis, brought about by blockage of the lumen of that organ by worms, has been frequently reported. Edema of the rectum, produced by numbers of worms embedded in that area, is responsible for rectal prolapse. The blood loss per worm is apparently slight. Layrisse et al. (1967), using radioisotope techniques, calculated it as approximately 0.005 ml. of blood per worm daily and estimated that infections of 800 worms or more are necessary to produce anemia in children. They did not consider it likely that adults would become anemic from whipworm infections. As in hookworm disease, it is probable that nutritional factors are of such paramount importance that in certain areas relatively low levels of infection may lead to overt anemia.

TREATMENT. Mebendazole (Vermox) is the first drug to be relatively effective against *Trichuris*. At a dose of 100 mg. twice daily for 4 days (children and adults) approximately two-thirds of infections will be cured; the remainder will exhibit an egg reduction of approximately 90 per cent (Sargent et al., 1974). Thiabendazole, given in the usual dosage of 25 mg. per Kg. of body weight, twice daily for two days, will usually result in elimination of about one-half of the worm burden. Repeated courses may be administered, but in many cases treatment is unnecessary.

Trichostrongylus Species

The genus *Trichostrongylus* contains a number of species that are primarily parasites of herbivores, and are found throughout the world. Human infections have been reported on occasion from many regions, and are accidental. *Trichostrongylus orientalis* is fairly common in Japan, Korea, China including Taiwan, and Armenia; a number of other species have also been reported from man in the Soviet Union. The larvae develop in the soil, but do not penetrate the skin; they are ingested with contaminated vegetation.

Trichostrongyles are related to the hookworms, and the adults are rather similar in appearance. The various species reported from man are smaller than the hookworms, but their eggs are larger. Identification of the various species of *Trichostrongylus* from the eggs is difficult, but differentiation of the eggs from those of hookworm can be readily accomplished. Trichostrongyle eggs (Fig. 110, 7 and 8) are symmetrical and thin shelled, and differ from hookworm eggs in their size, and in having more pointed ends. The size range is from 73 to 95 microns in length, and 40 to 50 microns in breadth.

SYMPTOMATOLOGY AND PATHOGENESIS. The larvae attach themselves to the intestinal mucosa and grow to adults in three to four weeks. They ingest blood, but only in rather heavy infections is the blood loss of clinical significance. Heavily infected patients may become emaciated.

TREATMENT. Light infections do not warrant treatment. Thiabendazole, in the dosage used in ascariasis, hookworm infection, and strongyloidiasis, is effective in treatment of trichostrongyliasis as well (Markell, 1968). Bephenium is apparently effective in a single oral dose of 5 gm.

LARVAL NEMATODES ACQUIRED FROM FISH

Anisakiasis

Marine fish frequently are infected with roundworm larvae belonging to the genera *Anisakis*, *Phocanema*, or related genera. In the area of the North Sea, around Japan, and on both coasts of the United States (Little and Most, 1973; Kates et al., 1973; Chitwood, 1975), infections have been reported following consumption of such fish, either raw or pickled. The worms may cause acute nausea and vomiting, or penetrate into the wall of the digestive tract, where they give rise to eosinophilic granulomas in the stomach or small intestine. These infections are frequently misdiagnosed as gastric or duodenal ulcer, carcinoma, appendicitis, or other surgical conditions, depending upon their location.

Granulomatous tissue obtained at surgery contains nematode larvae which in most instances appear to belong to the genus *Anisakis*. The adult worms occur in marine mammals, which acquire the infection by eating fish. As far as is known, the larvae do not mature in man.

The disease in man is accompanied by a low grade eosinophilia, usually less than 10 per cent; occult blood is generally present in gastric juice or stools.

A presumptive diagnosis can be made on the basis of the patient's food habits. Definitive diagnosis rests upon the demonstration of worms in specimens obtained at surgery (Little and MacPhail, 1972) (Fig. 126). Prevention of the disease is by thorough cooking of marine food fishes. A comprehensive review of Anisakiasis in Japan, including clinical aspects and treatment, is given by Oshima (1972).

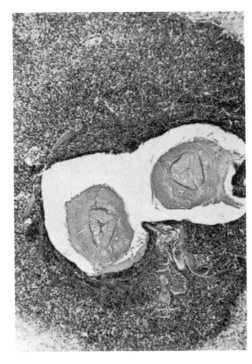

FIGURE 126. Cross section of larval *Anisakis* in eosinophilic abscess in submucosa of stomach. (Courtesy Dr. Muneo Yokogawa, Chiba University, Japan.)

REFERENCES

Beaver, P. P. C., Kriz, J. J., and Lau, T. J. 1973. Pulmonary nodule caused by *Enterobius vermicularis*. Amer. J. Trop. Med. & Hyg., *22*:711–713.

Botero, D., and Castaño, A. 1973. Comparative study of pyrantel pamoate, bephenium hydroxynaphthoate, and tetrachloroethylene in the treatment of *Necator americanus* infections. Amer. J. Trop. Med. & Hyg., *22*:45–52.

Brooks, T. J., Jr., Goetz, C. C., and Plauché, W. C. 1962. Pelvic granuloma due to *Enterobius vermicularis*. J.A.M.A., *179*:492–494.

Cahill, K. M. 1967. Thiabendazole in massive strongyloidiasis. Amer. J. Trop. Med. & Hyg., *16*:451–453.

Chitwood, M. 1975. *Phocanema*-type larval nematode coughed up by a boy in California. Amer. J. Trop. Med. & Hyg., *24*:710–711.

Cross, J. H., Banzon, T., Murrell, K. D., Watten, R. H., and Dizon, J. J. 1970. *A New Epidemic Diarrheal Disease Caused by the Nematode Capillaria philippinensis. Industry and Tropical Health.* Vol. 7. Industrial Council for Tropical Health, Harvard School of Public Health, Boston.

Cruz, T., Reboucas, G., and Rocha, H. 1966. Fatal strongyloidiasis in patients receiving corticosteroids. New Eng. J. Med., *275*:1093–1906.

Dauz, U., Cabrera, B. D., and Canlas, B., Jr. 1967. Human intestinal capillariasis. I. Clinical features. Acta Med. Philip., *4*:72–83.

Farid, Z., Nichols, J. H., Bassily, S., and Schulert, A. R. 1965. Blood loss in pure *Ancylostoma duodenale* infection in Egyptian farmers. Amer. J. Trop. Med. & Hyg., *14*:375–378.

Fresh, J. W., Cross, J. H., Reyes, V., Whalen, G. E., Uylangco, C. V., and Dizon, J. J. 1972. Necropsy findings in intestinal capillariasis. Amer. J. Trop. Med. & Hyg., *21*:169–173.

Gelpi, A. P., and Mustafa, A. 1967. Seasonal pneumonitis with eosinophilia. A study of larval ascariasis in Saudi Arabs. Amer. J. Trop. Med. & Hyg., *16*:646–657.

Georgi, J. R., and Sprinkle, C. L. 1974. A case of human strongyloidosis apparently contracted from asymptomatic colony dogs. Amer. J. Trop. Med. & Hyg., *23*:899–901.

Gloor, R. F., Breylery, E. R., and Martinez, I. G. 1970. Hookworm infection in a rural Kentucky county. Amer. J. Trop. Med. & Hyg., *19*:1007–1009.

Grové, S. S., and Elsdon-Dew, R. 1958. Internal auto-infection with *Strongyloides stercoralis*. S. Afr. J. Lab. & Clin. Med., *4*:55–63.

Johansson, S. G. O., Mellbin, T., and Vahlquist, B. 1968. Immunoglobulin levels in Ethiopian preschool children with special reference to high concentrations of immunoglobulin E (IgND). Lancet, *1*:1118–1121.

Kates, S., Wright, K. A., and Wright, R. 1973. A case of human infection with the cod nematode *Phocanema* sp. Amer. J. Trop. Med. & Hyg., *22*:606–608.

Layrisse, M., Aparcedo, L., Martinez-Torres, C., and Roche, M. 1967. Blood loss due to infection with *Trichuris trichiura*. Amer. J. Trop. Med. & Hyg., *16*:613–619.

Little, M. D., Cuello, C. J., and D'Alessandro, A. 1973. Granuloma of the liver due to *Enterobius vermicularis*. Amer. J. Trop. Med. & Hyg., *22*:567–569.

Little, M. D., and MacPhail, J. C. 1972. Large nematode larva from the abdominal cavity of a man in Massachusetts. Amer. J. Trop. Med. & Hyg., *21*:948–950.

Little, M. D., and Most, H. 1973. Anisakid larva from the throat of a woman in New York. Amer. J. Trop. Med. & Hyg., *22*:609–612.

Markell, E. K. 1968. Pseudohookworm infection—Trichostrongyliasis. Treatment with thiabendazole. New Eng. J. Med., *278*:831–832.

Martin, L. K. 1972. Hookworm in Georgia. I. Survey of intestinal helminth infections and anemia in rural school children. Amer. J. Trop. Med. & Hyg., *21*:919–929.

Nawalinski, T. A., and Schad, G. A. 1974. Arrested development in *Ancylostoma duodenale:* course of a self-induced infection in man. Amer. J. Trop. Med. & Hyg., *23*:895–898.

O'Brien, W. 1975. Intestinal malabsorption in acute infection with *Strongyloides stercoralis*. Trans. Roy. Soc. Trop. Med. & Hyg., *69*:69–77.

Oshima, T. 1972. *Anisakis* and Anisakiasis in Japan and adjacent area. Prog. Med. Parasitol. Jap., vol. 4, pp. 303–393. Meguro Parasitological Museum, Tokyo.

Roche, M., and Layrisse, M. 1966. The nature and causes of "hookworm anemia". Amer. J. Trop. Med. & Hyg., *15* 1031–1102.

Rogers, W. A., Jr., and Nelson, B. 1966. Strongyloidiasis and malignant lymphoma. J.A.M.A., *195*:685–687.

Sargent, R. G., Savory, A. M., Mina, A., and Lee, P. R. 1974. A clinical evaluation of mebendazole in the treatment of trichuriasis. Amer. J. Trop. Med. & Hyg., *23*:375–377.

Seabury, J. H., Abadie, S., and Savoy, F., Jr. 1971. Pulmonary strongyloidiasis with lung abscess. Ineffectiveness of thiabendazole therapy. Amer. J. Trop. Med. & Hyg., *20*:209–211.

Schüffner, W., and Swellengrebel, N. H. 1949. Retrofection in oxyuriasis. A newly discovered mode of infection with *Enterobius vermicularis*. J. Parasit., *35*:138–146.

Stemmerman, G. N. 1967. Strongyloidiasis in migrants. Pathological and clinical considerations. Gastroenterology, *53*:59–70.

Stoll, N. R. 1947. This wormy world. J. Parasit., *33* 1–18.

Villarejos, V. M., Arguedas-Gamboa, J. A., Eduarte, E., and Swartzelder, J. C. 1971. Experiences with the antibiotic pyrantel pamoate. Amer. J. Trop. Med. & Hyg., *20*:842–845.

Watten, R. H., Beckner, W. M., Cross, J. H., Gunning, J.-J., and Jarimillo, J. 1972. Clinical studies of capillariasis philippinensis. Trans. Roy. Soc. Trop. Med. & Hyg., *66*:828–834.

Whalen, G. E., Rosenberg, E. B., Gutman, R. A., Cross, J., Fresh, J. W., Strickland, T., and Uylangco, C. 1971. Treatment of intestinal capillariasis with thiabendazole, bithionol and bephenium. Amer. J. Trop. Med. & Hyg., *20*:95–100.

11

The Blood- and Tissue-Dwelling Nematodes

THE FILARIAE

The filariae are long, thread-like nematodes. In man, various species inhabit portions of the lymphatic system and of the subcutaneous and deep connective tissues. Five of the species known to infect man produce microfilariae, which appear in the circulating blood. Microfilariae of a sixth species, *Onchocerca volvulus,* do not usually enter the circulation but migrate freely in the subcutaneous tissues and dermis.

In addition to these six species, a number of filariae, primarily parasites of other animals, are reported occasionally from man.

Wuchereria bancrofti

Bancroftian filariasis is very widely distributed throughout the tropics and subtropics. It is found through much of Central Africa, in Malagasy and along the African coast of the Mediterranean. Scattered cases have been reported from Spain, Italy, Yugoslavia, Hungary and Turkey. In Asia, the disease may be found along the Arabian seacoast, in India, Pakistan, Burma, Thailand, Southeast Asia and the Philippines, as well as the southern parts of China, Korea and Japan. It occurs extensively throughout the Pacific islands, and used to be seen on the northern and eastern coasts of Australia, but is now very rare in those areas. In the New World, it is found in the West Indies, Central America, and in Venezuela, the Guianas, Brazil and Colombia. An

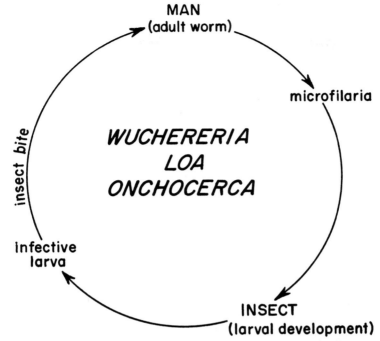

FIGURE 127. Schematic representation of life cycle of the human filarial worms.

endemic focus formerly occurred in the region of Charleston, South Carolina.

The life cycle of *Wuchereria bancrofti* (Fig. 127) is of more than usual interest, as Manson's discovery, in 1878, of the transmission of this parasite by mosquitoes was the first demonstration of an arthropod as vector of a parasitic organism. The mosquito Manson found infected in China was *Culex fatigans;* since then it has been found that various species of *Aedes* or *Anopheles* are the important vectors in some other parts of the world. The mosquito is more than a simple agent of transmission of the parasite; an essential developmental cycle takes place within the body of the insect. The mosquito, upon biting an infected person, may ingest microfilariae with its blood meal. The microfilariae bore through the stomach wall to enter the body cavity of the insect. There they migrate to the thoracic musculature for a period of growth. During the next ten days or so the larvae grow and molt to become infective stage larvae. During this period they have increased in length from about 300 microns to 1.5 to 2 mm. The infective larvae enter the proboscis of the mosquito, and when the next blood meal is taken, escape from the proboscis onto the skin. They enter through the puncture hole left by the mosquito, to infect their new host. The subsequent development in man is not as completely known. Infective larvae gain access to the peripheral lymphatics and thence to the regional lymph nodes and larger lymph vessels. They may mature in the lymph nodes or vessels, and if male and female worms are present in the same area they will mate, and microfilariae will be produced. The length of time necessary for the worms to grow to sexual maturity is probably several months; the adult worms are known to live for some years. Adults are thread-like white worms. The males measure 2.5 to 4 cm. in length, and the females 5 to 10 cm.

Microfilariae of *Wuchereria bancrofti* (Fig. 128) are said to be sheathed. The "sheath" is actually the egg shell, which is very thin and delicate, and surrounds the embryo as it circulates in the blood; it is not lost until it is digested away in the stomach of the mosquito. In thick blood films, microfilariae range in length from about 245 to nearly 300 microns. A large number of distinct nuclei can be seen in the body of well-stained specimens, as well as the rudiments of some organs of the adult worm. There is no alimentary canal. The cylindrical body is

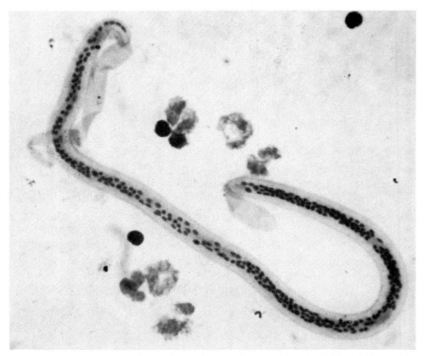

FIGURE 128. Microfilaria of *Wuchereria bancrofti* in thick blood film. (Photomicrograph by Zane Price.)

bluntly rounded anteriorly; posteriorly it tapers to a point. Nuclei are not seen in the posterior portion of the tail, and this characteristic serves to differentiate microfilariae of this species from other sheathed microfilariae. A key to the microfilariae found in the blood is given at the end of this section.

In most parts of the world where filariasis is endemic, the infection is seen in its so-called periodic form. Microfilariae, present in very low numbers in the circulating blood during the daytime hours, and often virtually undetectable then, appear at their greatest density at night, generally between the hours of 10 P.M. and 2 to 4 A.M. The subperiodic form of filariasis occurs throughout the Pacific islands. Persons infected with this strain exhibit at all times a microfilaremia, but the organisms are present in greatest numbers between noon and 8 P.M. The subperiodic form has also been found in some areas of Vietnam. The suggestion has been made that the subperiodic form be recognized as a separate variety, *Wuchereria bancrofti* var. *pacifica*, or that it should form a distinct species, *W. pacifica*. There has not been wide acceptance of either proposal, as the morphological differences reported between adult worms of the periodic and non-periodic forms are extremely minor, and microfilariae of the two sorts appear to be identical.

The basis of filarial periodicity remains largely unknown; it may be altered by a change in the habits of the host, if the waking and sleeping hours are transposed. It takes about a week for such reversal to be effected, suggesting that sleeping and waking as such do not affect the periodicity, but that the entire 24-hour rhythm of the host is in some way responsible for this phenomenon. When absent from the peripheral circulation, the microfilariae are found primarily in the capillaries and small vessels of the lungs. Some of the factors influencing migration of microfilariae of the periodic strain of *W. bancrofti* to the lungs are increased pulmonary pO_2 and increased exertion (McFadzean and Hawking, 1956). Obviously, while normal daily activity can in this manner influence migration of the nocturnally periodic or common strain of *W. bancrofti*, it must affect the Pacific or subperiodic strain differently. Presumably other factors are also important in influencing the larval migration which determines periodicity. In general, it has been noted that where the non-periodic disease occurs the vectors bite during the day, and that in areas of the periodic disease the mosquitoes are night-biters. It should not be assumed from this, as some have done, that the biting habits of the mosquito host have affected development of periodicity in the filariae. It is more likely that microfilarial periodicity, plus the biting habits of the mosquito, have influenced distribution of the disease.

Diagnosis of filarial infection is frequently made on strict clinical grounds, particularly in endemic areas, but demonstration of microfilariae in the circulating blood is the only means by which one may make a certain diagnosis. The microfilariae may be found by examination of a fresh blood film, where their movements make them conspicuous. If they are present in small numbers, it may be necessary to prepare a thick blood film, or a concentrate of a larger volume of venous blood, to detect them. The Knott concentration and membrane filtration techniques used for this purpose, are given in Chapter 15. The sensitivity of the membrane filtration technique has been clearly demonstrated (Desowitz and Hitchcock, 1974). Microfilariae of strains normally exhibiting nocturnal periodicity can be demonstrated in the blood during the day, in numbers approximating one third of the nocturnal levels,

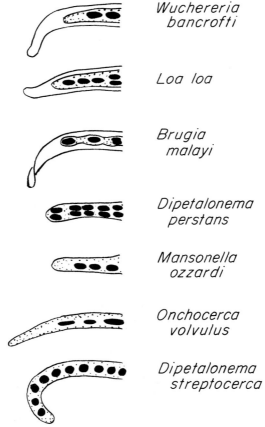

Wuchereria
bancrofti

Loa loa

Brugia
malayi

Dipetalonema
perstans

Mansonella
ozzardi

Onchocerca
volvulus

Dipetalonema
streptocerca

FIGURE 129.   Differentiation of the species of microfilaria found in the human blood, on the basis of posterior ends of the larvae. Note the distribution of nuclei and their presence or absence in the extreme caudal portion, and the presence or absence of a sheath.

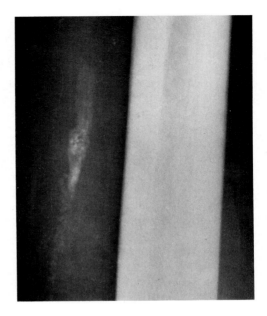

FIGURE 130. Calcified *Wuchereria bancrofti* in tissue.

three-quarters to two or more hours after the administration of an oral dose of 100 mg. of diethylcarbamazine (Manson-Bahr and Wijers, 1972). In areas where more than one kind of filarial disease exists, well-stained slides are essential, as the different filarial infections are distinguished by differences in structure of the microfilariae (Fig. 129). A skin test, using an extract of the dog heartworm, *Dirofilaria immitis*, is group-specific for filarial infections, as are various serologic tests (Chapter 16).

X-ray evidence of infection can at times be detected (Fig. 130), as the worms die and become calcified. Lymphangiography may demonstrate characteristic changes in filarial elephantiasis.

SYMPTOMATOLOGY. Clinical manifestations of infection are variable, and probably depend upon constitutional factors in the host, numbers of infecting organisms and possibly upon strain differences in the parasite itself. "Constitutional" factors are probably of paramount importance, as some individuals may become heavily infected without ever showing any signs of disease other than large numbers of microfilariae in the circulating blood. It is probable that in other individuals the presence of even a few worms will provoke severe reactions.

Frequent early manifestations of filariasis are fever, lymphangitis and lymphadenitis. Febrile attacks may be seen with or without associated lymphangitis, although the latter are less common. These attacks are sometimes referred to as "elephantoid fever." In either case the attack usually begins with a chill, the fever remains high for one or two days, and gradually subsides over the following two to five day period.

Lymphangitis commonly affects the limbs, but may occur in the breast, scrotum or elsewhere. When seen on the limbs it is usually centrifugal in development, starting in the region of a lymph node and progressing along the lymphatic channel in a distal direction. The affected lymphatic vessel is distended and acutely tender, with the overlying skin tense, erythematous and hot. The surrounding area is frequently edematous. Attacks of lymphangitis recur periodically. Occasionally they are accompanied by abscess formation, either along the course of the lymphatic or at a lymph node. When such abscesses are opened, or drain spontaneously, remnants of adult worms are sometimes found in the pus. Lymphadenitis, either alone or in combination with periodic lymphangitis attacks, is frequently seen. The lymph nodes most commonly affected are the femorals and epitrochlears; once enlarged, they tend to remain so. They are firm, discrete, and somewhat tender. Enlargement of the epitrochlear lymph nodes occurs early in the subperiodic form of filariasis, while it is relatively much less common in the periodic form.

Scrotal involvement may occur early, and sometimes in the absence of other signs or symptoms. Orchitis and inflammation of the spermatic cord are common, and some permanent thickening of the cord is seen in a high percentage of cases. Lymph varix of the cord may appear and rupture into the scrotal sac, leading to a condition known as lymphocele. Lymphocele is one type of hydrocele, a condition which may also develop gradually as a result of recurrent attacks of orchitis. Microfilariae may be found in the hydrocele fluid if it is wholly or partially made up of lymph. Hydrocele is a very common finding in patients who have had filariasis for a number of years. Rupture of lymph varices into any part of the urinary tract will lead to the passage of lymph in the urine, or chyluria. Chyluria usually comes on suddenly, and lasts for a few days. There may be repeated episodes, separated by long intervals. Microfilariae may be found in the chylous urine.

Elephantiasis, enlargement of one or more limbs, scrotum, breasts or vulva, with dermal hypertrophy and verrucous changes, is a relatively uncommon and late complication of filariasis (Fig. 131). It must be emphasized that elephantiasis is by no means the inevitable end-result of filarial infection. Even in endemic areas where the population is exposed to infection during their entire lives, many persons who become infected never develop symptoms or signs other than a microfilaremia. Others develop a lymphadenopathy, or may have recurrent attacks of fever and lymphangitis, but the disease does not progress to elephantiasis. The two most serious sequelae of filarial infection, elephantiasis and hydrocele, affect only a portion of those people who have been exposed to repeated infection over a period of years.

Beaver (1970) emphasizes that filarial infection may occur without

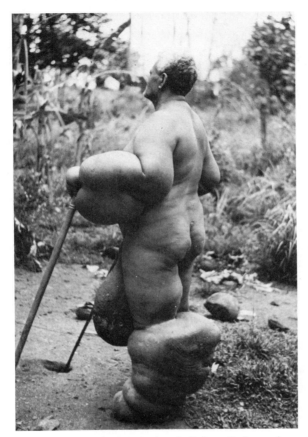

FIGURE 131. Extreme elephantiasis of all four limbs and scrotum. (Photograph courtesy of Dr. John F. Kessel.)

detectable microfilaremia. Eosinophilic lung, and Meyers and Kouwenaar's syndrome (lymphadenopathy with splenomegaly, transient pulmonary infiltrates and hypereosinophilia) are most frequently seen in individuals from nonendemic areas. Various reports indicate that such individuals may actually have very low levels of circulating microfilariae, which may be detected by membrane filtration techniques (Chapter 15).

PATHOGENESIS. Obstruction of lymphatic drainage, seen in an acute form in lymphangitis attacks, may become chronic. Formerly, it was considered that the permanent obstruction was largely mechanical, the result of blockage of the lymphatics by the bodies of living or dead adult filariae. This seems unlikely, and it is now believed that tissue reactions of an allergic nature, occurring around the worms, produce the obstruction. Variations in allergic responsiveness of different individuals explain why some persons develop lymphatic obstruction, while others with apparent equal exposure to the worms fail to do so. The effects of obstructed lymph drainage may be seen in the extremities, the breasts, scrotum or labia.

Chronic obstruction of scrotal lymph flow may lead to the development of varices on the grossly dilated lymph channels of that organ, both internally and also close to the surface of the skin. Transudation of fluid into the tissues leads to edema and subsequent fibrous tissue proliferation, while those lymph varices near the surface of the scrotum form small blebs which may rupture and ooze continuously. This condition is known as lymph scrotum. With progressive hyperplasia of the connective tissue elements and thickening of the skin, the organ may become greatly enlarged, and the edema becomes hard and non-pitting. The skin may develop folds and verrucous growths. This chronic enlargement, with associated hyperplastic changes, is known as elephantiasis (Figs. 131, 132). It does not necessarily develop as a sequel to lymph scrotum, but that organ may become elephantoid without the formation and rupture of surface lymph varices.

Elephantiasis may develop in any limb, and in women elephantiasis of the breasts and vulva is sometimes seen. Elephantiasis is a disfiguring, and frequently a disabling, condition and an elephantoid limb or organ, in which circulation is badly impaired, is in constant danger of secondary bacterial infection.

EPIDEMIOLOGY. While *W. bancrofti* is capable of larval development in a large number of species of mosquitoes, only a rather small number of anthropophilic species are important as vectors. As there are no reservoir hosts for this species, endemicity of the infection demands

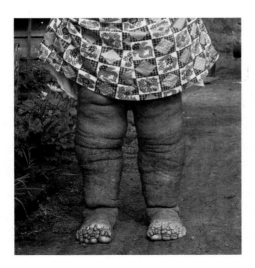

FIGURE 132. Moderately advanced elephantiasis involving both legs. Note verrucous hyperplasia of skin over toes.

both an adequate human reservoir, and sufficient numbers of circulating microfilariae in the blood of those infected. The importance of these two criteria lies in the fact that transmission of the disease may be interrupted when either the number of persons infected in a given area, or the microfilaria level in those infected, falls below a critical level. Of course, measures directed against the adult mosquitoes or their larvae are also important in control of the disease. The incidence of demonstrable infection is low in young children, but in endemic areas probably remains constant after the first few years of life (Desowitz and Hitchcock, 1974). In many areas, clinical infection appears more common in males than females; this may have a physiologic basis, as Ash (1971) has found it to be true in experimental infections with the filaria *Brugia pahangi.*

TREATMENT. Attacks of filarial lymphangitis usually respond to the administration of antihistaminics such as promethazine hydrochloride (Phenergan), 25 mg. four times daily, with acetylsalicylic acid in conventional doses. Diethylcarbamazine (Hetrazan) is an effective microfilaricidal drug, but it eliminates the adult worms more slowly. It is generally administered at the rate of 2 mg. per Kg. of body weight, three times daily for two to four weeks. Allergic reactions may occur early in treatment; these reactions consist of fever, urticaria and lymphangitis and are usually well controlled with promethazine. Later, bullous reactions may be seen requiring at the onset corticosteroids in doses equivalent to 20 mg. of prednisone daily. These are also thought to be allergic in nature. Filarial abscesses, which may occur at any point along a lymphatic chain, denote death of the adult worm and a hypersensitivity reaction to its remains. Portions of the dead worm can at times be distinguished when the abscess is drained. Generalized malaise, vertigo, headache, nausea and vomiting are occasional non-specific side effects of diethylcarbamazine administration.

In mass treatment programs (Kessel, 1967), diethylcarbamazine may be given at the rate of 6 mg. per Kg. of body weight once a month for 12 to 18 months. In such programs, as with individual treatment, periodic re-examination must be carried out by means of thick blood films, with retreatment as necessary.

Surgical procedures for treatment of scrotal elephantiasis are generally satisfactory; hydrocele may be treated by the accepted surgical means, or by injection of sclerosing solutions such as sodium psylliate or sodium morrhuate. Surgical treatment of elephantiasis of the extremities is seldom successful. The use of elastic bandages or Unna's paste boots may gradually reduce the size of affected limbs. Corticosteroids may be used in conjunction with pressure bandages to reduce induration of the affected tissues, but it must not be given in the presence of bacterial infection, and it must always be administered with caution.

Cortisone, at the rate of 100 mg. daily, or prednisone in equivalent doses, given over a period of several weeks, results in a marked softening of the woody induration of the elephantoid tissues.

Brugia malayi

The Malayan form of filariasis has a distribution centering roughly around the Malay peninsula. In addition to Malaysia, it occurs in India, Sri Lanka, Indonesia, New Guinea, Thailand, Vietnam and in certain parts of China, Korea and the island of Hachijo-shima in Japan. The distribution of this species obviously overlaps that of *Wuchereria bancrofti*.

The life cycle of *Brugia malayi* is similar to that of *W. bancrofti*, except that in most areas the principal mosquito vectors belong to the genus *Mansonia*. In some areas, *Anopheles* may be an important or the only vector, and on Hachijo-shima the vector is a species of *Aedes*. While there is no evidence of any reservoir hosts for *W. bancrofti*, monkeys, dogs and cats have been found naturally infected with parasites similar to *B. malayi*. Recent experimental work has shown that parasites from man can be transmitted to monkeys, domestic cats, and civet cats. Thus, the presence of different mammalian reservoir hosts must be considered in the control of Malayan filariasis.

The microfilariae were until recently believed to be exclusively of the periodic type, but a strain occurring in the eastern part of the Malay peninsula exhibits little periodicity. The larvae are sheathed, averaging 175 to 230 microns in length; the body nuclei extend almost to the tip of the tail, whereas in *W. bancrofti* larvae the tail contains no nuclei. Two terminal nuclei are distinctly separate from the others in the tail, and this characteristic serves further to differentiate the microfilariae from those of *Loa loa*, to be discussed below. Adults of *B. malayi* seem to be somewhat smaller than those of *W. bancrofti*, although few as yet have been recovered. Laboratory diagnosis is accomplished by examination of blood films, stained to demonstrate the differential morphological features of the microfilariae (Fig. 129).

SYMPTOMATOLOGY AND PATHOGENESIS. Clinical features of malayan filariasis are similar to those seen in bancroftian infections. Elephantiasis affects primarily the legs, and is not often so severe as that seen in *W. bancrofti* infections. There is rarely any genital involvement, and chyluria is also very uncommon.

Pulmonary nodules, seen on x-ray and surgically explored, have not infrequently been found to contain filarial worms. Beaver et al. (1971) reported such a nodule containing an immature live *Brugia* (presumably *B. malayi*), thought to have been acquired in India. Beaver and Cran

(1974) identified a *Wuchereria* (probably *W. bancrofti*) in a pulmonary infarct.

TREATMENT. Treatment is the same as that used in filariasis bancrofti. Allergic reactions tend to be severe in filariasis malayi, and treatment with diethylcarbamazine may be initiated with smaller doses, or antihistamines may be administered as a routine measure.

NON-FILARIAL ELEPHANTIASIS. An elephantiasis of non-filarial origin is seen not uncommonly in Northern and Central East Africa (Ethiopia, Uganda, Kenya, Tanzania, and the Sudan), where its range overlaps that of Bancroftian filariasis. It seems to be confined to areas where the soil contains large quantities of the clay, kaolinite, and iron and aluminum salts. Persons affected go barefoot all or much of the time, and are thought to absorb these materials through abrasions on the feet. Crystals of silicates, with iron and aluminum salts are found in the hypertrophied lymphatics of these individuals. Some 100,000 persons are said to be victims of this disease in Ethiopia, where the average age at onset is 18. Onset is generally distal, and it proceeds upwards on the leg, rarely extending above the knees. (See Heather and Price, 1972; Price, 1972, 1974, 1975.)

Loa loa

The African eye worm, *Loa loa*, migrates actively throughout the subcutaneous tissues, and derives its popular name from the fact that it is most conspicuous and irritating when crossing the conjunctiva. The scientific name comes from a native name for this worm, which is found throughout the rain-forest areas of the Sudan, the basin of the Congo and West Africa. In some of these areas it is encountered in a very high percentage of the population.

Adult males of *Loa loa* are from 2 to 3.5 cm. in length, and the females generally 5 to 7 cm; they are 0.5 mm. or less in width. The microfilariae, which are 250 to 300 microns long, and sheathed, differ from the microfilariae of *Wuchereria* and *Brugia* in having the body nuclei continuous to the tip of the tail. While adult worms migrate through the subcutaneous and deeper connective tissues, the microfilariae make their way into the blood stream, where they circulate and may be ingested by any of several species of mango flies. The mango fly, *Chrysops*, is large, with mouth parts which can produce a painful bite. The microfilariae undergo a developmental cycle in the thoracic musculature of the fly similar to that of *Wuchereria* in the mosquito, and after ten to twelve days have reached the infective stage. When the fly bites, the infective larvae migrate out onto the surface of the skin, and then enter through the bite.

Diagnosis of loiasis is most frequently made on the basis of a history of Calabar swellings, or the appearance of the worm in the conjunctivae, since microfilariae frequently do not appear in the blood until years after the worms, or the results of their activities, become apparent. At times, circulating microfilariae (Fig. 129) will be found quite early in the disease.

SYMPTOMATOLOGY. Migration of the adult worms through the tissues is not painful, and seldom noticed except when they happen to pass through the conjunctival tissue across the eyeball, or over the bridge of the nose. While they migrate rapidly, they can often be caught and excised while passing through the conjunctiva. There may be some edema of conjunctiva and lids when the worms are in that area. At other times, patches of localized subcutaneous edema, known as Calabar swellings, may appear anywhere on the body. The swellings may be several inches in diameter, and are often preceded by localized pain and pruritus. They last for several days to weeks, and subside slowly. It is thought that these Calabar swellings are a type of allergic reaction to the metabolic products of the worms, or to dead worms. A worm is not necessarily present in the area in which a Calabar swelling forms at the time it appears.

PATHOGENESIS. There is little to suggest that *Loa* produces any lasting damage to its host. Its quite rapid migration through subcutaneous tissue (at about 1 cm. per minute) may be completely painless in areas other than the face. An eosinophilia of 50 to 70 per cent is frequently noted, especially when Calabar swellings are present.

EPIDEMIOLOGY. Several species of African monkeys harbor a *Loa* morphologically indistinguishable from *Loa loa* of man. However, the monkey strain exhibits a nocturnal periodicity and is carried by species of *Chrysops* which are arboreal and night-biting. The human infection has been experimentally transmitted to monkeys, but the possibility that the reverse occurs in nature remains unproven. The two strains of *Loa* probably represent a relatively early stage in a "radiative evolution," which might ultimately result in morphologically distinguishable species.

Of possible public health concern is the report by Orihel and Lowrie (1975) that *Loa loa* will develop in the American deerfly, *Chrysops atlanticus,* and is infective for monkeys after development in this insect.

The infection is long-lived, and the pre-patent period may in some cases be as long as ten years, although it is generally perhaps closer to one year.

TREATMENT. Surgical removal of the migrating adult worms, most readily effected when they are found crossing the bridge of the nose or in the conjunctiva, is a relatively simple matter. However, diethylcarbamazine is so effective in elimination of both microfilariae and adult worms that its use seems preferable. It is administered as in filariasis bancrofti, for a period of two to three weeks. Doses as small as 2 mg. per Kg. of body weight daily may be effective. Allergic reactions are common during the course of treatment. Prophylactic antihistaminics may be given, or the reactions may be treated with corticosteroids.

Diethylcarbamazine has been demonstrated to be of value in the prophylaxis of loiasis (Duke, 1963). For this purpose, the dosage in adults is 200 mg. daily for three consecutive days, once a month.

Dipetalonema streptocerca

Dipetalonema streptocerca is found in the Congo basin in both monkeys and man. Microfilariae are found primarily in the skin, where they must be distinguished from those of *Onchocerca volvulus,* but also in the blood. Differential morphologic features of the microfilariae are shown in Figure 129.

Infection in man is characterized by a pruritic dermatitis with hypopigmented macules, and inguinal adenopathy (Meyers et al., 1972). Treatment with diethylcarbamazine (3 mg. per Kg. of body weight daily) is accompanied by pruritus. Papules which appear during treatment may on biopsy be found to contain adult worms. A description of the adult worm is given by Neafie et al. (1975). Small midges, belonging to the genus *Culicoides,* transmit this filaria.

Dipetalonema perstans and Mansonella ozzardi

There are two, and possibly more, filarial parasites of man, which, while affecting large numbers of people, seem to produce little or no damage. *Dipetalonema perstans* is a common parasite of man and apes in wide areas of Africa. It is also found in Panama, and in South America from Venezuela to the Argentine. The adult worms, similar in size to the other filariae which have been discussed, live in the deep connective tissues. Their unsheathed larvae are found in the peripheral blood, where they exhibit no periodicity. These microfilariae (Fig. 129) are characterized by nuclei which extend to the tip of the tail. This filaria is also transmitted by *Culicoides.*

Mansonella ozzardi is found in the West Indies, in the state of Yucatan in Mexico, in Panama, the Guianas and Argentina. The adults inhabit the mesenteries and visceral fat; the unsheathed, non-periodic larvae are found in the blood. The nuclei of the body of the microfilaria (Fig. 129) do not extend to the tip of the tail. *M. ozzardi* is likewise transmitted by *Culicoides.*

While both of these species are considered non-pathogenic, there have been some reports of allergic symptoms associated with infection by each of them. It seems very probable that death of the adult worms would provoke such symptoms, even if none was associated with the presence of the living filariae.

TREATMENT. Treatment is probably unnecessary in most cases. Diethylcarbamazine is apparently ineffective against *Mansonella,* but it has been used in standard dosages in the treatment of *Dipetalonema* infections with apparent success.

Onchocerca volvulus

The microfilariae of *Onchocerca volvulus,* as well as the adult worms, are found in the dermis and subcutaneous tissues, thus distinguishing this species from the filariae discussed previously except for *Dipetalonema streptocerca.*

O. volvulus is widely distributed throughout Central Africa. It is also present in the Yemen and in the Western Hemisphere in restricted areas of Mexico, Guatemala, Venezuela and Colombia. It is generally considered to have been introduced into the Americas by the slave trade.

The intermediate host and vector of *Onchocerca volvulus* may be one of a number of species of *Simulium,* the black fly or buffalo gnat. These minute insects are widespread in their distribution, but only certain species are suitable vectors, possibly because of their feeding habits, or perhaps for other reasons. The simuliid, upon biting an infected person, ingests microfilariae which have a developmental cycle in the insect similar to that undergone by other filarial larvae (Fig. 127), transforming into infective forms which may enter a new host when the simuliid again takes a blood meal. After introduction into the new host, the developing worms wander through the subcutaneous tissues, but settle down, usually in groups of two or more; most worms finally become encapsulated. Nodules, produced by encapsulation of the adult worms in a fibrous tissue tumor-like mass, usually form within a year after infection. They are most frequently subcutaneous, but may occur in connective tissues deeper in the body. The nodules vary in size from a few millimeters to several centimeters in diameter and may be numerous. In Venezuela and in Africa the majority of nodules are located on the trunk or limbs and few form on the head, while in Mexico and Guatemala they are frequently seen in the scalp (Fig. 133), and less often in other parts of the body. The reason for this difference in distribution of lesions is by no means apparent but may be related to the biting habits of the several vectors. Studies by De Leon and

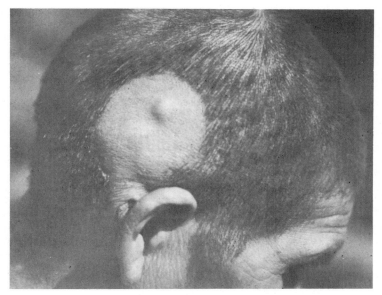

FIGURE 133. *Onchocerca volvulus* nodules on scalp. Note also thickened, wrinkled skin in front of ear. (Courtesy of Ash and Spitz, Pathology of Tropical Diseases, Armed Forces Institute of Pathology, #79,133 D.)

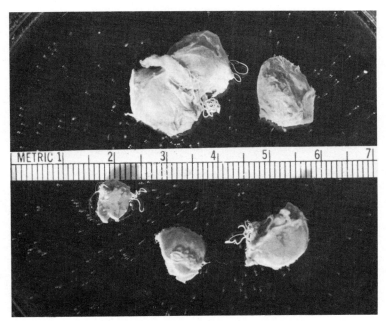

FIGURE 134. *Onchocerca volvulus* nodules. Portions of contained adult worms protruding. (Photograph by Zane Price.)

Duke (1966) suggest that the African and American strains are distinct; it is possible that there are several distinct strains in Africa.

The adult worms lie coiled within the fibrous tissue capsules (Fig. 134), and are wire-like and whitish. The female may be as long as 50 cm., though less than 0.5 mm. in diameter. Males are considerably smaller, reaching a length of under 5 cm. Microfilariae make their way out of the nodules, and migrate actively through the dermis and in the connective tissues not only in the vicinity of the nodules but at some distance from them. As seen in skin biopsies, the larvae are unsheathed, and from 150 to over 350 microns in length.

Diagnosis is by identification of the microfilariae found in "skin snips" (Fig. 135). The bits of tissue needed for diagnosis may be secured by two different techniques. After suitable preparation of the skin with a volatile antiseptic agent, a fold of skin may be squeezed between thumb and forefinger of one hand, while a thin slice of skin is removed with a razor blade held in the other. Or, a needle may be used to catch and raise a small "cone" of skin, which is then removed with scissors or a razor blade. The tissue is then placed in saline, and may be teased to facilitate liberation of the microfilariae. It may be necessary to take multiple skin snips in light infections. In Africa, they are customarily taken from the buttock region, and in Mexico and Guatemala, from the shoulders.

Although microfilariae are more commonly found in the skin than elsewhere, microfilaruria is not uncommon. In an area in Guatemala where infection is seen in virtually 100 per cent of the population, 80 per cent had microfilariae in skin snips, and 17 to 30 per cent of those 10 years or more of age had microfilaruria (Fazen et al., 1975). The num-

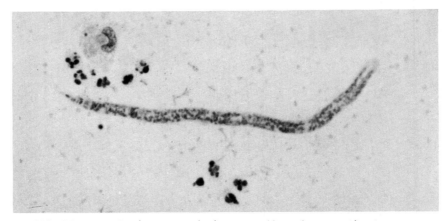

FIGURE 135. *Onchocerca volvulus,* microfilaria from scarification preparation. (Photomicrograph by Zane Price.)

bers of microfilariae in the urine may be increased following the admini-istration of an oral dose of 50 mg. of diethylcarbamazine, and they may also be found in the blood and sputum (Anderson et al., 1975a). The same authors (1975b) note a diurnal periodicity of microfilariae in the skin.

In the tropical rain forest of Africa, microfilariae of *Dipetalonema streptocerca* may also be found in skin snips. They are generally smaller than those of *O. volvulus*, but for differentiation, the microfilariae should be stained. In stained smears, nuclei will be seen to extend to the tip of the tail of *D. streptocerca*, while the tail of *O. volvulus* is free of nuclei.

Biopsy of the onchocercomas may be undertaken not only for therapeutic but for diagnostic purposes, and sections of these nodules reveal a characteristic picture (Fig. 136).

SYMPTOMATOLOGY.   The nodules, while sometimes disfiguring, are not painful, and the importance of the infection lies not in the adult worms but the effects which may be produced by their larvae. In Mexico and Guatemala an acute inflammatory reaction, involving usually the face, eyes, ears, neck or shoulders, but sometimes found elsewhere on the body, may occur spontaneously. The skin is hot, edematous and often painful. There may be associated pruritus. The inflammation subsides slowly, and may recur many times, eventually resulting in permanent thickening of the skin, which may also assume a violaceous color. This reaction is thought to be caused by death of

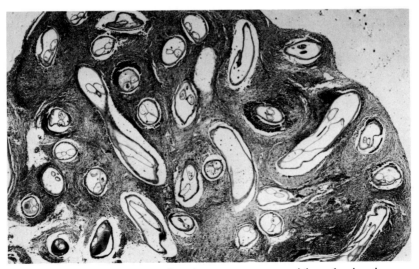

FIGURE 136.   Section of onchocercoma removed from forehead.

microfilariae in the skin, and liberation of antigenic materials from them. It may be provoked by administration of drugs known to kill the microfilariae, and prevented by administration of cortisone and similar drugs. Onchodermatitis seems to assume somewhat distinct forms in different areas. In Mexico and Central America the patchy purplish or reddish eruption characterizing acute attacks is known as "mal morado" or "erysipela de la costa." Chronically infected skin is atrophic and wrinkled, with subcutaneous thickening. In Africa atrophy of the skin and subcutaneous lymphedema are also seen, along with depigmentation producing a "leopard skin" appearance, and the presence of papular to pustular nodules up to 1 cm. in diameter, caused by inflammatory reactions to localized collections of microfilariae in the skin. These lesions are locally referred to as "craw-craw."

The infected skin loses its elasticity and becomes deeply wrinkled and atrophic. In Mexico and Guatemala, this is seen mainly in the head and neck region, producing an appearance of premature senility and sometimes a rather leonine facies. In Africa, the same process occurring around the hip region is responsible for the spectacular complication known as "hanging groin" (Fig. 137), a condition in which a sac of tissue forms in the inguinal region (Nelson, 1970). It may contain inguinal or femoral lymph glands, and hang down as far as the knees. Lymphedema of the external genitalia and scrotal elephantiasis are seen as complications of onchocerciasis in some areas of Africa.

As a measure of the severity of the eye lesions in onchocerciasis, it has been estimated that while blindness is two to four times as prevalent in an area where trachoma is endemic than in a control area, such as Europe, it is at least six times more commonly seen in areas of high *Onchocerca* endemicity. Anderson et al. (1974a,b) in their studies in the Cameroon note quite different degrees of eye involvement in different areas. In the rain forest, some 80 to 90 per cent of children in the five to nine year old group are infected, and of these about 2 per cent are blind, while in the savanna areas only 60 to 70 per cent of a comparable age group are infected, but 5 per cent are blind. Among persons over forty, the figures for the two areas become 4.2 per cent and 14.4 per cent for the two areas.

PATHOGENESIS. Encapsulation in the characteristic onchocercomas is by no means the universal fate of adult *Onchocerca volvulus*. Some worms, especially during the early stages of the disease in young children and in lightly infected individuals, produce no apparent tissue reaction; these worms are found free in the tissues. The dermal lesions are without doubt of an allergic nature, and can be exactly duplicated by administration of small doses of diethylcarbamazine, resulting in the death of large numbers of microfilariae in the skin. Such acute reactions, occurring either spontaneously or as the result of therapy, can be suppressed by the administration of corticosteroids. The loss of elastic-

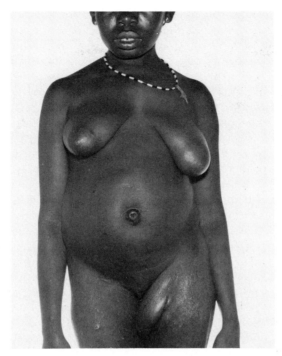

FIGURE 137. Patient with hanging groin caused by underlying obstructive onchocercal lymphadenitis and loss of dermal elasticity. Note also onchodermatitis. (Photograph by Dr. Daniel H. Connor, Armed Forces Institute of Pathology, #68–10066–1).

ity of the skin of the pelvic region, seen in chronic African onchocerciasis, results not only in the "hanging groin" mentioned earlier but in a high prevalence of inguinal and femoral hernias.

Differences in frequency of the various ophthalmologic lesions between the African and American strains of *Onchocerca* have been noted (Woodruff et al., 1966), but are not well explained. Choyce (1966) has made careful studies of the ophthalmologic complications of onchocerciasis. The earliest lesions noted consist of a punctate keratitis; at this time microfilariae may be found within the cornea and in the anterior chamber. These opacities may coalesce, usually in the lower portions of the cornea; there may be inflammation of the limbus of the cornea and of the adjacent scleral tissue, as well as the formation of pterygia which grow out over the cornea. Iridocyclitis appears somewhat later than the corneal changes; posterior synechiae frequently displace the pupil, which becomes fixed and sometimes distorted. An exudate may form and cover the pupillary area, finally leading to blindness. These lesions of the cornea, anterior chamber and iris are seen both in African and American onchocerciasis, but they tend to be more severe in the latter. Lesions of the posterior chamber are less common in both areas. Microfilariae are not seen adherent to or within the lens substance, or in the posterior chamber. Onchocercal chorioretinitis and optic atrophy are seen, but they cannot readily be distinguished from those caused by toxoplasmosis or other etiologies.

EPIDEMIOLOGY. As has previously been noted, African and American onchocerciasis exhibit certain differences, some of which may be related to vector biting habits (localization of the onchocercomas), and some to strain or other as yet unexplained differences (rain forest vs. savanna). Onchocerciasis was presumably introduced to the Americas by the slave trade, and observations of Trapido et al. (1971) in Colombia are of some interest as regards present-day distribution of the disease in that country. The simuliid vectors in Colombia are zoophilic, and where domestic livestock is found the human infection has died out, to persist only in areas where no large domestic animals are kept. Onchocerciasis has been sporadically reported from many non-endemic areas, such as Great Britain, and some at least of these cases represent zoonotic infections (Beaver et al., 1974) with onchocercas from horses or other domestic animals.

Simuliid gnats have larval stages which are aquatic, most of them requiring swiftly-flowing streams in which the larvae and pupae attach to submerged rocks or vegetation. Some species develop in more quiet waters, and certain African species attach to freshwater crabs. It follows that endemic areas generally follow the course of rivers or streams, whence the common name of "river blindness" for the disease.

TREATMENT. Diethylcarbamazine is a very effective microfilaricide, as in other filarial infections. Death of the microfilariae may lead to severe dermal reactions, necessitating the use of antihistaminics or corticosteroids. Severe generalized reactions, while uncommon, have been reported, with respiratory distress, collapse and even loss of consciousness (Fuglsang and Anderson, 1974). On the other hand, adult worms are unaffected by standard doses of diethylcarbamazine. Suramin* is effective against both adult worms and microfilariae but is quite toxic. In practice, a combination of the two drugs is both effective and reasonably well-tolerated. Diethylcarbamazine may be given first, starting with a single oral dose of 25 mg. daily for the first three days. Antihistamines or steroids may be given in conventional doses to lessen allergic reactions to the death of microfilariae. The daily dose is doubled for the next three days, and doubled again (to 100 mg. daily) for the seventh to ninth day of therapy. For the next 12 days, 150 mg. is given

---

*Available in the United States from the Parasitic Disease Service, Center for Disease Control, U.S. Public Health Service, Atlanta, Ga. 30333.

daily. At the end of the course of diethylcarbamazine, treatment with suramin is instituted with an intravenous test dose of 100 mg. If hypersensitivity to the drug (with nausea, vomiting and loss of consciousness) does not occur, it may be continued with weekly intravenous injections of 1 gm. (10 to 15 mg. per Kg. of body weight in children) for an additional five weeks. Frequent side reactions include vomiting, pruritus, paresthesias and hyperesthesias, and photophobia. Effects of treatment may be monitored by skin snips and visual field determinations before and at intervals after treatment. Topical diethylcarbamazine has been suggested (Lazar et al., 1970) for the treatment of ocular onchocerciasis, but Anderson and Fuglsang (1973) caution that it may cause an anterior uveitis.

Other Filarial Infections in Man

Zoonotic filarial infections are reported sporadically from man in various parts of the world, and it is of interest that about half of these have originated in the United States (Beaver and Orihel, 1965). The most common type is that found in nodules in the subcutaneous tissues, generally identified as *Dirofilaria conjunctivae*. These are usually immature, but some mature microfilaria-containing worms found in the subcutaneous tissues have been identified as *D. tenuis*, which is commonly found in the subcutaneous tissues of raccoons. Next most common is *Dirofilaria immitis*, the heartworm of dogs, found in the heart and lungs of man. Some have been found alive at autopsy; more frequently they have been first noted as solitary pulmonary nodules ("coin lesions"), and their true nature discovered only after surgery (Tannehill and Hatch, 1968; Spear et al., 1968). Pulmonary infarction has been described secondary to the presence of *Dirofilaria* in the pulmonary artery (Goodman and Gore, 1964) or elsewhere in the lungs (Yoshimura and Yokogawa, 1970). Transmission of these *Dirofilaria* infections to man is without doubt by the agency of the same mosquitoes which infect their usual hosts.

Key to Microfilariae Commonly Found in the Blood

a. Larvae possess sheath .... b
   Larvae unsheathed .... d
b. Nuclei found in tip of tail.. c
   Nuclei do not extend to tip..*Wuchereria bancrofti*
c. Nuclei form continuous row in tail .... *Loa loa*
   Nuclei not continuous, two at tip of tail .... *Brugia malayi*
d. Nuclei found in tip of tail.. e
   Nuclei do not extend to tip..*Mansonella ozzardi*
e. Nuclei often in double row....................................*Dipetalonema perstans*
   Nuclei in single row, tail curved..*D. streptocerca*

Eosinophilic lung disease (tropical eosinophilia), characterized by persistent hypereosinophilia and pulmonary symptoms, has been known frequently to respond to the administration of diethylcarbamazine. Studies by Danaraj et al. (1966) have shown that microfilariae can be found in biopsies of lung tissue from affected individuals, in whom they could not be demonstrated in the peripheral blood. Joshi et al. (1969) also found microfilariae in lung biopsies from patients with tropical eosinophilia, but consider that certain non-filarial parasites may also play a role in the etiology of this condition.

THE GUINEA WORM

Dracunculus medinensis

The guinea worm, *Dracunculus medinensis,* is of imposing antiquity among known agents of human disease. It is thought that the fiery serpents which plagued the Israelites by the Red Sea were *Dracunculus;* the disease which they cause was recognized and named by Galen.

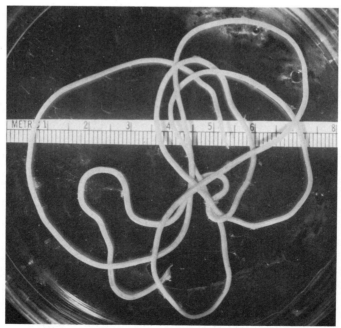

FIGURE 138. *Dracunculus medinensis,* female worm removed surgically. (Photograph by Zane Price.)

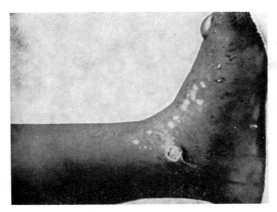

FIGURE 139. *Dracunculus medinensis,* uterus of female worm protruding from ulcerated lesion over ankle. On dorsum of foot may be seen a vesicle produced by another worm about to break through skin. (Courtesy of Dr. E. C. Smith, Nigeria.)

The guinea worm is an important parasite in Asia from the Arabian peninsula to central India, and is found in Africa in the Nile Valley from Egypt to the Sudan, scattered through central Equatorial Africa, and on the west coast. It is seen in southeastern Russia, in parts of Indonesia, and was once found in the West Indies, the Guianas and Brazil, but apparently no longer occurs in the Western Hemisphere except in reservoir hosts. It is a parasite of dogs and other carnivores in North America, and of a number of different mammalian hosts in the areas from which human infections are reported.

While sometimes classed with the filarial worms, *Dracunculus* is not a true filaria. The worms are elongate (Fig. 138), females measuring up to a meter or slightly more in length, but averaging under 1 meter, and with a diameter of less than 2 mm. The little-known male worm is inconspicuous, and 2 cm. or less in length. Worms develop to maturity in the body cavity or deeper connective tissues, and the females migrate to the subcutaneous tissues when they become gravid. The body of the fully gravid female worm is almost completely filled by uterus distended with larvae. A papule is produced in the skin where the head of the female lies just under the dermis, and this becomes vesicular and finally ulcerates, exposing the worm. A loop of uterus becomes prolapsed through the body wall of the worm, to lie in the ulcer opening (Fig. 139); when the ulcer is immersed in water larvae are discharged in large numbers. These larvae are unlike microfilariae, having a well-developed digestive tract, and are never found in the blood or tissues of the host, being discharged directly into water. If ingested (Fig. 140) by copepods, belonging to various species of the genus *Cyclops,* the

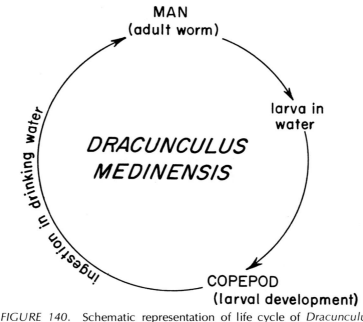

FIGURE 140. Schematic representation of life cycle of *Dracunculus medinensis.*

larvae will mature into infective forms within that host in about three weeks. Frequently, wells, streams or other sources of drinking water contain large numbers of copepods; whenever the ulcer of an infected person is immersed in water, larvae are liberated, so that in endemic areas a high proportion of copepods may be infected. If such copepods are swallowed, the contained larvae will be liberated to penetrate through the digestive tract, entering the deep connective tissues where they mature. Maturation apparently takes a period of approximately one year.

Diagnosis usually presents no problems in endemic areas, as the development of the local lesion is quite characteristic. Once the ulcer is formed, larvae may be obtained for diagnostic purposes by flooding the area with water.

SYMPTOMATOLOGY AND PATHOGENESIS. One or many worms may be seen at one time, in any part of the body, but most commonly on the legs or feet. The majority of infections consists of a single worm, but in endemic areas repeated reinfection is the general rule. The presence of maturing worms gives rise to no symptoms until they are ready to discharge their larvae. When the gravid female seeks a position close to the skin, there may be some localized erythema and tenderness in the area where the ulcer will form. The patient frequently exhibits some generalized symptoms at this time, with pruritus, sometimes nausea, vomiting or diarrhea, or asthmatic attacks. These symptoms usually disappear with the appearance of the ulcer, the drainage of fluid which has formed around the female worm and the initial discharge of larvae. A localized reaction, often quite painful, remains around the site of the ulcer during the entire period while the worm continues to discharge its larvae. Discharge is intermittent, whenever the affected part comes in contact with water, and may take as long as three weeks to be complete. After the uterus is emptied, the worm may withdraw into the tissues and become resorbed, or may be expelled. If the lesion does not become secondarily infected, healing is rapid after all larvae have been discharged. If the worms are removed surgically, the wound will heal promptly. When, in the process of its removal, the worm is broken, secondary infection almost inevitably sets in. A rare complication of infection is invasion of the extradural space by the guinea worm, leading in two reported cases (Mitra and Haddock, 1970) to abscess formation and paraplegia.

The calcified remains of worms which have died in the subcutaneous tissues may be found on x-ray examination. They may appear as linear calcific densities up to 25 cm. in length, as tightly coiled bodies, or as rather dense, usually somewhat elongate nodules (Reinhard, 1961).

TREATMENT. Niridazole (Ambilhar) is reported to be effective in treatment of dracunculiasis. It is given by mouth, the dosage being 25 mg. per Kg. of body weight daily for seven days. Niridazole may cause nausea and vomiting, diarrhea, cramps, dizziness and headache, rash, insomnia, paresthesias and electrocardiographic changes which are apparently transitory. It may cause a hemolytic anemia in glucose-6-phosphate dehydrogenase (G-6-PD) deficient individuals, and rarely gives rise to convulsions or psychoses. It is not available in the United States, but it is manufactured by Ciba in Switzerland. Diethylcarbamazine has some activity against the adult Guinea worm and is apparently of value when taken prophylactically. There are conflicting reports as to the usefulness of metronidazole. Antani et al. (1972) gave 200 mg. orally three times daily for 7 days, with results which they considered superior to those obtained with niridazole, thiabendazole, or diethylcarbamazine. Mebendazole is considered ineffective by Kale (1975).

OTHER TISSUE NEMATODES

Trichinella spiralis

Discussed here because of the importance of the tissue phase of its life cycle, *Trichinella spiralis* might equally well be considered with the intestinal helminths. The intestinal infection, in which adult worms are found in the mucosa, is transitory and usually asymptomatic or nearly so, whereas the phase of migration and encystment of larvae in the muscles is prolonged and frequently accompanied by serious symptoms.

T. spiralis is a parasite of carnivorous mammals, showing little if any host specificity. It is especially common in rats, and in swine fed uncooked garbage and slaughterhouse scraps. It may occur in man whenever uncooked pork is consumed, and is most commonly seen in those groups making a practice of the consumption of raw pork products, such as various types of salami and wurst. Bears are heavily infected, as numerous hunters have learned to their sorrow. *Trichinella* is cosmopolitan in its distribution, but much more common in man in those areas where uncooked garbage containing pork scraps is fed to hogs. It was once very common in many European countries, but enlightened sanitary practices have resulted in a marked lowering of the rate in many areas, so that at the present time the United States is said to enjoy the doubtful distinction of having three times as much trichinosis as the rest of the world combined. Incidence of trichina infection in this country was estimated on the basis of autopsy findings covering the years 1931 to 1942, and was in the vicinity of 16 per cent of the population; it has been stated that approximately 4 per cent of these infections were sufficiently heavy to cause symptoms. Many states have adopted or are adopting laws requiring the sterilization of garbage fed to hogs; a lower incidence of infection will undoubtedly result.

Infection is initiated by the consumption of raw or insufficiently cooked pork or other meat containing the encysted larvae (Fig. 141). The larvae excyst after the cysts are digested, and penetrate into the intestinal mucosa, developing to adult worms within the short space of thirty to forty hours. Male worms are generally under 2 mm. in length, while females may reach a length of almost 5 mm. Mating may take place as soon as the worms are mature, and larvae may be produced within three days after fertilization. Thus, within about five days the larvae grow to maturity and begin the stage of larval deposition, which continues for as long as the female worms remain in the intestine. The duration of the intestinal infection probably depends upon a number of factors, including the number of worms present in the intestine and the immune status of the host as determined by previous infections. The intestinal phase persists in congenitally athymic (nude) mice much longer than in those heterozygous for the athymic gene, indicating that T-cell dependent antigen is necessary for protection against the intestinal phase of the infection (Ruitenberg and Steerenberg, 1974). Human intestinal infections have been known to persist for as long as fifty-four days; the average duration is probably less than that period.

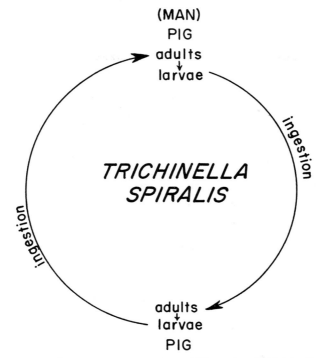

FIGURE 141.   Schematic representation of life cycle of *Trichinella spiralis*.

Upon their deposition in the mucosa, the larvae enter lymphatic vessels and from them gain access to the general circulation. They are 80 to 120 microns long, and 5 or 6 microns in diameter, and so are readily transported throughout the body. They leave the capillaries in striated muscle to penetrate through the sheaths of the muscle fibers. Degenerative and inflammatory changes are seen in infected muscle fibers, and within about a month the larvae have reached their full growth (Fig. 142). They are coiled in a spiral and gradually become surrounded by a sheath derived from the muscle fiber. The fully developed larva measures about 1 mm. in length. Encysted trichinae may remain viable for many years, even after calcification of the capsule has taken place.

The diagnosis may be fairly obvious on the basis of clinical symptoms and history, but should be confirmed by laboratory examination or skin testing. The Bachman skin test consists of the intracutaneous administration of 0.1 ml. of an extract of dried and powdered *Trichinella* larvae. The test substance is also known as trichinellin, and after the first two weeks of infection most patients will give a positive reaction, of the immediate type. Positive skin reactions may be elicited for a

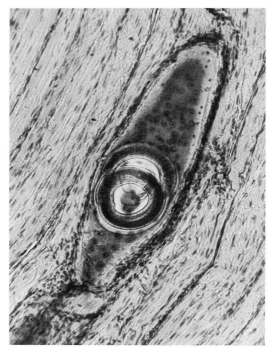

FIGURE 142. *Trichinella spiralis,* larva in muscle. (Photomicrograph by Zane Price.)

number of years following infection, and do not necessarily indicate an active disease process. Several serological tests, of which the simplest are precipitin reactions, are also described; an antigen is now commercially available. Biopsy of skeletal muscle, usually gastrocnemius, may reveal the encysting larvae at any time after the first week of infection. Knott concentrates of venous blood taken during the period of larval migration may demonstrate these organisms (see Chapter 15).

SYMPTOMATOLOGY. Symptoms during the intestinal phase may be so minor in nature as not to be noticed, or may be of moderate severity. If present, they usually appear suddenly, and are those of a non-specific gastroenteritis. Diagnosis of the disease is seldom made at this stage, but an epidemic outbreak of gastroenteritis, from two to seven days after ingestion of uncooked pork products by a group, should make one suspect trichinosis. Diarrhea, with or without abdominal pain, may last for several weeks.

During the stage of muscle invasion, symptoms will vary again according to the intensity of infection. Fever and eosinophilia are rather consistently seen when the infection is sufficiently severe to produce any symptoms, and eosinophilia probably accompanies even asymptomatic cases. It usually reaches its height in the third or fourth week, and at that time may range from 10 per cent or less to 90 per cent. In some overwhelming infections, eosinophilia may not appear. Characteristically, the eosinophilia increases rapidly during the early stages of the disease, and gradually declines thereafter over a period of some months. Leukocytosis is common, but not always present. Myositis appears early, and with it almost invariably occurs the classical sign of trichinosis, circumorbital edema. This sign is rarely absent in patients who develop clinical symptoms of infection; it is thought to be related to the vasculitis responsible for the production of splinter hemorrhages. Edema of the eyelids appears as early as the seventh day of infection, but may come on much later. It may extend to involve the cheeks or pre-auricular regions. In some patients, photophobia, diplopia or other visual disturbances may occur. Muscular pain may be severe, and usually reaches its height from the twelfth to twentieth days of infection. Muscles are often sensitive to pressure. Splinter hemorrhages beneath the nails are seen in a high percentage of patients. Central nervous system involvement, with symptoms suggestive of an acute psychosis, meningoencephalitis, cerebral vascular accident or brain tumor, is seen in a small percentage of patients with clinical trichinosis. In moderate infections, symptoms usually begin to lessen during the fifth or sixth week. In severe cases, death may occur four to six weeks after infection.

PATHOGENESIS. The intestinal phase of a *Trichinella* infection ends when the adult worms are rejected because of the development of local tissue immunity. The development of immunity can be suppressed and the intestinal phase can be prolonged by the administration of corticosteroids; these facts must be borne in mind if these drugs are used in therapy. The primary pathogenic effect of *Trichinella* comes from destruction of the striated muscle fibers in which it encysts. A vasculitis may accompany the migration of the larvae, accounting for the splinter hemorrhages and perhaps the periorbital edema. Certain of the neurologic manifestations of trichinosis may also be due to vasculitis; granulomas which sometimes contain *Trichinella* larvae have also been found in the brains of patients dying of this infection (Kennedy and Rege, 1966). Clinically apparent trichinal myocarditis is rare, but death has been ascribed to this cause.

EPIDEMIOLOGY. In the 1930's it was estimated that one out of every six persons in the United States became infected with *Trichinella spiralis* during his lifetime; recent studies indicate that the infection rate has declined to approximately one in twenty-five (Zimmermann et al., 1973). From 150,000 to 300,000 infections are estimated to occur each year in the United States, but the number of clinical cases reported is only a minute fraction of this amount (average of 113.4 during 1966–70). Among the factors responsible for this decline are legislative measures requiring heat treatment of garbage used as hog food, low temperature storage of pork (refrigeration at −15°C. for 20 days or more or quick freezing at −37°C.). public awareness of the danger involved in eating undercooked pork, and perhaps a decline in the consumption of pork and pork products. Sporadic outbreaks are still seen, generally associated with the consumption of homemade sausage.

Of the many flesh-eating mammals which may become infected with *T. spiralis,* only two are of epidemiologic importance in addition to swine. The rat may become infected by feeding on scraps of infected pork, or through cannibalism, and forms a sometimes important source of infection for hogs. Bears are frequently infected and are a source of occasional outbreaks of the disease (Maynard and Kagan, 1964).

TREATMENT. In severely symptomatic infections, corticosteroids are beneficial and may at times be lifesaving. Recognition that, as mentioned previously, the intestinal phase of the infection may be prolonged by their use suggests that they should be reserved for cases in which there is considerable toxicity. The initial dose may be 20 to 40 mg. of prednisone, or its equivalent, reduced after the first few days to the lowest dosage which will alleviate symptoms and then gradually discontinued. The use of thiabendazole in this infection is still debated. Thiabendazole in conventional dosage (25 mg. per Kg. of body weight, twice daily), even when given for five to seven days, has failed to kill larvae in the tissues (Kean and Hoskins, 1964), but numerous reports indicate that this drug affords symptomatic relief.

Visceral Larva Migrans

Eggs of non-human ascarids such as *Toxocara canis* or *T. cati* are capable of undergoing a limited development in the human host. The adult worms, similar to *Ascaris lumbricoides* in appearance but only one-quarter to one-half its size, live in the small intestine of dogs and cats. Their eggs, which require a period of maturation outside the host, are infective for dogs, cats and man. In all of these hosts, infective eggs hatch in the intestine and liberate larvae which burrow into the wall of the intestine. In puppies less than five weeks of age, the larvae complete a migratory and developmental cycle similar to that of *Ascaris lumbricoides* in man and become mature *Toxocara* in the intestinal tract. In older puppies or adult dogs, the larvae are unable to complete their development. They may wander for some time in the tissues, finally encysting as second stage larvae. By some mechanism not yet understood, these larvae may excyst in a pregnant bitch and cross the placenta, to grow to adult worms in the pups. Eggs of *T. cati,* ingested by cats, apparently complete their developmental cycle and become adult worms in the intestine.

If man or a variety of other animals ingest infective ova of *T. canis* or *T. cati,* development will proceed only as far as the second stage larvae, which after a period of migration encyst in the tissues. If rats or mice so infected are eaten by dogs or cats, the contained larvae will finish their development in the new host, becoming adult worms in the intestine.

Diagnosis of visceral larva migrans in man is generally made on clinical grounds. Chronic eosinophilia, especially in a young child who has been exposed to ascarid-infected pets, accompanied by hepatomegaly or chronic non-specific pulmonary disease, is suggestive of this condition. A skin test and various serologic tests have been described; the skin test and hemagglutination test seem to be of reasonable specificity (Wiseman and Woodruff, 1970; Krupp, 1974). Needle biopsy is not an effective method of diagnosing hepatic infection.

SYMPTOMATOLOGY.   Visceral larva migrans affects primarily children, probably because they are more likely to come in contact with dog and cat ascarid ova in the soil. Eosinophilia is very common; hepatomegaly may be seen, and some cases present symptoms of chronic pulmonary inflammation, with cough and fever. In rare cases pulmonary involvement has been sufficiently severe to lead to considerable respiratory embarrassment, and deaths have been reported from this condition. Visual difficulties may indicate a toxocaral chorioretinitis or peripheral retinitis (Hogan et al., 1965); such involvement would be expected to be unilateral. Epilepsy and myocarditis have also been associated with *Toxocara* infections in man.

PATHOGENESIS.   Wandering of the second stage larvae through the tissues produces tracks marked by hemorrhage, necrosis, and infiltration of round cells and eosinophils. Granulomatous foci are produced around dead larvae. Woodruff (1970) and Khalil et al. (1971) suggest that *Toxocara* larvae may carry with them in their migration from intestinal tract to central nervous system the virus of poliomyelitis and perhaps other viruses or bacteria, and point to the higher prevalence of serologic evidence of infection with *Toxocara* in children with poliomyelitis.

TREATMENT.   The disease is self-limited, frequently coming first to the attention of the physician at a time when the symptoms are at their worst. Watchful waiting is advised, and corticosteroids (employed as in trichinosis) are reserved for patients who are severely symptomatic. Both thiabendazole (25 mg. per Kg. of body weight twice daily until symptoms abate or significant side effects are noted) and diethylcarbamazine (2 mg. per Kg. of body weight, three times daily for 30 days) are reported to be effective in treatment of this infection.

Angiostrongylus cantonensis

Epidemic outbreaks, as well as sporadic occurrences of a generally self-limited meningitis, characterized by a pleocytosis with marked eosinophilia, have been noted throughout the Pacific area for many years. Thailand and Taiwan are heavily endemic areas. Sporadic cases have also been reported from Central America. Only recently has it been possible to relate this condition to infection with a nematode parasite, *Angiostrongylus cantonensis*, a lungworm of rats. *A. cantonensis* is a slender worm, up to 25 mm. long. Larval stages develop in slugs and land snails. When eaten by rats, the larvae migrate to the meninges and develop in the brain for about a month. Young adults then migrate to the pulmonary artery and attain maturity. The incidence of this infection in rats and snails may be quite high in endemic areas.

Sources of human infection are slugs, land snails, or fresh-water prawns and other paratenic (transport) hosts, which are often consumed raw in islands of the Pacific (Rosen et al., 1967), in Thailand and in Vietnam. Raw prawns are a frequent article of diet in Tahiti, and larvae found in them are infective to white rats. The contamination of fresh vegetables by carnivorous land planarians which have fed on infected snails appears to be another important means of infection in New Caledonia and perhaps elsewhere.

A presumptive diagnosis can be made in patients from areas where the disease is endemic on the basis of meningitis with eosinophilia of blood and spinal fluid.

SYMPTOMATOLOGY. The incubation period of the disease varies and apparently can be as long as 47 days. Infection in man is usually benign and self-limited, although fatalities have occurred. Symptoms of meningitis or meningoencephalitis—headache and stiff neck, often with sensorial changes—are of abrupt onset. The spinal fluid usually contains from 100 to 1000 white blood cells per cubic millimeter, generally accompanied by a marked eosinophilia.

PATHOGENESIS. Little is known concerning the effects of this parasite on the central nervous system, since most patients recover uneventfully. Autopsy findings in a single case have been recorded by Rosen et al. (1962). Sections of immature *Angiostrongylus* were seen in the cerebrum and cerebellum, associated with infiltrates of eosinophils, monocytes and foreign-body giant cells. Marked tissue necrosis was seen in some areas in connection with dead worms. Immature worms have been found in spinal fluid obtained by lumbar puncture; adult worms have been found in the eye and the pulmonary artery.

TREATMENT. Trials of specific therapy are still inconclusive. For a detailed discussion of this infection, see Alicata and Jindrak (1970).

Angiostrongylus costaricensis

The adult of *A. costaricensis* ordinarily inhabits the mesenteric arteries of the cotton rat (*Sigmodon hispidus*) and several other species of wild rodents. It has been encountered as a human parasite primarily in Costa Rica, though additional cases have been reported from most other parts of Central America, from Mexico (Yucatan) and from Brazil (Saõ Paulo). Most such infections have been found in children (Morera and Céspedes, 1971; Morera, 1973).

Egg-laying takes place in arterioles of the intestinal wall of the rodent host; the eggs hatch to produce larvae which migrate through the intestinal wall to appear in the feces. First stage larvae, ingested by the slug *Vaginulus plebeius*, grow and undergo two molts, after which they are infectious to rats or man. Children are likely to become infected while playing in the grassy areas infested by these slugs; infection has also been traced to contaminated salad vegetables. Physid snails may also serve as intermediate hosts.

In man, the worms cause an inflammatory lesion of the bowel wall (Fig. 143). Most frequently involved is the appendix, but they may also be found in the terminal ileum, cecum, ascending colon and regional

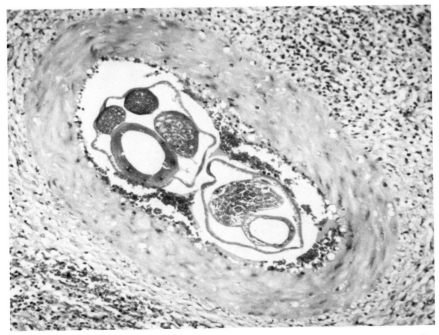

FIGURE 143. Angiostrongylus costaricensis in section of human appendix. (Microphotograph by Zane Price, from material furnished by Dr. Pedro Morera.)

lymph nodes. Inflammation, thrombosis and regional necrosis may mark the presence of the worms in mesenteric arteries, and an inflammatory reaction surrounds the eggs in the wall of the intestine, which becomes thickened even to the point of obstruction. X-rays may mimic malignancy of the large bowel. Light infections may run a chronic course, but heavy ones are frequently accompanied by pain in the right iliac fossa or flank, fever, anorexia and vomiting. There is sometimes a palpable intra-abdominal mass, or a mass can be palpated on rectal examination. A leucocytosis of 10–50,000 may be seen, with an eosinophilia of about 10 to 80 or more per cent.

A skin test antigen has been prepared, and is reported to give good results. Diagnosis is generally made by surgery, which is the only available form of treatment. Eggs and larvae do not appear in the stools of man.

Gnathostomiasis

Larval stages of roundworms belonging to the genus *Gnathostoma* are acquired by man through ingestion of raw or improperly cooked fresh-water fish. While many species of *Gnathostoma* have been described, only *G. spinigerum* is of medical importance. Human infections with this parasite are fairly common in Japan, and have also been reported from China, Thailand, the Philippines, and other areas where raw or pickled fish are a part of the diet.

The life cycle of *G. spinigerum* involves two intermediate hosts; the

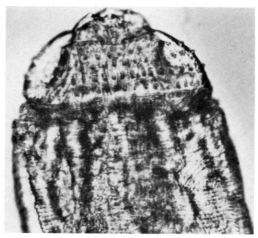

FIGURE 144. Head portion of larva of *Gnathostoma spinigerum*.

first is a copepod, the second is any of a number of fresh-water food fish, frogs, snakes or birds. The larval worms, about 4 mm. long, with numerous spines on the head and body (Fig. 144), encyst in the second intermediate host. Adult worms are normally found in dogs and cats, where they live coiled in the wall of the alimentary tract. Ingested by man, the larvae do not mature but migrate throughout the body.

SYMPTOMATOLOGY AND PATHOGENESIS. A few days after ingestion, migration of the larvae through the intestinal wall and into the abdominal cavity may produce epigastric pain, fever, vomiting and anorexia, which may persist for several weeks. These symptoms clear up when the characteristic cutaneous manifestations begin. Circumscribed patches of edema, usually on the abdomen, may last a few days and recur at different sites, depending on the path of the migrating worm. The edematous areas may be the size of a fist, slightly erythematous, and accompanied by pruritus, rash and stabbing pain. They may also produce lesions similar to those seen in cutaneous larva migrans. Ocular damage, blindness and cerebral involvement have been reported. An eosinophilia between 35 and 80 per cent is reported in patients with cutaneous involvement.

Presumptive diagnosis may be made on the basis of clinical symptoms and the patient's history in relation to food habits and residence. The differential diagnosis may include sparganosis, cutaneous paragonimiasis, cutaneous larva migrans, and myiasis. Definitive diagnosis rests on the recovery and identification of the worm. Nitidandhaprabas et al. (1975a,b) report cases in which worms have been found in the urine and sputum.

TREATMENT involves the surgical removal of the worms from subcutaneous or other accessible loci. Mebendazole, given at the rate of 200 mg. orally every 3 hours for 6 days, has been reported to give good results in skin and eye lesions. The infection is prevented by thorough cooking of food fishes. Consumption of pickled or marinated fish should be discouraged in endemic areas. For discussions of gnathostomiasis see Miyazaki (1966) and Chitanondh and Rosen (1967).

REFERENCES

Alicata, J. E., and Jindrak, K. 1970. *Angiostrongylosis in the Pacific and Southeast Asia*. 105 pp. Charles C Thomas, Springfield, Illinois.

Anderson, J., and Fuglsang, H. 1973. Topical diethylcarbamazine in ocular onchocerciasis. Trans. Roy. Soc. Trop. Med. & Hyg., 67:710–717.

Anderson, J., Fuglsang, H., Hamilton, P. J. S., and Marshall, T. F. deE. C. 1974a. Studies on onchocerciasis in the United Cameroon Republic. I. Comparison of populations with and without *Onchocerca volvulus*. Trans. Roy. Soc. Trop. Med. & Hyg., 68:190–208.

Anderson, J., Fuglsang, H., Hamilton, P. J. S., and Marshall, T. F. deE. C. 1974b. Studies on onchocerciasis in the United Cameroon Republic. II. Comparison of onchocerciasis in rain-forest and Sudan-savanna. Trans. Roy. Soc. Trop. Med. & Hyg., *68*:209–222.

Anderson, R. I., Fazen, L. E., and Buck, A. A. 1975a. Onchocerciasis in Guatemala. II. Microfilariae in urine, blood and sputum after diethylcarbamazine. Amer. J. Trop. Med. & Hyg., *24*:58–61.

Anderson, R. I., Fazen, L. E., and Buck, A. A. 1975b. Onchocerciasis in Guatemala. III. Daytime periodicity of microfilariae in skin. Amer. J. Trop. Med. & Hyg., *24*:62–65.

Antani, J. A., Srinivas, H. V., Krishnamurthy, K. R., and Borgaonkar, A. N. 1972. Metronidazole in dracunculiasis. Report of further trials. Amer. J. Trop. Med. & Hyg., *21*:178–181.

Ash, L. R. 1971. Preferential susceptibility of male jirds (*Meriones unguiculatus*) to infection with *Brugia pahangi*. J. Parasitol. *57*:777–780.

Beaver, P. C., and Orihel, T. C. 1965. Human infection with the filariae of animals in the United States. Amer. J. Trop. Med. & Hyg., *14*:1010–1029.

Beaver, P. C. 1970. Filariasis without microfilaremia. Amer. J. Trop. Med. & Hyg., *19*:181–189.

Beaver, P. C., Fallon, M., and Smith, G. H. 1971. Pulmonary nodule caused by a living *Brugia malayi*-like filaria in an artery. Amer. J. Trop. Med. & Hyg., *20*:661–666.

Beaver, P. C., and Cran, I. R. 1974. *Wuchereria*-like filaria in an artery, associated with pulmonary infarction. Amer. J. Trop. Med. & Hyg., *23*:869–876.

Beaver, P. C., Horner, G. S., and Bilos, J. Z. 1974. Zoonotic onchocerciasis in a resident of Illinois and observations on the identification of *Onchocerca* species. Amer. J. Trop. Med. & Hyg., *23*:595–607.

Chitanondh, H., and Rosen, L. 1967. Fatal eosinophilic encephalomyelitis caused by the nematode *Gnathostoma spinigerum*. Amer. J. Trop. Med. & Hyg., *16*:638–645.

Choyce, D.P. 1966. Onchocerciasis: Ophthalmic aspects. Trans. Roy. Soc. Trop. Med. & Hyg., *60*:720–726.

Danaraj, T. J., Pacheco, G., Shanmugaratnam, K., and Beaver, P. C. 1966. The etiology and pathology of eosinophilic lung (tropical eosinophilia). Amer. J. Trop. Med. & Hyg., *15*:183–189.

De Leon, R. J., and Duke, B. O. L. 1966. Experimental studies on the transmission of Guatemalan and West African strains of *Onchocerca volvulus* by *Simulium ochraceum, S. metallicum* and *S. callidum*. Trans. Roy. Soc. Trop. Med. & Hyg., *60*:735–752.

Desowitz, R. S., and Hitchcock, J. C. 1974. Hyperendemic bancroftian filariasis in the kingdom of Tonga: the application of the membrane filter concentration technique to an age-stratified blood survey. Amer. J. Trop. Med. & Hyg., *23*:877–879.

Duke, B. O. L. 1963. Studies on chemoprophylaxis of loiasis. II. Observations on diethylcarbamazine citrate (Banocide) as a prophylactic in man. Ann. Trop. Med. Parasit., *57*:82–96.

Fazen, L. E., Anderson, R. I., Figueroa Marriquin, H., Arthes, F. G., and Buck, A. A. 1975. Onchocerciasis in Guatemala. I. Epidemiological studies of microfilaruria. Amer. J. Trop. Med. & Hyg., *24*:52–57.

Fuglsang, H., and Anderson, J. 1974. Collapse during treatment of onchocerciasis with diethylcarbamazine. Trans. Roy. Soc. Trop. Med. & Hyg., *68*:72–73.

Goodman, M. L., and Gore, I. 1964. Pulmonary infarct secondary to Dirofilaria larva. Arch. Intern. Med., *113*:702–705.

Heather, C. J., and Price, E. W. 1972. Non-filarial elephantiasis in Ethiopia. Analytical study of inorganic material in lymph nodes. Trans. Roy. Soc. Trop. Med. & Hyg., *66*:450–458.

Hogan, M. J., Kimura, S. J., and Spencer, W. H. 1965. Visceral larva migrans and peripheral retinitis. J.A.M.A., *194*:1345–1347.

Joshi, V. V., Udwadia, F. E., and Gadgil, R. K. 1969. Etiology of tropical eosinophilia. A study of lung biopsies and review of published papers. Amer. J. Trop. Med. & Hyg., *18*:231–240.

Kale, O. O. 1975. Mebendazole in the treatment of dracontiasis. Amer. J. Trop. Med. & Hyg., *24*:600–605.

Kean, B. H., and Hoskins, D. W. 1964. Treatment of trichinosis with thiabendazole. A preliminary report. J.A.M.A., *190*:852–853.

Kennedy, F. B., and Rege, V. B. 1966. Trichinosis. Hemiplegia and liver involvement. Arch. Intern. Med., *117*:108–112.

Kessel, J. F. 1967. Diethylcarbamazine in filariasis control. Proceedings and papers of the 35th Annual Congress. California Mosquito Control Association, American Mosquito Control Association, pp. 17–22.

Khalil, H. M., Khattab, A. K., El-Fattah, S. M. A., Khalad, M. L., Awaad, S., and Rifaat, M. A. 1971. Interrelationships between poliomyelitis and *Toxocara* infection. Trans. Roy. Soc. Trop. Med. & Hyg., *65*:599–605.

Krupp, I. M. 1974. Hemagglutination test for the detection of antibodies specific for *Ascaris* and *Toxocara* antigens in patients with suspected visceral larva migrans. Amer. J. Trop. Med. & Hyg., *23*:378–384.

Lazar, M., Lieberman, T. W., and Leopold, I. H. 1970. Topical diethylcarbamazine in the treatment of ocular onchocerciasis. Amer. J. Trop. Med. & Hyg., *19*:232–233.

Manson-Bahr, P. E. C., and Wijers, D. J. B. 1972. The effect of a small dose of diethylcarbamazine on the circulation in the blood of microfilariae of *W. bancrofti*. Trans. Roy. Soc. Trop. Med. & Hyg., *66*:18.

Maynard, J. E., and Kagan, I. G. 1964. Intradermal test in the detection of trichinosis. Further observations on two outbreaks due to bear meat in Alaska. New Eng. J. Med., *270*:3–7.

McFadzean, J. A., and Hawking, F. 1956. The periodicity of microfilariae. V. Stimuli affecting the periodic migration of the microfilariae of *Wuchereria bancrofti* and of *Loa loa* in man. Trans. Roy. Soc. Trop. Med. & Hyg., *50*:543–562.

Meyers, W. M., Connor, D. H., Harman, L. E., Fleshman, K., Moris, R., and Neafie, R. C. 1972. Human streptocerciasis. A clinico-pathologic study of 40 Africans (Zairians) including identification of the adult filaria. Amer. J. Trop. Med. & Hyg., *21*:528–545.

Mitra, A. K., and Haddock, D. R. W. 1970. Paraplegia due to guinea-worm infection. Trans. Roy. Soc. Trop. Med. & Hyg., *64*:102–106.

Miyazaki, J. 1966. *Gnathostoma* and gnathostomiasis in Japan. Progress of medical parasitology in Japan. Meguro Parasitological Museum. Vol. 3. pp. 531–586.

Morera, P., and Céspedes, R. 1971. *Angiostrongylus costaricensis* n. sp. (Nematoda: Metastrongyloidea), a new lungworm occurring in man in Costa Rica. Rev. Biol. Trop., *18*:173–185.

Morera, P. 1973. Life history and redescription of *Angiostrongylus costaricensis* Morera and Céspedes, 1971. Amer. J. Trop. Med. & Hyg., *22*:613–621.

Neafie, R. C., Connor, D. H., and Meyers, W. M. 1975. *Dipetalonema streptocerca* (Macfie and Corson, 1922): description of the adult female. Amer. J. Trop. Med. & Hyg., *24*:264–267.

Nelson, G. S. 1970. Onchocerciasis. *In*: Dawes, B. (Ed.) *Advances in Parasitology*. Vol. 8. pp. 173–224. Academic Press, New York.

Nitidandhaprabas, P., Sirikarra, A., Harnsomburana, K., and Thepsitthar, P. 1975a. Human urinary gnathostomiasis: a case report from Thailand. Amer. J. Trop. Med. & Hyg., *24*:49–51.

Nitidandhaprabas, P., Handchansin, S., and Vongsloesvidhya, Y. 1975b. A case of expectoration of *Gnathostoma spinigerum* in Thailand. Amer. J. Trop. Med. & Hyg., *24*:547–548.

Orihel, T. C., and Lowrie, R. C. 1975. *Loa loa:* development to the infective stage in an American deerfly, *Chrysops atlanticus*. Amer. J. Trop. Med. & Hyg., *24*:610–615.

Price, E. W. 1972. The pathology of non-filarial elephantiasis of the lower legs. Trans. Roy. Soc. Trop. Med. & Hyg., *66*:150–159.

Price, E. W. 1974. Endemic elephantiasis of lower legs—natural history and clinical study. Trans. Roy. Soc. Trop. Med. & Hyg., *68*:44–52.

Price, E. W. 1975. The mechanism of lymphatic obstruction in endemic elephantiasis of the lower legs. Trans. Roy. Soc. Trop. Med. & Hyg., *69*:177–179.

Reinhard, M. C., Jr. 1961. Calcified guinea worm simulating intrapulmonary calcification. J.A.M.A., *175*:53–55.

Rosen, L., Chappell, R., Laqueur, G. L., Wallace, G. D., and Weinstein, P. P. 1962. Eosinophilic meningoencephalitis caused by a metastrongylid lungworm of rats. J.A.M.A., *179*:620–624.

Rosen, L., Loison, G., Laigret, J., and Wallace, G. D. 1967. Studies on eosinophilic meningitis. 3. Epidemiologic and clinical observations on Pacific islands and the possible etiologic role of *Angiostrongylus cantonensis*. Amer. J. Epidem., *85*:17–44.

Ruitenberg, E. J., and Steerenberg, P. A. 1974. Intestinal phase of *Trichinella spiralis* in congenitally athymic (nude) mice. J. Parasitol., *60*:1056–1057.

Spear, H. C., Daughtry, D. C., Chesney, J. G., Gentsch, T. O., and Larsen, P. B. 1968. Solitary pulmonary lesion due to *Dirofilaria*. New Eng. J. Med., *278*:832–833.

Tannehill, A. W., Jr., and Hatch, H. B., Jr. 1968. Coin lesions of the lung due to *Dirofilaria immitis*. Report of a case. Dis. Chest., *53*:369–371.

Trapido, H., D'Alessandro, A., and Little, M. D. 1971. Onchocerciasis in Colombia. Historical background and ecologic observations. Amer. J. Trop. Med. & Hyg., *20*:104–108.

Wiseman, R. A., and Woodruff, A. W. 1970. Evaluation of a skin sensitivity test for the diagnosis of toxocariasis. Trans. Roy. Soc. Trop. Med. & Hyg., *64*:239–245.

Woodruff, A. W., Choyce, D. P., Muci-Mendoza, F., Hills, M., and Petit, L. E. 1966. Onchocerciasis in Guatemala. A clinical and parasitological study with comparisons between the disease there and in East Africa. Trans. Roy. Soc. Trop. Med. & Hyg., *60*:707–719.

Woodruff, A. W. 1970. Toxocariasis. Brit. Med. J., *3*:663–669.

Yoshimura, H., and Yokogawa, M. 1970. *Dirofilaria* causing infarct in human lung. Amer. J. Trop. Med. & Hyg., *19*:63–67.

Zimmermann, W. J., Steele, J. H., and Kagan, I. G. 1973. Trichiniasis in the U.S. population, 1966–70. Health Services Rep., *88*:606–623.

12
Arthropods and Human Disease

Arthropods are as intimately associated with man's welfare as are any animals. The economic importance of this group to agriculture, in terms both of beneficial and of destructive effects, can hardly be over-emphasized. In addition, many species have a direct relationship to human health and well-being. It is not our purpose to consider this in detail, but we will discuss a few of the more important roles assumed by arthropods in their relation to disease in man. The majority of arthropods function indirectly in human disease, which they transmit but do not produce; some species are true parasites while others may inflict direct injury by their bites, stings or other activities. Some species are both parasites and vectors of disease. For the purposes of discussion one may conveniently divide the arthropods of medical importance into two groups, those which are true parasites and all others which in different ways affect health or well-being.

ARTHROPODS AS PARASITES

The Itch Mite

Sarcoptes scabiei

The itch mite, *Sarcoptes scabiei* (Fig. 145), is cosmopolitan in distribution, and thoroughly democratic in its choice of victims. It parasitizes both domestic animals and man, causing a disease known as scabies in man and mange in animals. The female mite is larger than the male,

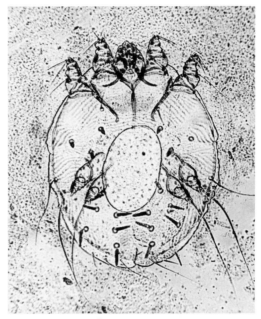

FIGURE 145. *Sarcoptes scabiei,* adult female. (Photomicrograph by Zane Price.)

and measures a little less than 0.5 mm. in length. The adult mites enter the skin, digging sinuous burrows in the upper layers of the epidermis. Eggs (Fig. 146) deposited in the burrows hatch after three or four days into larvae, which excavate new burrows and mature in about four

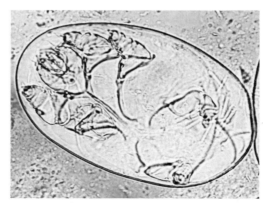

FIGURE 146. *Sarcoptes scabiei* egg, containing fully developed larva. (Photomicrograph by Zane Price.)

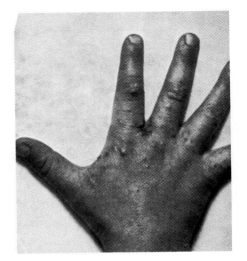

FIGURE 147. Scabies lesions on hand. (Courtesy of Dr. Hamnett A. Dixon.)

days. Preferred sites of infestation are the interdigital (Fig. 147) and popliteal folds, the groin and the inframammary folds. Many other parts of the body may also be involved. The activites and secretions of the mites cause intense itching of the affected areas. Very small vesicles may be seen on the skin surface. Scratching may result in bleeding and scab formation, frequently followed by secondary bacterial infection. Transmission of the mites is accomplished by direct contact with infected persons or with their clothing or bedding. Spread of the infection to different parts of the body occurs through scratching and manual transfer of the mite by the afflicted individual. The infection may also be acquired from infected domestic animals but there appear to be different strains of the mite, having distinct host preferences, so that an infection acquired from domestic animals is usually of short duration in man.

While infection with *Sarcoptes scabiei* may end spontaneously after a few months, chronic cases do occur; in such cases the parasites are less numerous and consequently more difficult to find. The only way in which a definitive diagnosis of scabies can be made is by finding the parasites or their eggs. Because of their location under the surface of the skin, scrapings must be made of the infected areas. Before scrapings are made it is best to examine the skin surface with a hand lens so as to find the minute burrows of the mite. While eggs may be found in any portion of a recent excavation, the adult mite is most frequently recovered from the terminal parts of a fresh burrow. It is therefore best to make scrapings in these regions. The material obtained in this fashion is placed on a microscope slide, cleared by adding one or two drops of a 20 per cent solution of potassium hydroxide, covered with a coverslip, and examined under the low power of the microscope. Rarely one may see very severe atypical infections. The parasites are not found in burrows but rather under adherent crusts. Patients do not complain of itching. These severe infections are often associated with unsanitary conditions and mental dullness (Kurtin and Leider, 1968). For detailed accounts of scabies and other mite infestations see Heilesen (1946) and Baker et al. (1956).

TREATMENT. Infestation with the itch mite can be eradicated by use of 1 per cent gamma benzene hexachloride in a lotion base. The medication should be applied in the evening after the lesions have been cleaned and softened by soaking in warm water and should be left on overnight. One or two additional applications, at weekly intervals, may be necessary to kill those mites which hatch subsequent to the initial treatment.

Lice

Pediculus humanus

The human body or head louse (Fig. 148) is found wherever personal or general hygiene is at a low level. Lice are dorsoventrally

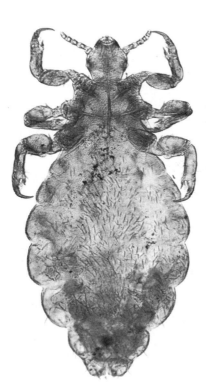

FIGURE 148. Pediculus humanus. (Photomicrograph by Zane Price.)

flattened insects, sufficiently large to be detected easily with the naked eye. Males are about 2 mm., females 3 mm. long. The whole life cycle occurs on the human host. Two sub-species, or biological races, are commonly recognized. *Pediculus humanus capitis* infests the scalp. The female lice deposit their eggs on the hairs where they are firmly attached. The eggs or nits are quite small and glistening white, and may be seen with the naked eye. About ten days after deposition, they hatch into nymphs which are structurally quite similar to the adults and mature in about two weeks. Both larvae and adults feed on blood obtained by their piercing mouth parts and a pumping device located in the pharyngeal region.

The body louse, *P. humanus humanus* (frequently called *P. humanus corporis*), lives on the protected parts of the body. Its life history is similar to that of the head louse which it closely resembles in appearance. While distinct habitat preferences characterize these two varieties, the lice may be found on other parts, particularly in cases of heavy infestation. When searching for body lice it is best to examine the clothing rather than the skin surface since the lice will remain on clothing when the latter is removed or discarded.

Head or body lice are transferred from one person to the next by direct contact or by contact with clothing, hats, or hairs from "lousy" individuals. The body louse may survive for more than a week in discarded clothing. Cloth-covered seats in theaters, railway carriages and other public places may be a source of infestation. Lice are quite sensitive to high environmental temperatures and will leave if their host has a fever. The importance of this in relation to the transmission of louse-borne diseases, listed in Table 7, is obvious.

TREATMENT. Benzene hexachloride is effective in treatment of head louse infestation. The hair is first thoroughly washed with soap, rinsed, and excess water is removed. One ounce or more of the benzene hexachloride lotion is then applied to the hair and thoroughly worked into the scalp. It is left on overnight; the hair is then washed and combed to remove loosened nits. A second application one week later will kill any lice which have hatched in the interim.

The nits of body lice will be destroyed if gamma benzene hexachloride lotion is applied to the entire body and allowed to remain for 24 hours. The adult lice, found in the clothing, may be killed by dusting with a 10 per cent benzene hexachloride (Lindane) powder or by heat. Lindane powder can be used for dusting in mass treatment programs and can be applied beneath the clothing.

Phthirus pubis

The pubic or crab louse (Fig. 149) usually is found on the hairs of the genital region, but may occur elsewhere on the body. *Phthirus* is

Text continued on page 313

Table 7. Some Important Diseases Transmitted by Arthropods

Arthropod Group	Disease	Vector or Intermediate Host	Vertebrate Reservoir of Disease**	Disease Distribution
Crustacea				
Copepods	Diphyllobothriasis	*Cyclops* spp.	Dog, bear	Scandinavia, northern United States, Finland, Russia
	Dracunculosis	*Cyclops* spp.	Carnivores probably	Africa, India, Middle East
Crabs, crayfish	Paragonimiasis	Fresh-water crabs, crayfish	Carnivores?	Asia, Africa, Philippines, Pacific Islands, South America
Arachnida				
Mites	Scrub typhus (Tsutsugamushi disease)	*Trombicula* spp.	Rodents	Far East, Southwest Pacific, Philippines
	Rickettsialpox	*Allodermanyssus*	Mice	United States
Ticks	Tularemia	*Dermacentor* spp.	Rabbits	North America, Europe, Japan
	Rocky Mountain spotted fever	*Dermacentor* spp. and other ixodid ticks	None	Canada, United States, Central and South America
	Q-fever	*Dermacentor*, *Boophilus*	Cattle, sheep, goats, bandicoot	Probably world-wide
	Colorado tick fever	*Dermacentor*	Wild rodents, porcupine	Western United States
	Tick-borne viral encephalitis	*Ixodes*	Various mammals and birds	Northern Europe and Asia
	Relapsing fever	*Ornithodorus*	Monkeys, squirrels, rats	Africa, Asia, America, Europe

Insecta				
Lice	Epidemic typhus	*Pediculus humanus*	None	Europe, Asia, Africa, Central America, United States
	Trench fever	*Pediculus humanus*	None	Central Europe
	Louse-borne relapsing fever	*Pediculus humanus*	None	Europe, Asia, Africa
Fleas	Plague	*Xenopsylla cheopis*, other rodent fleas	Rodents	World-wide
	Murine typhus	*Xenopsylla cheopis*	Rats and other rodents	Tropics and subtropics
	Dipylidiasis	Cat and dog fleas	Cats, dogs	World-wide
Bugs	Chagas' disease (South American trypanosomiasis)	*Triatoma, Panstrongylus*	Carnivores, rodents, armadillo	South America, Central America, North America
Beetles	Hymenolepiasis	Flour beetle*	Mice, rats	World-wide
Flies, gnats	African sleeping sickness	*Glossina* spp. (tsetse flies)	Herbivores?	Africa
	Onchocerciasis	*Simulium* spp. (Black flies)	None	Africa, Mexico, Central and South America
	Tularemia	*Chrysops* (Deer flies)	Rabbits	North America, Europe, Japan
	Loiasis	*Chrysops* spp.	Monkeys	Tropical Africa
	Leishmaniasis (all kinds)	*Phlebotomus* spp. (Sandfly)	Dogs and cats in various areas	Asia, Mediterranean, East Africa, southern Mexico, Central and South America
	Bartonellosis (Verruga peruana)	*Phlebotomus* spp. (Sandfly)	?	Peru, Colombia, Ecuador (1700–10,000 feet)

Table 7 *continued on the following page.*

Table 7. Some Important Diseases Transmitted by Arthropods (Continued)

Mosquitoes	Malaria	*Anopheles* spp.	None	World-wide
	Yellow fever	*Aedes aegypti**	Monkeys	Africa, Central and South America
	Dengue fever	*Aedes* spp.	?	Tropics and subtropics
	Western equine ⎫ encephalomyelitis	*Culex* spp.	Birds, horses	United States, southern Canada, Argentina
	Venezuelan equine ⎪	" "	Rodents, horses	Southern U.S., Central & South America
	St. Louis ⎬	*Culex* spp.	Birds, horses	United States
	Eastern equine ⎪	*Aedes* and *Mansonia* spp.	Birds, horses	United States, Canada, West Indies, Central America
	Japanese B ⎭	*Culex* spp.	Birds, domestic animals	Far East
	Filariasis, bancroftian	*Culex, Aedes, Anopheles*	?	Tropical Africa, South Pacific, Australia, Asia
	Filariasis, malayan	*Anopheles, Mansonia*	Monkeys? Cats?	India, Malaysia

*Important but not only vector
**Other than man

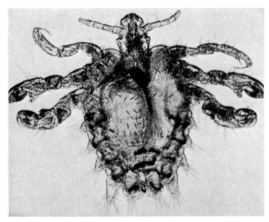

FIGURE 149. *Phthirus pubis.* (Courtesy of Army Medical Museum.)

somewhat shorter and broader than *Pediculus,* measuring up to 2 mm. in length. It possesses powerful legs, especially adapted to attachment to the hair, on which the eggs are laid. The entire life is spent on the host, and the life cycle is completed in from thirty to forty days. Transmission is by contact with infested individuals or their clothing. While the head louse moves about rapidly, the pubic louse is much more sedentary in its habits.

TREATMENT. Treatment consists of application of benzene hexachloride lotion as in the treatment of head louse infestation; it is to be remembered that the crab louse may infest not only the pubic area, but any hairy part of the body, especially the axillae and eyebrows.

Infestation with lice is usually referred to as pediculosis. Some people are very sensitive to the bites, which produce macular swellings and a great deal of pruritus. In person who have had lice for long periods the skin may become thickened, and show spots of hyperpigmentation, the maculae caeruleae. These skin changes have been referred to as vagabond's disease. Body lice are important vectors of disease, transmitting epidemic typhus, trench fever, and the louseborne variety of relapsing fever. The role of head lice in this regard is apparently negligible, while the pubic louse has not been incriminated in disease transmission.

Myiasis

Myiasis, or infestation with fly larvae, is commonly seen in domestic and wild mammals all over the world. In man, myiasis is of relatively frequent occurrence in rural regions where people are in close contact with domestic animals. Many different species of flies produce myiasis. While some of them require a host for larval development, many are opportunists only, being able to develop in living animals if occasion presents itself. Infection with fly larvae may occur when flies deposit eggs or first-stage larvae on the body or its apertures. The portions of the body affected will vary with the habits and preferences of the species of fly, and may depend also on other factors. An open wound or lesion, for example, may attract certain flies which will then deposit their eggs or larvae in the area of injury. They will develop and grow, thus establishing an infection. Larvae of certain other species invade the unbroken skin. Some will gain access to the body via the nose or ears. If eggs are deposited on the lips, within the mouth or on food, they may be swallowed and develop in the stomach or intestine, giving rise to gastric or intestinal myiasis. Genitourinary myiasis may occur when certain flies have the opportunity to oviposit on the genitourinary apertures.

In view of the large number of different myiasis-producing flies and because of the diversity in life cycle requirements, it seems best to discuss the more important species only, emphasizing their host-relations and sites of predilection rather than their taxonomic affinities. One may conveniently assign the various species to three groups or categories: The first of these, the so-called specific group, includes species which require a host for completion of larval development; the second or semi-specific group includes those species which will develop in a host if entry is facilitated by the presence of wounds or sores but which can complete development without a host. The third category includes accidental invaders which usually complete larval development without a host but may in rare instances develop in one.

Specific Myiasis

Flies which require a host for the development of their larval stages belong to a large number of different species which habitually parasitize animals. Important among them are the various botflies, including the human bot, *Dermatobia hominis,* found in humid areas of Mexico and Central and South America. The adult fly may deposit eggs on the abdomen of bloodsucking flies or mosquitoes which in turn distribute these eggs while getting a blood meal from an animal or from man. Upon deposition, the eggs hatch and the young larvae bore through the skin. As the larva grows, a lesion develops (Fig. 150) which may be quite painful. Between forty and fifty days elapse from the time of entry to full growth. The larva then leaves the host to pupate. Several other insects as well as ticks have been shown to carry eggs of *D. hominis* and to transport them to man or domestic animals.

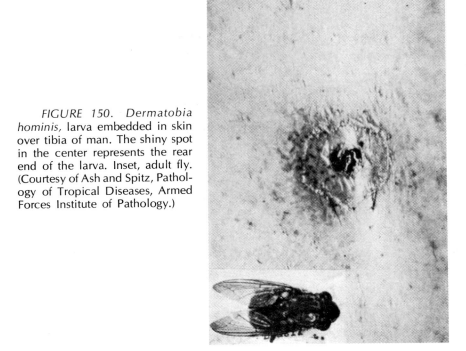

FIGURE 150. *Dermatobia hominis*, larva embedded in skin over tibia of man. The shiny spot in the center represents the rear end of the larva. Inset, adult fly. (Courtesy of Ash and Spitz, Pathology of Tropical Diseases, Armed Forces Institute of Pathology.)

Another important species is the sheep botfly, *Oestrus ovis*. Worldwide in distribution, it is prevalent in sheep-raising areas. The fly deposits living larvae in the nostrils or on the eyes of sheep and goats; and in man they may develop in the conjunctival sac, producing ophthalmomyiasis. Larval development in the host requires several months.

Species of *Hypoderma*, the cattle botflies or ox warbles, are also world-wide in distribution. Eggs are deposited on the skin and hatch into larvae which, after having penetrated the skin, migrate throughout the body. Eventually they come to lie beneath the skin, producing a local swelling.

Horses also have botflies, which belong to the genus *Gasterophilus*. The fly deposits eggs on the hair, skin or lips. After hatching, the larvae either penetrate the skin or are swallowed. In animals these larvae normally develop in the intestinal tract; in man they more frequently wander beneath the skin where they give rise to lesions similar to those produced by migration of the larvae of dog hookworms.

Some other forms producing specific myiasis are the screw worm flies. Of these, *Callitroga* (*Cochliomyia*) *americana* is prevalent in the

Western Hemisphere. This fly normally parasitizes animals, depositing eggs on the unbroken skin, on the nose and ears or on wounds. The larvae are able to burrow deeply into healthy tissue and may even penetrate bone. Infection with this species is dangerous because of the vigorous activity of the larvae, which may enter the middle ear, nasal sinuses or brain of man. Larval development is usually completed within ten days. Premature death of the host does not necessarily interrupt larval development which may proceed within the dead body of the host.

One of the most interesting although medically not nearly as important species is *Auchmeromyia luteola* of tropical Africa, known as the Congo floor maggot. The adult fly lays her eggs on sand or on the floor of native huts. The larvae become active at night, crawling about in search of food. If they come upon an animal or person sleeping on the ground they will suck blood, and after the blood meal detach and hide in the soil until another meal is needed. While blood meals are necessary for the development of these larvae, their procurement seems more a predatory than a parasitic activity.

Semi-specific Myiasis

Among the flies which cause what is known as semi-specific myiasis are some species which normally lay their eggs in decaying animal or vegetable matter. Prominent representatives of this group are species of *Phaenicia (Lacilia)*, the green-bottle flies, *Callitroga* or blue-bottle flies, and black-bottles belonging to the genus *Phormia*. All of these are world-wide in distribution, frequenting areas of human habitation. They occasionally will lay their eggs on open sores of animals or man, especially if necrotic and malodorous. Large numbers of these flies congregate near slaughterhouses and other unclean places.

Another group which causes intestinal and other types of myiasis in man is the flesh flies or sarcophagids. Species of *Sarcophaga* are world-wide in distribution. They normally breed in carrion or other decomposing matter and may deposit their eggs on various foods such as meat or fruit. Thus, ingestion of contaminated food may be a source of infection.

Accidental Myiasis

Flies producing accidental myiasis have no requirement or even preference for development in a host. However, eggs may be deposited accidentally on oral or genitourinary openings and the larvae gain

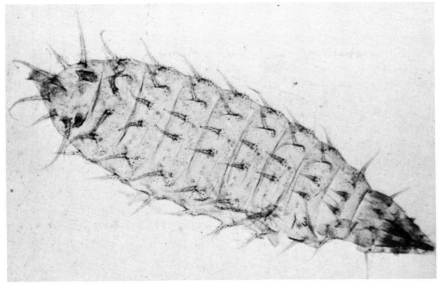

FIGURE 151. Larva of Fannia, a latrine fly.

entrance to the intestinal or genitourinary tract. The housefly, *Musca domestica, Fannia* or latrine flies (Fig. 151), certain species of flesh flies, green- or blue-bottle flies and many others may produce accidental myiasis.

One of the more striking species, *Tubifera tenax,* usually deposits eggs in manure, in rotting animal matter, or about privies. The larvae, known as rat-tailed maggots, have a long, slender tail and by their peculiar appearance frequently attract attention. Human cases of intestinal and other types of myiasis due to this fly are on record. However, the presence of rat-tailed maggots in stool specimens may also be the result of contamination after the specimen has been passed.

Diagnosis of Myiasis

In view of the different types of myiasis caused by many diverse species of flies it is impractical to present an adequate description of all the signs and symptoms of human infection. The clinical aspects of myiasis will vary with the regions affected, with the species of fly involved and with the numbers of maggots present. The possibility of maggot infection or infestation is frequently overlooked. The symptoms of intestinal myiasis are not specific, and neither are those of urinary myiasis. Cutaneous myiasis should be suspected in a patient with painful, indolent ulcers or furuncle-like sores of long standing. In addition, certain botfly larvae may give rise to dermal lesions similar to those of creeping eruption.

Nasal myiasis will often cause obstruction of the nasal passages, severe irritation and in some cases facial edema and fever. Fatal termination is not uncommon. Equally dangerous is aural myiasis in which the patient may complain of crawling sensations and buzzing noises. A foul-smelling, purulent discharge may be present. If located in the middle ear, the larvae may find their way into the brain. Ophthalmo-myiasis is not uncommon and is accompanied by severe irritation and pain.

A definitive diagnosis of myiasis can be made only upon finding the larvae, which should be removed and kept for identification. If live maggots are obtained, they should be placed on a dish of raw meat in a glass jar containing moist sand to a height of 5 cm. or more. The jar is

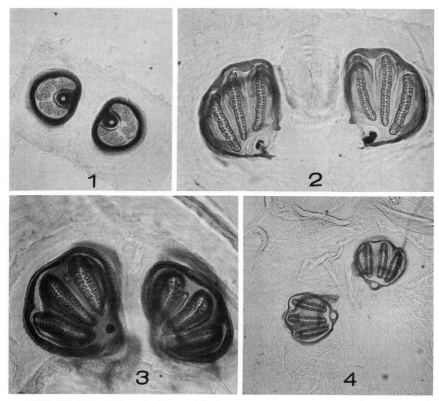

FIGURE 152. Stigmal plates of fly larvae. 1. *Musca;* 2. *Sarcophaga;* 3. *Cochliomyia;* 4. *Phaenicia.* (Photographs from material furnished by Dr. Ralph Barr.)

then tightly plugged with cotton and allowed to stand at room temperature. The maggots will burrow into the meat and remain there for some time, depending on their stage of development. They will eventually leave the meat and enter the sand in order to pupate. At this time, the meat should be removed and the jar examined periodically for the presence of emerged flies. A good substitute, usually available in a hospital laboratory, is a Petri dish containing blood agar in which maggots seem to thrive. Precise specific identification necessitates examination of the adult fly and, as a rule, cannot be made on larvae alone. Familial, and in some cases, generic determination can be accomplished on the basis of larval morphology. Important differential characters are provided by a pair of dark colored chitinous plates situated at the posterior end of the larva. These are the stigmal plates (Fig. 152) which contain the respiratory apertures or spiracles, arranged in a pattern characteristic for the different groups of flies. If stigmal plates are to be examined, they must be cut off with a sharp scalpel or razor blade, placed on a slide, and their structure observed under the microscope. While a good deal of information can thus be obtained by relatively inexperienced workers, it is always desirable to refer specimens of larvae or even adult flies to an experienced entomologist for identification.

The Use of Maggots in Medicine

A discussion of myiasis should not fail to include mention of the medicinal use of fly maggots. During World War I it was noted that maggot-infested wounds healed more readily than others. This was explained by the fact that maggots consumed devitalized tissues, in this manner perhaps reducing bacterial activity and the chance of secondary infection. Blowfly maggots were used frequently for the debridement of deep wounds in soldiers, and after the war for similar purposes in civilian practice. Eventually, flies were reared under sterile conditions and used in the treatment of chronic osteomyelitis.

The Chigoe Flea

Tunga penetrans

The chigoe flea, *Tunga penetrans* (Fig. 153), parasitizes many different kinds of warm-blooded animals including man. It is found in tropical and subtropical regions of America, as well as Africa and the Far East where it has been introduced from the New World. Chigoe fleas are relatively small, measuring no more than 1 mm. in length. While the males and virgin females behave in the usual manner of

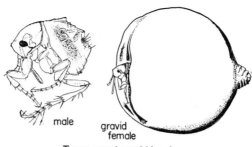

male   gravid
female

Tunga penetrans (chigoe)

W.L. Brudon '44

FIGURE 153.   *Tunga penetrans,* male and female. (Courtesy of Hunter, G. W., Swartzwelder, J. C., and Clyde, D. F. 1976. Tropical Medicine. 5th Ed. W. B. Saunders Company, Philadelphia.)

fleas, the fertilized female has the distressing habit of burrowing into the skin, preferably under the toe nails (Fig. 154) or between the toes, where she feeds on blood. As the eggs develop, the embedded female becomes progressively larger until the abdomen assumes a nearly spherical shape. At this time, a part of the abdomen is seen to protrude slightly beyond the skin surface. Mature eggs, sometimes as many as

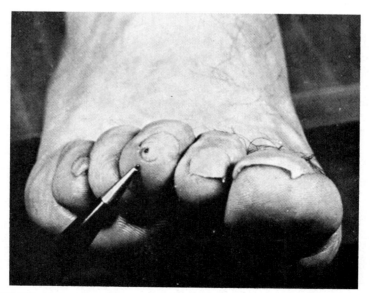

FIGURE 154.   The chigoe flea, *Tunga penetrans,* embedded in skin below nail. (Courtesy of Dr. T. H. G. Aitken.)

one hundred, are expelled to the outside and continue their development in the soil. The female eventually drops out of the host.

Infection with chigoe fleas is extremely irritating and usually produces inflammation and ulceration, the latter primarily due to development of secondary infection. Diagnosis is made by detecting the dark portion of the abdomen of the flea on the skin surface. Surgical removal of the flea is indicated.

ARTHROPODS AND DISEASE TRANSMISSION

Arthropods are of great importance as transmitters of disease-producing agents to man and other animals. Disease transmission can be accomplished in two general ways. It may be mechanical, which means that the arthropod carries an infectious organism from one person or object to the next without serving as a host for the development or multiplication of this organism. Transmission may also be biological, in which case the infectious organism develops or multiplies within the arthropod host, and is only then transmitted to the vertebrate host. Table 7 lists some of the arthropods of importance in disease transmission. The role of arthropods in transmission of viruses is discussed by Taylor (1967); a bibliography of ticks and the diseases they transmit was published by Hoogstraal (1970–1972).

Among those diseases which may be transmitted in a mechanical manner are the bacterial enteritides. Enteric organisms may be carried by flies feeding on fecal material to foods destined for human consumption. Pathogenic bacteria may be found on the mouth parts, legs or intestinal contents of flies feeding on excreta; it is possible that some protozoan cysts may be carried in a like manner. Flies have long been thought to play a role in the mechanical transmission of those viral diseases in which the organisms are passed in the feces. Certain gnats are mechanical vectors of yaws, and it is possible that trachoma is also spread from person to person in this manner.

Some infectious organisms require an arthropod host for completion of their life cycle, and also utilize this host as a vector. Most arthropod-borne diseases are carried in this fashion, reaching the vertebrate host through the agency of the bite of the vector. As examples may be mentioned malaria and filariasis. An arthropod may serve as intermediate host for an organism which is acquired by the vertebrate host when that host ingests the infected arthropod. Direct ingestion of the invertebrate host takes place in the life cycle of *Dracunculus medinensis;* in *Diphyllobothrium* infections the arthropod host is ingested by a vertebrate second intermediate host, which in turn is eaten to pass the infection to man or another definitive host.

HARMFUL EFFECTS OF ARTHROPODS

Stings and Bites

A discussion of arthropods in relation to disease would not be complete without mention of their obvious and annoying activities of stinging and biting. The bites of fleas, mosquitoes, bedbugs, and the like, while always irritating, do not affect every person in the same manner. Some people do not suffer any appreciable harm; others react very strongly to the bites of certain arthropods, exhibiting various allergic manifestations and generalized as well as local effects (Frazier, 1969). It is common knowledge that some individuals will not be unduly affected by flea bites but may be very sensitive to the bites of mosquitoes, for example. Conversely, insects of a given kind seem to prefer certain individuals to others. In general, it may be said that the reaction to bites and to stings of certain arthropods will vary with the species of arthropod and with each individual person. Insects such as bees, for instance, while inflicting a painful sting may not produce any further damage. However, in a person sensitized to bee venom, bee stings may have serious consequences and may even lead to death. It is of interest that bee stings were once used in the treatment of arthritis; the beneficial effects ascribed to this form of therapy may possibly have been due to increased secretion of steroid hormones.

The sting of certain species of scorpions, the bites of centipedes, and of spiders such as *Latrodectus mactans*, the black widow, may be quite dangerous (Dreisbach, 1974; Horen, 1972). The reaction to these stings and bites will vary with the amount of venom injected, and with the body size and general health of the afflicted individual. While a healthy adult will usually recover, small children or weakened individuals will suffer considerably and may die if proper care is not instituted immediately.

TREATMENT. Hospitalization is advisable for known or suspected black widow spider bites. Muscle spasms may be severe and may require the intravenous administration of calcium gluconate or other muscle relaxant agents. A specific antivenin is available and is valuable if given early. It is prepared from the serum of hyperimmunized horses, and patients must be tested for horse-serum sensitivity before use.

Necrotic arachnidism

The bites of certain spiders may cause the appearance of necrotizing skin lesions of varying extent and severity, depending on the species involved. Most important are spiders of the genus *Loxosceles*,

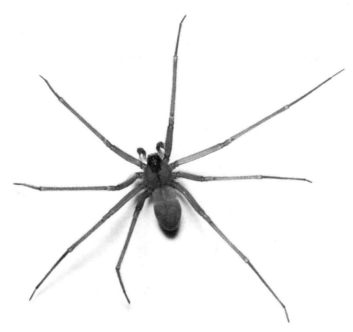

FIGURE 155. Violin spider (*Loxosceles sp.*); actual body length excluding legs is about 7 mm. (Courtesy of Dr. Findlay E. Russell, University of Southern California.)

commonly known as the brown spider and violin spider (Fig. 155). They are found in South and Central America, and several species occur in the United States. The spiders have relatively long legs and a brown body 5 to 10 mm. long (Russell et al., 1969); some species have a fiddle.shaped marking on the dorsal side. They are found under lumber or under rocks and also near or inside human dwellings.

While the bite is fairly painless, mild to severe pain develops within a few hours, accompanied by erythema, vesicle formation, and itching at the site. This is frequently followed by chills, headache and nausea. The bite of *Loxosceles laetae* may result in kidney damage and death. The initial lesion ulcerates (Fig. 156), becomes necrotic and, unless promptly treated, does not heal but continues to spread for weeks or months. It is very important that treatment be initiated as soon as possible after the bite.

TREATMENT. The prompt systemic administration of corticosteroids may prevent the development of local necrosis and of systemic reactions. Surgical excision of the lesion and at times skin grafting is required in neglected cases. For case histories, treatment, and illustrations of lesions see Russell et al. (1969).

A report by Spielman and Levi (1970) indicates that bites of the

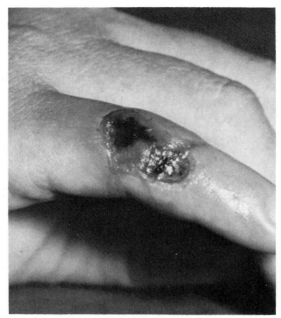

FIGURE 156. Local necrosis of finger following the bite of the brown recluse spider, *Loxosceles reclusa.* (Courtesy of Hunter, G. W., Swartzwelder, J. C., and Clyde, D. F. 1976. Tropical Medicine. 5th Ed. W. B. Saunders Company, Philadelphia.)

spider *Chiracanthium mildei,* commonly found in houses, also may produce necrotizing, painful lesions which, however, heal within a few weeks, are far less extensive than those caused by the brown spider, and are not accompanied by systemic manifestations.

It should be emphasized that the incrimination of a species of spider is not possible from the appearance of the lesion alone; the spider must be identified and, in the absence of a specimen, a description should be obtained from the patient as soon as possible.

Tick Paralysis

A condition known as tick paralysis may be induced by the bite of certain ticks. Tick paralysis has been observed in dogs, sheep and human beings in the United States and elsewhere. In North America, the occurrence of this disease coincides with the distribution of the tick *Dermacentor andersoni,* although other species have been incriminated as well. If the tick lodges in the occipital (or other) region of man or animal to obtain a blood meal, an acute ascending paralysis which can terminate in death may ensue. Prompt removal of the engorging tick will usually prevent progression of the paralysis, and recovery will take place in a few days. As far as is known, only the engorging adult female tick will cause tick paralysis. The etiological mechanism of this paralysis is entirely unknown.

Lepidopterism and Erucism

The hairs of some butterflies and moths are associated with cells or glands which secrete substances causing severe dermatitis when the hairs are deposited on the skin. Intense itching shortly after contact is followed by papule formation, swelling and induration. In South America, lepidopterism may occur in epidemic form during the time of year when large numbers of moths are airborne.

Erucism is caused by contact with the poison hairs of different kinds of caterpillars (Fig. 157). Erythema and swelling is accompanied by burning and itching, and occasionally by nausea and fever. Usually, these symptoms disappear after twenty-four hours, but the lesions may persist for several days.

Fire Ant

Fire ants are numerous in the Southeastern United States. Their stings are painful and result in flares and wheals of an inch or more in diameter, followed by the formation of fluid-filled vesicles which may

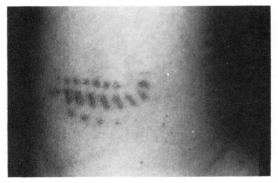

FIGURE 157.   Lesions on arm from contact with puss caterpillar. (Courtesy of Hunter, G. W., Swartzwelder, J. C., and Clyde, D. F. 1976. Tropical Medicine. 5th Ed. W. B. Saunders Company, Philadelphia.)

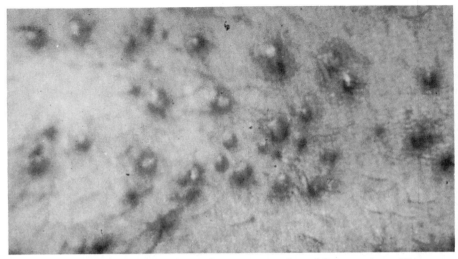

FIGURE 158. Clusters of pustules on arm at sites of fire ant stings. (Courtesy of Hunter, G. W., Swartzwelder, J. C., and Clyde, D. F. 1976. Tropical Medicine. 5th Ed. W. B. Saunders Company, Philadelphia.)

become purulent after twenty-four hours (Fig. 158). A necrotizing toxin, solenamine, has been identified as the probable active substance of fire ant venom. The skin response was studied by Jung et al. (1963). Systemic reactions to the stings may include fever, urticaria and localized edema.

Entomophobia

Fear of insects carried to a pathological degree is sometimes seen. Mentally disturbed patients will sometimes report insect infestation to their physicians, describing the presence of minute insects on or in the skin, which give rise to biting or crawling sensations. The skin may be extensively excoriated by the continuous scratching of these patients, who can usually be benefited only by proper psychiatric treatment.

Spanish Fly and Other Beetles

Among the many arthropods of interest from a medical point of view must be mentioned *Lytta vesicatoria*, the Spanish fly. This renowned insect is actually not a fly, but a beetle. It occurs in some abundance in Spain and southern France, where it is collected to be killed and ground into a powder, known as cantharidin. Cantharidin is highly irritant, producing blisters when applied to the skin. Its aphrodisiac properties have long been known, and exaggerated; they depend upon similar irritation of the genital tract.

Many other beetles may release fluids which cause mild to fairly severe skin irritation, with erythema and vesicle formation. These symptoms usually disappear within a week.

REFERENCES

Baker, E. W., Evans, T. M., Gould, D. J., Hull, W. B., and Keegan, H. L. 1956. *A Manual of Parasitic Mites of Medical or Economic Importance*. 170 pp. National Pest Control Association, Inc., Technical Publication.

Dreisbach, R. H. 1974. *Handbook of Poisoning*. 8th Ed. 517 pp. Lange Medical Publications, Los Altos, California.

Frazier, C. A. 1969. *Insect Allergy: Allergic Reactions to Bites of Insects and Other Arthropods*. 493 pp. Warren H. Green, Inc., St. Louis, Missouri.

Heilesen, B. 1946. Studies on *Acarus scabiei* and scabies. Acta Dermato Vener., *26*(Suppl. 14):1–370.

Hoogstraal, H. 1971–1974. *Bibliography of Ticks and Tickborne Diseases*. U.S. Naval Med. Res. Unit 3, Cairo, Egypt. Vols. 1–5.

Horen, P. W. 1972. Insect and scorpion sting. J.A.M.A., *221*:894–898.

James, M. T. 1947. *The Flies that Cause Myiasis in Man*. 175 pp. U.S. Department of Agriculture, Miscellaneous Publication No. 631.

James, M. T., and Harwood, R. F. 1969. *Herms' Medical Entomology*. 6th Ed. 484 pp. Macmillan, New York.

Jung, R. C., Derbes, V. J., and Burch, A. D. 1963. Skin response to a solenamine, a hemolytic component of fire ant venom. Dermatol. Trop., *2*:241–244.

Kurtin, S. B., and Leider, M. 1968. Norwegian scabies — Report and lessons of a case. New Eng. J. Med., *278*:1099–1100.

Russel, F. E., Waldron, W. G., and Madon, M. B. 1969. Bites by the brown spiders *Loxosceles unicolor* and *Loxosceles arizonica* in California and Arizona. Toxicon, *7*:109–117.

Spielman, A., and Levi, H. W. 1970. Probable envenomation by *Chiracanthium mildei;* a spider found in houses. Amer. J. Trop. Med. & Hyg., *19*:729–732.

Smith, K. G. V., Ed. 1973. *Insects and Other Arthropods of Medical Importance*. 561 pp. British Museum (Natural History), London.

Taylor, R. M. 1967. *Catalogue of Arthropod-borne Viruses of the World*. 898 pp. U.S. Department of Health Education & Welfare, Public Health Service Publication 1760.

13
Signs and Symptoms of Parasitic Disease

Very few of the signs or symptoms evoked by infection with parasitic organisms can be said to deserve that much-abused term pathognomonic. There are but a limited number of ways in which the body is able to react to altered conditions, and therefore, it is not surprising that few of these reactions are specific. However, the presence of certain signs and symptoms should alert the clinician to corresponding diagnostic possibilities, while various constellations of symptoms, or syndromes, are to a greater or lesser degree diagnostic.

It must be emphasized that the following is not intended as a complete differential diagnosis of any of the symptoms discussed. Limitations of space do not permit even mention of the various non-parasitic etiologies of many of these conditions.

ABSCESS, AMEBIC.   Amebic invasion of the liver is characterized by tenderness and enlargement of that organ, progressive malaise, an irregularly spiking fever with night sweats, leukocytosis, elevation and fixation of the right diaphragm, and sometimes development of a right lower lobe pneumonitis. With abscess formation, pain becomes more intense and may be referred to the tip of the right (less commonly the left) scapula.

ABSCESS, FILARIAL.   Abscesses may develop spontaneously or appear shortly after antifilarial treatment is begun. They occur along the course of lymphatics, or at lymph nodes, and may be distinguished from pyogenic abscesses by the fact that they are generally sterile when first opened, and that fragments of the adult worms may be found in the abscess drainage.

328

ANEMIA. Most frequently associated with malaria, hookworm, and broad fish tapeworm infections, anemia may be seen in kala-azar, trypanosomiasis, schistosomiasis, fasciolopsiasis and trichuriasis. In falciparum malaria the red count may fall to 2.5 to 4.0 million in cases of average severity, and under 1.0 million in severe infections. Anemia in vivax malaria is usually not severe, and is still less pronounced in quartan infections. The characteristic microcytic hypochromic anemia of hookworm infection is the result of blood loss, and is thus proportional to the severity of infection, although adequate dietary intake of iron may prevent its development in light or moderate infections. The small amount of blood ingested per *Trichuris* makes anemia rare in other than massive infections. Persons infected with *Diphyllobothrium latum* may develop a macrocytic hyperchromic anemia on the basis of vitamin B_{12} deprivation if the worm is attached to the jejunal wall. In kala-azar, and possibly also in Chagas' disease, anemia may be a consequence of proliferation of infected reticuloendothelial cells in the bone marrow. In the other trypanosomiases, schistosomiasis, and in certain intestinal helminthic infections such as fasciolopsiasis, anemia may result in part from nutritional causes.

APPENDICITIS. Amebic ulceration involving the cecal area or appendix may simulate acute appendicitis; surgical intervention in the face of extensive cecal ulceration may be disastrous. *Ascaris* may block the lumen of the appendix and give rise to appendicitis; this is reported also for *Trichuris. Angiostrongylus costaricensis* infection may also mimic appendicitis.

ASCITES. Circumoval tissue proliferation leading to extensive fibrosis of the liver in *Schistosoma mansoni* and *S. japonicum* infections may lead eventually to a condition clinically very similar to Laennec cirrhosis, with portal hypertension, splenomegaly and ascites. Although hepatomegaly and splenomegaly occur early in kala-azar, ascites is uncommon. It may occur in chronic cases, probably secondary to a nutritional cirrhosis.

ASTHMA, BRONCHIAL. Asthmatic attacks may occur in *Ascaris* infection during the stage of migration through the lungs, or later in the course of the infection because of hypersensitization to the absorbed worm antigens. It is not uncommon in visceral larva migrans infections, in which there is usually an accompanying hepatomegaly and marked eosinophilia. See also tropical eosinophilia, under EOSINOPHILIA.

BLACKWATER FEVER. See HEMOGLOBINURIA.

CALABAR SWELLINGS. Circumscribed subcutaneous swellings are seen in loiasis. They are usually intensely pruritic, and if they develop in areas where there is little loose subcutaneous tissue, may be quite painful. They appear rapidly, developing within an hour or so to a diameter of several centimeters, and persist for several days, or if in an area subject to repeated trauma may last for a week or longer.

CALCIFICATIONS, CEREBRAL. Calcification of areas of intracerebral infection in congenital toxoplasmosis may be seen on x-ray, and when intracerebral calcifications are found in a patient who has chorioretinitis, a diagnosis of toxoplasmosis is highly probable. Calcified cysts of *Cysticercus cellulosae* within the brain may be distinguished by their size and uniform rounded or oval shape.

CHAGOMA. The hard, reddened, raised primary lesion in *Trypanosoma cruzi* infection. It usually develops on the head or neck, sometimes on the abdomen or limbs, and may persist for two or three months. Although it may occur on or about the eye, the chagoma is not to be confused with the unilateral palpebral edema of Romaña's sign (q.v.).

CHORIORETINITIS. Infection of the retina and choroid by *Toxoplasma* or (rarely) *Entamoeba histolytica* may produce visual disturbances, which can be profound if the macula is involved. On ophthalmoscopic examination, a grayish or yellow-white area surrounded by exudate is seen early; with healing this leaves a white atrophic patch, bordered by pigment deposits.

CHYLURIA. The formation of lymphatic varices, consequent upon repeated attacks of filarial lymphangitis and obstruction of lymphatic drainage, may lead to the passage of lymphatic fluid in the urine, if varices rupture into any part of the urinary tract. Chyluria usually occurs in attacks lasting a few days; the urine may have a milky white color and contain microfilariae.

COMA. The sudden onset of coma in a patient known to be suffering from falciparum malaria, or in an apparently healthy person in, or recently returned from, a malarious area, should always suggest cerebral malaria, and requires emergency treatment. While most common as a complication of falciparum malaria, it may occur with other types of malaria. In African trypanosomiasis, coma develops after a protracted period of increasing symptoms of meningoencephalitis. It is also seen in primary amebic meningoencephalitis, in which a history of rapidly developing fever, meningeal signs, confusion and coma, and of recent swimming or diving in fresh water will often be elicited.

CONJUNCTIVITIS. Chronic conjunctivitis is seen in onchocercal infections, with hyperpigmentation of the conjunctiva, photophobia and gradual development of corneal opacities; acute exacerbations of conjunctivitis and photophobia may be associated with attacks of onchocercal dermatitis (q.v.). The sheep botfly, *Oestrus ovis*, may lay its eggs in the conjunctivae, and development of the larva in the conjunctival sac is accompanied by considerable pain, localized swelling and conjunctivitis.

CONVULSIONS. Focal convulsive seizures of the jacksonian type are seen in a number of parasitic infections that involve the central nervous system. These are discussed under NEUROLOGIC SYMPTOMS. Convulsions also may be seen in the malarial paroxysm, in acute toxoplasmosis occurring in newborn children and in *Ascaris* infection in children.

DERMATITIS. Dermal leishmanoid is a secondary cutaneous manifestation of *Leishmania donovani* infection, occurring a year or so after supposed successful treatment of kala-azar. The lesions may be flattened or depressed depigmented macules, or erythematous nodules which, on the face, often occur in a butterfly distribution reminiscent of lupus erythematosus. Leishmanial organisms are found in the lesions.

Penetration of schistosome cercariae through the skin causes a localized edema and pruritus, mild in the case of the human schistosomes, more severe in the "swimmer's itch" caused by bird schistosome cercariae. A similar localized pruritic reaction occurs with penetration of *Strongyloides* larvae through the skin; the reaction to penetration of hookworm larvae is somewhat more severe, often with the formation of papules or vesicles; it may last for a couple of weeks or longer if secondarily infected. The cutaneous larva migrans reaction caused by larvae of *Ancylostoma braziliense* is characterized by a reddened papule at the site of entry; the larva forms a reddened serpiginous tunnel, at first covered with vesicles, later dry and crusted, which advances at the rate of a few millimeters to centimeters a day. The area itches intensely; without treatment infection may persist for several weeks or months.

Presence of adult *Loa loa* beneath the skin may be indicated by a thin raised reddened line, a few centimeters in length. The adult female *Dracunculus* also may be visible beneath the skin, but usually produces no reaction until about to larviposit, when a vesicle forms over the point at which the worm is about to break through the skin. In onchocerciasis, presence of microfilariae in the skin at times elicits an acute pruritic inflammatory reaction resembling erysipelas and usually confined to the face, neck and ears; repeated acute attacks may result in a chronic lichenification, with hyperpigmentation and fissuring.

The migration of *Sarcoptes scabiei* through the skin produces lesions resembling those of cutaneous larva migrans, but frequently seen in parts of the body that have no contact with soil, such as the axilla, groin, inner aspects of the thighs, the waist, small of the back and shoulder blades. The larvae of the horse botfly, *Gasterophilus*, produce similar cutaneous lesions in man. Pediculosis in hypersensitive persons, usually as a result of repeated exposure, may give rise to a severe localized reaction, with reddish papules at the feeding site, and surrounding vesiculation and a weeping dermatitis. Bronzing of the affected area may persist following healing. The chigoe flea, *Tunga penetrans*, produces local pruritus as it lies partly buried in the skin of the toes or elsewhere on the body; secondary infections by clostridia are not uncommon. See also RASH.

DIARRHEA. Diarrhea in parasitic diseases may be of diverse etiologies. In kala-azar, infiltration of the submucosa with leishmania-containing macrophages may lead to mucosal ulceration and diarrhea. Plugging of the mucosal capillaries with parasitized red blood cells may lead, in falciparum malaria, to a watery diarrhea so profuse as to suggest cholera. Blood, containing parasitized red cells, may be found in the stools. The diarrhea or dysentery is usually accompanied by nausea and vomiting. Mucosal ulceration in amebiasis or balantidiasis may produce diarrhea or, if more extensive, dysentery (q.v.). *Isospora* develops within the epithelial cells of the lower ileum and cecum. Infection is self-limited, lasting usually a month or less, and often asymptomatic. In some cases there is mild abdominal pain, nausea and vomiting, and diarrhea. *Giardia* infections may be asymptomatic, accompanied by a mild mucoid diarrhea or, like *Isospora,* may give rise to a full-blown malabsorption syndrome, with steatorrhea.

Development of the cysticercoids of *Hymenolepis nana* within the intestinal villi may elicit a mucous diarrhea. Maturation of *Trichinella* within the wall of the duodenum and jejunum produces nausea, vomiting, colicky abdominal pain and diarrhea, starting about 24 hours after infection and lasting up to 5 days. In *Strongyloides* infections there may be mild diarrhea, alternating with periods of constipation, or the diarrhea may be severe and prostrating. In heavy infections ulceration and sloughing of the intestinal mucosa may take place, with dysentery and, often, with secondary bacterial infection and fever. *Capillaria philippinensis* infections may result in profuse diarrhea, malabsorption, and a protein-wasting enteropathy.

In schistosomiasis mansoni and japonicum, there is a diarrhea presumably of toxic origin, and associated with nausea, vomiting, hepatic tenderness, fever, eosinophilia and an urticarial rash, during the period while the worms are maturing in the liver sinusoids. Somewhat later, with the beginning of egg deposition in the intestinal wall, there may be a profuse diarrhea or dysentery.

In persons previously uninfected, the onset of a heavy hookworm infection may be marked by nausea, vomiting, epigastric or midabdominal tenderness, and diarrhea. The diarrhea is presumably on the basis of toxicity or hypersensitivity, although mechanical irritation may play some part. The same may be said of the diarrhea in heavy whipworm infections. In fasciolopsiasis, diarrhea, which usually has its onset about a month after infection takes place, is characterized by the passage of stools containing much undigested food; severe infections are accompanied by symptoms of severe malnutrition, with edema of the face, abdominal wall and lower extremities, ascites and prostration.

The diarrhea sometimes seen in *Taenia* and broad fish tapeworm infections and in infections with the smaller intestinal flukes may be related to local irritation.

DYSENTERY. Acute amebic dysentery is characterized by the passage of six to eight or sometimes a dozen or more mucoid blood-flecked stools a day. There may be generalized abdominal pain and tenderness if the entire colon is involved, tenderness over McBurney's point, nausea and vomiting with cecal infection, or tenesmus, with relief of the accompanying pain after evacuation if the rectosigmoid is the main diseased area. An untreated attack lasts a few days to several weeks, usually subsides spontaneously to recur after an interval of some days to several years. Between attacks the patient may be constipated. Balantidial dysentery is similar to amebic, and as in the latter disease, many infections are asymptomatic. Dysentery accompanying kala-azar, falciparum malaria infections, strongyloidiasis and schistosomiasis is mentioned in the discussion of DIARRHEA.

EDEMA. Circumorbital edema, possibly the result of a vasculitis provoked by the migrating larvae, is frequently seen in the early stages of trichinosis; there also may be edema of the hands. Unilateral circumorbital edema, with local pruritus and sometimes intense pain, results from passage of the adult *Loa loa* across the eyeball or lid. Passage of the worm across the eyeball takes from less than half a minute to as long as ten minutes; the resulting inflammatory changes usually persist for several days. Calabar swellings (q.v.) are also seen in loiasis, while localized edema of the face, neck, ears, etc., accompanied by an intense pruritus and erythema, may be recurrent in onchocerciasis. Ocular sparganosis is not uncommon in some areas, the result of poulticing eye lesions with split raw infected frogs. In the subcutaneous tissues around the eye, the sparganum produces a violent tissue reaction with edema; retrobulbar development of the sparganum may cause protrusion of the eyeball and consequent corneal ulceration. Areas of localized hard edema, of uncertain etiology, are frequently seen in Chagas' disease, occurring after appearance of the chagoma (q.v.) The most common type is unilateral edema of the eyelids (Romaña's sign) (q.v.). Edematous patches may develop elsewhere on the body, especially involving the abdominal wall, pubic area, scrotum and legs. Of equally obscure origin is the edema of the hips, legs, hands and face that may accompany the acute stage of African sleeping sickness. Edema of the face and legs, with a protuberant abdomen, is seen in severe hookworm infections, fasciolopsiasis and diphyllobothriasis, and may be related to malnutrition.

ELEPHANTIASIS. Filarial elephantiasis is a chronic enlargement of a limb, the scrotum, breast or vulva, with hyperplasia of the connective tissue and skin, a woody nonpitting edema, and thickened, coarsened skin, often with verrucous changes. In Malayan filariasis, elephantiasis is less severe, and generally is confined to the lower limbs. Elephantiasis of the external genitalia in both sexes, and hypertrophy of the femoral lymph nodes, producing a peculiar condition known as "hanging groin," have been reported from some areas in Africa where bancroftian filariasis is unknown, and are ascribed to onchocercal infection. In schistosomiasis haematobium, extensive egg deposition may lead to fibrosis blocking the lymphatic drainage, and to elephantiasis of the penis.

EOSINOPHILIA. Eosinophilia is a consistent finding in helminth infections, though it may be quite variable in degree. In general, tissue parasites provoke a higher eosinophilia than those that live only in the lumen of the bowel.

A marked eosinophilia (20 to 70 per cent or higher) is most frequently seen in trichinosis, strongyloidiasis, hookworm infection, visceral larva migrans, filariasis, schistosomiasis, and fasciolopsiasis. Moderate eosinophilia (6 to 20 per cent) often accompanies trichuriasis, ascariasis, paragonimiasis, taeniasis, and eosinophilic meningitis. It must be realized that eosinophilia is an index of host reaction to the parasite; therefore, it will vary considerably from one patient to another.

Eosinophilia is not characteristic of any of the protozoan infections.

Tropical eosinophilia or eosinophilic lung disease is characterized by symptoms of chronic bronchitis or asthma, a marked eosinophilia, elevated erythrocyte sedimentation rate, paroxysmal cough or wheezing, malaise, easy fatiguability, anorexia and weight loss. The chest film may show diffuse patchy mottling and transverse branching striations, most prominent in the midlung and basal lung fields, with enlargement of the hilar shadows. Occasionally there may be unilateral densities in the upper lung field, suggestive of the picture seen in pulmonary tuberculosis. The disease is reported from such areas as India, Pakistan, Sri Lanka, China, Burma, Thailand, the Philippines, Malaysia and Indonesia, tropical Africa and the West Indies. Its etiology may be diverse. Filarial infection, with human or non-human species, is considered to be a common cause of this condition. Other agents may be the pulmonary stages of *Ascaris, Strongyloides, Toxocara,* or other helminths. Treatment with conventional doses of diethylcarbamazine is often effective; antimonial (stibophen) or arsenical drugs (neoarsphenamine) are sometimes effective when there is no response to diethylcarbamazine.

EPIDIDYMITIS. An early complication of filarial infection, often associated with orchitis, and with or without accompanying lymphangitis and fever.

FEVER. Patterns of fever may be characteristic in malaria and kala-azar, but it is a mistake to suppose that they must conform to the "textbook" pattern. A *quotidian fever* is often seen in the initial attack of vivax malaria, with two or more broods of parasites completing their exoerythrocytic cycle at different times, so that there may be a daily fever peak, corresponding to rupture of the infected red cells and liberation of merozoites. Daily fever peaks usually are seen only for a few days; apparently within this time all broods of parasites become synchronized, and thereafter the fever cycle will exhibit a tertian periodicity. Quartan and falciparum malaria may likewise exhibit a quotidian or irregular periodicity during the first few days of the primary attack. *Tertian fever* is characteristic of vivax and ovale malaria. The paroxysm has an abrupt onset, usually initiated with a chill, which varies from a moderate sensation of cold to the intense "bed-shaking" chill usually thought typical of malaria. The chill lasts up to an hour, fever (to 104 or 105°) for two hours or longer, followed by a profuse sweat, during the course of which the temperature falls to normal over a period of an hour or so. The sweating stage usually is followed by sleep, and when the patient awakens he usually feels well. The next paroxysm is initiated approximately 48 hours after the onset of the previous one. *Subtertian fever,* seen in falciparum malaria, is so called because the cycle may more nearly approach 36 than 48 hours. There is usually no frank chill, and the febrile stage is prolonged, though the fever is not usually so high as in vivax; it may not fall to normal even in the intervals between paroxysms. There may be double peaks of fever in each 24 hours, resembling the fever curve in kala-azar. There is often no well defined sweating stage, though sweating may be continuous, periodic or completely absent. *Quartan fever* is seen in malaria caused by *Plasmodium malariae.* There is often a regular periodicity from the start; the paroxysms recur at 72-hour intervals; while similar to those of vivax malaria, generally they are more severe. The hot stage often lasts several hours, and is frequently accompanied by nausea and vomiting; the sweating stage may be followed by prostration. *Hyperpyrexia* may develop as part of an attack of cerebral malaria, or in the course of an apparently uncomplicated attack of falciparum malaria; as the result of injury to the heat-control center in the hypothalamus there is a rapid rise in temperature to 107° or higher, and death quickly ensues.

A *doubly remittent* or *"dromedary" fever* is frequently found in kala-azar. Febrile attacks, which last a few days to several weeks, are separated by afebrile periods of equal irregularity. At some time during the course of a febrile attack, there will usually be one or more days during which a double or triple rise to 103 to 105° can be demonstrated during a 24-hour period.

An irregularly spiking fever with hepatic tenderness, suggestive of cholangitis, may be seen in amebic hepatitis, fascioliasis, and in acute *Opisthorchis* infections. The initial period of schistosome infection is likewise marked by irregular fever and hepatic tenderness, with nausea and vomiting, diarrhea and giant hives. An irregular fever, usually with evening peaks and night sweats, is an early finding in African trypanosomiasis, and a high remittent fever, lasting for several weeks, occurs early in Chagas' disease. A remittent fever, with temperature to 104 or 105°, frequently marks the stage of larval migration in trichinosis. *Filarial fever* may occur very early in the course of a filarial infection. There is usually a sudden onset, with fever ranging in the neighborhood of 102 to 104° and remaining elevated for several hours to a couple of days, and gradually subsiding in the next several days. Attacks of lymphangitis and lymphadenitis (q.v.) usually accompany the febrile episodes.

FUNICULITIS. Inflammation of the spermatic cord is frequently an early symptom of filariasis.

HEMATURIA. In *Schistosoma haematobium* infections, beginning as soon as three months after infection, or sometimes not until several years later, there may be intermittent hematuria. There is no dysuria, but there may be some frequency and also bladder pain following urination. Hematuria is often referred to as terminal, being limited to the last few drops of urine, blood being forced out as the bladder wall contracts.

HEMOGLOBINURIA. Blackwater fever usually is seen in conjunction with an attack of falciparum malaria, generally in patients who have had previous attacks of malaria. The passage of reddish or red-brown urine signals a bout of intravascular hemolysis, which may occur once or repeatedly, and may lead to severe renal tubular damage and anuria. The cause of blackwater fever is unknown; hypotheses include quinine sensitivity, glucose-6-phosphate dehydrogenase deficiency in persons treated with primaquine and related drugs, and autohemolysis on the basis of antibodies formed against altered infected red cells.

HEPATITIS. Amebic hepatitis has already been described under the heading of ABSCESS, AMEBIC.

In kala-azar the liver is usually relatively less enlarged than the spleen, though the reverse occasionally may be true. The liver parenchyma is unaffected and the Küppfer cells are greatly increased and usually heavily infected. The liver is nontender, and reverts to normal size after effective treatment. Tenderness and moderate enlargement of the liver may be seen in cases of falciparum malaria with gastrointestinal symptoms and jaundice. Hepatomegaly also is seen in Chagas' disease, especially in children, in acute toxoplasmosis occurring in the neonatal period, and in visceral larva migrans. Hepatomegaly also may result from hydatid infections of that organ.

Infection with the liver flukes *Dicrocoelium, Fasciola,* and *Opisthorchis* likewise results in hepatic tenderness and enlargement, with an irregularly spiking fever. These worms probably produce few or no chronic symptoms unless present in large numbers. The hepatomegaly and tenderness that characterize early schistosome infections subside after the worms have become established in the veins of the intestinal wall or bladder, but in *Schistosoma mansoni* and *japonicum* infections ova carried to the liver produce a fibrotic reaction, which ultimately results in a clinical picture similar to Laennec cirrhosis.

HIVES. Giant hives and other allergic symptoms, such as bronchial asthma, are commonly seen in ascariasis, and hives often appear during the first few weeks of schistosome infections.

HYDATID THRILL. In large unilocular echinococcus cysts of the abdominal viscera, situated close to the abdominal wall, a characteristic thrill may be elicited by quick palpation or percussion.

HYDROCELE. This is a common finding in areas where filariasis is endemic, developing as a sequel to repeated attacks of orchitis. If lymphatic varices develop in the cord and rupture into the scrotal sac, a condition known as lymphocele results.

HYDROCEPHALUS. Although not so intimately associated with congenital toxoplasmosis as are chorioretinitis and cerebral calcifications, hydrocephalus or microcephaly are commonly seen in this condition.

HYPERPIGMENTATION. Kala-azar derives its name from intensification of the pigmentation of the skin over the cheeks, temples, and around the mouth. It is most obvious in dark-skinned races. In onchocerciasis repeated attacks of allergic dermatitis may result in hyperpigmentation of the area, usually on the face, neck, or ears. A bronzing and induration of the affected skin areas may occur in chronic pediculosis (vagabond's disease).

JAUNDICE. Obstructive jaundice may be seen in severe liver fluke infections, but is not characteristic of light infections or those of moderate intensity. The symptoms of the falciparum malaria syndrome known as *bilious remittent fever* include acute epigastric pain, nausea and vomiting, marked enlargement and tenderness of the liver, with jaundice appearing on about the second day. Diarrhea, a high remittent fever and oliguria are usually seen, and death may result from renal or hepatic failure.

KERANDEL'S SIGN. Noted in the stage of central nervous system involvement in African sleeping sickness, this sign may be elicited by pressure on the palm of the hand or over the ulnar nerve, and consists of severe pain which occurs shortly after the pressure has been relieved.

LEUKOCYTOSIS. Leukocytosis seldom is maintained throughout the course of any of the parasitic infections. In amebic hepatitis or abscess there may be a white blood cell count of 25,000 to 30,000, with 70 to 80 per cent polymorphonuclear neutrophils. In visceral larva migrans a leukocytosis of up to 80,000 has been reported, with an eosinophilia of 20 to 80 per cent. Trichinosis may be characterized by a white count of 30,000 early in the infection, and strongyloidiasis by one nearly as elevated; these usually decline, and may be followed by leukopenia. Leukocytosis early in the course of infection, followed by leukopenia with a relative monocytosis, is common to many protozoan and helminth infections.

LEUKOPENIA. A white cell count of 4000 or less, with a relative monocytosis, generally is seen throughout the course of kala-azar, sometimes terminating in agranulocytosis.

In malaria, a leukopenia of 3000 to 6000, with a relative monocytosis, characterizes the afebrile periods, while there may be a leukocytosis during the paroxysm.

LYMPHADENITIS. In filariasis the femoral and epitrochlear nodes are most commonly involved, also the axillary and inguinals. The nodes are enlarged, painful and tender during an acute attack of lymphangitis, and tend to remain enlarged between attacks. A condition resembling infectious mononucleosis sometimes is seen in the acute stage of toxoplasmosis, with fever, weakness, malaise, generalized adenopathy, and sometimes a rash. There may be generalized lymphadenitis without fever or other symptoms. In the early stages of African trypanosomiasis there may be generalized adenopathy; the glands of the posterior cervical triangle are most conspicuously affected (Winterbottom's sign). Generalized adenopathy is seen in the acute stage of Chagas' disease.

LYMPHANGITIS. Acute lymphangitis is an early symptom of filarial infection. It usually is accompanied by fever, and may affect the limbs, breast or scrotum. When it occurs on a limb, it is usually centrifugal in development, starting at a lymph node and progressing distally. The course of the lymphatic is readily seen because of local distention and erythema. Centrifugal spread of the lymphangitis is the reverse of that seen in bacterial lymphangitis (blood poisoning), in which the infection extends proximally from the point of origin.

LYMPHOCYTOSIS. A relative or absolute lymphocytosis, unusual in parasitic infections, is, however, generally seen in Chagas' disease. Initially there may be a slight leukocytosis, usually followed by leukopenia.

LYMPH VARICES. Dilatations of the lymphatic vessels may occur secondary to lymphatic blockage in filariasis. They are most frequently seen in the inguinal and femoral areas, or other lymphatic tracts may be affected. The soft lobulated swellings may rupture and drain. When this occurs on the scrotum, a chronic condition known as *lymph scrotum* may develop.

MENINGOENCEPHALITIS. Invasion of the central nervous system by trypanosomes is characterized in African sleeping sickness by increasing symptoms of meningoencephalitis. There may be quite variable sensory and motor changes, personality disorders, headache, confusion, drowsiness and finally coma. Similar but milder symptoms are seen in Chagas' disease. Minor neurologic symptoms are seen during almost any attack of malaria (i.e., headache, disorientation), and cerebral malaria may develop as a complication of any type of malaria. It is characteristic of falciparum malaria, however, and may develop slowly with increasing headache and drowsiness over several days, or present as a sudden coma or other acute mental disturbance. There may be signs of meningeal irritation; symptomatology is quite varied, depending upon the brain areas affected. If the cord is affected, symptoms may be suggestive of multiple sclerosis.

Amebic meningoencephalitis, caused by invasion of the central nervous system by ordinarily free-living ameboflagellates of the genus *Naegleria* and possibly other amebae, is an acute, rapidly progressive infection, apparently acquired while swimming or diving in fresh-water lakes or pools. It is characterized by fever, headache, mental confusion and coma, and death frequently occurs within a few days of onset.

Eosinophilic meningoencephalitis, seen in various parts of the Pacific area in recent years, is believed, on strong epidemiologic grounds, to be symptomatic of infection with *Angiostrongylus cantonensis*, and thus a form of larva migrans infection. It is characterized by fever, headache, stiff neck, and increased cells (mainly eosinophils) in the spinal fluid. It is generally a mild and self-limited infection.

MICROCEPHALUS. See HYDROCEPHALUS.

MONOCYTOSIS. A relative or absolute monocytosis is a frequent finding in both protozoal and helminthic infections.

MYOCARDITIS. Myocardial infection is characteristic of Chagas' disease, and is seen in about 50 per cent of chronic cases. Cardiac failure may come on slowly, although in infants it tends to occur in the early acute stage. There may be pericardial effusion. Congestive heart failure also has been reported in African trypanosomiasis, probably in the Rhodesian form of the disease. In African trypanosomiasis the etiology of the heart failure is not as apparent. Myocarditis, occasionally severe enough to cause death, has been reported in trichinosis. It is the result of migration of the larvae through the myocardium, in which they do not encyst. Myocarditis also may be seen in acute toxoplasmosis in both infants and adults, the result of invasion of the myocardium.

MYOSITIS. While a nonspecific symptom of many febrile illnesses, severe myositis is characteristic of the stage of larval migration in trichinosis. If accompanied by circumorbital edema, eosinophilia and a history of consumption of improperly cooked pork, the diagnosis may be made with some certainty. Myositis, usually involving a single muscle group, may also be seen in *Sarcocystis* infection.

NEUROLOGIC SYMPTOMS. Neurologic symptoms in trypanosomiasis, malaria, amebic and eosinophilic meningoencephalitis are discussed under MENINGOENCEPHALITIS. Variable neurologic symptoms may occur in schistosomiasis when eggs, carried by the bloodstream to the central nervous system, lodge there and provoke a granulomatous reaction. Neurologic and other symptoms caused by embolization of eggs are more common in *Schistosoma japonicum* infection than in the other two species, while in *S. mansoni* and *S. haematobium* eggs are found more frequently in the spinal cord than in the brain, perhaps because of ectopic wanderings of the adult worms. In *S. japonicum* infection, there may be severe neurologic symptoms, including coma and paresis, during the incubation period or first few weeks after infection. Transitory neurologic symptoms of a variable nature may be caused by the migration of ascarid and trichina larvae in the central nervous system; hemiplegia and focal epileptic attacks have been reported in trichinosis. Hydatid and coenurus cysts may develop within the central nervous system, where they may produce symptoms related to a space-occupying lesion, or if within the ventricular system, internal hydrocephalus. Cysticercus larvae seldom cause trouble while living, but after death may give rise to epileptiform seizures, as may *Sparganum proliferum* and adults of *Paragonimus westermani* that have gone astray.

NODULES, SUBCUTANEOUS. Lipoma-like subcutaneous nodules include onchocercomas (q.v.) and cysticercus and coenurus larvae. The cysticercus larva of *Taenia solium* develops most frequently in the subcutaneous tissues, where it forms nodules 0.5 to 3.0 centimeters in diameter. In almost half the recorded human cases of coenurus infection, the larvae have been found in the subcutaneous tissues; others have been recorded from the brain, spinal cord and eye. *Echinococcus* cysts also may be found in the subcutaneous tissues. Spargana also form subcutaneous nodules, somewhat elongate and several centimeters in length, which may resemble lipomas, but may move through the subcutaneous tissues at irregular intervals and are often painful. *Sparganum proliferum* may develop as branched or multiple nodules, and invade the viscera. (See also EDEMA for a discussion of ocular sparganosis.) Larvae of the botfly *Hypoderma* migrate through the subcutaneous tissues, finally coming to rest beneath the skin, where they produce elongate nodules, several centimeters in length. Considerable pain may accompany migration, but the resting nodule is seldom painful or pruritic. The human botfly, *Dermatobia hominis,* burrows into the skin and subcutaneous tissues, producing an intensely pruritic papular lesion, which has the appearance of a furuncle. There is a small central opening, from which comes a serous exudate, and through which the posterior end of the larva may protrude from time to time. Secondary infection is common.

OBSTRUCTION, INTESTINAL. *Ascaris*, especially in children, may produce complete intestinal obstruction, with accompanying abdominal pain, vomiting, distention and hyperperistalsis. Partial or complete intestinal obstruction may also characterize infection by *Angiostrongylus costaricensis*.

OCULAR SYMPTOMS. See CONJUNCTIVITIS, EDEMA and VISUAL DIFFICULTIES.

ONCHOCERCOMA. Adult worms of *Onchocerca volvulus* lie in coiled masses beneath the skin, completely enclosed in a fibrous tissue capsule. They are from a few millimeters to several centimeters in diameter, generally freely moveable, and resemble lipomas. In Mexico and Guatemala they frequently occur beneath the scalp, while in Africa most of them occur on other parts of the body.

ORCHITIS. Filarial orchitis may occur early in the disease, and at times in the absence of lymphangitis or fever; repeated attacks lead to hydrocele.

PAIN. Abdominal pain, generally of a vague or ill-defined nature, is said to accompany many of the intestinal parasitic infections. The presence or absence of such tenuous pains is of no value from a diagnostic standpoint. Epigastric pain, sometimes with nausea and vomiting, may be seen in giardiasis, trichinosis and strongyloidiasis, and is related to the duodenitis and jejunitis provoked by these infections. Moderate to severe abdominal pain is seen in acute amebic colitis; it may be confined to the cecal area, or generalized. *Angiostrongylus costaricensis* may give rise to similar symptoms. In ascariasis severe pain may signal intestine obstruction (q.v.), perforation and peritonitis (q.v.) or bile duct blockage.

Muscle pain in trichinosis is discussed under MYOSITIS, and the delayed pain sensation seen in African trypanosomiasis under the heading of KERANDEL'S SIGN.

PERITONITIS. Penetration of *Ascaris* through the wall of the intestine usually leads to generalized peritonitis, with pain, marked distention, generalized abdominal tenderness and free air under the diaphragm, detectable by x-ray. In severe amebic dysentery ulcers may erode through the wall of the intestine to initiate peritonitis.

PNEUMONITIS. Pneumonitis is characteristic of severe *Ascaris* infection, and is caused when the worm larvae break out of the capillaries into the alveoli, whence they are coughed up to be swallowed and initiate the intestinal phase of the disease. Symptoms are first noted one to five days after the eggs are ingested and consist of cough, fever, respiratory distress and the physical and x-ray signs of a bronchopneumonia; in severe cases there may be complete consolidation of one or more lobes. The pneumonitis usually clears within a week or two; it may be accompanied by high eosinophilia and an urticarial rash. Similar symptoms may accompany the corresponding stage in strongyloides infection, although the pneumonitis is generally not so severe. In hookworm infection there is seldom a clear-cut pneumonitis at this stage, but a cough is frequently present. In schistosomiasis there may likewise be a transitory cough, sometimes with hemoptysis and frequently with dyspnea, during the stage of migration through the lungs.

Pneumocystis carinii causes an interstitial plasma cell pneumonia, mainly seen in newborn and young children. Some cases have been reported in adults. The x-ray picture is that of bronchopneumonia. Pneumonitis may be a part of acute toxoplasmosis in the neonatal period, and more rarely in the adult. Atelectatic pneumonitis may be seen in amebic abscess, the result of pressure from the elevated right diaphragm. The abscess may erode through the diaphragm to produce a right lower lobe infection; infrequently an abscess may develop primarily in the lung. If there is erosion into a bronchus, there may be expectoration of abscess material, a light, reddish brown or "anchovy paste" color.

PROTEINURIA.   In falciparum malaria, proteinuria, with hyaline and granular casts in the urine, is common. Rarely there may be oliguria or anuria, usually accompanying an attack of blackwater fever (q.v.). The nephrotic syndrome, with proteinuria, is sometimes seen in quartan malaria.

PRURITUS ANI.   The nocturnal pruritus that accompanies pinworm infection varies considerably in degree, probably depending upon hypersensitivity of the host. In some persons there is no noticeable itching, whereas in others it may be sufficiently severe to interfere with rest. Anal pruritus may be associated with active migration of gravid proglottids of *Taenia saginata* out of the anus.

PULMONARY SYMPTOMS, CHRONIC.   In all three types of schistosomiasis, but especially in *S. haematobium* infections, ova may be carried to the lungs, where pseudotubercle formation around them may produce a radiologic picture suggestive of miliary tuberculosis, and increasing fibrosis may lead to cor pulmonale. Paragonimiasis is characterized by chronic cough, the production of thick blood-flecked sputum or sometimes frank hemoptysis, and increasing dyspnea. X-rays may show patchy infiltrates, rounded shadows suggestive of coin lesions, calcifications and pleural thickening or effusion. In pulmonary echinococcosis, cough is usually the first symptom. There may be increasing dyspnea; with erosion of blood vessels there will be hemoptysis, and with obstruction there results secondary bacterial infection and fever. If the cyst ruptures into a bronchus, the contents may be coughed up, or the patient become asphyxiated.

RASH.   An allergic urticarial rash or hives (q.v.) is often seen in the early stages of schistosome infection, and in ascariasis. A macular or maculopapular eruption may occur early in the course of a trichina infection, and one of the variants of acute toxoplasmosis is a typhus-like fever, with a macular rash, prostration, and sometimes stupor and cardiac decompensation. During attacks of fever in the early stages of African trypanosomiasis there may be an irregular blotchy rash, often annular in appearance. The individual patches may be several inches across, they tend to fade in a few hours, and reappear at irregular intervals.

RETINOCHOROIDITIS. See CHORIORETINITIS.

ROMAÑA'S SIGN. Unilateral palpebral edema, involving both upper and lower eyelids, appears early in the course of an infection with T. cruzi. The edema is hard and non-pitting; it may remain confined to the eyelids or may spread down to involve the cheek and neck. It may subside promptly or persist for weeks or months.

SHOCK. When shock complicates falciparum malaria, the patient is pale, with a cold and clammy skin, thin fast pulse and low blood pressure. There is often acute abdominal pain, vomiting and diarrhea. The etiology may be one of primary adrenal failure, through parasite-induced ischemia or infarction, or secondary to reduced blood volume and blood pressure, caused by widespread vascular injury. Rupture of an echinococcus cyst may lead to anaphylactic shock.

SPLENOMEGALY. As part of the generalized lymphoid hyperplasia in both African and American trypanosomiasis, splenomegaly may be observed. In kala-azar the spleen is said to enlarge downward about an inch per month, and may extend into the pelvis. It is nontender, and reverts to normal size after effective therapy. The spleen enlarges during an acute attack of malaria, and is usually palpable within two weeks of onset. Between attacks it may regress in size, and in adults become fibrotic and smaller than normal. In children, repeated attacks may lead to great enlargement of the organ, which may reach the pelvis. The "splenic index," as a guide to endemicity of malaria, as obtained by examination of a population for evidence of enlarged spleens, obviously must be derived only through examination of children. The spleen is usually tender during an acute attack of malaria, and tenderness may be apparent before the organ can be palpated. Splenic infarction or rupture occur rarely. In Schistosoma mansoni and S. japonicum infections, splenomegaly is secondary to hepatic fibrosis brought about by egg deposition in the liver, and portal hypertension.

SPLINTER HEMORRHAGES. Sometimes occurring during the stage of active larval migration in trichinosis, these hemorrhages are a sign of vascular injury.

TACHYCARDIA. A fast pulse is noted early in both African and American trypanosomiasis. In Chagas' disease it persists into the sub-acute and chronic stages, where it may be associated with heart block, Stokes-Adams syndrome and fibrillation.

ULCERS, CUTANEOUS. In leishmanial and trypanosomal diseases

there is a primary multiplication at the site of infection. In *Leishmania tropica*-complex infections there is first a papule at the site of infection, which gradually transforms into a shallow ulcer with raised edges. The Chiclero ulcer of Southern Mexico and Central America is similar to oriental sore, except when it occurs on the ear, where it may erode the pinna. *L. braziliensis* first produces cutaneous ulcerations, which may either through extension or metastasis come to involve the nasal mucosa, the soft and hard palate, nasal septum, pharynx, and larynx. In blacks, granulomatous rather than ulcerative lesions are generally seen. In African sleeping sickness there may be a firm tender raised lesion, up to 2 cm. or more in diameter, at the site of infection. This "trypanosomal chancre" is painful or pruritic, but like the chagoma (q.v.) does not apparently ulcerate unless secondarily infected. Ulcerative cutaneous lesions rarely are seen in amebiasis, either in the perianal region or in the skin surrounding fistulas or surgical drainage incisions from hepatic abscesses. A rounded ulcer, 2 mm. to several centimeters in diameter, marks the place at which the guinea worm discharges its larvae. In the center of the ulcer, a portion of the worm may be visible. There is often secondary infection, and a painful localized reaction may persist until discharge of the larvae is completed.

URETHRITIS. *Trichomonas vaginalis* has been found in up to one-third of cases of "nonspecific" urethritis in the male.

VAGINITIS. A prolific, irritating green or yellowish, thin discharge is seen in *Trichomonas vaginalis* infection; the vagina may be diffusely congested, or punctate hemorrhagic spots may be seen. The organisms may be present in asymptomatic individuals. Pinworms may migrate from the anus and enter the vagina, where they produce a temporary, intense pruritus in some children.

VISUAL DIFFICULTIES associated with parasitic disease include circumorbital edema (q.v.), conjunctivitis (q.v.) and chorioretinitis (q.v.). Ascarid larvae (both those of *Ascaris lumbricoides* and *Toxocara*) may invade the eye, producing iritis or other symptoms. Patients infected with *Onchocerca* actually may be aware of the intraocular movement of the microfilariae, and lesions of the anterior chamber, iris, ciliary body, choroid, and retina, developing in this condition, may lead to diminution of vision or total blindness. Cysticercus and coenurus larvae may develop within the eye. Ophthalmomyiasis may occur.

WINTERBOTTOM'S SIGN. See LYMPHADENITIS.

X-RAY EVIDENCE OF PARASITIC DISEASE. *Amebiasis:* Amebic granulomas of the large bowel simulate carcinoma in barium enema studies. Cecal amebiasis tends to produce a funnel-shaped deformity of that portion of the bowel as seen in barium enema studies. In amebic abscess of the liver there may be elevation of the right diaphragm, and sometimes right lower lobe pneumonitis. Intravenous sodium diatrizoate (Hypaque) infusion and tomography of the liver may demonstrate the wall of the amebic abscess. *Giardiasis*: Evidence of intestinal malabsorption. *Toxoplasmosis:* Intracerebral calcifications. *Pneumocystosis;* Pneumonitis, typically sparing lateral margins of the bases. *Dracunculiasis, filariasis,* and *loiasis:* Calcified worms may be seen in the tissues. *Ascariasis:* Pneumonitis. Adult worms may be seen as cylindrical empty spaces in the barium-filled bowel in a small bowel series. *Stronglyoidiasis* and *hookworm infection:* Pneumonitis. Loss of mucosal markings and a tubular deformity of the duodenum and jejunum may be seen in small bowel studies on patients with strongyloidiasis. *Cysticercosis:* Calcified cysts in the subcutaneous tissues, muscles, brain. *Echinococcosis:* Well defined, rounded masses may be seen in the lung parenchyma; sometimes a fluid level is visible within them. Hepatic cysts are visible only if calcification of the wall has taken place. Sometimes calcified daughter cysts are seen. (Hepatic photoscanning, with the use of radioactive isotopes, will reveal noncalcified cysts as well.) Hydatid cysts of bone produce extensive intramedullary erosion, demonstrable by x-ray. *Paragonimiasis;* Patchy infiltrates or rounded densities in the parenchyma, pleural thickening, or fluid. *Schistosomiasis:* Pulmonary fibrosis, or a picture suggestive of miliary tuberculosis. Cor pulmonale with dilatation of the pulmonary artery and its main branches, right ventricular hypertrophy. *S. haematobium* infections: Calcification in the wall of the bladder, hydronephrosis, hydroureter.

14

Pseudoparasites and Pitfalls

It is common experience that the beginner almost as frequently misidentifies a yeast or other plant cell as an ameba, or a platelet as a malarial parasite, as he fails to identify the parasitic organisms actually present in the material examined. A wide variety of objects which resemble parasites may be found in stool specimens or other materials. It would be impractical as well as unprofitable to attempt a complete listing of these diagnostic pitfalls, but a number of the more important types will be briefly considered.

A pseudoparasite is an object which resembles a parasite or the egg of a parasite, but is either not a parasite at all or is not parasitic in the host under consideration. "Pseudosymbiont" might be a better term; pseudoparasite has been used by some to designate commensal organisms, such as *Entamoeba coli*. While *E. coli* is not in the strict sense a parasite, it hardly seems necessary to call it a pseudoparasite and thus accuse it of sailing under false colors.

Even inorganic materials may occur in such forms as to suggest parasitic organisms to the unwary. Oil droplets, present in the stool because of diet, disease or drug administration, may be small and surprisingly uniform in size. If their lack of internal structure is disregarded, they may suggest amebic cysts. A fat stain will reveal their true nature, and fatty materials will be eliminated by the ether used in both of the concentration methods described in Chapter 15. Many kinds of yeasts are normally present in the stool, and may be confused with cysts of some of the intestinal protozoa. Figure 159 indicates some of the

346

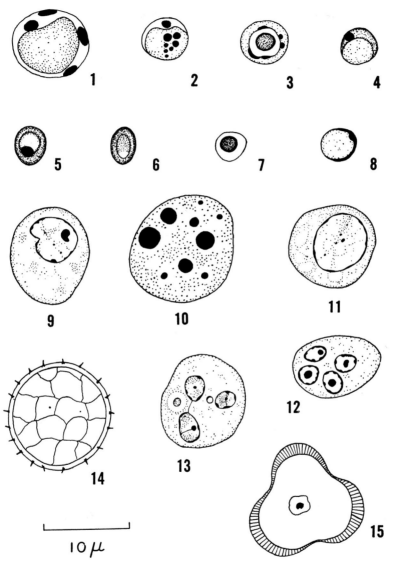

FIGURE 159. Various structures which may be seen in stool preparations: 1, 2, 4, Blastocystis hominis; 3, 5, 6, 7, 8, various yeasts; 9, 11, squamous cells from rectal mucosa; 10, deteriorated macrophage without nucleus; 12, 13, polymorphonuclear leukocytes; 14, 15, "pollen grains."

more common types. Yeasts are quite variable in size and shape, although the majority are ovoid and most fall within the size range of the various protozoan cysts. The nuclei of yeast cells are solid, without obvious internal structure, and stain blue-black or black with hematoxylin stains, and dark red when stained with trichrome. It is generally assumed that intestinal yeasts are harmless, but it must be remembered that *Candida* and, rarely, *Blastomyces* may occur in the feces. However, these organisms, like the pathogenic intestinal bacteria, cannot be recognized morphologically, and must be isolated and identified by specialized techniques when indicated. One of the larger non-pathogenic yeasts is of special importance to the parasitologist. *Blastocystis hominis* (Figs. 29 and 159) has a spherical form and ranges from 5 to 30 microns in diameter. It thus resembles amebic cysts in both size and shape, but differs from them sharply in internal organization. A large central fluid-filled vacuole is surrounded by a layer of cytoplasm containing the nuclei. In iodine preparations, the central area does not stain, but the peripheral layer is light yellowish in color, and the peripheral position of the one or more nuclei is clearly indicated. With permanent stains, the central material may take an intense stain, stain lightly or not stain at all; the nuclei stain darkly and may be seen to be embedded in the peripheral layer of cytoplasm. Some people believe that *Blastocystis* belongs to the Protozoa, but this claim requires additional documentation.

Two interesting fungi are occasionally seen as parasites of intestinal amebae. *Sphaerita* invades the cytoplasm, and *Nucleophaga* destroys the nucleus of the ameba. Individual organisms are spherical and about 0.5 to 1 micron in diameter. They usually occur in closely-packed

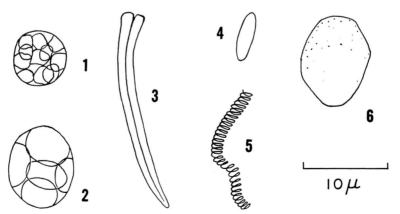

FIGURE 160. Plant structures seen in the stool: *1, 2,* aggregates of starch granules; *3,* plant hair; *4, 6,* amorphous vegetable materials, superficially resembling ova or protozoan cysts; *5,* vegetable spiral.

masses of varying size. These two organisms seem to be rather invasive, as a high proportion of amebae will be found infected when either organism is found in the stool. The obvious practical utilization of this phenomenon has unfortunately failed to materialize!

A variety of other plant materials regularly found in the feces may cause confusion. Some more common plant cells, hairs and fibers are shown in Figure 160. Pollen grains (Fig. 159) and similar structures are very regular in size, and often present in large numbers. Their regularity and abundance may suggest that they are some form of animal parasite, although their structure is quite unlike that of any of the parasitic forms. Vegetable fibers often have a spiral structure, and frequently a regularly sculptured surface. Plant cells may be recognized by their thick and frequently smooth walls. Some are of about the same size and shape as certain helminth ova, but seldom possess the regularity of shape which characterizes the ova. Vegetable hairs may be confused with larval nematodes, but will be seen to have a homogeneous thick refractile wall, and a minute central canal extending the whole length of the structure. Starch granules may be spherical, and if undigested can be seen to be composed of concentric layers of white homogeneous material. Potato starch frequently occurs in irregular sack-like aggregates of granules. When undigested, starch will be stained blue when iodine is added to the fecal suspension; when partially digested it will stain red. A frequent source of confusion is the presence in the feces of undigested citrus fruit vesicles, the small spindle-shaped individual components of sections of oranges or grapefruit. These resemble in size and general outline the gravid female pinworm. Close observation will show that they do not possess any obvious internal structure.

While intestinal myiasis, or the development of fly larvae in the intestinal tract, may occur in man (Chapter 12), more frequently body parts or whole larval or adult insects seen in the stool are present as the result of their ingestion with food. If live larvae are seen in a stool specimen, they may indicate either myiasis or contamination of the specimen. It is important in such cases to ascertain the method of collection of the specimen, particularly if it was obtained outside the laboratory or hospital.

Even if one finds unmistakable helminth eggs in a stool specimen, this does not necessarily indicate infection. Occasionally eggs of the roundworm *Capillaria,* and of certain trematodes such as *Fasciola,* may be accidentally ingested and pass through the gastrointestinal tract unchanged. The livers of cattle and sheep infected with *Fasciola* are not approved for human consumption if the infection is detected, but if the meat is not inspected, or the infection is light and escapes detection, the adult worms may be ingested and their eggs appear in the stools. When there is any question of the possibility of pseudoparasitism of this sort, one should request another specimen, obtained after the diet has been controlled to eliminate any chance of such contamination. Eggs of plant-parasitic roundworms may be ingested with root vegetables, and subsequently appear in the feces. One of these, *Heterodera,* is not un-common, and is listed in the key to helminth eggs which appears at the end of Chapter 3.

Mentally disturbed or malingering patients may attempt to feign parasitism by placing various objects in their stools. Earthworms seem to be widely favored for this purpose. The earthworm is an annelid, with a well-developed circulatory system, and the presence of blood vessels can usually be detected under the low power of the microscope. They do bear a superficial resemblance to ascarid nematodes, but are generally of a reddish-brown color, whereas ascarids are white or pinkish white. The reproductive openings of the earthworm are marked by an annular enlargement of the body, extending for several segments, which is not seen in nematodes.

Various cellular elements in the stool may be mistaken for intesti-nal amebae. Most important in this regard are polymorphonuclear leukocytes, macrophages, columnar epithelial cells from the intestinal mucosa or squamous cells from the anal mucosa (Fig. 159). Identifica-tion of these cells depends upon observation of structure and relative size of the nuclei in relation to the cytoplasm. Polymorphonuclear leukocytes, when stained, may show a nucleus divided into four appar-ently separate spheres, each with peripheral chromatin and an apparent karyosome. However, the nuclear material is larger in proportion to the amount of cytoplasm than in amebic cysts of comparable size, and the shape of the nuclei is usually more variable. Macrophages may be dif-ferentiated from the intestinal amebae by the possession of numerous inclusions within the darkly staining cytoplasm. The nucleus does not appear to have a karyosome, but instead has a fine network of chromatin as well as larger particles scattered throughout the nucleus. Degenerate macrophages which have lost their nuclei may also be seen.

In the examination of thin blood smears for malarial parasites, the novice is often misled by the superimposition of platelets on red cells. These may be said to have a vague resemblance to young trophozoites of *Plasmodium,* but if the slide is correctly stained, their color will be altogether different. While a malarial parasite has blue cytoplasm and red chromatin, the platelet stains in varying shades of purple. Platelets are rather fuzzy in outline, whereas the malarial parasite will usually be quite sharp. Careful focusing will help to distinguish the extracellular platelets from intracytoplasmic malarial parasites. Various abnormali-ties of the red cells, such as the presence of Howell-Jolly bodies or Cabot's rings, may also be superficially misleading, but again do not stain in the same manner as the malarial parasites.

15
Special Procedures

ANIMAL INOCULATION

By comparison with the rather extensive use of animal inoculation in the identification of the other infectious agents of disease, little use is made of this method with the animal parasites. In part, this is because many animal parasites are readily identified on the basis of morphology, obviating the need for more lengthy and costly procedures. In many cases, too, there is such a degree of host specificity among the protozoa and helminths that it is impossible or difficult to carry out animal inoculations.

Various laboratory animals are susceptible to infection with *Entamoeba histolytica*. Dogs, rabbits, guinea pigs, rats and hamsters can all be infected, but it is frequently necessary to inject the organisms intracecally or intrahepatically. Rectal injection of kittens with fecal material suspected of containing *E. histolytica* was once used to a limited extent as a diagnostic tool, but has been long outmoded.

Trypanosoma brucei brucei, from which *T. brucei gambiense* and *T. brucei rhodesiense* are thought to have evolved, has a wide host range, and so it is not surprising that infections with the latter two parasites can be established in a number of laboratory animals. White rats, white mice and guinea pigs are most useful for diagnosis and the maintenance of laboratory strains. Young animals are most readily infected, and *T. brucei rhodesiense* is more virulent than *T. brucei gambiense*. Rats infected with *T. brucei gambiense* will survive for several months, with a low-grade parasitemia; infected with *T. brucei rhodesiense*, they die within a short time with an overwhelming parasitemia. As mentioned in Chapter 7, posterior nucleated forms of *T. brucei rhodesiense* sometimes are seen in laboratory animals infected with this parasite, but never in those infected with the

Gambian form. *T. rangeli* multiplies in the common laboratory animals, but does not cause apparent disease. Young white rats and white mice can be infected with *T. cruzi;* the white mouse is best for diagnostic inoculation. When first isolated this trypanosome is quite virulent, but after repeated animal passage it loses its virulence, and may become noninfective. Intraperitoneal or subcutaneous inoculation should be used; inject amounts up to 2 ml. of blood, depending upon the size of the animal used. It is important to check rats for the presence of their common parasite, *T. lewisi*, before inoculation.

For isolation of leishmanias, the hamster is most satisfactory; other laboratory animals are infected with difficulty. Following intraperitoneal or intratesticular inoculation, hamsters will develop a generalized infection with any form of *Leishmania*, and the organisms may be demonstrated in spleen impression smears, or testicular aspirates. The infection develops slowly, and culture methods are generally regarded as superior for diagnostic use.

Toxoplasma gondii, a parasite which shows little host specificity, will infect all common laboratory animals. White rats and mice are generally used; rats develop a chronic infection and are good for maintenance of the strain, while intraperitoneal infection of mice results in tremendous proliferation of the organisms in the ascitic fluid, and death of the mice within a few days. Mouse peritoneal fluid, rich in organisms, is used as a source of toxoplasmas for the dye test and other diagnostic procedures.

Xenodiagnosis may be considered a special case of animal inoculation; the term means host diagnosis and was originally applied to the diagnosis of Chagas' disease by feeding uninfected reduviid bugs on a patient suspected of having the disease. Subsequent examination of the bugs will reveal developmental stages of the parasites, if the test is positive. While a rather esoteric-sounding procedure, it is very convenient for use in the field, and reduviid bugs are raised for this purpose by certain South American governmental laboratories, and supplied to physicians who return the bugs to the laboratory for examination after having allowed them to feed on patients suspected of having trypanosomiasis. Recently the term "xenodiagnosis" has been used for diagnosis of trichinosis by feeding muscle tissue from patients suspected of having the infection to rats.

BIOPSY AND ASPIRATION

Spleen, liver and bone marrow biopsies are extensively used in the diagnosis of visceral leishmaniasis. Organisms may be demonstrated directly in the biopsy material, which may also be used for culture or animal inoculation. Sternal marrow aspiration is approximately as productive as the more hazardous splenic or hepatic biopsies. *Leishmania tropica* cannot be recovered from the surface of an oriental sore; if a hypodermic syringe is introduced from the side of the ulcer, below the ulcer bed, intracellular parasites may be demonstrated in the fluid which is withdrawn after instillation of a few drops of normal saline. Aspiration of enlarged posterior cervical or other involved lymph nodes will at times reveal trypanosomes when the blood is apparently free. The lymph nodes are less often involved in Rhodesian sleeping sickness than in the Gambian form, or in Chagas' disease. Biopsy of enlarged nodes from patients having the latter disease may reveal intracellular (leishmanial) forms of the parasite.

Aspiration of fluid from a hydatid cyst—a dangerous procedure unless done as part of an open surgical operation—will frequently reveal hydatid sand, but it must be remembered that certain hydatid cysts are sterile, so that the absence of scolices or hooklets in the centrifuged sediment is not evidence against the parasitic nature of the cyst. Aspiration of an amebic abscess will often demonstrate a thick reddish-brown fluid, but amebae are seldom seen as they occur chiefly in the tissue surrounding the abscess cavity.

Eggs of *Schistosoma mansoni* may be found in tissue taken from the rectal mucosa when they cannot be recovered from the stools; mucosa from the bladder wall, taken at cystoscopy, may likewise reveal eggs of *Schistosoma haematobium*. Larval *Trichinella spiralis* may be found in any voluntary muscle, but biopsies are usually taken from the gastrocnemius. Larvae are usually most abundant in the diaphragm, and a search may be made for them in this muscle at autopsy.

Examination of duodenal contents.

Sampling and examination of duodenal contents is probably the most reliable means of recovery of *Strongyloides* larvae and of other parasites of the small intestine. Until recently intestinal intubation, entailing discomfort to the patient, was the only procedure used. A new technique, the capsule method, (Beal et al., 1970) causes little, if any, distress to the patient and is convenient for the physician. A number 00 gelatin capsule containing a 90 cm. line, composed of a 20 cm. silicon rubber-covered thread and 70 cm. soft nylon yarn, is swallowed by the patient while the thread, which protrudes from a hole in the capsule, is held firmly. The capsule also contains a 1 gram lead weight which eventually helps carry the thread into the duodenum. The end of the line is taped to the back of the patient's neck, and after 4 hours it is pulled up and the bile-stained mucus adhering to it is examined under the microscope. The lead weight becomes disengaged in the intestine at the time the thread is withdrawn. Further details of this procedure may be found in Beal et al. (1970).

CONCENTRATION METHODS

Concentration of stool specimens to demonstrate cysts and eggs present in small numbers should be a routine part of the parasitologic examination. Special techniques have been devised for the concentration of leishmanias, trypanosomes and microfilariae in the blood, and nematode larvae in the stool. These are rather simple to perform, and should be used whenever the presence of any of these parasites is suspected, if they cannot be demonstrated by more direct forms of examination.

Modified zinc-sulfate flotation.

> Zinc sulfate, USP ....330 gm.
> Distilled water, to make...................1 liter

This is only an approximation of the correct solution, which should have a specific gravity of 1.180. A reliable battery hydrometer must be used in adjusting to the correct specific gravity by the addition of zinc sulfate or water. Specific gravity must be checked frequently. The procedure for use is as follows:

1. Prepare a fecal suspension of approximately 1 cc. of feces (more if dilute) in ten to fifteen times its volume of tap water.

2. Strain through two layers of wet gauze in a funnel, into a small test tube. Add 1 to 2 ml. of ether, cork or use thumb as stopper, shake (with caution), then fill with water to about 1 cm. from top of tube.

3. Centrifuge for forty-five seconds at approximately 2500 rpm. Break up any "plug" which may have formed at the top, and decant supernatant.

4. Add 2 to 3 ml. of tap water, shake or tap tube to resuspend sediment, and fill tube with tap water to 1 cm. from top. Centrifuge as before.

5. Decant supernatant, add 2 to 3 ml. zinc-sulfate solution, resuspend, and fill tube with zinc sulfate solution to about 0.5 cm. from top.

6. Centrifuge at 2500 rpm for two minutes. Do not "brake" the centrifuge or jar the tubes.

7. Without removing tubes from centrifuge, remove several loopfuls of material floating on surface (be careful not to go below surface film with wire loop), place on a slide with a drop of iodine solution, and cover with a coverslip.

Ritchie formalin-ether concentration.

1. Emulsify approximately 1 gm. of feces in 10 to 12 ml. of normal saline.

2. Filter through two layers of moist gauze into a centrifuge tube.

3. Centrifuge one minute at 1500 rpm; pour off supernatant, and resuspend in fresh saline.

4. Centrifuge one minute at 1500 rpm; if supernatant is still cloudy, repeat.

5. Add 10 ml. of 10 per cent formalin to sediment, and allow to stand for five minutes.

6. Add 3 ml. of ether, shake vigorously.

7. Centrifuge one and one half minutes at 1500 rpm, loosen "plug" between formalin and ether layer, decant supernatant, and examine sediment.

Baermann apparatus for recovery of *Strongyloides* larvae.

The Baermann technique gives a good concentration of the *living Strongyloides* larvae in a large volume of feces. It is too cumbersome a method for routine use, but is an excellent method for following the results of therapy.

1. A glass funnel with a diameter of 4 inches or greater is set up in a ring stand, with a short piece of rubber tubing attached to its stem, and a pinchcock closing the tubing.

2. A wire circle, of slightly smaller diameter than the top of the funnel, is covered with two layers of gauze. The edges of the gauze are folded under the ring, which is fitted into the funnel.

3. The funnel is filled with lukewarm water to a level just covering the gauze, and a specimen of stool is placed on the gauze, partially in contact with the water.

4. Allow apparatus to stand at room temperature for 8–12 hours, then draw off a few drops of fluid through the tubing into a small glass dish.

5. Examine for larvae under low power of the microscope.

Knott concentration for microfilariae (modified)

This technique hemolyses the red cells, and concentrates leukocytes and microfilariae.

1. Obtain 1 ml. of blood by venipuncture, and deliver it directly into a centrifuge tube containing 10 ml. of 2 per cent formalin. Mix thoroughly.

2. Centrifuge at 1500 rpm for one minute.

3. Decant supernatant, spread sediment out to approximate thickness of thick films on a slide or slides. Dry thoroughly.

4. Stain with Wright's or Giemsa's stain.

Membrane filtration method for microfilariae (Dennis and Kean, 1971).

1. Blood is collected in tubes containing 3.8 per cent sodium citrate (20 per cent by volume of blood specimen).

2. A Nuclepore* filter of 5 micron pore size is placed in a Swinney adapter; a 20–50 ml. disposable plastic syringe is attached to the adapter.

3. Several milliliters of physiologic saline are added to the upright barrel.

4. About 2 to 4 ml. of the blood specimen are added to the saline, and the mixture of blood and saline is forced through the filter.

5. Following several washes of small amounts of saline or distilled water, the filter may be removed from the adapter, placed on a microscope slide, and examined for the presence of living microfilariae; it can also be dried, fixed and stained as for a thin blood film.

Gradient centrifugation technique for concentration of microfilariae (Jones et al., 1975).

1. Thirty ml. of 50 per cent Hypaque are mixed with 14 ml. of distilled water; 1 part of this mixture is added to 2.4 parts of 9 per cent Ficoll.

2. Four ml. of the Ficoll-Hypaque mixture is placed in a 17 × 100 mm. plastic centrifuge tube, and overlayed with 4 ml. of heparinized venous blood.

3. The tube is centrifuged at 1200 rpm for forty minutes.

4. Microfilariae will be found in the middle Ficoll-Hypaque layer, which separates the overlying plasma and white cell layers from the underlying red cells.

Buffycoat films for leishmanias.

This method is useful for the detection of *Leishmania donovani* if present in the circulation, and will also reveal *Histoplasma capsulatum*, a fungus similar in size and shape to *Leishmania*, but which can be differentiated by details of internal structure.

1. Obtain 5 ml. of blood and deliver into a tube containing oxalate crystals (prepared as for the Wintrobe hematocrit method).

2. Transfer blood with a capillary pipette into a Wintrobe tube. Cap to prevent evaporation and centrifuge for thirty minutes at 3000 rpm.

3. With a fine capillary pipette, withdraw the cells of the "buffy coat" which lies between the packed red cells and the overlying plasma.

4. Spread out as thin film, dry, and stain with Wright's or Giemsa's stain.

---

*This method is unsatisfactory for the isolation of *D. perstans* microfilariae, because of their small size. Other filters of similar pore size are not as satisfactory as the Nuclepore.

Triple centrifugation method for trypanosomes.

1. Deliver 9 ml. of blood, obtained by venipuncture, into a centrifuge tube containing 1 ml. of 6 per cent citrate solution.

2. Centrifuge at 1000 rpm for ten minutes.

3. Remove supernatant fluid to another centrifuge tube, recentrifuge at 1500 rpm for ten minutes.

4. Remove supernatant fluid once more to a clean centrifuge tube; centrifuge at 2500 rpm for ten minutes.

5. Examine sediment as a wet film, or make into a thin film and stain with Wright's or Giemsa's stain.

SPECIAL METHODS FOR RECOVERY OF HELMINTHS AND HELMINTH EGGS

All helminth eggs can be concentrated by one or the other of the two techniques given above. However, eggs of *Enterobius* frequently do not appear in the feces, but must be recovered from the perianal region, and when eggs of *Schistosoma mansoni* or *S. japonicum* are scarce, their presence is perhaps most easily detected by allowing them to hatch and examining for the free-swimming miracidia.

Graham Scotch Tape swab for *Enterobius* and *Taenia* eggs.

1. Fold together sticky surfaces of a piece of Scotch Tape, 1 by 8 cm. in length, for about 1 cm. at each end.

2. Stretch tape, sticky side out, over butt end of a test tube, holding non-sticky ends firmly with thumb and forefinger.

3. Apply tape to anal area, rocking back and forth to cover as much of the mucosa and mucocutaneous area as possible.

4. Remove tape and apply to microscope slide, sticky side down. Press firmly into position.

5. Examine for eggs under low power of microscope. Pinworm eggs, which are generally deposited at night, will be found scattered around the perianal region. The examination should be made in the morning, before the patient has washed or defecated.

Schistosomal hatching test.

If urine or feces containing viable schistosome eggs are diluted with approximately 10 volumes of water, the eggs will hatch within a few hours, releasing miracidia. There is seldom any point in using this technique for schistosome eggs in urine, as they are readily concentrated by centrifugation. The miracidia are positively phototropic, and advantage is taken of this characteristic in the following procedure:

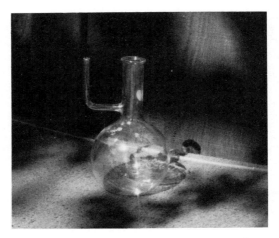

FIGURE 161. Side-arm flask used in hatching of miracidia.

1. A stool specimen is homogenized by shaking in normal saline and is then strained through two layers of gauze.

2. The material is allowed to sediment, the supernatant decanted and the sediment resuspended in saline. This process is repeated at least twice.

3. The saline is decanted and replaced with distilled water, and the suspension is placed in a side-arm (Fig. 161) or Erlenmeyer flask. The side-arm flask is covered with black paper, aluminum foil, or black paint, except for the side arm. If an Erlenmeyer flask is used, it is covered to 1 cm. below the level of fluid in the neck of the flask. Additional water is added if necessary.

4. The flask is allowed to stand at room temperature for several hours in subdued light.

5. The side arm, or water in the neck of the flask, is then illuminated strongly from the side.

6. The illuminated area is then examined with a magnifying glass to detect the presence of free-swimming miracidia.

Filter paper strip procedure for recovery of *Strongyloides* or *Trichostrongylus* larvae.

This technique, originally described by Harada and Mori (1955), is essentially a concentration method. A 20 × 13 mm. filter paper strip, smeared in the center with 0.5 to 1.0 gm. of feces, is inserted into a 15 ml. centrifuge tube containing 3 to 4 ml. distilled water.

The tube is kept at room temperature in a rack or in a slightly slanted position for about 10 days. The filter paper should keep moist by capillary flow. Water can be added as needed to maintain the original fluid level. A detailed discussion of this procedure is contained in the World Health Organization Technical Report, Series No. 255, 1963.

After 10 days a small amount of fluid is withdrawn from the bottom of the tube and examined for larvae.

Recovery and identification of *Taenia* from stool specimens.

Two simple and useful techniques may be adopted in the examination of stool specimens containing pork or beef tapeworms. Search for scolices in patients who have been treated with quinacrine may be accomplished with a Wood's light, as used by dermatologists for the detection of ringworm. The worms, having absorbed the dye, fluoresce brilliantly on exposure to this wavelength (3600 Å). Search for the scolex may thus be facilitated and accomplished more quickly (Dawson, 1963).

If gravid proglottids are found in a stool specimen they should be rinsed in tap water and placed between two microscope slides which are separated at the edges by thin pieces of cardboard. The preparation may then be fastened by means of rubber bands at each end of the slides so that the segments become somewhat flattened. The uterine branches should be clearly visible under the low power of a dissecting microscope.

Species identification on the basis of uterine structure of gravid segments may be greatly facilitated by injection of segments with india ink. A little ink is drawn into a 1 ml. tuberculin syringe, a No. 26 hypodermic needle is inserted in the distal end of the proglottid or in the central uterine stem, and a small amount of ink is slowly injected. The branches of the uterus will become black and can be easily counted. This procedure works best with fresh specimens but may also be successful with formalin-fixed segments.

Methods for Estimation of Worm Burden

Estimates of daily egg output have been made for a number of hepatic and intestinal worms. If these estimates have any degree of accuracy, and if one can further estimate with some precision the total number of eggs in a twenty-four-hour stool specimen, it should be possible to calculate the approximate number of adult worms present. There are various circumstances under which this may be advantageous. One can follow the results of therapy in a somewhat quantitative manner by periodic egg counts, which perhaps afford a more solid basis for comparison of the efficacy of various medications. An estimation of the total number of worms present may be of value as a guide in deciding whether or not to treat a particular patient for a worm infection which may be of no clinical significance. It is estimated, for example, that twenty-five hookworms are necessary to produce clinical symptoms in an individual who is receiving an adequate diet, and who is otherwise normal. Each *Necator* adult in the intestine will be represented by approximately 6750 eggs in each twenty-four-hour stool specimen, and each *Ancylostoma* by about twice that number.

A number of methods have been devised for calculation of the total egg count in a specimen. Of these, the Stoll count is perhaps most widely used, and will be given here.

Stoll egg-counting technique.

1. Save entire twenty-four-hour stool specimen, and determine weight in grams.
2. Weigh out accurately 4 gm. of feces.
3. Place feces in calibrated bottle or large test tube, add sufficient N/10 NaOH to bring volume to 60 ml.
4. Add a few glass beads and shake vigorously to make a uniform suspension. If specimen is hard, the mixture may be placed in a refrigerator overnight, before shaking, to aid in its comminution.
5. With a pipette, remove immediately 0.15 ml. of the suspension, and drain onto a slide.
6. Do not coverslip; place slide on mechanical stage and count all the eggs.
7. Multiply egg count by 100 to obtain the number of eggs per gram of feces, and by weight of specimen to get total number of eggs per twenty-four-hour specimen.

Estimates on numbers of eggs laid per female worm vary considerably (see Muller, 1975) and depend to some extent on the numbers of worms present. The Chinese liver fluke may lay 2400 or so eggs within 24 hours, and an *Ascaris* female about 200,000 during the same time period. Thus, from 1000–2000 eggs would be found per gram of feces in a 24-hour specimen from a patient infected with one pair of *Ascaris.* The egg-laying capacity of a single *Necator* female may vary from 12–44 eggs per gram of feces in a 24 hour period, and less than 2100 eggs per gram usually represents a subclinical infection. *Ancylostoma* females lay about twice as many eggs as *Necator. Trichuris* females presumably lay about 14,000 eggs in 24 hours, but egg laying capacity seems to vary inversely with total numbers of worms present.

The Kato thick-smear technique.

This technique is useful for the estimation of worm burdens. According to Martin and Beaver (1968), whose detailed evaluation and modification should be consulted, this method entails the examination of a standard sample (50 mg.) of fresh feces pressed between a microscope slide and a strip of cellophane that has been soaked in glycerin. After the fecal film has cleared, eggs in the entire film are counted.

Materials recommended by Martin and Beaver are wettable, medium thickness cellophane coverslips, 22 × 30 mm. They are soaked for at least 24 hours in a solution of 100 ml. pure glycerin, 100 ml. water, and 1 ml. 3 per cent malachite green (the latter is optional).

Feces are transferred to a clean slide and covered with a presoaked cellophane coverslip. The slide is inverted and pressed against an absorbent surface until the fecal mass covers an area 20 to 25 mm. in diameter. The preparation is then left for one hour at room temperature to allow clearing of the fecal material (but *not* of the eggs) and should then be examined promptly.

Method for estimating numbers of malaria parasites in blood.

Determine the white and red blood cell counts of the patient. On a thick blood smear, count the number of parasites seen per 100 white blood cells; the total number per cu. mm. of blood can be determined and should be expressed as a percentage of the total red cell count.

CULTURE METHODS

Relatively few of the protozoa, and none of the helminth parasites, can be cultured in such a manner as to be useful in laboratory identification. Other than as strictly research techniques, the only culture methods in general use are for the isolation of *Entamoeba histolytica*, the leishmanias, *Trypanosoma cruzi* and *Trichomonas vaginalis*.

Balamuth's aqueous egg yolk infusion medium for amebae (modification as used in Dr. Balamuth's laboratory).

Phosphate buffer:
    Tribasic potassium phosphate
        K_3PO_4 ....212.27 gm.
        Distilled water...1 liter
    Monobasic potassium phosphate
        KH_2PO_4...136.092 gm.
        Distilled water ....1 liter

Mix above in a ratio of 3 parts tribasic to 2 parts monobasic to make 1M phosphate buffer stock. Dilute stock buffer to M/15 for use.

Whole liver concentrate solution:

> Liver concentrate powder (Wilson or Lilly) ... 5 gm.
> Distilled water ....100 ml.

Suspend powder in cold water and autoclave. Filter through Buchner funnel to remove heavy sediment, tube in measured amounts, and autoclave again.

The medium is prepared as follows:

1. Blend twelve absolutely fresh hard-boiled egg yolks with 375 ml. 0.8 per cent NaCl, using a Waring Blendor.

2. Autoclave at seven pounds pressure for ten minutes, remove pressure slowly, and stir.

3. Autoclave again for forty-five minutes at same pressure.

4. Cool slightly, add distilled water to offset evaporation loss, if any. Transfer to muslin bag, press maximum fluid portion through this. Return volume to 375 ml. with 0.8 per cent saline.

5. Autoclave for twenty minutes at fifteen pounds, then refrigerate to approximately 5° C. Do not agitate at this point or during filtration.

6. Decant fluid carefully through gauze into Buchner funnel with Whatman No. 3 filter paper. Replace papers as required.

7. Measure filtrate, add equal quantity of M/15 phosphate buffer; autoclave for twenty minutes at fifteen pounds, and when cool add sufficient stock liver concentrate solution to give final concentration of 0.5 per cent liver extract (1 part stock concentrate to 9 parts medium).

8. After preliminary refrigeration decant into sterile flasks, in which medium is stored and dispense into tubes as required.

Tubes are prepared containing 6 to 8 ml. of completed medium, and should be incubated for four days to check sterility. A loopful of sterile rice starch or powder is added to each tube before inoculation. Inoculate with portion of stool the size of a small pea, break up well in medium, and incubate at 37° C. The cultures should be examined after two, three and four days' incubation, by removing approximately 0.1 ml. of sediment with a pipette. The fluid is transferred to a slide, covered, and examined under low power of the microscope. Characteristic motility should be observed in the amebae. Primary isolation may yield few organisms, while subsequent transfers show a considerable increase in numbers.

Boeck and Drbohlav's Locke-egg-serum (L.E.S.) *medium* for amebae.

Locke's solution:

> NaCl.....................................9.0 gm.
> CaCl$_2$... 0.2 gm.
> KCl... 0.4 gm.
> NaHCO$_3$ .... 0.2 gm.
> Glucose..................................... 2.5 gm.
> Distilled water ....1000.0 ml.

This solution should be autoclaved before storage. L.E.S. medium is prepared as follows:

1. Wash four eggs, brush with alcohol to sterilize, and break into a sterile flask containing glass beads.

2. Add 50 ml. Locke's solution; shake until homogeneous.

3. Dispense in test tubes sufficient quantity to produce a 1 to 1½ inch slant in bottom of tube.

4. Slant plugged tubes and place in inspissator at 70° C. until slants are solidified. If an inspissator is not available, a substitute may be devised by leaving the door of the autoclave partly open.

5. When slants are solidified, autoclave at fifteen pounds pressure for twenty minutes. If any slants are badly broken, discard them.

6. Cover slants to depth of about 1 cm. with mixture of 8 parts of sterile Locke's solution to 1 part sterile inactivated human blood serum. Sterility of mixture of Locke's solution and serum should be insured by filtration sterilization followed by incubation at 37° C. for 24 hours or longer before use.

Tubes are inoculated in the same manner as Balamuth's medium; rice powder is added before inoculation.

Acanthamoeba medium.

For the isolation of *Acanthamoeba* from tissues or soil samples, Culbertson et al. (1965) recommend the following procedure:

Materials.

1. a. Prepare a neomycin sulfate solution, 0.56 per cent in sterile distilled water.

   b. Prepare sterile nystatin suspension in distilled water containing 1500 units per ml.

2. Prepare agar stock, 3 gm. of Bacto-Agar per 100 ml. of 1.7 per cent NaCl.

3. Prepare suspension of *Aerobacter aerogenes* in trypticase soy broth, giving 40 per cent transmission on a Coleman Junior spectrophotometer against uninoculated broth. Since both live as well as killed bacteria are to be used in medium preparation, place at least 5 ml. of the suspension in a sealed ampule and immerse in a water bath at 65° C. for 30 minutes to kill the organisms. Keep refrigerated until use.

Procedure.

1. To a mixture consisting of
   a. 5 ml. of each antibiotic solution,
   b. 5 ml. of killed bacterial suspension, and
   c. 85 ml. of sterile distilled water

add 100 ml. of melted and cooled 3 per cent agar and combine all ingredients at 56° C. in water bath.

2. Pour mixture into Petri plates, 8 ml. per plate; allow excess moisture to evaporate by inverting bottom plate and resting it at a slight angle.

3. Place 0.05 ml. of live *Aerobacter* suspension in center of plate and spread over an area 25 to 40 mm. in diameter. Allow surface to dry at room temperature or at 4° C. overnight.

Inoculation.

Place drops of fluid or small pieces of tissue suspected of containing amebae near center of plate. Check for presence of amebae at edges of inoculum during the following 4 or 5 days.

Novy-MacNeal-Nicolle or *N.N.N. medium* for *Leishmania.*

Agar base

Agar	14 gm.
NaCl	6 gm.
Distilled water	900 ml.

The water is brought to the boiling point and the salt and agar added and dissolved in it. It is then distributed in test tubes, filled to about one-third capacity. The test tubes are plugged and sterilized in the autoclave in the usual manner. Tubes containing the agar base may be stored in the refrigerator and used as needed.

For use, the tubes are placed in hot water to melt the agar, after which they are cooled to 48 to 50° C. To each tube is added approximately one-third as much sterile defibrinated rabbit's blood as the volume of agar. The blood and agar are thoroughly mixed by rapid rotation of the tube, and the tube is then placed in a slanting position, on ice, and cooled. After the tubes are cool, they are placed in an upright position and incubated for twenty-four hours at 37° C. to determine sterility.

Blood may be obtained from the rabbit by cardiac puncture, sterile precautions being observed. The blood so obtained is placed in a sterile flask containing glass beads and defibrinated by shaking.

Peripheral blood, or material obtained from biopsy, marrow aspiration or from cutaneous ulcers may be cultured on this medium, which gives excellent results. The tubes are kept at room temperature, as close to 22° C. as possible. The organisms develop in the water of condensation which collects at the bottom of the slanted agar. Cultures should be examined every other day for a month before being discarded as negative. If leishmanias are present in the inoculum in some numbers, culture forms will usually be found within two to ten days, but if scarce may require much longer to develop in sufficient numbers to be detected. Leishmanias will not grow in the presence of bacterial contamination.

Lash's casein hydrolysate-serum medium for *Trichomonas.*

Dissolve in 500 ml. distilled water:
Casamino acids (Difco)...................14 gm.
Maltose.......................................1.5 gm.
Dextrose....................................2.0 gm.
Sodium lactate 60 per cent solution...0.5 gm.
Add to above solution:
NaCl...6.0 gm.
KCl..0.1 gm.
CaCl$_2$.. 0.1 gm.

Adjust pH of solution to 6.0, using phosphoric acid, dispense in 5 ml. aliquots in test tubes, plug with cotton and sterilize by autoclaving at fifteen pounds pressure for fifteen minutes.

A serum solution is prepared as follows:

Whole beef blood serum ....200 ml.
Distilled water ....300 ml.
NaHCO$_3$.....................................0.1 gm.

The serum solution is sterilized by filtration. The completed medium is prepared by the addition of 5 ml. of the serum solution to each 5 ml. of the basic solution. *Trichomonas vaginalis* multiplies well in this medium. Cultures are best maintained at 37.5° C. and may be examined at twenty-four and forty-eight hours after inoculation.

REFERENCES

Beal, C. B., Viens, P., Grant, R. G. L., and Hughes, J. M. 1970. A new technique for sampling duodenal contents. Demonstration of upper small-bowel pathogens. Amer. J. Trop. Med. & Hyg., *19*:349–352.

Culbertson, C. G., Ensminger, P. W., and Overton, W. M. 1965. The isolation of additional strains of pathogenic *Hartmanella* sp. *(Acanthamoeba).* Proposed culture method for application to biological material. Amer. J. Clin. Path., *43*:383–387.

Dawson, J. B. 1963. Taenia in expulsis. Lancet, *1*:24.

Dennis, D. T. and Kean, B. H. 1971. Isolation of microfilariae: Report of a new method. J. Parasit., *57*:1146–1147.

Jones, T. C., Mott, K., and Pedrosa, L. C. 1975. A technique for isolating and concentrating microfilariae from peripheral blood by gradient centrifugation. Trans. Roy. Soc. Trop. Med. & Hyg., *69*:243–246.

Martin, L. K., and Beaver, P. C. 1968. Evaluation of Kato thick-smear technique for quantitative diagnosis of helminth infections. Amer. J. Trop. Med. & Hyg., *17*:382–391.

Muller, R. 1975. *A Manual of Medical Helminthology.* William Heinemann Medical Books, Ltd., London, 161 pp.

16
Intradermal Tests and Serologic Methods

A number of dermal sensitivity reactions, or skin tests, have been devised for the diagnosis of protozoan and helminth diseases. The majority are research procedures, since the antigens utilized are prepared with some difficulty, and are not commercially obtainable. Among these may be mentioned the group-specific intradermal test for leishmaniasis, using as antigenic material culture forms of any one of these parasites. It is said that this antigen does not give cross reactions in trypanosomal infections. The reaction, induration and erythema at the injection site, generally of the delayed type, appears twenty-four hours after inoculation of the test material. A skin test for cutaneous and mucocutaneous leishmaniasis, called the Montenegro reaction, involves the use of formalinized leptomonad stages obtained from culture. Positive reactions to the antigen may also occur in treated, though not in active, cases of kala-azar.

Antigens have been prepared for intradermal testing in schistosomiasis, using extracts of adult worms, cercariae and eggs. It is interesting that active cases usually do not react to the extract of eggs, but may become reactive after treatment. In this disease, reactions are of the immediate type, with production of a wheal and surrounding erythematous zone within half an hour after the injection.

More readily obtainable than the above are skin test antigens for filariasis and echinococcosis. A group-specific intradermal reaction is elicited when an antigen prepared from the dog heartworm, *Dirofilaria immitis*, is injected into patients infected with any of the filarial worms. The dog heartworm is common in some areas in this country, and worms may usually be obtained for preparation of the antigen. The worms are washed thoroughly and dried, and the antigen is prepared as follows:

1. 0.5 gm. of dried adult *Dirofilaria* is powdered in a mortar and added to 50 ml. of normal saline in a stoppered bottle or test tube.

2. The powdered worms are extracted in the saline for two hours at 37° C. Shake by hand from time to time during the extraction process.

3. The extract is filtered through Whatman No. 1 paper, a Buchner funnel, and finally sterilized by filtration. It is kept in dark vials or bottles, under refrigeration. It gradually loses its potency after some months.

The test is performed by the injection of 0.1 ml. of antigen intradermally in the forearm, in the manner of a tuberculin test. A saline control injection should be made in the other forearm. Both immediate and delayed reactions may be obtained. The antigen should be standardized on known infected and non-infected patients, but either immediate or delayed reactions with a wheal and erythema 1 cm. or more in diameter may be considered presumptively positive. False positive reactions are sometimes encountered. More satisfactory antigens have been prepared by fractionation of the saline extract.

The Casoni test utilizes hydatid fluid from human or animal infections in the diagnosis of echinococcosis. Fluid is obtained aseptically, and is sterilized by filtration. Kept in dark vials under refrigeration, it will remain useful for approximately a year. It should be tested, both when made up and periodically thereafter, against both normal persons and infected individuals, to determine its specificity and potency. The test consists of the administration of 0.1 ml. of antigen, intradermally, and the reaction is of the immediate variety. Cross reactions may be seen in cysticercosis. While the standard Casoni test is generally of a high order of reliability, a more sensitive antigen can be prepared from hydatid sand or from the germinal layer of the hydatid cyst. Also, sensitivity of the test is enhanced by the use of boiled hydatid fluid, standardized to contain 10 μg. of nitrogen per ml. (Yarzábel et al., 1975).

Skin test antigens have in the past been available commercially for diagnosis of *Toxoplasma* and *Trichinella* infections. A larval extract of trichina is known as trichinellin, and the test is sometimes referred to as the Bachman reaction. It is highly specific but variable in potency, and the antigen should be tested on a known positive individual. Early in infection the reaction may be of the delayed type, while later an immediate reaction will be elicited. As in many infections, dermal sensitivity to the test antigen may be demonstrated for many years after the active phase of the disease. Also available, although at present for research purposes only, is toxoplasmin, an antigen prepared from the peritoneal fluid of mice infected with *Toxoplasma gondii*. The reaction is of the delayed type, and is of a high order of specificity.

SEROLOGICAL METHODS

Most of the standard bacteriologic and viral serologic procedures have been used in the diagnosis of protozoan and helminth infections.

At the present time, serologic techniques are most widely used in the diagnosis of amebiasis, toxoplasmosis, leishmaniasis, Chagas' disease, schistosomiasis, cysticercosis, hydatid disease and trichinosis. Kessel et al. (1965) have demonstrated the usefulness of serologic procedures in the diagnosis of clinical amebiasis. The hemagglutination test developed by these authors is quite sensitive. An evaluation of serologic procedures in amebiasis has been made by Healy (1968), and an improved method of preparing sensitized cells was described by Farshy and Healy (1974). The indirect fluorescent antibody test appears to be nearly as sensitive (Kagan and Norman, 1974).

Complement fixation and hemagglutination tests have been long used for the diagnosis of toxoplasmosis. Toxoplasmas recovered from the peritoneal exudate of mice infected with this parasite are employed as a source of antigen. The most commonly used serologic procedure was for many years the Sabin-Feldman dye test. This procedure will not be described in detail because its performance requires the maintenance of a strain of live *Toxoplasma* in mice, and special equipment beyond the scope of the average laboratory. In recent years, the indirect hemagglutination and indirect immunofluorescence tests have been used in preference to the dye test because they are simpler and safer to perform as well as being of comparable sensitivity.

Useful serologic tests for the diagnosis of malaria include an indirect hemagglutination test and indirect fluorescent antibody tests. Both procedures appear to be highly sensitive as well as specific (Kagan et al., 1969; Sulzer et al., 1969). Wilson et al. (1975) compared the efficiency of complement fixation, indirect immunofluorescence, and indirect hemagglutination tests and noted that sensitivities of all three are comparable within two months after onset of symptoms while seven and twelve months after onset, positive results are obtained only with the hemagglutination test. They also found that sensitivity of all three tests was decreased with sera from heroin addicts who had developed needle-induced *P. vivax* infections.

The aldehyde or formol-gel test devised by Napier for the diagnosis of kala-azar is actually a test for increased serum euglobulin, and similar reactions may be seen in some other diseases, including malaria, tuberculosis, leprosy, trypanosomiasis and schistosomiasis. It is, nevertheless, of value as a screening test in an endemic area, as approximately 85 per cent of patients with active infection of at least four months' duration will give a positive reaction. The test is performed by adding 1 drop of commercial formaldehyde solution to 1 ml. of the patient's serum in a small test tube. A positive reaction is seen when the serum becomes opaque and assumes a stiff jelly-like consistency in three to thirty minutes. If no reaction occurs within twenty-four hours, it is considered negative. The development of opacity is the important part of the reaction, and a test that shows opacity but no solidification within twenty-four hours may be read as weakly positive. Other, more specific tests for the diagnosis of the leishmaniases are the indirect fluorescent antibody test (Walton et al., 1972) for American cutaneous leishmaniasis; and the direct agglutination test, especially sensitive in cases of acute leishmaniasis (Allain and Kagan, 1975). The direct agglutination test is group specific in that it apparently does not differentiate among the species of *Leishmania,* showing high cross-reactivity with the three antigens used.

The Machado test for the diagnosis of Chagas' disease is a complement fixation reaction, using as antigen an extract of the spleen of puppies severely infected with *Trypanosoma cruzi.* This test is used extensively in the endemic areas of South America, and gives a high percentage of positive reactions in patients in the chronic stage of the disease. A direct agglutination test (Vattuone and Yanovsky, 1971) is a very sensitive method for the diagnosis of acute cases. Cossio et al. (1974) demonstrated the presence of a gamma globulin factor (the EVI antibody) which reacts with endocardium, muscle interstitium and vascular structures, especially in patients with chagasic cardiomyopathy. This should be a useful finding in the serology of Chagas' disease.

Various antigenic extracts of adult schistosomes and their cercariae, or the livers of snails infected with larval stages of these worms, have been prepared for use in complement fixation and precipitation reactions. More interesting, perhaps, and simpler to perform are certain other types of serologic reactions. A "Cercarienhüllenreaktion," conveniently abbreviated as CHR phenomenon, is seen when the cercariae of *Schistosoma mansoni* (or presumably of other species), obtained from snails infected in the laboratory, are placed in the serum of infected individuals. A granular precipitate forms about the cercaria, forming a complete envelope or shell from which the cercaria may gradually break away. The shell is sufficiently hardened to retain its form after the cercaria has broken away from it. A "circumoval" precipitate may be formed when the eggs of schistosomes raised in the labora-

Table 8. Immunodiagnostic Tests for Parasitic Disease*

Parasitic Diseases	Intradermal	Complement Fixation	Bentonite Flocculation	Indirect Hemagglutination	Latex	Indirect Fluorescent Antibody	Precipitin
Amebiasis	▲	●	▲	●	●	▲	○
Chagas'	○	●		●	○	●	○
African trypanosomiasis		▲		○		▲	●
Leishmaniasis	●	●		●	○	▲	●
Malaria		▲		▲	○	●	●
Pneumocystis						●	○
Toxoplasmosis	●	▲		●	○	○	
Ancylostomiasis	▲	●		▲	▲	▲	
Ascariasis	▲	○	●	▲		▲	▲
Filariasis	▲	○	●	●	○	▲	
Toxocariasis	●	●	●	●		●	○
Trichinellosis	●	●	●	●	●		●
Clonorchiasis	▲	●		●		▲	○
Fascioliasis	●	●		●			○
Paragonimiasis	●	●	○	●			
Schistosomiasis	○	●	▲	○	○	●	○
Cysticercosis		●			○	▲	○
Echinococcosis	●	●	●	●	●	●	▲

● Evaluated
▲ Experimental test
○ Reported in the literature
*Courtesy, Dr. Irving Kagan, Center for Disease Control, Atlanta, Georgia.

tory are incubated in serum from infected individuals. The effectiveness of many other serologic tests is being studied at present. Currently in use for diagnostic purposes are bentonite flocculation, cholesterol-lecithin flocculation, complement fixation and indirect immunofluorescence. For a review of the serologic diagnosis of schistosomiasis see Kagan (1968, 1974).

Many serologic tests are currently in use in the serologic diagnosis of hydatid disease (Table 8). According to Kagan and Norman (1974) the tests of choice are indirect hemagglutination, indirect fluorescence and immunoelectrophoresis. It should be noted that hydatid cysts of the lung are detected less frequently than those of the liver by serologic means.

A review on immunity and serology in hydatid disease was published by Kagan (1963), and an evaluation of these tests with reference to location of the cysts and cross reactions has been made by Kagan et al. (1966). In the diagnosis of acute trichinosis, bentonite flocculation, complement fixation tests, indirect immunofluorescence and latex agglutination tests have proved to be useful (Norman and Kagan, 1963). The indirect immunofluorescence is especially valuable in light infections. Reagents for some of these tests are commercially available.

In summary, there are now available fairly reliable and sensitive serologic tests for many of the major parasitic diseases (Tables 8 and 9,

Table 9. Serologic Tests Performed For the Diagnosis of Parasitic Diseases (Parasitology Division, Center for Disease Control)*

Diseases	Tests	Diagnostic Titers
Amebiasis	IHA	$\geq 1{:}128$
Chagas' disease	CF[1], DAT[2], IHA[3]	$\geq 1{:}32$[1], $\geq 1{:}128$[2], $\geq 1{:}128$[3]
Leishmaniasis	IHA, DAT	$\geq 1{:}64$, $\geq 1{:}64$
Malaria	IIF	$\geq 1{:}64$
Pneumocystosis	IIF	$\geq 1{:}16$
Toxoplasmosis	IIF, (IgM–IIF), IHA	$\geq 1{:}256$, $\geq 1{:}16$, $\geq 1{:}128$
Ascariasis	IHA, BFT**	$\geq 1{:}128$, $\geq 1{:}5$
Filariasis	IHA, BFT**	$\geq 1{:}128$, $\geq 1{:}5$
Toxocariasis	IHA, BFT**	$\geq 1{:}128$, $\geq 1{:}5$
Strongyloidiasis	IHA	$\geq 1{:}64$
Trichinellosis	BFT	$\geq 1{:}5$
Paragonimiasis	CF	$\geq 1{:}16$
Schistosomiasis	CF, IIF	$\geq 1{:}8$, $\geq 1{:}16$
Cysticercosis	IHA, BFT**	$\geq 1{:}128$, $\geq 1{:}5$
Echinococcosis	IHA, BFT**	$\geq 1{:}128$, $\geq 1{:}5$

IHA — indirect microhemagglutination
CF — complement fixation
DAT — direct agglutination
IIF — indirect immunofluorescence
BFT — bentonite flocculation
*Courtesy, Dr. Irving Kagan, Center for Disease Control, Atlanta, Georgia.
**Both tests must be positive for clinical diagnostic purposes.

and Kagan and Norman, 1974). Most of these tests are performed at the Center for Disease Control, Atlanta, Georgia. Commerical antigens and diagnostic kits for some diseases are also available in the United States and elsewhere. A recent list of these is given by Kagan (1974) who stresses the variability of the results obtained with the different reagents.

REFERENCES

Allain, D. S., and Kagan, I. G. 1975. A direct agglutination test for Leishmaniasis. Amer. J. Trop. Med. & Hyg., *24*:232–236.

Cossio, P. M., Diez, C. Szarfman, A., Kreutzer, E., Candiolo, B., and Arana, R. M. 1974. Chagasic cardiopathy. Demonstration of a serum gamma globulin factor which reacts with endocardium and vascular structures. Circulation, *49*:13–21.

Farshy, D., and Healy, G. R. 1974. Use of stable, sensitized cells in indirect microhemagglutination test for amebiasis. Appl. Microbiol., *27*:11–15.

Healy, G. R. 1968. Use of and limitations to the indirect hemagglutination test in the diagnosis of intestinal amebiasis. Health Lab. Sci., *5*:174–179.

Kagan, I. G. 1963. Seminar on immunity to parasitic helminths. VI. Hydatid disease. Exp. Parasit., *13*:57–71.

Kagan, I. G., Osimani, J. J., Varela, J. C., and Allain, D. S. 1966. Evaluation of intradermal and serologic tests for the diagnosis of hydatid disease. Amer. J. Trop. Med. & Hyg., *15*:172–179.

Kagan, I. G. 1968. Serologic diagnosis of schistosomiasis. Bull. N.Y. Acad. Med., 2nd series, *44*:262–277.

Kagan, I. G., Mathews, H., and Sulzer, A. J. 1969. The serology of malaria: Recent applications. Bull. N.Y. Acad. Med., 2nd series, *45*:1027–1042.

Kagan, I. G. 1974. Advances in the immunodiagnosis of parasitic infections. Z. Parasitenk., *45*:163–195.

Kagan, I. G., and Norman, L. 1974. Serodiagnosis of parasitic disease. *In* Lennette, E. H., Spaulding, E. H., and Truant, J. P. (Eds.): *Manual of Clinical Microbiology*, 2nd Ed. pp. 645–663. American Society for Microbiology, Washington, D.C.

Kessel, J. F., Lewis, W. P., Pasquel, C. M., and Turner, J. A. 1965. Indirect hemagglutination and complement fixation tests in amebiasis. Amer. J. Trop. Med. & Hyg., *14*: 540–550.

Norman, L., and Kagan, I. G. 1963. Bentonite, latex, and cholesterol flocculation tests for the diagnosis of trichinosis. Pub. Health Rep., *78*:227–232.

Sulzer, A. J., Wilson, M., and Hall, E. C. 1969. Indirect fluorescent-antibody tests for parasitic diseases. V. An evaluation of a thick-smear antigen in the IFA test for malaria antibodies. Amer. J. Trop. Med. & Hyg., *18*:199–205.

Vattuone, N. H., and Yanovsky, J. F. 1971. *Trypanosoma cruzi:* Agglutination activity of enzyme treated epimastigotes. Exp. Parasit., *30*:349–355.

Wilson, M., Fyfe, E. H., Jr., Mathews, H. M., and Sulzer, A. J. 1975. Comparison of the complement fixation, indirect immunofluorescence, and indirect hemagglutination tests for malaria. Amer. J. Trop. Med. & Hyg., *24*:755–759.

Yarzábal, L. A., Schantz, P. M., and López-Lemes, M. H. 1975. Comparative sensitivity and specificity of the Casoni intradermal and the immunoelectrophoresis tests for the diagnosis of hydatid disease. Amer. J. Trop. Med. & Hyg., *24*:843–848.

17

Fixatives, Stains, and Preservatives

INTESTINAL PROTOZOA AND HELMINTHS

Fixatives

Bouin's fluid.

Picric acid, saturated aqueous.................................... 75 parts
Formaldehyde .... 25 parts
Glacial acetic acid .... 5 parts

For best results, the acetic acid should be added just prior to use to the picric acid-formaldehyde mixture, which may be made up and stored indefinitely.

PVA fixative solution.*

This fixative, which consists of polyvinyl alcohol, glycerin, glacial acetic acid and Schaudinn's solution, will keep indefinitely but must not be subjected to extremes of temperature. It is convenient to dispense the PVA fixative solution in screw-capped bottles, in approximately 5 ml. quantities. To this volume of fixative, approximately 1 gm. of feces may be added. It must be well broken up and thoroughly mixed with the preservative solution. The solution preserves both trophozoites and cysts of protozoa, and some eggs are recognizable after PVA preserva-

---

*Obtainable from Delkote Incorporated, 76 S. Virginia Ave., Penns Grove. New Jersey 08069.

373

tion. Protozoa remain stainable for about one month. To prepare slides for staining, shake well or mix contents with two applicator sticks. Pour some of the PVA mixture onto a paper towel and allow to stand for a few minutes. Apply stool material to slide and dry for several hours at 37°C, or overnight at room temperature, then stain with trichrome. This method is particularly useful because outpatients may be given vials containing PVA fixative and instructions on how to fix their own stool specimens immediately after passage. If desirable, an entire series of specimens may be brought in at one time after all have been collected.

Schaudinn's solution.

> Mercuric chloride, saturated aqueous........................ 2 parts
> Ethyl alcohol, 95 per cent...................................... 1 part

Glacial acetic acid is added to Schaudinn's solution in the proportion of 1 part acetic to 19 parts of stock immediately before use. Doubling the amount of acetic acid is sometimes advisable, as in the fixation of *Dientamoeba;* for general use the lower strength is preferable.

Stains for Direct Smears

Modified D'Antoni's iodine.

> Distilled water .... 100 ml.
> Potassium iodine.. 1 gm.
> Powdered iodine crystals .... 1.5 gm.

The potassium iodide solution should be saturated with iodine, with some excess remaining in the bottle. Store in brown glass-stoppered bottles, in dark. Solution is ready for use after four days, and sufficient for daily use is decanted into brown glass dropping bottle, and discarded after one day. Stock solution remains good as long as an excess of iodine remains in the bottle.

Lugol's solution.

> Distilled water .... 100 ml.
> Potassium iodide.. 10 gm.
> Iodine crystals .... 5 gm.

Gram's iodine.

> Lugol's solution .... 1 part
> Distilled water .... 14 parts

MIF stain (for direct smears).

Lugol's solution.. 0.10 ml.
Formaldehyde solution... 0.125 ml.
Tincture of Merthiolate... 0.775 ml.

Combine in Kahn tube, to make sufficient quantity for twenty-five or thirty preparations. Must be made fresh daily, and when used in these proportions Lugol's solution should not be over one week old. Lugol's solution up to three weeks old may be used by adjusting quantities. (See Sapero and Lawless, 1953.) To use the stain, add a small quantity of feces to 1 drop of MIF solution and 1 drop of distilled water, mix thoroughly, and cover with a cover-glass.

MIF stain-preservative solution.

Stock MF solution:
Distilled water .... 250 ml.
Tincture of Merthiolate...200 ml.
Formaldehyde .... 25 ml.
Glycerin... 5 ml.

This solution is stored in brown glass bottles. For use, it is combined with fresh Lugol's solution (not over one week old) in the following manner:
1. Measure 2.35 ml. of MF stock solution into a Kahn test tube and stopper with a cork.
2. Measure 0.15 ml. of Lugol's solution into a second tube and close with a rubber stopper.
The two solutions are combined immediately before addition of the fecal specimen. The amount of fecal material to be added to this volume of preservative should be about 0.25 gm. Break up the specimen in the MIF solution and mix thoroughly. The specimen may be examined immediately or stored in a well-stoppered tube; it will retain a good stain for some months. After storage, it will be found that most protozoa and helminth eggs occur in the upper layers of sedimented feces. A drop of mixed supernatant fluid and feces is withdrawn, placed on a slide, and covered with a coverslip.

Gomori's trichrome stain.

Chromotrope 2R*... 0.6 gm.
Light green SF*... 0.3 gm.
Phosphotungstic acid.. 0.7 gm.

*Manufactured by National Aniline Division, Allied Chemical and Dye Corp., New York, N.Y.

Allow to stand for 30–60 minutes, then add
Acetic acid, glacial... 1.0 ml.
Distilled water .... 100.0 ml.

Slides are prepared for trichrome staining, from either fresh or PVA-preserved specimens. They are then processed as follows:

1. Fix in Schaudinn's solution with acetic acid added... 30 minutes
2. Wash in 70 per cent alcohol............................. 15 minutes
3. Wash in 70 per cent alcohol to which sufficient iodine has been added to produce a port-wine color .... 3 minutes
4. Wash in 70 per cent alcohol, two changes, each..... 1 minute
5. Stain in Gomori's trichrome .... 8 to 15 minutes
6. Rinse in 90 per cent alcohol with 1 per cent acetic acid.. 1–2 seconds
7. Dip twice in 100 per cent alcohol
8. Dehydrate in second change of 100 per cent alcohol.. 30 seconds
9. Place in xylol... 1 minute
10. Mount in Permount, or other mounting medium.

If PVA-preserved material is used, steps 1 and 2 should be omitted.

Lawless acid-fuchsin light-green stain.

Mix together:
Acetone... 50 ml.
Glacial acetic acid... 50 ml.
Formaldehyde .... 10 ml.
Schaudinn's solution... 890 ml.

Add to above:
Acid fuchsin.. 2.5 gm.
Fast green FCF... 1.0 gm.

Store in tightly stoppered glass bottles. Fecal films are prepared in the same manner as for trichrome staining, from fresh material only. The combined fixation-staining procedure is as follows:
1. Using a medicine dropper or dropping bottle, immediately cover all parts of the fecal film with the prepared solution.
2. Gently heat the stain-covered film over an alcohol lamp or

laboratory burner until steam is first observed. Two or three slow passes of the slide above the flame are usually sufficient; do not boil and do not allow staining solution to flame.

3. As soon as steaming occurs, wash gently under running tap water.

4. Place in 50 per cent and 70 per cent alcohol for thirty seconds each, 95 per cent and 100 per cent alcohol for fifteen seconds each, and clear in xylol for one minute.

5. Mount in Permount and examine.

The times given for dehydration are minimal, and it will be found safer to double them, using 50 per cent and 70 per cent alcohol for one minute each, and 95 per cent and 100 per cent alcohol for thirty seconds each.

BLOOD FILMS AND TISSUE IMPRESSION SMEARS

Field's stain.

Solution A:

Methylene blue	0.8 gm.
Azure I	0.5 gm.
Na_2HPO_4 anhydrous	5.0 gm.
KH_2PO_4 anhydrous	6.25 gm.
Distilled water	500 ml.

Solution B

Eosin	1.0 gm.
Na_2HPO_4 anhydrous	5.0 gm.
KH_2PO_4	6.25 gm.
Distilled water	500 ml.

Dissolve salts first, then add the stains, after grinding the azure I in a mortar. Let the solutions stand for twenty-four hours, then filter. If a scum forms or dye precipitates, filter again. The same solutions may be used for many weeks, but the eosin should be renewed when it becomes greenish. The staining procedure is as follows:

1. Dip slides in solution A.. 1 second
2. Rinse by immersion in water, waving gently for
   a few seconds until stain ceases to flow from film.
3. Dip slides in solution B.. 1 second
4. Rinse as before for two or three seconds.
5. Place vertically against a rack to drain and dry.

Giemsa's stain.

Giemsa's stain is sold commercially as a concentrated stock solution. The product is quite variable, and each new lot should be thoroughly tested before being put into use. In general, if the coloration of the red and white cells seems satisfactory, it can be assumed that the stain will be adequate for the demonstration of malarial and other parasites. The procedure for use of Giemsa's stain with thin films is as follows:

1. Fix blood films in absolute methyl alcohol for one minute.
2. Allow slides to dry.
3. Immerse slides in a solution of 1 part of Giemsa stock to 30 to 50 parts of buffered water (pH 6.8 to 7.2). Stain thirty minutes to one hour.
4. Dip slides briefly in buffered water, drain quickly and thoroughly, and air-dry.

The procedure to be used with thick films is the same, except that steps 1 and 2 are omitted. If the slide has a thick film at one end and a thin film at the other, fix only the thin portion, then stain both parts of the film simultaneously.

Wright's stain.

Wright's stain may be obtained in powder or tablet form. A product bearing certification of the Biological Stain Commission should be employed.

Wright's stain	0.3	gm.
Glycerin	3.0	ml.
Methyl alcohol, absolute	97.0	ml.

Grind the stain and glycerin together, and then add alcohol. Place in stoppered brown bottle, let stand for two or three weeks, filter, and use. The procedure for staining is as follows:

1. Cover blood film with a measured number of drops of Wright's stain; allow to remain for one minute.
2. Add an equal number of drops of buffered water (pH 6.8 to 7.2); blow on slide to mix water with stain.
3. Stain for three to five minutes; for malarial parasites up to fifteen minutes may give better results.
4. Flood off the stain with buffered water, drain quickly and thoroughly, and air-dry.

This method is suitable for thin films only.

Saponin technique for hemolysis of thick-films (Umlas and Fallon, 1971).

1. Prepare a solution of 0.5 per cent saponin* in normal saline.
2. Prepare thick blood films in the usual manner, and allow to dry thoroughly.
3. Lyse the thick film by the addition of approximately 3 drops of saponin solution.
4. Agitate slide gently until saponin solution becomes pink-tinged (approximately five seconds).
5. Allow films to drain by gravity and dry for about ten minutes (need not be completely dry).
6. Stain with Giemsa or Wright-Giemsa stain.

PRESERVATION AND SHIPMENT OF SPECIMENS

The importance of proper initial handling and examination of specimens has been stressed in preceding chapters. At times it may be necessary or desirable to refer specimens to various experts for identification. Adequate preservation and shipment of such specimens is equally important, and will greatly facilitate subsequent examination.

Stool specimens which have been fixed in PVA solution should be shipped in tightly stoppered vials, preferably by surface mail. Each vial should be labeled as follows: patient's name or identifying number, date of collection, and name of laboratory or hospital from which shipment is made. If PVA-preserved specimens are to be examined by a laboratory some distance away, shipment should be made as soon as possible, since best staining results are obtained within a few weeks after fixation. If several vials are shipped in one container, each vial should be wrapped in cotton or soft paper to prevent breakage during transit.

Shipment of other specimens requires similar care and attention. If fixatives other than PVA are used, this information should be added to the data on the label. When vials containing arthropod or worm parasites are sent to specialists for identification, the location of the parasite in or on the host should be given, as well as a clinical summary.

If stool specimens containing cysts are to be preserved for more than a few weeks, a 10 per cent formalin solution should be used for preservation. Specimens containing eggs should also be preserved in 10 per cent formalin. When large amounts of stool containing cysts or eggs are to be preserved in formalin, it is advantageous to prepare a concentrate. Concentration of the specimen will eliminate much debris and fatty materials, making the parasites correspondingly easier to find. To make a concentration of a large volume of fecal material, proceed as follows:

---

*Saponin powder obtainable from Harleco, Philadelphia, Penna. 19143.

1. Make a homogeneous suspension of the specimen in several volumes of water.

2. Strain through two layers of gauze to eliminate large particulate material.

3. Place in large centrifuge tubes, add approximately 5 per cent of ether, and shake.

4. Centrifuge at 1500 rpm for one minute.

5. Loosen fatty material at top of tubes and decant, retaining only the sediment.

6. Preserve sediment in 10 volumes of 10 per cent formalin.

After a few days the formalin may be changed and its volume reduced.

Permanent stains cannot be made from formalin-fixed fecal specimens. Iodine will give almost as good results with formalin-preserved as with fresh protozoan cysts. The MIF stain-preservation technique may also be used for preservation of fairly large quantities of stool. Preserved material is generally not optimal for identification. If protozoa found in a stool specimen are to be referred to a specialist for identification, it is best to send him one or more trichrome-stained slides, as well as material preserved in PVA, if available.

Adult roundworms may be fixed and preserved in 10 per cent formalin or 70 per cent alcohol. Small roundworms are best fixed in hot 70 per cent alcohol, as this will kill them in an extended condition. For flatworms, Bouin's fluid is the fixative of choice. Specimens should be fixed in Bouin's fluid for twenty-four hours and then washed in several changes of 70 per cent alcohol, in which they may also be stored. Formalin-fixed helminths are best stored in 70 per cent ethyl or isopropyl alcohol. Fly larvae, lice, fleas and other arthropods may be fixed in 80 or 90 per cent alcohol. Snails should be fixed and preserved in 70 per cent alcohol, but not in formalin. Snail shells may also be preserved dry for identification; species determination sometimes requires reference to the soft parts of the snail, and some whole specimens should be preserved.

It is important to fix specimens as soon as possible after removal from the host. Worm parasites may be cleaned by washing in tap water or saline; they should not be kept in tap water for longer than one hour, and in warm climates they should be refrigerated unless they are fixed immediately. Deterioration of internal structures frequently prevents proper staining and identification.

Although many clinical laboratories do not keep reference collections of their own, such a collection, built up over a period of years, will be of great interest, and is often extremely useful for training purposes. Stained slides, whether of stool or blood, will usually keep for many years if properly handled. In a moist climate, or if the slides are frequently used, it is advisable to cover blood films with a coverslip. All stained slides should be protected from exposure to light when not in use, to prevent fading. Many fine collections of specimens have been lost because of evaporation of the preservative fluid. A coat of melted paraffin applied over the corks or lids will help to prevent evaporation, but stored specimens should be checked periodically, and additional fluid added as necessary.

REFERENCES

Sapero, J. J., and Lawless, D. K. 1953. The "MIF" stain-preservative technic for the identification of intestinal protozoa. Amer. J. Trop. Med. & Hyg., 2:613–619.

Umlas, J., and Fallon, J. N. 1971. New thick film technique for malaria diagnosis. Use of saponin stromatolytic solution for lysis. Amer. J. Trop. Med. & Hyg., 20:527–529.

INDEX